Congenital Bleeding Disorders

Akbar Dorgalaleh
Editor

Congenital Bleeding Disorders

Diagnosis and Management

Springer

Editor
Akbar Dorgalaleh
Department of Hematology and Blood Transfusion
School of Allied Medicine
Iran University of Medical Sciences
Tehran
Iran

ISBN 978-3-030-09565-9 ISBN 978-3-319-76723-9 (eBook)
https://doi.org/10.1007/978-3-319-76723-9

Softcover re-print of the Hardcover 1st edition 2018

Printed on acid-free paper

This Springer imprint is published by the registered company Springer International Publishing AG part of Springer Nature
The registered company address is: Gewerbestrasse 11, 6330 Cham, Switzerland

Foreword

It is a privilege to be given the opportunity of preparing a brief foreword to this magisterial and comprehensive work by Dr. Dorgalaleh and his associates.

Indeed, it is not inappropriate for me to have been invited to provide these few words, as I have been a living witness, in the course of over half a century, of the astonishing evolution of the diagnosis and, most particularly, the care of patients suffering from inherited bleeding disorders, both in this country and the world.

Care has ranged, during this period, from the use of whole blood for the hemophilias in the 1950s to the current employment of recombinant products and the promise of a revolutionary bipolar monoclonal antibody in hemophilia A (HA), and the successful implementation of gene therapy in both HA and hemophilia B (HB).

Those among us who have lived through this astonishing clinical and scientific journey have witnessed a parade of phases in hemophilia care: the initial dearth of therapeutic options; the crippling effects of chronic joint bleeding; the scourge of blood-borne virus infection; and the affliction of inhibitors, which remains current, although a future resolution is within sight.

A few words about the early origins of these bleeding disorders are needed, in order to provide some historical context for this book.

The mutations giving rise to hemophilia are probably of great antiquity, because they occur in at least three orders of placental mammals: the Ungulata, the Carnivora, and the Primates. Hemophilia has been described in the horse, and nine breeds of dog, as well as in all races of man. The orders to which these groups belong may have been distinct from the end of the Cretaceous—say sixty five million years ago, and the mutations have probably recurred independently many times in all three, since they must be lethal in the wild state. The mutation rate has been estimated at about $1–4 \times 10^{-5}$.

The earliest references to what may have been human hemophilia are attributed to Jewish records of the second century A.D. A ruling of Rabbi Judah the Patriarch exempts a woman's third son from circumcision, if two older brothers had died of bleeding following the operation.

It is now well known that Queen Victoria herself (1819–1901) was a carrier of hemophilia B, affecting coagulation factor IX. No evidence of the disorder exists among her antecedents, so we must assume that the mutation occurred at spermatogenesis in her father, Edward, Duke of Kent. The disorder only manifested itself for the first time with the birth of her eighth child in 1853, when Leopold, Duke of

Albany, was born with hemophilia, which proved fatal when he died of a cerebral hemorrhage at the age of 31.

Leopold's sisters, Beatrice and Alice, were both carriers. Alice married the Grand Duke of Hesse, and two of her daughters, Irene and Alix, had hemophilic sons. Alix, better known as Alexandra (Queen Victoria's granddaughter), married Tsar Nicholas II of Russia, and their son, probably the most famous hemophiliac in the world, was Alexei, who was born in 1904. Alexei was also the most tragic example of the disorder, who created so much anguish in the Romanov family. It was through his successful treatment of Alexei's extreme pain by hypnosis, when he was 8 years old (probably due to a psoas muscle hemorrhage), that Rasputin, the charismatic monk, gained such a sinister influence upon the entire household of the Tsar.

The last known carrier of Queen Victoria's mutation was Princess Alice, wife of the Earl of Athlone, who represented the British Crown at the celebration in Tehran, of Crown Prince Mohammad Reza Pahlavi's marriage to Princess Fowziyeh, the sister of Malek Farouq, the king of Egypt, in 1941.

Until 1964, no one took any interest in the inherited bleeding disorders, such as the hemophilias, in Iran. These were truly clinical orphans, and those unfortunate children suffering from the severe form of hemophilia A, or B who had survived into adulthood, were already hopeless cripples. In addition, they had little recourse to treatment, as the sole available form of therapy was fresh whole blood, carrying infinitesimal quantities of the relevant coagulation factor.

At the newly established Tehran University Clinical Hematology Department at the 500-bed Pahlavi (now Emam Khomeini) Hospital, the small associated laboratory was only equipped to carry out blood counts and May-Grunwald staining and microscopy of patients' peripheral blood and bone marrow aspirates, at the time.

However, a personal grant of 18,000 pounds sterling from the Sir Henry Wellcome Trust enabled me to purchase all the equipment required to set up a modern clinical hematology laboratory.

While awaiting the delivery of all these myriad items of equipment from abroad, I became interested in the investigation of inherited bleeding disorders. Using the Thromboplastin Generation Test of Biggs and Douglas (1953), together with the classic Prothrombin Time test of Armand Quick, it became possible to distinguish hemophilia A from hemophilia B, then known as Christmas disease in the UK, and to carry out bioassays of these factors, using a broken 37° waterbath and hand-pulled Pasteur pipettes. Although it was exciting to have been able to actually demonstrate the hemostatic defect in the laboratory for the first time in Iran, this academic exercise was of little benefit to the wretched children affected by these bleeding disorders.

As a result of repeated acute hemarthroses, particularly affecting weight-bearing joints, such as knees and ankles, many of them were bedridden due to contractures and muscle wasting. Some had become drug addicted because of pain and despair. Mothers felt guilty for being carriers; sisters were in an agony of doubt as to whether or not they were carriers of the genetic disorder, and would pass it on to their sons. Indeed, in some cases, wives were ostracized and returned to their families, once the husband learned that his spouse was the cause of the disease. The education of affected boys is disrupted, resulting in unemployment and a sense of inadequacy. The cost of these inherited bleeding diatheses to society is enormous, not only because of the premature death of potentially useful members of society but also because, if left untreated, patients end up hopelessly crippled, and a burden upon their families, and the health facilities of their country.

Dr. Judith Graham Pool's discovery of cryoprecipitate allowed for the preparation of a crude, home-made concentrate of factor VIII in the Hematology Department laboratories. Bottles of cell-free fresh plasma were snap-frozen in a mixture of dry ice and alcohol, and subsequently thawed slowly at 4° C. A precipitate at the bottom of the bottles contained most of the FVIII, Fibrinogen, and FXIII from the original crude plasma, and was stockpiled in deep freeze cabinets for future use. The cryo-supernatant plasma was also stored for use in hemophilia B, burns, and hypovolemia.

Major orthopedic surgery, mainly arthrodesis of knees, was successfully carried out in the late 1960s, in cases of severe hemophilia A by a few intrepid surgeons in Tehran, such as Dr. Sheikh ol-Eslamzadeh or Dr. Gorgi, using only cryoprecipitate to prevent bleeding, and circulating FVIII levels were assayed daily, before and after each infusion for at least ten days. Soft tissue surgery, such as pyloroplasty and vagotomy for repeated hematemesis, or pulmonary lobectomy for hydatid cyst causing life-threatening hemoptyses was also undertaken with success by Dr. Kazemi, with similar replacement therapy.

It must be emphasized that in the mid-1960s, commercial preparations were not easily available anywhere in the world, with the sole exception of Fraction 1-O, pioneered by Birger and Margaretha Blomback at the Karolinska Institute in Stockholm, which was later manufactured on an industrial scale by Kabi. The only alternatives were bovine and porcine FVIII, produced in the UK, which, although they were potent, were dangerously antigenic. Indeed, one of the cases I treated with bovine FVIII developed both thrombocytopenia and a protein-losing nephropathy, probably caused by an immunogenic reaction to this fraction.

Baruch Blumberg had recently reported what came to be known as "Australian Antigen" or hepatitis B surface antigen, and since hemophilic patients had been repeatedly exposed to plasma, even though there had been no history of overt jaundice, it was felt that they should all be screened for the antigen by the Ouchterlony gel-immunodiffusion technique—the only method available at the time. This was the first application of a test for hepatitis B in Iran, and it was found that this viral infection was common among blood donors.

Inevitably, seeking treatment for hemophilic patients drew attention to the appalling state of blood transfusion in Iran. Virtually without exception, blood for transfusion, whether in private hospital practice or in government and university hospitals, was procured through disreputable dealers. Professional blood sellers exploited the poorest sectors of society, who were prey to malnutrition, anemia, and hepatitis, as well as drug addiction. This was also true of the transfusion services of the Red Lion & Sun Society, the Iranian affiliate of the International Red Cross, currently renamed the Red Crescent Society. Even the military hospitals relied solely upon soldiers—never officers—who were ordered to volunteer, in return for 72 h leave, ostensibly to allow for their recovery. In addition, modern advances in blood group serology and proper compatibility testing had made little impact upon the rudimentary, fragmented, and grossly commercialized blood services available at the time. Increasing population density and rapid advances in hospital surgery and medicine, together with the growing expectations of both the expanding middle classes and highly trained medical practitioners revealed the glaring inadequacies and dangers of the blood services, and set the scene for fundamental reforms in this vital sector of public health infrastructure.

The unsatisfactory state of blood transfusion services led to the conception of a plan, in 1972, for the establishment of a modern, centralized, national service for blood transfusion, based entirely upon the voluntary, unremunerated donation of blood by healthy members of the public. Implementation of such a program called for a veritable social revolution and a profound change in public attitudes, together with an extensive public education and recruitment campaign.

In 1974, the Iranian National Blood Transfusion Service achieved legal status, and within a relatively short time, a technically advanced service based entirely upon voluntary blood donation replaced the commercialism and inadequacies of the past.

In 1971, the World Federation of Hemophilia (WFH) agreed to hold their 7th international congress in Tehran—the first time such a meeting had been held outside of Europe or Canada. This was a groundbreaking meeting in other ways as well, in that the main thrust of the Congress emphasized the impossibility of providing adequate, comprehensive hemophilia care, without the close support of a safe, modern blood transfusion service, which formed an integral part of the national health services.

Even in the 1970s, it was clear that support for the hemophilic population could not remain confined to doctors and scientists alone. There had to be at least a minimal participation by parents of affected children, and the patients themselves. Early efforts to establish a viable Hemophilia Society remained unfulfilled for many years. It is a source of satisfaction that today a strong Iranian Hemophilia Society (IHS) has been established, which is devoted to the interests of patients and their families, which defends their rights as citizens, and acts as their advocate at both national and international levels. The IHS has not merely confined its efforts to the conventional range of activities typical of similar societies elsewhere in the world: social services, dormitory services for patients from the provinces, support for employment and education, counseling affected families, providing information booklets, etc.; it has gone much further by creating the first comprehensive, interdisciplinary hemophilia care center in Iran as well. The Iranian Comprehensive Hemophilia Care Center (ICHCC) in Tehran is officially affiliated to the World Federation of Hemophilia and was inaugurated in April 2001.

A network of hemophilia centers now exists throughout Iran, often affiliated to regional medical schools.

Registered patients suffering from inherited bleeding disorders are covered by a national insurance scheme under the aegis of the Ministry of Health, such that all their laboratory investigation expenses as well as replacement therapy with either plasma-derived or recombinant concentrates are provided free of charge.

In sum, the authors of this definitive reference book concerning both common and rare inherited hemostatic disorders meticulously bring together the clinical signs, symptoms, complications, the phenotypic and genotypic diagnoses in the laboratory, together with all the latest forms of treatment currently available, including physiological background, and molecular studies.

This will be an invaluable source of all the relevant, up-to-date and exhaustively reviewed evidence for postgraduate students, scientists, and research workers in the field.

(Some sections of this piece have been published in a modified form in: Arch. Iranian Medicine (2016); 19(3): 229–232)

Fereydoun Ala
Honorary President, The Iranian Comprehensive
Hemophilia Care Center, Tehran, Iran

Contents

Introduction

I did visit Iran at least twice before the Islamic Revolution. In 1971 the World Federation of Hemophilia held in Tehran its 7th World Congress and in September 1978 I organized in the same city a Hemophilia Workshop on behalf of the same international organization. During the two visits I was most impressed by the extraordinary and warm friendship that Iranian people expressed for foreign visitors, as well as by the high level of development in the country of blood transfusion services and the advanced degree of clinical and research knowledge in the field of bleeding disorders. The long, useless and bloody war with Iraq that lasted for a whole decade in the 1980s devastated Iran and made practically impossible for foreigners to visit the country. In addition many of the excellent scientists and clinicians left and went abroad. I returned to Tehran only in December 1995, prompted by the collaboration with Flora Peyvandi who, a native of Iran, had graduated in medicine at the University in Milan and then became a postgraduate hematology fellow with me. I noticed several changes in the lifestyle of Iranians compared with my previous experiences in the 1970s, but two positive aspects had remained unchanged: the spirit of friendship and collaboration with us foreigners and the high quality of medical services, including those dealing with inherited bleeding disorders. I remember distinctly that during my visit and clinical seminar at the Imam Khomeini hospital in Tehran my attention was drawn by a map of the whole country that identified with colored flags the patients with different inherited coagulation disorders. Together with my Italian colleague Alessandro Gringeri we were impressed to notice that the flags representing patients with hemophilia A and B were outnumbered by those identifying patients with recessively inherited coagulation disorders (RICD), with absolute numbers much higher than those that I knew for countries that like Italy and the United Kingdom had general populations not very different in size from that of the Islamic Republic of Iran. Cognizant that global knowledge about the molecular basis but also about the most prevailing symptoms of these disorders was rather limited, Flora, myself, and the whole staff of clinicians and scientists of the Angelo Bianchi Bonomi developed a strong collaboration program with Iranian clinicians and scientists with emphasis on RICD. This collaboration led to the publication of an array of manuscripts that contributed significantly to extend our general knowledge on these rare disorders. Needless to say these studies, which made Flora Peyvandi the main scientific authority in this field, were possible due to the enthusiastic collaboration of Iranian clinicians and scientists, of whom the most active at that time were Manijeh Lak, Sharifian, and Sirous Zeinali, the latter at the Tehran Pasteur Institute. Not surprisingly, the publications on Iranian patients with RICD attracted the attention and interest of international experts other than those from Milan. For instance, Tuddenham, one of the authors of this book, visited Iran during a summer period, and with the help of Flora Peyvandi managed to publish a seminal study on the molecular basis of the combined deficiency of coagulation factors V and VIII.

The seeds of the international scientific collaboration that Flora and myself put on the fertile soil of Iranian hematologists and pediatricians produced subsequently several additional fruits, and this book is clearly witnessing the role that Iran currently plays in the competitive global arena of hemostasis and thrombosis. At a personal level, it was with great pride that owing to my contributions to the advancement of medical sciences I was honored to receive in Teheran in 2008 the Khwarizmi International Award, a most prestigious international initiative of the Iranian Research Organization for Science and Technology, named after a famous Persian mathematician of the seventh century. Flora and myself are continuing to collaborate with Iranian scientists, who for sake of an example were recently major contributors to the landmark SIPPET study published in 2006. All in all, this excellent book and its contents demonstrate clearly the role prominent achieved by clinicians and scientists of the Islamic Republic in an important field of hematology such as that of inherited bleeding disorders.

Pier Mannuccio Mannucci
Emeritus Professor of Internal Medicine,
University of Milan and IRCCS Ca'
Granda Maggiore Policlinico Hospital Foundation
Milan, Italy

Part I

An Overview of Hemostasis and Congenital Bleeding Disorders

1 An Overview of Hemostasis

Akbar Dorgalaleh, Maryam Daneshi, Jamal Rashidpanah, and Elaheh Roshani Yasaghi

1.1 Introduction

The term hemostasis is derived from Greek roots "heme," which means blood, and "stasis," which means halt, and therefore the word means the halt of blood. The hemostasis is a physiological and well-controlled process in the body in which the integrity of the circulatory system is maintained after vascular injury. Several cellular and noncellular components are involved in this process. These components include coagulation system, platelets, vascular system, fibrinolysis system, kinin system, complement system, and serine protease inhibitors. From the other view, hemostasis has three main components including vascular system, cellular components, and noncellular components (Fig. 1.1).

1. Vascular system: Endothelial cells, smooth muscle, and connective tissue
2. Cellular components: Platelets, granulocytes, monocytes, and lymphocytes
3. Noncellular components: Coagulation factors, fibrinolysis system, serine protease inhibitors, complement system, and kinin system

Following vascular damage, these components work together in close relationship to stop bleeding and then remove the formed clot from the bloodstream. These hemostatic components have also important role in other processes such as wound

A. Dorgalaleh (✉) · M. Daneshi
Department of Hematology and Blood Transfusion, School of Allied Medicine, Iran University of Medical Sciences, Tehran, Iran

J. Rashidpanah
Tehran Heart Center, Tehran, Iran

E. Roshani Yasaghi
Independent researcher, Tehran, Iran

A. Dorgalaleh (ed.), *Congenital Bleeding Disorders*,
https://doi.org/10.1007/978-3-319-76723-9_1

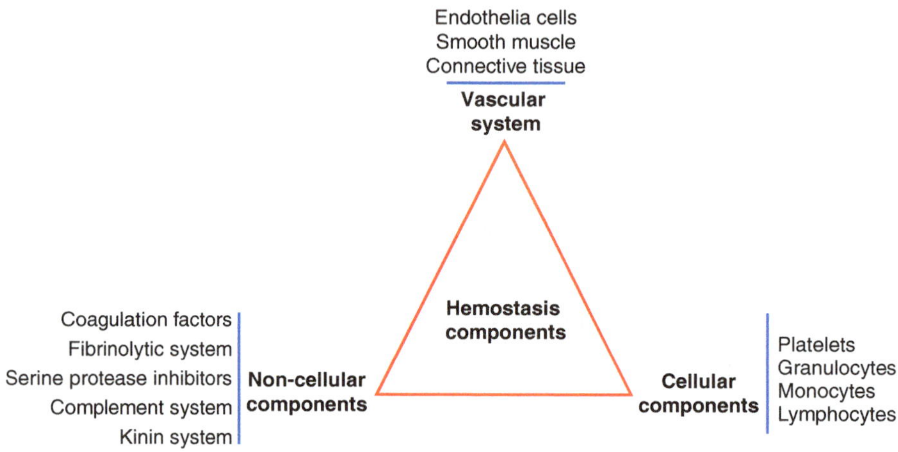

Fig. 1.1 Hemostasis has three main components including vascular system, cellular components, and noncellular components. These components closely work together to keep the hemostasis system in the best situation. Each of these three arms of hemostasis has several other components

healing and angiogenesis. The response of hemostasis system to vascular injury is prompt and well-controlled, and following vascular injury, three steps occur to stop the bleeding:

1. Vasoconstriction
2. Platelet plug formation
3. Blood coagulation [1–3]

Vasoconstriction occurs as the first response of vascular system injury. This process occurs almost promptly in the smooth muscle cells, via the sympathetic nervous system. This response occurred due to the direct damage in the smooth muscles as well as the release of endothelin-1 from the endothelial cells and platelets. This response leads to a decreased blood flow in the area of injury that reduces blood loss. In the second step, platelets adhere to the subendothelium of vasculature in the site of injury, a process known as adhesion. Platelet shape change occurs during the process, and platelet granules are released. This process leads to activation and recruitment of further platelets and induces platelet aggregation, resulting in platelet plug formation. In fact, with vascular injury, subendothelial elements, notably collagen I and III, laminin, and microfibrils, are exposed to the circulating blood. These elements cause platelet adhesion, activation, and secretion. Collagen is the main subendothelial element that allows platelet adhesion. Platelet adhesion to subendothelial collagen is performed by the two main platelet glycoproteins (GP), namely, GPIa/IIa (integrin $\alpha2\beta1$, CD49b/CD29) and GPVI, which are the main platelet collagen receptors. GPVI is exclusively expressed on platelet/megakaryocyte lineage, while integrin $\alpha2\beta1$ is not restricted to this lineage. Deficiency

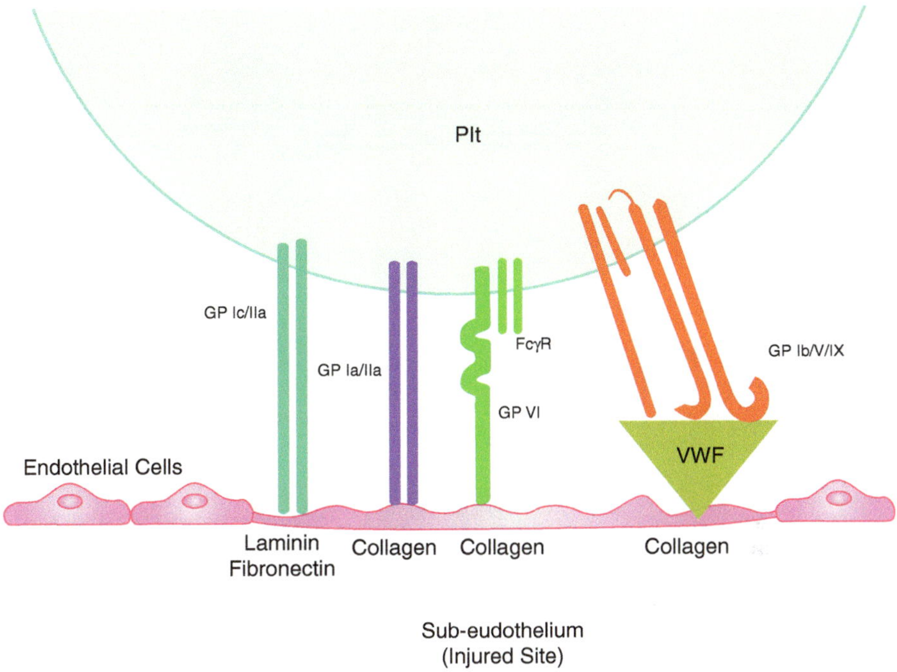

Fig. 1.2 Platelet adhesion, molecular mediations, and subendothelial factors. Glycoprotein (GP) Ic/IIa, GPIa/IIa, GPVI, and GPIb/V/IX are the most important GPs that mediate platelet adhesion. GPIc/IIa and GPIa/IIa directly bind to laminin/fibronectin and collagen, respectively, in the injured site. GPVI also binds to the subendothelial collagen directly, and FcγR has a main role in signal transduction. GPIb/V/IX is comprised of four chains: GPIbα, GPIbβ, GPV, and GPIX. Its binding to collagen is mediated by VWF. *Plt* platelet, *GP* glycoprotein, *VWF* von Willebrand factor

of both GPs leads to extremely rare and mild bleeding disorders. Primary platelet adhesion to the subendothelium at high shear is performed via binding of GPIb/V/IX (CD42a-c) to von Willebrand Factor (VWF) in the subendothelial matrix. This interaction helps in binding of other platelet surface GPs to collagen and other subendothelial elements, which results in firm adhesion of platelets to the injured site (Fig. 1.2) [4, 5].

Activated platelets have a considerable number of agonists that can activate other platelets. These components may be weak platelet stimuli, such as adenosine diphosphate (ADP) and epinephrine, or may be strong such as thrombin. These agonists lead to further activation and subsequent conformational changes of other platelets. Activation of integrin αIIbβ3 (GPIIb/IIIa) on activated platelets is one of the most important events in platelet response to vascular injury. Integrin αIIbβ3 as the most abundant platelet surface GP has a crucial role in platelet–platelet interaction and platelet plug formation at the site of injury. In this process, which is called aggregation, integrin αIIbβ3 and fibrinogen molecules have crucial role. In fact, fibrinogen is attached to integrin αIIbβ3 of neighboring platelets and mediates platelet–platelet interaction (Fig. 1.3) [6].

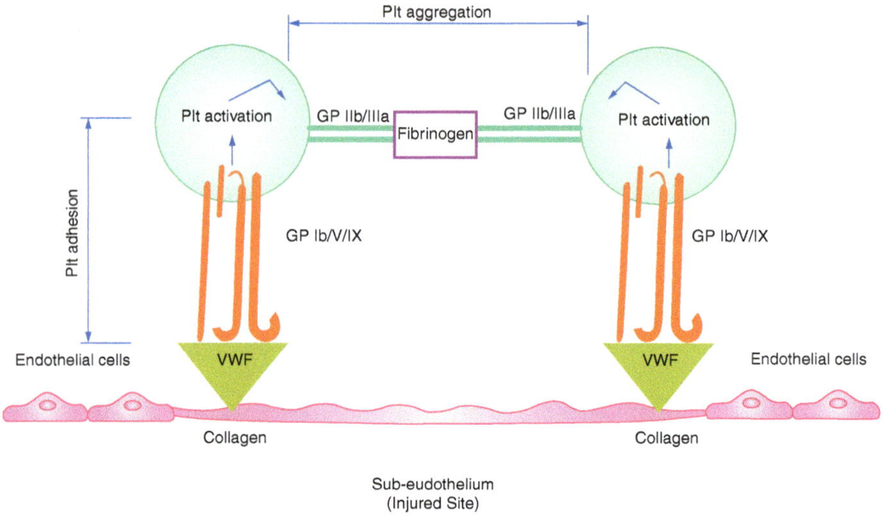

Fig. 1.3 Platelet activation and aggregation and their mediators. Glycoprotein (GP)Ib/V/IX and GPIIb/IIIa are the main GPs that mediate platelet adhesion and aggregation, respectively. Fibrinogen also has an important role in platelet aggregation. *Plt* platelet, *GP* glycoprotein, *VWF* von Willebrand factor

In fact, in addition to well-known role of most of these components in hemostasis, a considerable number of these components have vital roles in other body processes. The process of hemostasis is under precise regulation in the body. Any abnormality in this process can result in severe consequences. Bleeding and thrombotic complications are consequences of abnormalities in the process of hemostasis including missing or dysfunction of specific elements of hemostasis.

Hemostasis is categorized into two main categories, including primary and secondary hemostasis [7].

1.2 Platelets

Platelets are anucleated cells that, in addition to their well-known role in hemostasis, are involved in several other crucial processes in the body including inflammatory processes and tumor angiogenesis and have a role in defense against microbial infections. In normal circumstances, they don't have significant interaction with the vessel walls, but in vascular injury, they promptly interact with the subendothelial extracellular matrix at the injured site in order to stop bleeding. This adhesion leads to platelet activation and granule releases. Stable platelet adhesion at the site of injury occurs in a dynamic process, which includes platelet tethering, rolling, activation, and firm adhesion (Fig. 1.4) [8, 9].

Subendothelial extracellular matrix has several molecules; most of them are ligands for different platelet GPs. Among these adhesive macromolecules, collagen type I and III are the most important for platelet adhesion.

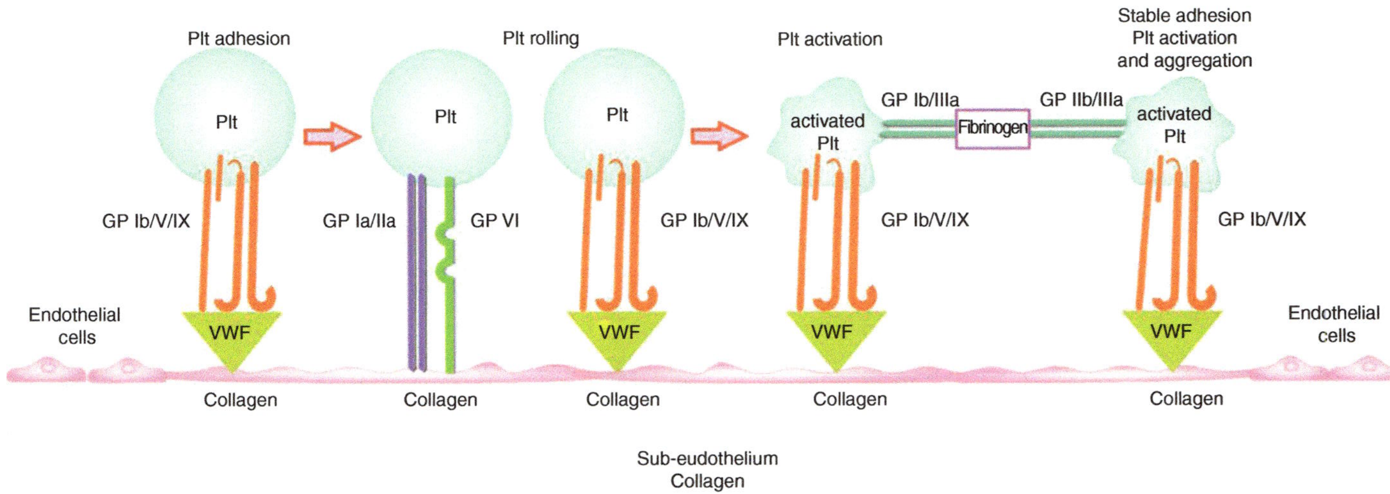

Fig. 1.4 Stable platelet adhesion at the site of injury occurs in a dynamic process that includes platelet tethering, rolling, activation, and firm adhesion. Firstly platelet adhesion is mediated by glycoprotein (GP)Ib/V/IX. This GP also has a role in platelet rolling accompanied with GPIa/IIa and GPVI. After platelet activation, firm adhesion has occurred. GPIIb/IIIa and fibrinogen are the main molecules in platelet aggregation. *Plt* platelet, *GP* glycoprotein, *VWF* von Willebrand factor

Although platelet adhesion is primarily mediated by interaction of GPIb/V/IX complex with VWF in subendothelial matrix, integrin α2β1 (GPIa/IIa) has a crucial role in adhesion process. Binding of integrin α2β1 to collagen leads to the promotion of intracellular process and subsequently platelet activation and firm adhesion to subendothelial.

Initially, integrin α2β1–collagen interaction results in inducing collagen and GPVI interaction. In addition, this interaction leads to the activation of integrin αIIbβ3. Although integrin αIIbβ3, in inactivated form, doesn't bind to fibrinogen, upon activation of platelets, conformational changes occur in this integrin, so the integrin gains the fibrinogen-binding ability. Therefore, integrin αIIbβ3 has a role in both adhesion and aggregation processes. The final stage of adhesion process is firm platelet adhesion to the extracellular matrix. This process requires activation of platelets and shifting integrin αIIbβ3 to its high affinity state. The mechanism of platelet adhesion is different in two conditions, that is, low (20–200 s^{-1}) and high shear (300–800 s^{-1}) conditions. In high shear, initial interaction of platelets GPIb/V/IX complex with VWF in the external subendothelial matrix is loose. This initial adhesion is firmed by integrin receptors and their ligands, including α5β1 (GPIc/IIa) and α2β1 (GPIa/IIa) integrins. In low shear, αIIbβ3 and α2β1 integrins interact with fibrinogen and collagen, respectively, directly initiating platelet adhesion. Following platelet adhesion and with the activation of integrin αIIbβ3 and platelet agonist release, platelet aggregation occurs and subsequently hemostatic plug is formed [10].

1.3 Platelet Surface Glycoproteins

1.3.1 Integrin $\alpha_{IIb}\beta_3$ (Glycoprotein IIb/IIIa) (CD41/CD61)

Out of 18 integrin α and 10 integrin β subunits, platelets express 4 members of β1 including α2β1, α5β1, α6β1, and α8β1 and both β3, αVβ3 and αIIbβ3 subfamilies. α2β1, α5β1, and α6β1 are collagen, fibronectin, and laminin receptors, respectively. Integrin αIIbβ3 is the receptor of several extracellular matrix elements such as collagen, VWF, fibronectin, and vitronectin. Although β1 family members have a crucial role in adhesion, they have a minor role in platelet aggregation, but they are unable to independently support this process (Table 1.1).

Integrin αIIbβ3 is the most abundant platelet integrin with 40,000 to 80,000 copies on unstimulated platelets plus exposable intracellular pool of this integrin. Integrin αIIbβ3 is the main platelet glycoprotein that is required for platelet aggregation and has an important role in the final step of adhesion, which is known as firm adhesion. Although platelet aggregation mainly is mediated by integrin αIIbβ3 and its ligands including VWF and fibrinogen, other molecules such as GPIb and VWF also have some roles.

Glanzmann thrombasthenia (GT) is a moderate to severe hemorrhagic disorder due to mutation in *ITGA2B* or *ITGB3* genes that leads to quantitative or qualitative defects

Table 1.1 Platelet glycoprotein properties

Glycoprotein	Alternative name	Number/cell	Function	Ligand	Prevalence of related defect	Bleeding tendency
GPIa/IIa	1. Integrin α2β1 2. VLA-2 3. CD49b/CD29	2000–4000	Adhesion	1. Collagen 2. Laminin 3. Vitronectin 4. Tenascin 5. Decorin	Extremely rare	Mild
GPIc/IIa	1. Integrin α5β1 2. VLA-5		Adhesion	1. Fibronectin 2. Denatured collagen 3. Laminin	Extremely rare	Mild
GPIb/V/IX	CD42 a–d	~25,000[a]	1. Platelet adhesion 2. Platelet-endothelial cell adhesion 3. Platelet-leukocyte adhesion	1. VWF 2. Mac-1 3. P-selectin 4. α-Thrombin 5. HMWK 6. FXI 7. FXIIa	Rare	Mild–moderate
GPIIb/IIIa	1. Integrin αIIbβ3 2. CD41/CD61	40,000–80,000	1. Aggregation 2. Adhesion	1. Fibrinogen 2. VWF	Rare	Moderate–severe
GPIV	GP IIIb, CD36		1. Adhesion 2. Aggregation signaling	1. Collagen	Extremely rare	Mild
GPVI	–		1. Adhesion	1. Collagen 2. Collagen-related peptide (CRP) 3. Convulxin	Extremely rare	Mild
GPα6/IIa	1. Integrin α6β1 2. VLA-6		Adhesion	1. Laminin 2. Epiligrin	Extremely rare	Mild
–	α8β1 CD29/CD49h		Adhesion	1. Fibronectin 2. Vitronectin 3. Tenascin 4. Laminin	Extremely rare	Mild
VR (vitronectin receptor)	1. αVβ3 2. CD51/CD61	A few hundreds	1. Adhesion 2. Aggregation	1. Collagen 2. Osteopontin 3. Tenascin 4. VWF	Rare	Mild

[a]Approximately 25,000 copies of the first three peptides including GP Ibα, GP Ibβ, and GP IX reside in the platelet surface along with half as many copies of GPV

in integrin αIIbβ3 with defect in platelet aggregation. In heterozygotes of GT, about 50% amount of integrin αIIbβ3 is present, which is sufficient for normal aggregation.

Integrin αIIbβ3 is present on platelets in both inactivated and activated conformations, but to prevent spontaneous aggregation, it is constrained to inactivated conformation on circulating platelets. Upon vascular injury, nearly immediate activation of integrin αIIbβ3 occurs via stimulation of platelet agonists such as thrombin and ADP [11, 12].

1.3.2 Glycoprotein Ib/V/IX (CD42 a–d)

GPIb/V/IX (CD42 a–d) is the major platelet adhesion GP that initiates platelet adhesion to the subendothelial matrix in high shear stress. In fact, adhesion process at high shear is initiated by interaction between GPIb/V/IX and VWF in extracellular matrix at the site of vascular injury. This initial interaction enables platelet arrests at high shear, inducing signal transduction and finally integrin-mediated platelet adhesion. α2β1 (GPIa/IIa), α5β1 (GPIc/IIa), and αIIbβ3 (GPIIb/IIIa) integrins are involved in firm platelet adhesion.

Following this adhesion, signal transduction leads to platelet shape change and activation, granule secretion, and inside-out integrin activation that promote platelet adhesion and aggregation. During this phase, platelet agonists such as ADP and thrombin are released. These agonists cause platelet activation and additional platelet recruitment at the site of injury. Signal transduction via GPIb/V/IX leads to activation of integrin αIIbβ3 on platelets, which is required for firm platelet adhesion and aggregation. GPIb/V/IX complex consists of several separated subunits, GPIbα (CD42bα), GPIbβ (CD42bβ/CD42c), GPIX (CD42a), and GPV (CD42d), in a ratio of 2:2:2:1, all of them are members of the leucine-rich repeat (LRR) family. GPIbα and GPIbβ are linked with each other with disulfide bond(s) while noncovalently associated with GPIX and GPV subunits.

The N-terminal of GPIbα has binding sites for VWF, Mac-1 (CD11b/CD18), P-selectin, α-thrombin, high-molecular-weight kininogen (HMWK), and coagulation factors including factor (F) XI and FXIIa. α-Thrombin binding to N-terminal of GPIbα leads to platelet activation by thrombin via protease-activated receptor-1 (PAR-1).

GPIbα can mediate platelet–endothelial and platelet–leukocyte adhesion by binding to P-selectin or leukocyte integrin, Mac-1. Platelet–endothelial adhesion also can be mediated by integrin αIIbβ3 on activated platelets and integrin αVβ3 on activated endothelial cells via adhesive molecules such as fibrinogen. Qualitative and quantitative defects in GPIbα, GPIbβ, and GPIX lead to the occurrence of Bernard–Soulier syndrome (BSS) [13, 14].

1.3.3 Integrin α2β1 (Glycoprotein Ia/IIa) (CD49b/CD29)

Integrin α2β1 is one of the main platelet surface collagen receptors that are expressed in different cell types. In fact, platelets have two receptors with definitive role in platelet–collagen interaction; integrin α2β1 is expressed on the platelet surface on low affinity state for collagen, but upon platelet activation, inside-out signaling leads to occurrence of conformational changes in this integrin and increasing its affinity. Initial adhesion of platelets by GPVI causes platelet activation, and inside-out signaling results in conformational change in integrin α2β1, increasing its affinity, that is, from low to high, which leads to stable platelet adhesion.

Integrin α2β1 and collagen binding has several consequences, including promoting GPVI and collagen interaction and activating integrin αIIbβ3. Integrin α2β1 deficiency is an extremely rare disorder with mild bleeding tendency [15].

1.3.4 Glycoprotein VI

GPVI is a member of immunoglobulin superfamily that initiates platelet activation and promotes integrin αIIbβ3 activation, which is required for platelet aggregation at the site of injury. GPVI is present on platelet surface in complex with Fc receptor (FcR) γ-chain. Extracellular region of GPVI has no affinity for collagen but in dimeric form (GPVI-FcR) has this affinity. This shows that dimeric structure of GPVI is necessary for the affinity of this receptor to collagen. Similar to GPIb/V/IX (CD42 a–d), GPVI is critical for the initial interaction of platelets with extracellular matrix at the site of vascular injury under high shear condition. GPVI deficiency is an extremely rare hemorrhagic disorder with mild bleeding tendency. One of the most important laboratory findings in these patients is lack of platelet aggregation in response to collagen with normal response to other agonists in aggregometry studies. Some patients have very low response to collagen, which is attributed to presence of other collagen receptors on the platelet surface including integrin α2β1 [16, 17].

1.3.5 Integrin α5β1 (Glycoprotein Ic/IIa)

Integrin α5β1 (GPIc/IIa) as the major platelet receptor of fibronectin has a supplemental role in platelet adhesion at the site of vascular injury.

1.3.6 Integrin αVβ3 (CD51/CD61)

Only a few hundreds of integrin αVβ3 (CD51/CD61) are presented on the platelet surface. The expression of this integrin is not restricted to megakaryocyte lineage. Similar to other integrins, αVβ3 (CD51/CD61) is presented in low affinity state on unstimulated platelet surface, while in other cells this integrin is presented in high affinity state. In fact, integrin αVβ3 (CD51/CD61) is presented in low affinity default state in circulating platelets, while in tissue cells, it is presented in high affinity default state [18–20].

1.4 Platelet Granules and Secretion

Platelet adhesion is accompanied with their activation and release of procoagulatory mediators such as ADP, thrombin, and prostaglandins. This process leads to thrombus formation that in addition to platelets, incorporates red blood cells (RBC) and leukocytes. In addition to lysosomes, platelets have two main types of secretory granules including α-granules and dense granules. These small, anucleated cells have more than 300 distinct molecules that have been detected in their releasates. α-granules and dense granules are lysosome-related organelles that are restricted to the platelets. α-granules with a frequency of 50–80 per platelet are the most frequent, while only 0–3 lysosome can be found in each platelet. This number is 3–8 per platelet for dense granules. The diameters of α-granules, dense granules, and lysosomes are 200–500, 200–300, and 200–250 nm, respectively. Platelet granules participate in a variety of body functions including the well-known process of hemostasis, inflammation, wound healing, and angiogenesis as well as malignancies and antimicrobial host defense. Most of these functions including thrombosis and hemostasis, inflammation, angiogenesis, wound healing, and antimicrobial host defense are related to α-granules. The majority of platelet α-granules constitutes are synthesized in megakaryocytes, while the minority including fibrinogen, FV, albumin, and immunoglobulins are captured and endocytosed by circulating platelets and transported to α-granules. Platelets serve as circulating reservoirs of these components and can rapidly release them at local sites after activation (Table 1.2) [21, 22].

α-granules are immediately exocytosed after platelet activation and enhance hemostasis and inflammation processes. α-granules express large amount of P-selectin that after platelet activation are moved to the surface of these cells for interaction with neutrophils, monocytes, endothelial cells, and other platelets.

This interaction between P-selectin and P-selectin glycoprotein ligand-1 (PSGL-1) leads to tethering of platelets, and rolling of them at the site of vascular injury allows firm platelet adhesion.

In addition to the relatively well-known role of platelets on trapping of pathogens, they have a crucial role in directly killing of some pathogens. After *Plasmodium falciparum* infection, activated platelets are attached to infected RBCs and released platelet factor 4 (PF4) from their α-granules. This chemokine inhibits the growth of pathogen and kills it. β-defensins are other platelet constitutes that have direct antimicrobial effects on *Staphylococcus aureus*. PF4 is also able to recruit cells to the inflamed site. Defensins are not located in the mentioned granules and are either cytosolic molecules or contents of other unidentified granules.

Dense granules, dense bodies, or δ-granules contain adenine nucleotides such as adenosine triphosphate (ATP) and ADP and serotonin that are involved in different platelet functions including vasoconstriction, pro-inflammatory cytokine production, inflammation, and platelet aggregation (Table 1.3) [23].

Lysosomes are less frequent than α-granules and dense granules, and contain several enzymes involved in the degradation of carbohydrates, proteins, and lipids. These include glycosidases, proteases, and cationic proteins such as β-glucuronidase,

Table 1.2 Contents of α-granules

	Contents
Hemostatic factors	1. Factor V 2. von Willebrand factor (VWF) 3. Fibrinogen 4. Factor XIII 5. Factor IX 6. Protein S 7. Tissue factor pathway inhibitor (TAFI) 8. Antithrombin 9. Plasminogen 10. Plasminogen activator inhibitor-1(PAI-1)
Growth factors	1. Platelet-derived growth factor (PDGF) 2. Vascular endothelial growth factor (VEGF) 3. Basic fibroblast growth factor (bFGF) 4. Epidermal growth factor (EGF) 5. Transforming growth factor-β (TGF-β) 6. Stromal cell-derived factor-1 α (SDF-1 α)
Proteases	1. Matrix metalloproteinase-2 (MMP-2) 2. Matrix metalloproteinase-9 (MMP-9)
Angiogenic factors	1. Angiogenin 2. Vascular endothelial growth factor (VEGF)
Anti-angiogenic factors	1. Angiostatin 2. Platelet factor-4 (PF-4)
Necrotic factors	1. Tumor necrosis factor-α (TNF-α) 2. Tumor necrosis factor-β (TNF-β)
Chemokines	1. Chemokine (C-X-C motif) ligand-1 (CXCL-1) 2. Chemokine (C-X-C motif) ligand-4 (CXCL-4) 3. Chemokine (C-X-C motif) ligand-5 (CXCL-5) 4. Chemokine (C-X-C motif) ligand-7 (CXCL-7) 5. Chemokine (C-X-C motif) ligand-8 (CXCL-8) 6. Chemokine (C-X-C motif) ligand-12 (CXCL-12) 7. Chemokine (C-C motif) ligand-2 (CCL-2) 8. Chemokine (C-C motif) ligand-3 (CCL-3) 9. Chemokine (C-C motif) ligand-5 (CCL-5)
Granule membrane-specific proteins	1. P-selectin 2. CD63 3. Platelet alpha-granule membrane protein (GMP-33)

Table 1.3 Contents of dense granules

	Contents
Nucleotides	1. Adenosine triphosphate (ATP) 2. Adenosine diphosphate (ADP) 3. Guanosine 5′-triphosphate (GTP) 4. Guanosine diphosphate (GDP)
Amines	1. Serotonin or 5-hydroxytryptamine (5-HT) 2. Histamine
Bivalent cations	1. Calcium 2. Magnesium

Table 1.4 Contents of the lysosomes

	Contents
Acid proteases	1. Carboxypeptidase A 2. Carboxypeptidase B 3. Cathepsin D 4. Cathepsin E 5. Acid phosphatase 6. Collagenase
Glycohydrolases	1. Heparinase 2. β-*N*-Acetyl-glucosaminidase 3. β-Glycerophosphatase 4. β-Glucuronidase 5. β-Galactosidase 6. α-D-Glucosidase 7. α-L-Fucosidase 8. β-D-Fucosidase

elastase, and collagenase with bactericidal activity. These enzymes can help in pathogen and platelet thrombi clearance, extracellular matrix degradation, and heparin inactivation (Table 1.4) [24].

When platelets become activated, anionic lipids such as phosphatidylserine are exposed on platelet surface. Then FV of platelet α-granules is released and bound to these anionic lipids. This FV is activated by initial, small amount of thrombin that is generated from the initial interaction between tissue factor (TF) and FVII at the site of vascular injury. Activated FV (FVa) accompanied with FXa, calcium, and anionic lipids form the prothrombinase complex. This complex cleaves prothrombin and changes it to thrombin (FIIa). FXa bounded to FV is relatively protected from inhibition by plasma inhibitors such as antithrombin. The main consequence of these events is the dramatic increase of thrombin generation on activated platelet surface, and this process is restricted to the site of vascular injury. In fact, platelets localize coagulation process to thrombus and protect coagulation enzymes from inhibition by plasma and platelet inhibitors, therefore preventing the occurrence of disseminated intravascular coagulation (DIC). In Scott syndrome, as an inherited platelet function disorder (IPFD) with mutated *TMEM16F* gene, this procoagulant activity of platelets is impaired. These issues show close relationship between activated platelets and coagulation factors [25].

1.5 Endothelium

The endothelium has been described as a barrier between circulatory blood and surrounding tissues. It is a dynamic organ that can regulate its environment and response to external stresses. Although the endothelium is less than 0.2 μm thick, it includes 6×10^3 endothelial cells that weigh about 1 kg in an average person and covers 4000–7000 m^2. The endothelium acts as a blood-compatible surface that maintains blood flow and regulates blood coagulation system [26].

Endothelial cells have several functions include vascular tone regulation, cellular adhesion, smooth muscle cell proliferation, and vascular inflammation. Endothelial cells have numerous functions that are specific to different vascular beds. The main function of the endothelium is to regulate systemic blood flow via change in vascular diameter. Furthermore, the endothelium acts as a barrier that controls fluid, ion, and macromolecule movement between the circulating blood and surrounding tissues selectively. Endothelium regulates recruitment and extravasation of procoagulation leukocytes in response to tissue injury and inflammation. Endothelial cells play a crucial role in the healing process after injury or inflammation. They also act as angiogenesis vector, which is necessary for tissue repair and obstructive fibrin clot recanalization. Endothelial cells accompanied with smooth muscle cells also regulate local blood pressure, because these cells are responsive to vasoactive agents. These cells can response to inflammatory cytokines and other stresses like hypoxia and metabolic stresses. Altogether, the endothelium expresses many molecules that regulate platelets and activate coagulation cascade that results in the prevention of post-vascular injury thrombosis development [27, 28].

Endothelial cells cover the arteries, veins, and microvessels. Shear stress, blood oxygenation, and smooth muscle cell density are different between these vessels, so endothelial cells differently response to procoagulation signals in different vascular beds. For instance, vasodilation regulation in the arteries is faster than in the veins. These cells adapt their phenotype according to the nature of the surrounding tissues and have abundant phenotypic heterogeneity.

Endothelial cells have an important role in clot development due to their position and are closely related to coagulation cascade. Intact endothelial cells express inhibitors to prevent thrombin synthesis and activation. When these cells are activated, they play a role in the initiation and development of thrombin production via procoagulation factor expression [29, 30].

Coagulation cascade can be activated via two pathways, intrinsic and extrinsic. Extrinsic and intrinsic pathways are initiated by converting FVII to FVIIa and FXII to FXIIa, respectively. Activated endothelial cells contribute to extrinsic pathway, expressing TF in response to vascular injury and inflammation. TF/FVIIa complex activates protease-activated receptor-2 (PAR-2) that induces a pro-inflammatory response. The endothelium regulates clot formation by PAR activation. Acute release of endothelial products is mostly mediated by PAR-1. PAR-1 plays an important role in response to procoagulation stimuli. It induces Weibel–Palade body (WPB) activation, and therefore VWF and tissue-type plasminogen activator (t-PA) are released. It also mediates nitric oxide (NO) and prostacyclin production, which reduces platelet activation. Finally, thrombin-mediated PAR-1 activation is related to surface TF exposure [31, 32].

It is observed that microvascular endothelial cells induce angiogenesis by releasing TF-rich microparticles.

Although activated endothelial cells are typically related to extrinsic pathway, they also may play a role in intrinsic pathway. The mechanism of endothelial cell function in intrinsic pathway is unclear, but there is a supposition that these cells prevent the inhibition of intrinsic pathway factors; for instance, FXIIa can be protected from C1 inhibition activity by the endothelial cells [33]. Investigations also have shown that these cells are the primary source of FVIII. Therefore, endothelial cells are probably the necessary component of both intrinsic and extrinsic coagulation pathways.

In addition to coagulation, endothelial cells have a main role in primary hemostasis. The interaction between platelets and endothelium is important for platelet activation and regulation. An intact endothelium prevents platelets from adhesion, while activated endothelial cells express molecules and receptors that enhance platelet adhesion to the injured site. WPB stores VWF, P-selectin, angiopoitin-2, t-PA, and endothelin-1 in endothelial cells which mediate platelet adhesion, leukocyte recruitment, inflammation regulation, fibrinolysis, and vasoconstriction, respectively.

VWF has two main roles in hemostasis: first, it is necessary for collagen to have platelet adhesion to GPIb/V/IX in the injured vascular sites and, second, it stabilizes plasma coagulation FVIII [34, 35].

Furthermore, an intact endothelium actively prevents thrombosis formation by suppressing platelet activation and adhesion. It expresses multiple anticoagulants such as tissue factor pathway inhibitor (TFPI), thrombomodulin, endothelial protein C receptor (EPCR), and heparin-like proteoglycans. There is an ectonucleotidase (CD39) on the endothelial cell surface that converts platelet stimulator ADP into adenosine. TFPI is one of the most important inhibitors of coagulation cascade. It inhibits coagulation cascade by direct inhibition of FXa and TF/FVIIa/FXa complex. Patients with less than 10% of the normal level of TFPI have increased risk of venous thrombosis and coronary heart disease. Thrombomodulin and EPCR catalyze thrombin-mediated protein C pathway activation. Activated protein C inactivates FVa and FVIIIa that results in reduced thrombin formation. Platelet activation is inhibited by prostacyclin and prostaglandin E2 (PGE2) which are released from the activated endothelium by vasoactive agents. NO enhances prostacyclin effect [36–38].

Endothelial cells are important components that contribute to clot destruction. In wound healing process, endothelial cells release proteofibrinolytic molecules, such as t-PA and urokinase-type plasminogen activator (u-PA), and metalloproteases for clot destruction. These cells also release ADAMTS13 and ADAMTS18 that mediate platelet aggregate dissolution [27, 39, 40]. The endothelial cells are one of the main parts of the blood vessels and can induce angiogenesis after stimulation. For instance, protein C can stimulate angiogenesis in the brain endothelium [41].

Endothelial disorders are responsible for inflammation and inappropriate clot formation and can be related to cardiovascular diseases.

1.6 Coagulation Factors

All coagulation factors are synthesized by the liver except for FVIII, which is produced by the endothelial cells. VWF is also synthesized in megakaryocytes, in addition to endothelial cells.

Initiation of blood coagulation is triggered by vascular injury and exposure of TF to bloodstream that leads to generation of small amount of thrombin. This thrombin is sufficient to activate platelets, FV, FVIII, and FXI and triggers consolidation pathway that leads to sufficient generation of thrombin. This thrombin is sufficient to convert fibrinogen to fibrin. Thrombin is the key coagulation enzyme that has two major functions in hemostasis including fibrinogen to fibrin conversion and activation of platelets.

From the initial theory of coagulation cascade by Macfarlane, Davie, and Ratnoff in 1964, which involved a series of enzymatic reactions by which initial small amount of stimulus was amplified and results in burst generation of thrombin that is sufficient for fibrinogen to fibrin conversion, extensive revision was made. Two alternative pathways, namely, intrinsic and extrinsic, have been introduced for the initiation of coagulation cascade (Table 1.5).

Coagulation cascade is a precise mechanism that leads to clot formation and blood loss prevention. In physiological status, this cascade is counterbalanced by anticoagulant system mechanisms. This exact regulation leads to prevent aberrant clot formation. In pathological status, due to hereditary or acquired defects, normal controlling mechanisms of coagulation system may be disrupted, which can result in pathological conditions such as thrombosis [42].

The Extrinsic Pathway Unlike intrinsic pathway, an external component of pathway, TF is present in this pathway. This pathway is initiated by a complex formation between plasma FVIIa with TF from the extravascular tissue. Although TF is not present in the bloodstream at high concentration, upon tissue injury, it's exposed to FVIIa. TF, as a cofactor of FVII, induces activation of FVII. This complex cleaves trace amount of FIX and FX to FIXa and FXa, respectively. FXa in combination with FVa, as a cofactor for FVa, forms the prothrombinase complex. This complex converts prothrombin (FII) into thrombin (FIIa), and thrombin converts fibrinogen into fibrin monomers. These fibrin monomers are unstable and cross-linked by FXIIIa to be stable.

The Intrinsic or Contact Activation Pathway This pathway is named intrinsic because all components are present in the blood, and this pathway is initiated by exposure of the blood to negatively charged surfaces. This pathway consists of several proteins including FXII that is activated by negatively charged surfaces. FXIIa converts prekallikrein into activated form, kallikrein. Kallikrein itself converts more

Table 1.5 Characteristics of blood coagulation factors

Coagulation factor	Alternative name	Structure	Function in coagulation cascade	Other functions	Plasma half–life	Hemostatic level	Normal range
Factor I	Fibrinogen	Heterotrimer	Clot formation	Platelet adhesion	72–120 h	20–30%	1.5–4.0 g/l
Factor II	Prothrombin	Monomer	Serine protease	Anticoagulant activity	60–70 h	20–40%	75–115 u/dl
Factor III	1. Tissue factor 2. Tissue thromboplastin 3. Tissue phospholipid 4. CD142	Extracellular, transmembrane, and intracellular zones	Cofactor	Arterial and vein thrombosis Myocardium infarction Angiogenesis	–	5–19 pM	–
Factor IV	Calcium	Ion	Cofactor	Role in proper muscle, nerve, and heart function	–	–	9–10.5 mg/dl
Factor V	1. Labile factor 2. Proaccelerin 3. Owern	Single-chain protein consists of six domains	Cofactor	Anticoagulant activity	36 h	10%	63–115 u/dl
Factor VII	Stable factor Proconvertin	FVII: single chain FVIIa: double chain	Serine protease	–	FVII: 4–6 h FVIIa: 2 h	10–15%	70–125 u/dl
Factor VIII	Antihemophilic factor	Non-covalent heterodimer	Cofactor	1. Essential blood-clotting protein 2. Association of factor VIIIa with factor IXa to form the intrinsic factor Xase complex 3. Increase the catalytic efficiency for factor Xa generation	17 h	30–60%	55–150 u/dl
Factor IX	Christmas	Monomer	Serine protease	Coagulation FX activator	24 h	20–30%	70–165 u/dl

Coagulation factor	Alternative name	Structure	Function in coagulation cascade	Other functions	Plasma half–life	Hemostatic level	Normal range
Factor X	Stuart Prower	Heterodimer of light and heavy chains	Serine protease	Coagulation factor II activator	30–40 h	20%	79–155 u/dl
Factor XI	Plasma thromboplastin antecedent	Homodimer (four apple domains with one catalytic domain in each subunit)	Serine protease	1. FIX activator 2. Thrombin generation 3. Antifibrinolysis	52 h	15–50%	65–135 u/dl
Factor XII	Hageman	Monomer (SP, fibronectin types I and II, kringle, proline reach, EGF1 and EGF2 like, catalytic, activating peptide, and lytic activator domains)	Serine protease	Activation of complement classic pathway	60 h	0–2%	60–125 u/dl
Factor XIII	1. Fibrin stabilizing factor 2. Laki–Lorand factor 3. Fibrinase 4. Fibrin polymerase 5. Protransglutaminase	Heterodimer (FXIII-A2B2)	Transglutaminase	1. Angiogenesis 2. Maintenance of pregnancy 3. Wound healing 4. Bone metabolism 5. Cardioprotection	9–12 days	2–5%	15 mg/dl
HMWK	Fitzgerald factor	Monomer	Cofactor	1. Fibrinogen adherence to phospholipid surfaces 2. Induce PGI2 and NO generation from the endothelium 3. Role in kinin system	9–10 h	0–2%	8 mg/dl

(continued)

Table 1.5 (continued)

Coagulation factor	Alternative name	Structure	Function in coagulation cascade	Other functions	Plasma half–life	Hemostatic level	Normal range
PKK	Fletcher factor	Dimer (SP, catalytic serine protease, activating peptide, hydrolytic, and four apple domains)	Serine protease	1. Inflammation 2. Pain 3. Smooth muscle cell dilatation 4. Vasodilation	35 h	0–2%	5 mg/dl
VWF	Von Willebrand factor	Monomer (D1, D2, D′, D3, A1, A2, A3, D4, B1, B2, B3, C1, C2, and CK domains)	Cofactor of FVIII Platelet adhesion, platelet aggregation, stabilization of circulating FVIII	1. Inflammation 2. Angiogenesis	12.4 h		50–150 u/dl

Mg milligram, *dl* deciliter, *pM* picomole, *SP* signal peptide, *EGF* epidermal growth factor, *PGI2* prostaglandin I2, *NO* nitric oxide, *HMWK* high molecular weight kininogen, *PKK* prekallikrein amounts of FXII into FXIIa, so there is a positive feedback for FXII activation. FXIIa activates FXI into FXIa. High-molecular-weight kininogen (HMWK) plays a cofactor role for all reactions. HMWK also converts to kininogen and then kinin, which causes vasodilation, swelling, erythema, pain, and local hypotension. On the other hand, high amounts of FXIIa created by kallikrein play a role as t-PA and plasminogen activator. Therefore, it prevents further clotting in non-injured areas by plasmin formation. In the following, FXIa with Ca^{2+} as cofactor activates FIX into FIXa. Finally the intrinsic tenase complex is composed of FIXa, FVIIIa, and Ca^{2+}, and phospholipid converts FX into FXa.

The rest of the path continues similar to the extrinsic pathway. This similar part between intrinsic and extrinsic pathways is called common pathway (Fig. 1.5).

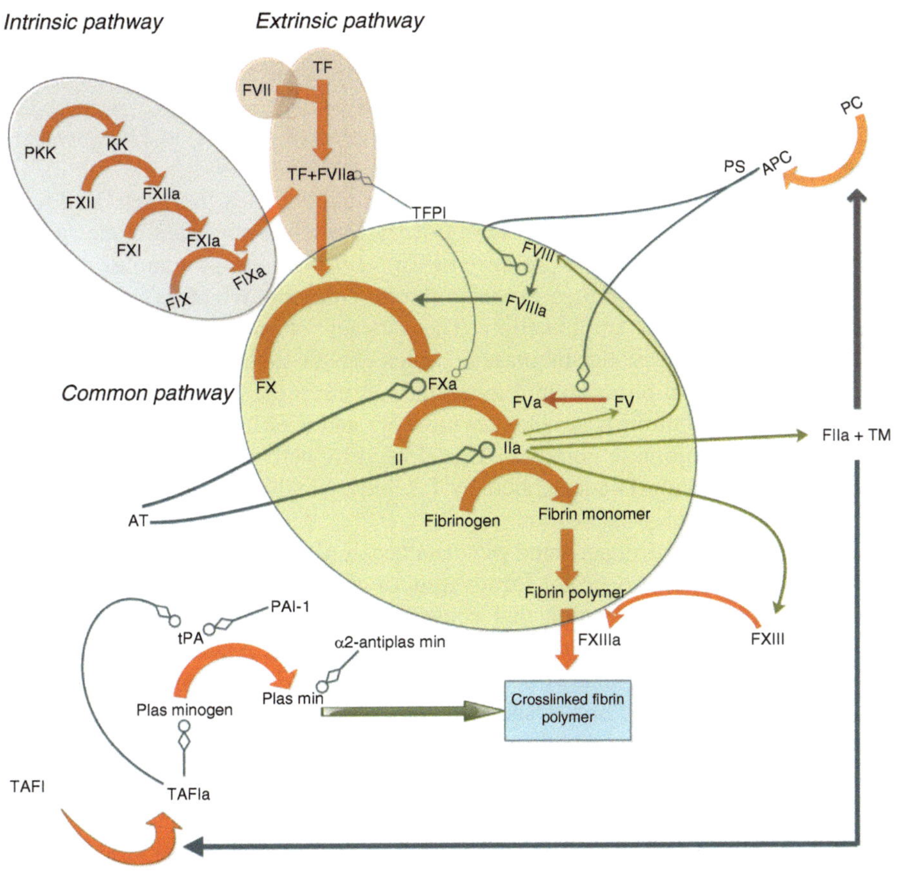

Fig. 1.5 Coagulation cascade and fibrinolysis system interaction

More recent concepts suggest that coagulation is composed of three phases (initiation, amplification, and propagation):

1. *Initiation phase* starts with TF exposure to coagulation factors caused by endothelial injury or activation. Endothelial cells can express TF in response to inflammatory stimulus such as exposure to bacterial lipopolysaccharide (LPS) in sepsis, adhesion molecules, inflammatory cytokines, and oxidized low-density lipoprotein (LDL).

   Because there is no human model of TF deficiency and murine model exhibits embryonic lethality in homozygous TF knockout mice, it seems that lack of TF is incompatible with life.

   TF forms a catalytic complex with FVIIa (TF/FVIIa complex), which is known as extrinsic tenase complex. This complex is placed on the phospholipid surface of cell membrane and converts FIX and FX into FIXa and FXa, respectively. Then FXa generates small amounts of FIIa (thrombin). The length of initiation phase depends on the concentration of TF/FVIIa complex and tissue factor pathway inhibitor (TFPI), which acts as FXa and TF/FVIIa complex neutralizer.

   Initiation phase is characterized by localization of process on TF-expressing cells and generation of thrombin in picomolar amounts.
2. In *amplification phase*, FIX forms intrinsic tenase complex in its activated form with FVIIIa (FIXa/FVIIIa) that is optimally formed on the membrane surface provided by platelets in the presence of Ca^{2+}. Intrinsic tenase complex activates FX 50–100-folds more than extrinsic tenase complex, which is necessary for coagulation process amplification. The efficacy of intrinsic tenase complex (FIXa/FVIIIa) and prothrombinase complex (FXa/FVa) is multiplied with their co-localization on phospholipid membrane in the presence of Ca^{2+}. Generated thrombin in initiation phase activates more FV and FVIII, which plays a cofactor role in prothrombinase complex. Therefore, FIX activates more FX, and prothrombin activation is accelerated by FX [43]. Finally, thrombin is generated adequately to form a stable clot.
3. In *propagation phase*, activated platelets accumulate in the injured site to provide phospholipid surface for localization of coagulation process. This leads to optimal thrombin generation that converts fibrinogen to fibrin. Soluble fibrin monomers are converted to stable polymer by covalent bonds. These bonds are generated by FXIIIa that is activated by thrombin. Thrombin also activates thrombin-activatable fibrinolysis inhibitor (TAFI) which acts as clot protector against fibrinolysis [44–47].

1.7 Anticoagulation Mechanisms

Fibrin clot formation is the end of coagulation process. Natural anticoagulations are necessary to limit clot formation process at the injured site. One of the most important anticoagulants is antithrombin (AT), which is the main inhibitor of thrombin. It is a vitamin K-independent serine protease that is synthetized in the liver. AT mainly inhibits thrombin and FXa, but it can also inhibit FIXa and FVIIa. Inhibitory effect of AT is enhanced in the presence of heparin. Heparan sulfate is also an AT activity enhancer located on the endothelial cell surface. Heparin cofactor II is another vitamin K-independent serine protease that specially inhibits thrombin. Its inhibitory activity is enhanced in the presence of dermatan sulfate. α_2-Macroglobulin and α_1-antitrypsin are other thrombin inhibitors. Protein C is a vitamin K-dependent serine protease which is activated by thrombin. Activated protein C (APC) is a potent anticoagulant that degrades FVa and FVIIIa using protein S as cofactor. Protein C inhibitor, α_2-macroglobulin, and α_1-antitrypsin limit APC activity. Thrombomodulin (TM) is a transmembrane receptor on the endothelial cell surface that binds to thrombin. Protein C activation is increased in the presence of TM–thrombin complex [48, 49].

EPCR is another transmembrane receptor on the endothelial cell surface that binds to protein C, resulting in more APC generation. In addition to these anticoagulants, TFPI is the main inhibitor of tissue factor pathway. TFPI has little, direct effect on FVa, but it binds to FXa at first and generates FXa–TFPI complex. Then this complex binds to TF–FVa complex and generates a complex that inactivates both FV and FX. Furthermore, there is a plasma enzyme named protein Z-dependent protease inhibitor (ZPI) that plays a role in FIXa, FXa, and FXIa inhibition [50, 51]. In addition, fibrinolysis system is one of the most important mechanisms that degrade formed clot.

1.8 Fibrinolysis System

Fibrinolysis system is necessary to degrade the clot that formed by hemostasis mechanisms. Plasminogen is the main enzyme of this system. It is not able to degrade fibrin clot, but it has affinity to fibrin, and thus it binds to the clot. Plasminogen is converted to its activated form, known as plasmin, by two activators: t-PA and u-PA. Plasmin as a serine protease cleaves the formed fibrin and also produces more t-PA and u-PA. Plasminogen activators have more effect on Lys-plasminogen. Plasmin converts Glu-plasminogen to Lys-plasminogen, which has more affinity to plasminogen activators. In fact, plasmin enhances its own production by positive feedback.

T-PA has little effect on plasminogen in the absence of fibrin. Both t-PA and plasminogen bind to fibrin. Generation of t-PA/plasminogen/fibrin complex is necessary to produce plasmin. Therefore, fibrin acts as cofactor for plasminogen activation and substrate for plasmin simultaneously [52].

Fibrinolysis is limited by plasminogen activator inhibitors (PAIs), which prevent plasminogen to plasmin conversion by t-PA and u-PA inhibition, and by plasmin inhibitors such as α_2-antiplasmin and α_2-macroglubulin and TAFI that inhibits plasmin effect on fibrin. Thrombin is a weak TAFI activator, but TM–thrombin complex enhances this activity several times. TAFI removes lysine and arginine residues from fibrin C-terminal. These residues are necessary for plasminogen and t-PA binding; thus TAFI causes decreased plasminogen activation by t-PA. It also decreases Glu-plasminogen conversion to Lys-plasminogen by plasmin. TAFI also increases direct inhibition of plasmin by α_2-antiplasmin [53–55].

References

1. Osaki T, Ichinose A. Current views of activating and regulatory mechanisms of blood coagulation. Nihon rinsho Japanese. J Clin Med. 2014;72(7):1206–11.
2. Davie EW. A brief historical review of the waterfall/cascade of blood coagulation. J Biol Chem. 2003;278(51):50819–32.
3. Butenas S, Mann K. Blood coagulation. Biochem Mosc. 2002;67(1):3–12.
4. Kasirer-Friede A, Shattil SJ. Regulation of platelet adhesion receptors. In: Platelets in thrombotic and non-thrombotic disorders. Cham: Springer; 2017. p. 69–84.
5. Feghhi S, Munday AD, Tooley WW, Rajsekar S, Fura AM, Kulman JD, et al. Glycoprotein Ib-IX-V complex transmits cytoskeletal forces that enhance platelet adhesion. Biophys J. 2016;111(3):601–8.
6. Bennett JS. Regulation of integrins in platelets. Peptide Sci. 2015;104(4):323–33.
7. Versteeg HH, Heemskerk JW, Levi M, Reitsma PH. New fundamentals in hemostasis. Physiol Rev. 2013;93(1):327–58.
8. Gremmel T, Frelinger AL III, Michelson AD. Platelet physiology. Semin Thromb Hemost. 2016;42(3):191–204.
9. Sorrentino S, Studt J-D, Medalia O, Sapra KT. Roll, adhere, spread and contract: structural mechanics of platelet function. Eur J Cell Biol. 2015;94(3):129–38.
10. Goto S, Hasebe T, Takagi S. Platelets: small in size but essential in the regulation of vascular homeostasis–translation from basic science to clinical medicine. Circ J. 2015;79(9):1871–81.
11. Coller B. αIIbβ3: structure and function. J Thromb Haemost. 2015;13(Suppl 1):S17–25.
12. Bledzka K, Smyth SS, Plow EF. Integrin αIIbβ3. Circ Res. 2013;112(8):1189–200.
13. López JA. The platelet glycoprotein Ib-IX-V complex. In: Gresele P, Kleiman N, Lopez J, Page C, editors. Platelets in thrombotic and non-thrombotic disorders. Cham: Springer; 2017. p. 85–97.
14. Li R, Emsley J. The organizing principle of the platelet glycoprotein Ib–IX–V complex. J Thromb Haemost. 2013;11(4):605–14.
15. Madamanchi A, Santoro SA, Zutter MM. α2β1 integrin. In: I domain integrins. Cham: Springer; 2014. p. 41–60.
16. Arman M, Krauel K. Human platelet IgG Fc receptor FcγRIIA in immunity and thrombosis. J Thromb Haemost. 2015;13(6):893–908.
17. Gawaz M, Vogel S, Pfannenberg C, Pichler B, Langer H, Bigalke B. Implications of glycoprotein VI for theranostics. Thromb Haemost. 2014;112(1):1–6.
18. Kunicki TJ. Platelet membrane glycoproteins and their function: an overview. Ann Hematol. 1989;59(1):30–4.
19. Nurden AT. Platelet membrane glycoproteins: a historical review. Semin Thromb Hemost. 2014;40:577–84.
20. George JN. Platelet membrane glycoproteins. Cham: Springer; 2013.
21. Koseoglu S, Flaumenhaft R. Advances in platelet granule biology. Curr Opin Hematol. 2013;20(5):464–71.
22. Heijnen H, Sluijs P. Platelet secretory behaviour: as diverse as the granules… or not? J Thromb Haemost. 2015;13(12):2141–51.
23. Sadeghian MH, Keramati MR, Badiei Z, Ravarian M, Ayatollahi H, Rafatpanah H, et al. Alloimmunization among transfusion-dependent thalassemia patients. Asian J Transfusion Sci. 2009;3(2):95.

24. Yadav S, Storrie B. The cellular basis of platelet secretion: emerging structure/function relationships. Platelets. 2017;28(2):108–18.
25. Golebiewska EM, Poole AW. Platelet secretion: from haemostasis to wound healing and beyond. Blood Rev. 2015;29(3):153–62.
26. Yau JW, Teoh H, Verma S. Endothelial cell control of thrombosis. BMC Cardiovasc Disord. 2015;15(1):130.
27. van Hinsbergh VW. Endothelium—role in regulation of coagulation and inflammation. Semin Immunopathol. 2012;34:93–106.
28. Monahan-Earley R, Dvorak AM, Aird WC. Evolutionary origins of the blood vascular system and endothelium. J Thromb Haemost. 2013;11(s1):46–66.
29. Dekker RJ, van Thienen JV, Rohlena J, de Jager SC, Elderkamp YW, Seppen J, et al. Endothelial KLF2 links local arterial shear stress levels to the expression of vascular tone-regulating genes. Am J Pathol. 2005;167(2):609–18.
30. Aird WC. Phenotypic heterogeneity of the endothelium: II. Representative vascular beds. Circ Res. 2007;100(2):174–90.
31. Bode M, Mackman N. Protective and pathological roles of tissue factor in the heart. Hamostaseologie. 2015;35(1):37–46.
32. Borissoff JI, Spronk HM, ten Cate H. The hemostatic system as a modulator of atherosclerosis. N Engl J Med. 2011;364(18):1746–60.
33. Schousboe I. Binding of activated Factor XII to endothelial cells affects its inactivation by the C1-esterase inhibitor. FEBS J. 2003;270(1):111–8.
34. Do H, Healey JF, Waller EK, Lollar P. Expression of factor VIII by murine liver sinusoidal endothelial cells. J Biol Chem. 1999;274(28):19587–92.
35. Dubois C, Panicot-Dubois L, Gainor JF, Furie BC, Furie B. Thrombin-initiated platelet activation in vivo is vWF independent during thrombus formation in a laser injury model. J Clin Investig. 2007;117(4):953.
36. Esmon CT, Esmon NL. The link between vascular features and thrombosis. Annu Rev Physiol. 2011;73:503–14.
37. Wood JP, Ellery PE, Maroney SA, Mast AE. Biology of tissue factor pathway inhibitor. Blood. 2014;123(19):2934–43.
38. Dahm A, van Hylckama Vlieg A, Bendz B, Rosendaal F, Bertina RM, Sandset PM. Low levels of tissue factor pathway inhibitor (TFPI) increase the risk of venous thrombosis. Blood. 2003;101(11):4387–92.
39. Collen D, Lijnen HR. The tissue-type plasminogen activator story. Arterioscler Thromb Vasc Biol. 2009;29(8):1151–5.
40. Chung DW, Fujikawa K. Processing of von Willebrand factor by ADAMTS-13. Biochemistry. 2002;41(37):11065–70.
41. Petraglia AL, Marky AH, Walker C, Thiyagarajan M, Zlokovic BV. Activated protein C is neuroprotective and mediates new blood vessel formation and neurogenesis after controlled cortical impact. Neurosurgery. 2010;66(1):165–72.
42. Adams RL, Bird RJ. coagulation cascade and therapeutics update: relevance to nephrology. Part 1: overview of coagulation, thrombophilias and history of anticoagulants. Nephrology. 2009;14(5):462–70.
43. Palta S, Saroa R, Palta A. Overview of the coagulation system. Indian J Anaesth. 2014;58(5):515.
44. Mann KG, Brummel-Ziedins K, Orfeo T, Butenas S. Models of blood coagulation. Blood Cell Mol Dis. 2006;36(2):108–17.
45. Grignani G, Maiolo A. Cytokines and hemostasis. Haematologica. 2000;85(9):967–72.
46. Mann KG, Butenas S, Brummel K. The dynamics of thrombin formation. Arterioscler Thromb Vasc Biol. 2003;23(1):17–25.
47. Lasne D, Jude B, Susen S. From normal to pathological hemostasis. Can J Anesth. 2006; 53(2):S2–S11.
48. Pike RN, Buckle AM, Le Bonniec BF, Church FC. Control of the coagulation system by serpins. FEBS J. 2005;272(19):4842–51.

49. Rigby AC, Grant MA. Protein S: a conduit between anticoagulation and inflammation. Crit Care Med. 2004;32(5):S336–41.
50. Dahm A, Sandset P, Rosendaal F. The association between protein S levels and anticoagulant activity of tissue factor pathway inhibitor type 1. J Thromb Haemost. 2008;6(2):393–5.
51. Corral J, González-Conejero R, Hernández-Espinosa D, Vicente V. Protein Z/Z-dependent protease inhibitor (PZ/ZPI) anticoagulant system and thrombosis. Br J Haematol. 2007;137(2):99–108.
52. Rijken D, Lijnen H. New insights into the molecular mechanisms of the fibrinolytic system. J Thromb Haemost. 2009;7(1):4–13.
53. Dellas C, Loskutoff DJ. Historical analysis of PAI-1 from its discovery to its potential role in cell motility and disease. Thromb Haemost. 2005;93(4):631–40.
54. Ezihe-Ejiofor JA, Hutchinson N. Anticlotting mechanisms 1: physiology and pathology. Contin Edu Anaesth Crit Care Pain. 2013;13(3):87–92.
55. Chapin JC, Hajjar KA. Fibrinolysis and the control of blood coagulation. Blood Rev. 2015;29(1):17–24.

Congenital Bleeding Disorders

2

Akbar Dorgalaleh and Fariba Rad

2.1 Congenital Bleeding Disorders

Congenital bleeding disorders (CBD) are heterogeneous group of hemorrhagic disorders with highly variable incidence, clinical presentations, and laboratory findings [1, 2]. Although in most of these disorders, precise incidence is not clear, these disorders can be as common as von Willebrand disease (VWD), with an incidence of ~1%, or be as rare as congenital factor (F) XIII and FII deficiencies with estimated incidence of 1 per 2 million [3, 4]. Although bleeding tendency is mild in most of inherited platelet function disorders (IPFD), severe life-threatening bleeds such as intracranial hemorrhage (ICH) are common in FXIII deficiency [5, 6]. Severe recurrent bleeds can also be observed in hemophilia A as the most common severe congenital bleeding disorder, hemophilia B and VWD, notably type 3. Timely diagnosis of CBD is crucial for appropriate management of these disorders [6]. Clinical presentations, family history, and appropriate laboratory approach are useful for timely diagnosis. Although diagnosis of most coagulation factor deficiencies is straightforward (except for FXIII deficiency and some qualitative fibrinogen disorders), diagnosis of most cases with IPFD is sophisticated and requires advanced laboratory tests (except for Glanzmann thrombasthenia (GT) and Bernard-Soulier syndrome (BSS)) [7]. Timely diagnosis and appropriate management of these disorders are crucial and can significantly improve the quality of life in these patients. Although most of the patients with IPFD have mild bleeding disorders, regular prophylaxis is recommended for patients with severe hemophilia A and B. Replacement therapy is the mainstay of treatment in patients with RBD [7, 8]. Most of the patients with RBD require "on-demand therapy", which means treatment of bleeding as soon as possible after onset; regular primary prophylaxis is mandatory for all patients with severe congenital FXIII deficiency from the time of diagnosis (Table 2.1) [8, 9].

A. Dorgalaleh (✉)
Department of Hematology and Blood Transfusion, School of Allied Medicine, Iran University of Medical Sciences, Tehran, Iran

F. Rad
Cellular and Molecular Research Center, Yasuj University of Medical Sciences, yasuj, Iran

A. Dorgalaleh (ed.), *Congenital Bleeding Disorders*,
https://doi.org/10.1007/978-3-319-76723-9_2

Table 2.1 Common features of congenital bleeding disorders

CBD			Gene defect	Inheritance	Prevalence	Bleeding tendency
Common bleeding disorder	VWD	VWD-type 1	*VWF (12p13.3)*	Autosomal dominant	1 per 1000	Mild
		VWD-type 2		Mainly autosomal dominant[a]	Undetermined	Moderate-severe
		VWD-type 3		Autosomal recessive	1 per 1 million	Severe
	Hemophilia A		*F8 (Xq28)*	X-linked recessive	1 per 10,000 male	Severe
	Hemophilia B		*F9 (Xq27.1)*	X-linked recessive	1 per 50,000 male	Severe
RBD	FI deficiency	Afibrinogenemia	*FGA, FGB, FGG (4q28)*	Autosomal recessive	1 per 1 million	Severe
		Hypofibrinogenemia		Mainly autosomal dominant	Undetermined	Mainly asymptomatic
		Dysfibrinogenemia		Mainly autosomal dominant	Undetermined	Mainly asymptomatic
		Hypodysfibrinogenemia		Mainly autosomal dominant	Undetermined	Mild
	FII deficiency		*F2* (11p11–q12)	Autosomal recessive	1 per 2 million	Moderate-severe
	FV deficiency		*F5* (1q24.2)	Autosomal recessive	1 per 1 million	Mild
	CFV-FVIII deficiency		*LMAN1* (18q21.3–q22) *MCFD2* (2p21–p16.3)	Autosomal recessive	1 per 1 million	Mild
	VKDCFD		*GGCX* (2p12) *VKORC1* (16p11.2)	Autosomal recessive	1 per 1 million	Moderate
	FVII deficiency		*F7* (13q34)	Autosomal recessive	1 per 500,000	Moderate-severe
	FX deficiency		*F10* (13q34)	Autosomal recessive	1 per 1 million	Moderate-severe
	FXI deficiency		*F11* (4q35.2)	Autosomal recessive	1 per 1 million	Mild
	FXIII deficiency		*F13A1 (6p24–p25)* *F13B (1q31–q32.1)*	Autosomal recessive	1 per 2 million	Severe

CBD		Gene defect	Inheritance	Prevalence	Bleeding tendency
IPFD	GT	*ITGA2B&ITGB3 (17q21.31–32)*	Autosomal recessive	1 per 1 million	Moderate-severe
	BSS	*GP1BA (17p13)* *GP1BB(22q11.21)* *GP9 (3q21)*	Biallelic: autosomal recessive Monoallelic: autosomal dominant	1 per 1 million	Biallelic: moderate-severe Monoallelic: mild
	GPS	*NBEAL* *GFI1B* *GATA1*	Mainly autosomal recessive	1 per 1 million	Mild

CBD congenital bleeding disorder, *VWD* von Willebrand disease, *RBD* rare bleeding disorders, *FI* factor I, *FII* factor II, *FV* factor V, *CFV-FVIII* combined factor V and factor VIII, *FVII* factor VII, *VKDCF* vitamin K-dependent coagulation factor, *FX* factor X, *FXI* factor XI, *FXIII* factor XIII, *IPFD* inherited platelet function disorder, *GT* Glanzmann thrombasthenia, *BSS* Bernard-Soulier syndrome, *PT-VWD* platelet-type von Willebrand disease, *QPD* Quebec platelet disorder, *GPS* gray platelet syndrome, *HPS* Hermansky-Pudlak syndrome, *WAS* Wiskott-Aldrich syndrome

[a]Some of type 2 VWD such as type 2N VWD are autosomal recessive

2.2 Clinical Manifestations

The pattern of bleeding is different among patients with CBD; mucocutaneous bleeding is common in patients with IPFD, while deep tissue hemorrhage is more common among patients with congenital coagulation factor deficiencies. Although mucocutaneous bleeds are common in IPFD, the frequency and severity of bleeding are variable among these patients. Bleeding tendency is variable among patients with IPFD, even in members of a family, especially in GT and BSS. Although most of the patients with IPFD have mild bleeding tendency, GT and BSS are considered as severe disorders of this group [6, 10, 11]. In patients with GT, gingival bleeding, purpura, and epistaxis, and among women, menorrhagia, are the constant presentations. Purpura commonly appears after minor trauma or pressure, and epistaxis is the most common cause of severe bleeding in GT [12, 13]. The severity of bleeding is more profound in patients with leukocyte adhesion deficiency-III/leukocyte adhesion deficiency-I variant (LAD-III/LAD-Iv) than GT and severe life-threatening bleeds, and recurrent infections are common among these patients. Myelofibrosis is a rare presentation of patients with gray platelet syndrome (GPS) due to high level of platelet-derived growth factors (PDGF). Oculocutaneous albinism is a key feature of Hermansky-Pudlak syndrome (HPS), while immunodeficiency is a distinguishing feature of HPS-2 [6].

In patients with hemophilia, the intensity of bleeding depends on the severity of factor deficiency, and spontaneous hemorrhages notably in soft tissues, joints, and muscles are common among patients with severe hemophilia (FVIII and FIX level <1%). Patients with mild and moderate hemophilia present posttraumatic or postsurgical bleeding. Hemarthrosis is the most common presentation and the most debilitative manifestation of hemophilia [14–17]. Among patients with RBD, severe bleeds can be observed among patients with afibrinogenemia, FII, FVII, FX, and FXIII deficiencies, while most of the patients with combined FV and FVIII (CFV-FVIII) deficiency are asymptomatic, and patients with FXI deficiency experience posttraumatic or postsurgical bleeding. Patients with FV deficiency have mild bleeding tendency [9, 18, 19]. Umbilical cord bleeding is the common clinical presentation of patients with afibrinogenemia (85%) and FXIII deficiency (>80%). Recurrent miscarriage is also common in patients with congenital fibrinogen disorders (CFD) and FXIII deficiency [20–22]. Although successful delivery was observed, it is believed that homozygote women with FXIII deficiency are unable to have successful delivery [23–25]. ICH with a frequency of ~30% is more common in patients with congenital FXIII deficiency than any other CBD. This diathesis is also relatively common in FVII deficiency and was also reported in afibrinogenemia and FII and FX deficiencies and rarely in FV deficiency. Neonatal ICH is relatively common in vitamin K-dependent clotting factor (VKDCF) deficiency [5, 26]. Thrombotic and obstetrical complications are common complications of patients with CFD, notably dysfibrinogenemia and hypodysfibrinogenemia [21, 27]. These complications can also be observed in patients with FII deficiency [28]. Although generally heterozygotes of CBD are asymptomatic, severe bleeding has been observed among some of heterozygotes of CBD including FXIII and FVII deficiencies [29–31]. Mucocutaneous bleeding including epistaxis and menorrhagia is the typical presentation of patients with VWD. Patients with type 3 VWD had severe presentations, while type 1 and type 2 are very heterogeneous and strictly related to functional VWF measured as ristocetin cofactor activity (WF:RCo). Epistaxis and bruising are the most common presentations of children with VWD, while in adults, hematoma, menorrhagia, and bleeding from minor wounds are the most frequent presentations (Table 2.2) [3, 32, 33].

2.3 Molecular Basis

Congenital coagulation factor deficiencies are due to mutation in genes encoding corresponding coagulation factors except for congenital combined FV and FVIII deficiency and VKDCF deficiency (VKCFD). Combined FV and FVIII deficiency is caused by mutation in proteins involving intracellular transport of FV and FVIII. These are *MCFD2* and *LMAN1* genes. In VKCFD, congenital defect in coagulation factors is due to mutation in genes encoding enzymes involving in posttranslational modification and vitamin K metabolism including *gamma-glutamyl carboxylase (GGCX)* and *vitamin K epoxide reductase (VKOR)*. Most of RBD have autosomal recessive manner of inheritance except for some cases with FXI deficiency and CFD (hypofibrinogenemia and dysfibrinogenemia) [9, 34–37]. The inheritance pattern of IPFD is autosomal manner, while in hemophilia A and hemophilia B, pattern of inheritance is X-linked recessive [6]. A considerable number of patients with hemophilia A and hemophilia B are due to de novo mutations in *F8* and *F9* genes [38]. Among CBD, recurrent mutations are rare, and the most common gene defects are intron 22 inversion that occurred in ~50% of patients with severe hemophilia A. The second common mutation is intron 1 inversion with a frequency of 1–5%. Screening for these mutations can be the first step in molecular diagnosis of patients with severe hemophilia A [39–41]. Such gene defects are rare for other CBD. According to some studies, *FGA* IVS 4 + 1G > T mutation can be the first mutation in the screening algorithm for new individuals with congenital afibrinogenemia of European origin, and *FGA* 11-kb deletion is the other common target for molecular diagnosis and the avoidance of diagnostic errors [21, 42]. In Iranian patients with congenital FXIII deficiency, Trp187Arg (c.559T > C) is recommended as first line in molecular diagnosis [4, 43].

Milder forms of hemophilia A are mostly due to missense mutations. In patients with congenital fibrinogen deficiency, missenses are the most common gene defects, and the bleeding severity is more profound in those with missense mutation. Some of these mutations are clustered in especial gene areas including clustering of missense mutations in the highly conserved βC of FGB. Most cases with CBD are due to new mutations that are restricted to a special family or special geographical areas mostly due to founder effect (Fig. 2.1) [44, 45].

A wide spectrum of mutations was identified throughout affected genes in CBD. In RBD, missense mutation with a frequency of >50% is the most common identified mutation [9]. In patients with GT, the disorder is due to homozygote and

Table 2.2 Clinical features of patients with congenital bleeding disorders

CBD		Common clinical presentations (%)	Less common presentations (%)	Rare clinical presentations (%)
Common bleeding disorder	VWD	Epistaxis (62) Menorrhagia (60) Bleeding from minor wounds (36) Post-extraction bleeding (51) Hematoma (49) Gum bleeding (35) Postsurgical bleeding (28) Postpartum bleeding (23)	GI bleeding (14) Hemarthrosis (8) Hematuria (7)	CNS bleeding (1)
	Hemophilia A	Hemarthrosis (86) Postdental extraction bleeding (84) Hematoma (82) Postoperative bleeding (76) Ecchymosis (71) Oral cavity bleeding (64) Epistaxis (59)	Hematuria (12) GI bleeding (10)	CNS bleeding (4) UCB (2)
	Hemophilia B	Postdental extraction bleeding (97) Hemarthrosis (73) Ecchymosis (57) Epistaxis (55)	GI bleeding (4) Hematuria (12)	CNS bleeding (5) Hematoma (4) UCB (5)

RBD	FI deficiency[a]	UCB (85) Epistaxis (80) Menorrhagia (70) Hemarthrosis (54) Gingival bleeding (70) Postoperative bleeding (40)	Thrombotic events (9)	CNS bleeding (5)
	FII deficiency	Hematoma (60) Hemarthrosis (42) Postdental extraction bleeding (36) Menorrhagia (20)	Postoperative bleeding (12)	GI bleeding (3) CNS bleeding (1)
	FV deficiency	Epistaxis (68) Menorrhagia (50) Postoperative bleeding (43) Oral cavity bleeding (31)	Hemarthrosis (18) Hematoma (60) GI bleeding (6)	UCB (3) CNS bleeding (1)
	CFV-FVIII deficiency	Postdental extraction bleeding (88) Postpartum hemorrhage (83) Excessive post-major surgical bleeding (75) Menorrhagia (63) Post-circumcision hemorrhage (56) Epistaxis (42.5) Gum bleeding (29) Ecchymosis/easy bruising (32)	Hemarthrosis (18) GI bleeding (7.5)	Hematuria (2) Hematoma (2) ICH (1)
	VKDCF deficiency	ICH (34) Ecchymosis/easy bruising (21)	UCB (17) Posttraumatic/postsurgical hemorrhage (17) Epistaxis (17) Gingival/oral bleeding (12)	Hemarthrosis (4)

(continued)

Table 2.2 (continued)

CBD		Common clinical presentations (%)	Less common presentations (%)	Rare clinical presentations (%)
	FVII deficiency	Epistaxis (60) Menorrhagia (69) Easy bruising (36) Gum bleeding (34) Hematoma (20)	Hemarthrosis (19) GI bleeding (14) Hematuria (6)	CNS bleeding (4)
	FX deficiency	Menorrhagia (71) Easy bruising (55) Hematoma (43) Epistaxis (36) Hemarthrosis (33) Gum bleeding (31)	GI bleeding (12) ICH (9) Hematuria (7)	Hemarthrosis (2)
	FXI deficiency	Postsurgical bleeding (66) Ecchymosis (28) Epistaxis (24) GI bleeding (15)	Menorrhagia (7)	Gum bleeding (1) Postdental extraction bleeding (3.5)
	FXIII deficiency	UCB (>80) Hematoma (53) Prolonged wound bleeding (31) Intracranial bleeding (~30) Postsurgical bleeding (19) Gum bleeding (17) Epistaxis (14) Miscarriage (~100)[b]	GI bleeding (10) Menorrhagia (10) Post-circumcision bleeding (4) Delayed postdental extraction bleeding (7)	Splenic rupture (<1)

IPFD	GT	Epistaxis (79) Menorrhagia (74) Gingival bleeding (68) Ecchymosis/easy bruising (43)	GI bleeding (7.4) Hematuria (7) Hematoma (6)	CNS bleeding (1.8) Excessive bleeding at time of delivery (0.5) UCB (0.3) Hemarthrosis (0.3)
	BSS	Postpartum hemorrhage (75) Epistaxis (64)	Ecchymosis (7) Gum bleeding (15.5) Postdental extraction bleeding (15) Menorrhagia (11.3)	GI bleeding (4.1) Hematoma (3) CNS bleeding (1)
	GPS	Epistaxis (53) Easy bruising (48) Menorrhagia (38) Splenomegaly (70)	Ecchymosis (7) Postsurgical bleeding (10) Postdental extraction bleeding (6)	ICH (1)

CBD congenital bleeding disorder, *VWD* von Willebrand disease, *RBD* rare bleeding disorders, *FI* factor I, *FII* factor II, *FV* factor V, *CFV-FVIII* combined factor V and factor VIII, *FVII* Factor VII, *VKCFD* vitamin K-dependent clotting factor deficiency, *FX* factor X, *FXI* factor XI, *FXIII* factor XIII, *IPFD* inherited platelet function disorder, *GT* Glanzmann thrombasthenia, *BSS* Bernard-Soulier syndrome, *PT-VWD* platelet-type von Willebrand disease, *QPD* Quebec platelet disorder, *GPS* gray platelet syndrome, *HPS* Hermansky-Pudlak syndrome, *WAD* Wiskott-Aldrich syndrome, *GI* gastrointestinal bleeding, *CNS* central nervous system, *UCB* umbilical cord bleeding, *ICH* intracranial hemorrhage

[a]Data were presented for afibrinogenemia

[b]Almost all untreated women with severe FXIII deficiency experience miscarriage

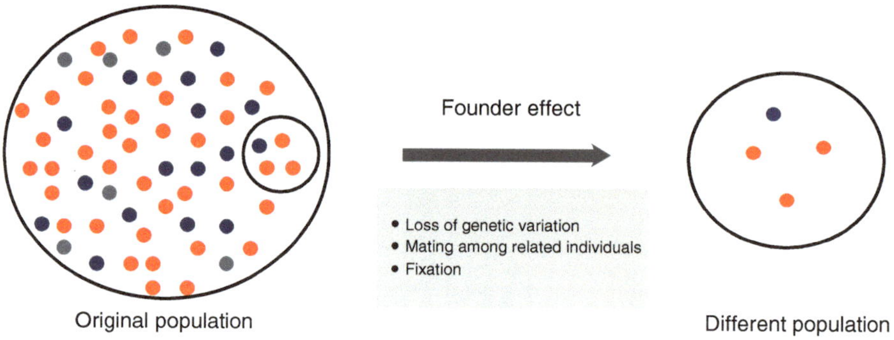

Fig. 2.1 Founder effect. A founder effect occurs when a new colony is started by a few members of the original population

double heterozygote mutations in *ITGA2B* and *ITGB3* genes [46, 47]. VWD has autosomal recessive/dominant pattern of inheritance. Although type 1 VWD is an autosomal recessive disorder, in ~30% of patients, underling mutation cannot be identified. Type 3 VWD that is the most severe form of disorder is due to homozygote or double heterozygotes mutations in *VWF* gene (Table 2.3) [48, 49].

2.4 Diagnosis

Diagnosis of CBD can be made based on clinical presentations, family history, and appropriate laboratory approach. A positive family history is an important clue for timely diagnosis of CBD; therefore previous to laboratory assessment, a proper family history should be taken [1, 2, 50]. In CBD with autosomal manner of inheritance, such as RBD, IPFD, and VWD, any family member can be affected, while in hemophilia A and B, due to X-linked manner of inheritance, males are affected. This issue should keep in mind that about one-third of patients with hemophilia have de novo mutations, and therefore absence of family history should not always lead to ruling out of CBD [6, 50–52]. In addition to this issue, in some patients with CBD including GT, BSS, and FX deficiency, even with same mutation in member of same family, the bleeding tendency is variable [9, 47]. The type of bleeding and severity of disorder can also help in diagnosis. Mucocutaneous hemorrhages are more frequent in patients with IPFD, while this type of bleeding is less common in coagulation factor deficiency, and hemorrhage in deep tissues is more frequent among these patients [10, 53]. Hemarthrosis is a hallmark of hemophilia, and those joints that bleed often are referred to as "target joints." The most common target joints are the knees and elbows and less frequently, the hip, wrist, and shoulder [54, 55]. Although hemarthrosis is common in hemophilia, it also can be observed in other CBD, including RBD and especially in type 3 VWD that is accompanied by significant decrease of FVIII (Table 2.4) [9, 56, 57].

Although a number of IPFD are severe bleeding disorders, including GT and BSS, most of the patients with IPFD have mild bleeding tendency and can be

Table 2.3 Molecular characteristics of congenital bleeding disorders

CBD			Gene defect	Defects	Type of mutation (%)	Number of mutation
Common bleeding disorder	VWD	VWD	*VWF*	–	Missense (59) Deletion (13) Nonsense (13) Others (15)	410
		VWD-type 1	*VWF*	–	Missense (72) Splice site (9) Deletion (8) Nonsense (5) Others (6) UDM (~30)[a]	>130
		VWD-type 2	*VWF*	–	Missense (89) Splice site (2) Deletion (3) Nonsense (2) Others (4)	Type 2: 160 Type 2A: 75 Type 2B: 25 Type 2N: 30 Type 2M:30
		VWD-type 3	*VWF*	–	Missense (18) Splice site (11) Deletion (30) Nonsense (31) Others (10)	120
	Hemophilia A		*F8*	–	Intron 22 inversion (~50) Intron 1 inversion (~2) Large deletion (1) Small deletion (10) Nonsense (9) Splice site (4)	2320
	Hemophilia B		*F9*	–	Missense/nonsense (64) Small insertion/deletion (18) Splice site (9) Large insertion/deletion (6) Regulatory (2) Complex rearrangement (1)	1113

Table 2.3 (continued)

CBD			Gene defect	Defects	Type of mutation (%)	Number of mutation
RBD	FI deficiency	Afibrinogenemia Hypofibrinogenemia	*FGA, FGB, FGG (4q28)*	FGA: 73 FGB: 61 FGG: 66	FGA (48 Ins/Del, 35 Nonsense, 17 Splicing) FGB (42 Missense, 5 Ins/Del, 24 Nonsense, 29 Splicing) FGG (58 Missense, 5 Ins/Del, 16 Nonsense, 21 Splicing) Large deletions are not frequency in quantitive Fibrinogenemia (5)	200
		Dysfibrinogenemia	*FGA, FGB, FGG (4q28)*	FGA: 40 FGB: 9 FGG: 39	Missense (85.2) Deletion/insertion 9.1 Frameshift (3.5) Nonsense (1.1) Intronic (1.1)	88
		Hypodysfibrinogenemia	*FGA, FGB, FGG (4q28)*	FGA: 10 FGB: 5 FGG: 17	Missense (66) Nonsense (12.5) Frameshift (12.5)	32
	FII deficiency		*F2 (11p11–q12)*			
	FV deficiency		*F5 (1q24.2)*		Missense (46.6) Small deletion (18.4) Nonsense (11.7) Splice site (10.7) Insertion (6.7) Small in-frame deletion (3.9) Major rearrangement (1) Large deletion (1)	150

	CFV-FVIII deficiency	*LMAN1 (18q21.3–q22)*		Frameshift (47) Splice site (24) Nonsense (18) Missense (5) Initiation codon (3) Deletion (3)	38
		MCFD2 (2p21–p16.3)		Missense (50) Frameshift (25) Splice site (15) Nonsense (5) Large deletion (5)	20
	VKDCF deficiency	*GGCX (2p11.2)*		Missense (61) Splice site (27.8) Frameshift (5.55) Deletion (5.55)	18
		VKORC1 (16p11.2)		Missense (100)	1
	FVII deficiency	*F7 (13q34)*	–	Missense (79) Small ins/del (9) Splice sites (8) Nonsense (4)	636
	FX deficiency	*F10 (13q34)*		Missense (80) Nonsense (7) Splice sites (5) Deletion/insertion (6.5) Frameshift (1.5)	141
	FXI deficiency	*F11 (4q35.2)*		Missense (71.6) Nonsense (10.9) Insertion/deletion (7.5) Splice sites (9) Promoter (0.7)	265
	FXIII deficiency	*F13A1 (6p24–p25)* *F13B (1q31–q32.1)*	F13A1: 156 F13B: 16		*F13A1*: 156 *F13B*: 16

(continued)

Table 2.3 (continued)

CBD		Gene defect	Defects	Type of mutation (%)	Number of mutation
IPFD	GT	*ITGA2B/ITGB3*	ITGA2B:221		335
			ITGB3:134		
	BSS	*GP1BA/GP1BB/GP9*	GP1BA/GP1BB/ GP9	Missense (45.5) Frameshift (28.6) Nonsense (17.9) Others (8)	112
			GP1BA: 45	Missense (22.2) Frameshift (46.7) Nonsense (22.2) Others (8.9)	
			GP1BB: 39	Missense (59) Frameshift (20.5) Nonsense (15.4) Others (5.1)	
			GP9: 28	Missense (64.3) Frameshift (10.7) Nonsense (14.3) Others (10.7)	
	GPS	*NBEAL* *GFI1B* *GATA1*		Missense (48) Nonsense (19) Deletion (19) Intronic (14)	21

CBD congenital bleeding disorder, *VWD* von Willebrand disease, *RBD* rare bleeding disorders, *FI* factor I, *FII* factor II, *FV* factor V, *CFV-FVIII* combined factor V and factor VIII, *FVII* factor VII, *VKDCF* vitamin K-dependent clotting factor, *FX* factor X, *FXI* factor XI, *FXIII* factor XIII, *IPFD* inherited platelet function disorder, *GT* Glanzmann thrombasthenia, *BSS* Bernard-Soulier syndrome, *PT-VWD* platelet-type von Willebrand disease, *QPD* Quebec platelet disorder, *GPS* gray platelet syndrome, *HPS* Hermansky-Pudlak syndrome, *WAD* Wiskott-Aldrich syndrome

[a]Some of type 2 VWD such as type 2 N VWD are autosomal recessive

Table 2.4 Main laboratory features of congenital bleeding disorders

CBD				Laboratory features	
Common bleeding disorder	VWD	VWD-type 1		VWF:Ag: ↓ to ↓↓ VWF:GPIb binding: ↓ to ↓↓ VWF:CB: ↓ to ↓↓ FVIII:C: N to ↓↓	Multimers: normal pattern but reduced intensity GPIb binding/Ag: > (0.5–0.7) CB/Ag: > (0.5–0.7) FVIII/VWF: > (0.5–0.7)
		VWD-type 2	2 A	VWF:Ag: N to ↓↓ VWF:GPIb binding: ↓↓ to ↓↓↓ VWF:CB: ↓↓ to ↓↓↓ FVIII:C: ↓ to ↓↓	Multimers: loss high MMW VWF GPIb binding /Ag: < (0.5–0.7) CB/Ag: < (0.5–0.7) FVIII/VWF: > (0.5–0.7)
			2 B	VWF:Ag: N to ↓↓ VWF:GPIb binding: ↓ to ↓↓↓ VWF:CB: ↓ to ↓↓↓ FVIII:C: N to ↓↓	Multimers: loss high MMW VWF GPIb binding/Ag: < (0.5–0.7) CB/Ag: < (0.5–0.7) FVIII/VWF: > (0.5–0.7)
			2 N	VWF:Ag: N to ↓↓ VWF:GPIb binding: N to ↓↓ VWF:CB: N to ↓↓ FVIII:C: ↓↓ to ↓↓↓	Multimers: normal pattern GPIb binding /Ag: > (0.5–0.7) CB/Ag: > (0.5–0.7) FVIII/VWF: < (0.5–0.7)
			2 M	VWF:Ag: N to ↓↓ VWF:GPIb binding: ↓ to ↓↓↓ VWF:CB: ↓ to ↓↓↓ FVIII:C: ↓ to ↓↓	Multimers: no loss of HMW VWF but some multimer defects may be present GPIb binding /Ag: < (0.5–0.7) CB/Ag: < (0.5–0.7) FVIII/VWF: > (0.5–0.7)
		VWD-type 3		VWF:Ag: ↓↓↓ (absent) VWF:GPIb binding: ↓↓↓ (absent) VWF:CB: ↓↓↓ (absent) FVIII:C: ↓↓↓	Multimers: no VWF present GPIb binding /Ag: NA CB/Ag: NA FVIII/VWF: NA
	Hemophilia A			PT: N aPTT: ↑↑↑ TT: N BT: N	FVIII: C: ↓↓↓ FVIII: Ag: ↓↓↓
	Hemophilia B			PT: N aPTT: ↑↑↑ TT: N BT: N	FIX: C: ↓↓↓ FIX: Ag: ↓↓↓

(continued)

Table 2.4 (continued)

CBD			Laboratory features	
RBD	FI deficiency	Afibrinogenemia	PT: ↑↑↑ aPTT: ↑↑↑ TT: ↑↑↑ RT: ↑↑↑	Fibrinogen activity: UD Fibrinogen antigen: UD Fibrinogen functional/antigenic ratio: NA
		Hypofibrinogenemia	PT: ↑ to ↑↑ depending on fibrinogen levels aPTT: ↑ to ↑↑ depending on fibrinogen levels TT: ↑ to ↑↑ depending on fibrinogen levels RT: ↑ to ↑↑ depending on fibrinogen levels	Fibrinogen activity: <1.5 g/L Fibrinogen antigen: <1.5 g/L Fibrinogen functional/antigenic ratio: > 0.7
		Dysfibrinogenemia	PT: usually ↑↑ aPTT: usually ↑↑ TT: usually ↑↑ RT: usually ↑↑	Fibrinogen activity: <1.5 g/L Fibrinogen antigen:< 1.5 g/L Fibrinogen functional/antigenic ratio: < 0.7
		Hypodysfibrinogenemia	PT: ↑ to ↑↑ depending on fibrinogen levels aPTT: ↑ to ↑↑ depending on fibrinogen levels TT: ↑ to ↑↑ depending on fibrinogen levels RT: ↑ to ↑↑ depending on fibrinogen levels	Fibrinogen activity: <1.5 g/L Fibrinogen antigen: <1.5 g/L Fibrinogen functional/antigenic ratio: <0.7

	FII deficiency	PT: ↑↑ to ↑↑↑ aPTT: ↑↑ to ↑↑↑ TT: N BT: N	FII:C: ↓↓↓ FII:Ag: ↓↓↓
	FV deficiency	PT: ↑↑ to ↑↑↑ aPTT: ↑↑ to ↑↑↑ TT: N BT: N	FV:C: ↓↓↓ FV:Ag: ↓↓↓
	CFV-FVIII deficiency	PT: ↑↑ to ↑↑↑ aPTT: ↑↑ to ↑↑↑ TT: N BT: N	FV:C: ↓↓ FV:Ag: ↓↓ FVIII: C: ↓↓ FVIII: Ag: ↓↓
	VKDCF deficiency	PT: ↑↑ to ↑↑↑ aPTT: ↑↑ to ↑↑↑ TT: N BT: N	FII: C: ↓↓ FII: Ag: ↓↓ FVII: C: ↓↓ FVII:Ag: ↓↓ FIX:C: ↓↓ FIX:Ag: ↓↓ FX:C: ↓↓ FX:Ag: ↓↓
	FVII deficiency	PT: ↑↑ to ↑↑↑ aPTT: N TT: N BT: N	FVII:C: ↓↓↓ FVII:Ag: ↓↓↓
	FX deficiency	PT: ↑↑ to ↑↑↑ aPTT: ↑↑ to ↑↑↑ RVVT: ↑↑ BT: N	FX:C: ↓↓↓ FX:Ag: ↓↓↓

(continued)

Table 2.4 (continued)

CBD			Laboratory features	
	FXI deficiency		PT: N aPTT: ↑↑ TT: N BT: N	FXI:C: ↓↓↓ FXI:Ag: ↓↓↓
	FXIII deficiency		PT: N aPTT: N TT: N BT: N	Clot solubility test: abnormal FXIII:C: ↓↓↓ FXIII:Ag: ↓↓↓
IPFD	GT	Type-I	Plt count: N Plt morphology: N PT: N aPTT: N TT: N BT/CT (PFA-100/200): ↑↑	CR: Absent Platelet integrin αIIbβ3 expression: UD or ↓↓↓ Platelet integrin αIIbβ3 (%) (Flow cytometry): < 5 Platelet aggregation: absent Platelet agglutination: N
		Type-II	Plt count: N Plt morphology: N PT: N aPTT: N TT: N BT/CT (PFA-100/200): ↑↑	CR: ↓ Platelet integrin αIIbβ3 expression: ↓↓↓ Platelet integrin αIIbβ3 (%) (Flow cytometry): 5–20 Platelet aggregation: absent Platelet agglutination: N
		Variant	Plt count: N Plt morphology: N PT: N aPTT: N TT: N BT/CT (PFA-100/200): ↑↑	CR: Variable Platelet integrin αIIbβ3 expression: N Platelet integrin αIIbβ3 (%) (Flow cytometry): > 20 Platelet aggregation: absent/abnormal Platelet agglutination: N

	BSS	Plt count: thrombocytopenia Plt morphology: large platelet (monoallelic), giant platelet (biallelic) PT: N aPTT: N TT: N BT/CT (PFA-100/200): ↑↑ or ↑↑↑	RIPA: defective Platelet aggregation: response to collagen, arachidonic acid, and thromboxane analogues is normal. Decrease in response to low dose but no high dose of thrombin Flow cytometry: GP1b-IX-V (CD42a-d)
	GPS	Plt count: usually <100 × 109/L Plt morphology: macrothrombocytopenia, gray and pale platelet PT: N aPTT: N TT: N BT: ↑	TEM: ↓↓ α-granules LTA: normal for ADP, epinephrine, arachidonic acid, and ristocetin and defective in response to thrombin and collagen B12 concentration: in half of patients ↑↑↑

CBD congenital bleeding disorder, *VWD* von Willebrand disease, *RBD* rare bleeding disorders, *FI* factor I, *FII* factor II, *FV* factor V, *CFV-FVIII* combined factor V and factor VIII, *FVII* factor VII, *VKDCF* vitamin K-dependent clotting factor, *FX* factor X, *FXI* factor XI, *FXIII* factor XIII, *IPFD* inherited platelet function disorder, *GT* Glanzmann thrombasthenia, *BSS* Bernard-Soulier syndrome, *PT-VWD* platelet-type von Willebrand disease, *QPD* Quebec platelet disorder, *GPS* gray platelet syndrome, *HPS* Hermansky-Pudlak syndrome, *WAD* Wiskott-Aldrich syndrome, *UD* undetectable, *NA* not applicable, *PT* prothrombin time, *aPTT* activated partial thromboplastin time, *TT* thrombin time, *RT* reptilase time, *BT* bleeding time, *Plt* platelet, *CT* closure time, *TEM* thromboelastometry, *LTA* light transmission aggregometry, *ADP* adenosine diphosphate, *PFA* platelet function analysis, *CR* clot retraction, *RVVT* Russell's viper venom time, *VWF:CB* von Willebrand Factor collagen binding, *Ag* antigen undiagnosed during the patient's life. In such cases, due to mild phenotype of disorder, both family history and bleeding episodes may be undetectable [6]. Some especial hemorrhages can be considered as important diagnostic clues in CBD. These include umbilical cord bleeding that is common in patients with afibrinogenemia and FXIII deficiency. Miscarriage is also common in both of these disorders. ICH as a severe life-threatening hemorrhage is more common in FXIII deficiency than any other CBD [22, 58, 59]. Among patients with CFD, most of the patients with hypofibrinogenemia and dysfibrinogenemia are asymptomatic, while hemorrhage is more common in afibrinogenemia. Thrombotic events are relatively common in patients with CFD [21].

Diagnosis of CFD is based on the assessment of antigenic and functional fibrinogen levels. Although a considerable number of functional and antigenic assays are available, for routine clinical use, the Clauss functional assay is recommended. Genotype helps to confirm the diagnosis [21, 60]. In patients with FXIII deficiency, all routine coagulation tests are normal. Although functional FXIII assay is recommended as first-line screening test, clot solubility test remained as the only diagnostic test in a considerable number of countries [61]. In coagulation factor deficiencies that are involved in common pathway of coagulation cascade, based on severity of deficiency, both prothrombin time and activated partial thromboplastin time (aPTT) can be prolonged [9, 62].

Different methods are available for factor assay in patients with hemophilia, but chromogenic assay was suggested by International Society of Thrombosis and Hemostasis (ISTH) as a reference method for FVIII coagulant activity (FVIII:C) assay in plasma and in concentrate. In ~30% of mild hemophilia A, the discrepancy between one stage assay and chromogenic assay can be observed, and in 5–10% of mild hemophilia A, FVIII:C assay is placed within normal range while lower FVIII:C assay with other method. In such patients, if only one assay be used, diagnosis may be missed; thus simultaneous use of one stage and chromogenic assays is recommended for diagnosis of mild hemophilia A [63–66]. Although in a number of patients with IPFD including GT and BSS diagnosis of disorder is straightforward, diagnosis of most cases with IPFD is sophisticated and requires precise and sometime sophisticated laboratory assessments [6]. In routine practice, the rate of misdiagnosis is relatively high and because of this, platelet physiology subcommittee of the ISTH proposed a standard algorithm for proper diagnosis of IPFD. Based on this guideline, first step in diagnosis of IPFD should include blood smear examination, light transmission aggregometry (LTA) with a limited number of agonists, platelet granules release, and flow cytometric analysis of major platelet glycoproteins (Fig. 2.2) [67, 68].

GT is a severe IPFD that is accompanied by mucocutaneous hemorrhage with impaired aggregation studies with all physiological agonists, while ristocetin-induced platelet agglutination is normal. All routine coagulation tests are normal in GT except for BT. Platelet count and morphology is also normal [47, 69]. Diagnosis

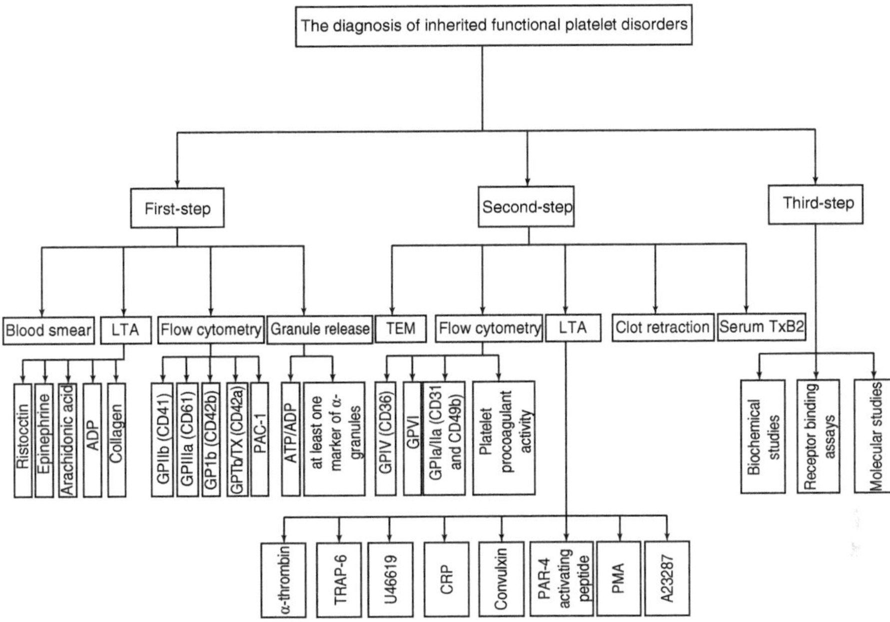

Fig. 2.2 International Society of Thrombosis and Haemostasis (ISTH) suggested algorithm for diagnosis of inherited platelet function disorders

of VWD most often is a difficult process and requires precise and sometime sophisticated laboratory assessment. Three main criteria were introduced for diagnosis of VWD including decreased VWF level, bleeding symptoms, and inheritance; among them clinical manifestation is the most important one [70, 71].

2.5 Treatment

Due to variability in severity of bleeding symptoms in patients with CBD, management of these disorders is highly variable. A considerable number of patients with IPFD never experience significant bleeding episodes, and therefore most of them never require medical intervention [6]. On the other hand, in some severe bleeding disorders such as FXIII deficiency, regular primary prophylaxis is mandatory from the time of diagnosis. This is due to high rate of life-threatening episodes such as ICH in these patients [5]. In patients with hemophilia, two main treatment strategies are used, including on-demand treatment, which means stopping bleeding as soon as possible after onset of hemorrhage, and prophylaxis. Although on-demand therapy is the main therapeutic option in a considerable number of countries, mostly due to limited resources and low economic situation, prophylaxis treatment is the treatment of choice for patients with severe hemophilia, particularly in children [72, 73]. Although in RBD, except for FXIII deficiency, on-demand treatment is used, in some cases with severe life-threatening bleeds especially those with severe FVII deficiency, FX deficiency, and afibrinogenemia, regular secondary prophylaxis could be considered [19, 74]. Although in patients with VWD, on-demand therapy is the traditional treatment choice, long-term prophylaxis should be considered for those patients with type 3 VWD and recurrent hemarthrosis, recurrent GI bleeding, and frequent epistaxis (Table 2.5) [75].

Different therapeutic choices are available for patients with CBD, including traditional choices, fresh frozen plasma (FFP), cryoprecipitate and platelet concentrate, and more recently factor concentrate and recombinant products. FFP can be used for all coagulation factor deficiencies, but the risk of blood-borne disease transmission is an important obstacle. In spite of this limitation, in countries with limited resources, FFP is the only therapeutic choice, and in such areas, virus-inactivated form of product is better to be considered. Cryoprecipitate is another therapeutic choice which can be used for patients with CFD, hemophilia A, FXIII deficiency, and VWD [76, 77]. Due to lack of inactivated form of cryoprecipitate, this product is not recommended in these patients. In patients with CBD, factor concentrate is available for patients with FI, FVII, FVIII, FX, FIX, and FXIII deficiencies, VWD, and more recently for FV deficiency (Clinical study), while recombinant products are available for FVII, FVIII, FIX, and FXIII deficiencies and VWF [78]. On the whole, management of bleeding depends on the severity of disease, type of bleeding episode, and minimal residual activity in patients' plasma [19].

Table 2.5 Therapeutic options in congenital bleeding disorders

CBD		Kind of treatment	Replacement therapy	Non-replacement therapy
Common bleeding disorder	VWD	On-demand[a]	FFP Cryoprecipitate FVIII/VWF concentrate rVWF	Platelet [b]Desmopressin
	Hemophilia A	Prophylaxis	PdFVIII rFVIII EHL FVIII	Concizumab (anti-TFPI) Fitusiran (siRNA) Emicizumab
	Hemophilia B		PdFIX rFIX EHL FIX	Concizumab (anti-TFPI) Fitusiran (siRNA)

Table 2.5 (continued)

CBD		Kind of treatment	Replacement therapy	Non-replacement therapy
RBD	FI deficiency	On-demand	FFP Cryoprecipitate Pd Fibrinogen	NA
	FII deficiency	On-demand	PCC FFP	NA
	FV deficiency	On-demand	FFP pdFV (clinical study)	Platelet transfusion
	CFV-FVIII deficiency	On-demand	FFP rFVIII	Desmopressin
	VKDCF deficiency	On-demand	Vitamin K PCC FFP	NA
	FVII deficiency	On-demand	rFVIIa PCC FFP PdFVII	NA
	FX deficiency	On-demand	PCC PdFX	NA
	FXI deficiency	On-demand	PdFXI	NA
	FXIII deficiency	Prophylaxis	rFXIII A subunit PdFXIII FFP Cryoprecipitate	NA
IPFD	GT	On-demand	Platelet transfusion	Tranexamic acid Epsilon-aminocaproic acid Topical thrombin rFVII
	BSS	On-demand	Platelet transfusion	Tranexamic acid Epsilon-aminocaproic acid rFVII
	GPS	On-demand	Platelet transfusion	Tranexamic acid Epsilon-aminocaproic acid Desmopressin

CBD congenital bleeding disorder, *VWD* von Willebrand disease, *RBD* rare bleeding disorders, *FI* factor I, *FII* factor II, *FV* factor V, *CFV-FVIII* combined factor V and factor VIII, *FVII* factor VII, *VKDCF* vitamin K-dependent clotting factor, *FX* factor X, *FXI* factor XI, *FXIII* factor XIII, *IPFD* inherited platelet function disorder, *GT* Glanzmann thrombasthenia, *BSS* Bernard-Soulier syndrome, *PT-VWD* Platelet-type von Willebrand disease, *QPD* Quebec platelet disorder, *GPS* gray platelet syndrome, *HPS* Hermansky-Pudlak syndrome, *WAD* Wiskott-Aldrich syndrome

[a]For patients with severe presentations, especially type 3 VWD, prophylaxis treatment can be used

[b]Desmopressin cannot be used for type 3VWD and most cases with type 2 VWD

References

1. Rick ME, Walsh CE, Key NS. Congenital bleeding disorders. ASH Education Program Book. 2003;2003(1):559–74.
2. Brown DL. Congenital bleeding disorders. Curr Probl Pediatr Adolesc Health Care. 2005;35(2):38–62.
3. Sadler J, Budde U, Eikenboom J, Favaloro E, Hill F, Holmberg L, et al. Update on the pathophysiology and classification of von Willebrand disease: a report of the Subcommittee on von Willebrand Factor. J Thromb Haemost. 2006;4(10):2103–14.
4. Dorgalaleh A, Tabibian S, Hosseini S, Shamsizadeh M. Guidelines for laboratory diagnosis of factor XIII deficiency. Blood Coagul Fibrinolysis. 2016;27(4):361–4.
5. Alavi SER, Jalalvand M, Assadollahi V, Tabibian S, Dorgalaleh A. Intracranial hemorrhage: a devastating outcome of congenital bleeding disorders—prevalence, diagnosis, and management, with a special focus on congenital factor XIII deficiency. Semin Thromb Hemost. 2017. https://doi.org/10.1055/s-0037-1604109.
6. Dorgalaleh A, Tabibian S, Shamsizadeh M. Inherited platelet function disorders (IPFDs). Clin Lab. 2017;63(1):1–13.
7. Gresele P. Diagnosis of inherited platelet function disorders: guidance from the SSC of the ISTH. J Thromb Haemost. 2015;13(2):314–22.
8. Naderi M, Dorgalaleh A, Alizadeh S, Tabibian S, Hosseini S, Shamsizadeh M, et al. Clinical manifestations and management of life-threatening bleeding in the largest group of patients with severe factor XIII deficiency. Int J Hematol. 2014;100(5):443–9.
9. Palla R, Peyvandi F, Shapiro AD. Rare bleeding disorders: diagnosis and treatment. Blood. 2015;125:2052–61.
10. Biss T, Blanchette V, Clark D, Wakefield C, James P, Rand M. Use of a quantitative pediatric bleeding questionnaire to assess mucocutaneous bleeding symptoms in children with a platelet function disorder. J Thromb Haemost. 2010;8(6):1416–9.
11. Lowe GC, Lordkipanidzé M, Watson SP. Utility of the ISTH bleeding assessment tool in predicting platelet defects in participants with suspected inherited platelet function disorders. J Thromb Haemost. 2013;11(9):1663–8.
12. Toygar HU, Guzeldemir E. Excessive gingival bleeding in two patients with Glanzmann thrombasthenia. J Periodontol. 2007;78(6):1154–8.
13. Poon M-C, Di Minno G, d'Oiron R, Zotz R. New insights into the treatment of Glanzmann thrombasthenia. Transfus Med Rev. 2016;30(2):92–9.
14. Santagostino E, Mancuso M, Tripodi A, Chantarangkul V, Clerici M, Garagiola I, et al. Severe hemophilia with mild bleeding phenotype: molecular characterization and global coagulation profile. J Thromb Haemost. 2010;8(4):737–43.
15. Stieltjes N, Calvez T, Demiguel V, Torchet M, Briquel M, Fressinaud E, et al. Intracranial haemorrhages in French haemophilia patients (1991–2001): clinical presentation, management and prognosis factors for death. Haemophilia. 2005;11(5):452–8.
16. Den Uijl I, Fischer K, Van Der Bom J, Grobbee D, Rosendaal F, Plug I. Clinical outcome of moderate haemophilia compared with severe and mild haemophilia. Haemophilia. 2009;15(1):83–90.
17. Van den Berg H, de Groot P, Fischer K. Phenotypic heterogeneity in severe hemophilia. J Thromb Haemost. 2007;5(s1):151–6.
18. Peyvandi F, Palla R, Menegatti M, Siboni S, Halimeh S, Faeser B, et al. Coagulation factor activity and clinical bleeding severity in rare bleeding disorders: results from the European Network of Rare Bleeding Disorders. J Thromb Haemost. 2012;10(4):615–21.
19. Dorgalaleh A, Alavi SER, Tabibian S, Soori S, Moradi EH, Bamedi T, et al. Diagnosis, clinical manifestations and management of rare bleeding disorders in Iran. Hematology. 2017;22(4):224–30.
20. De Moerloose P, Neerman-Arbez M. Congenital fibrinogen disorders. Semin Thromb Hemost. 2009;35:356–66.

21. De Moerloose P, Casini A, Neerman-Arbez M. Congenital fibrinogen disorders: an update. Semin Thromb Hemost. 2013;39:585–95.
22. Inbal A, Muszbek L. Coagulation factor deficiencies and pregnancy loss. Semin Thromb Hemost. 2003;29:171–4.
23. Anwar R, Miloszewski KJ. Factor XIII deficiency. Br J Haematol. 1999;107(3):468–84.
24. Coopland A, Alkjaersig N, Fletcher AP. Reduction in plasma factor XIII (fibrin stabilizing factor) concentration during pregnancy. J Lab Clin Med. 1969;73(1):144–53.
25. Padmanabhan L, Mhaskar R, Mhaskar A, Ross C. Factor XIII deficiency: a rare cause of repeated abortions. Singap Med J. 2004;45(4):186–7.
26. Dorgalaleh A, Naderi M, Shamsizadeh M. Morbidity and mortality in a large number of Iranian patients with severe congenital factor XIII deficiency. Ann Hematol. 2016;95(3):451–5.
27. Mosesson MW. Dysfibrinogenemia and thrombosis. Semin Thromb Hemost. 1999;25:311–9.
28. Girolami A, Ferrari S, Cosi E, Girolami B, Lombardi AM. Congenital prothrombin defects: they are not only associated with bleeding but also with thrombosis: a new classification is needed. Hematology. 2018;23(2):105–10.
29. Cramer TJ, Anderson K, Navaz K, Brown JM, Mosnier LO, von Drygalski A. Heterozygous congenital Factor VII deficiency with the 9729del4 mutation, associated with severe spontaneous intracranial bleeding in an adolescent male. Blood Cell Mol Dis. 2016;57:8–12.
30. Girolami A, Cosi E, Ferrari S, Girolami B, Lombardi AM. Bleeding manifestations in heterozygotes with congenital FVII deficiency: a comparison with unaffected family members during a long observation period. Hematology. 2017;22(6):375–9.
31. Dorgalaleh A, Rashidpanah J. Blood coagulation factor XIII and factor XIII deficiency. Blood Rev. 2016;30(6):461–75.
32. Federici AB, Bucciarelli P, Castaman G, Mazzucconi MG, Morfini M, Rocino A, et al. The bleeding score predicts clinical outcomes and replacement therapy in adults with von Willebrand disease. Blood. 2014;123(26):4037–44.
33. Makris M. Gastrointestinal bleeding in von Willebrand disease. Thromb Res. 2006;118:S13–S7.
34. Neerman-Arbez M, Johnson K, Morris MA, McVey J, Peyvandi F, Nichols W, et al. Molecular analysis of the ERGIC-53 gene in 35 families with combined factor V-factor VIII deficiency. Blood. 1999;93(7):2253–60.
35. Zhang B, McGee B, Yamaoka JS, Guglielmone H, Downes KA, Minoldo S, et al. Combined deficiency of factor V and factor VIII is due to mutations in either LMAN1 or MCFD2. Blood. 2006;107(5):1903–7.
36. Brenner B, Sánchez-Vega B, Wu S-M, Lanir N, Stafford DW, Solera J. A missense mutation in γ-glutamyl carboxylase gene causes combined deficiency of all vitamin K-dependent blood coagulation factors. Blood. 1998;92(12):4554–9.
37. Oldenburg J, Von Brederlow B, Fregin A, Rost S, Wolz W, Eberl W, et al. Congenital deficiency of vitamin K-dependent coagulation factors in two families presents as a genetic defect of the vitamin K-epoxide-reductase-complex. Thromb Haemost-stuttgart. 2000;84(6):937–41.
38. Dorgalaleh A, Dadashizadeh G, Bamedi T. Hemophilia in Iran. Hematology. 2016;21(5):300–10.
39. Bagnall RD, Waseem N, Green PM, Giannelli F. Recurrent inversion breaking intron 1 of the factor VIII gene is a frequent cause of severe hemophilia A. Blood. 2002;99(1):168–74.
40. Jenkins P, Collins P, Goldman E, McCraw A, Riddell A, Lee C, et al. Analysis of intron 22 inversions of the factor VIII gene in severe hemophilia A: implications for genetic counseling. Blood. 1994;84(7):2197–201.
41. Antonarakis SE, Rossiter J, Young M, Horst J, De Moerloose P, Sommer S, et al. Factor VIII gene inversions in severe hemophilia A: results of an international consortium study. Blood. 1995;86(6):2206–12.
42. Asselta R, Duga S, Tenchini M. The molecular basis of quantitative fibrinogen disorders. J Thromb Haemost. 2006;4(10):2115–29.
43. Dorgalaleh A, Tabibian S, Bamedi T, Tamaddon G, Naderi M, Varmaghani B, et al. Molecular genetic analysis of ten unrelated Iranian patients with congenital factor XIII deficiency. Int J Lab Hematol. 2016;39(2):e33–6

44. Vu D, Neerman-Arbez M. Molecular mechanisms accounting for fibrinogen deficiency: from large deletions to intracellular retention of misfolded proteins. J Thromb Haemost. 2007;5(s1):125–31.
45. Neerman-Arbez M. The molecular basis of inherited afibrinogenaemia. Thromb Haemost. 2001;86(1):154–63.
46. Bellucci S, Caen J. Molecular basis of Glanzmann's thrombasthenia and current strategies in treatment. Blood Rev. 2002;16(3):193–202.
47. Nurden AT. Glanzmann thrombasthenia. Orphanet J Rare Dis. 2006;1(1):10.
48. Favaloro EJ. Von Willebrand disease: local diagnosis and management of a globally distributed bleeding disorder. Semin Thromb Hemost. 2011;37:440–55.
49. Favaloro EJ. Diagnosis and classification of von Willebrand disease: a review of the differential utility of various functional von Willebrand factor assays. Blood Coagul Fibrinolysis. 2011;22(7):553–64.
50. Martinez M, Graf L, Tsakiris DA. Congenital bleeding disorders. In: Marcucci C, Schoettker P, editors. Perioperative hemostasis. Berlin: Springer; 2015. p. 71–87.
51. Levinson B, Lehesjoki A, De La Chapelle A, Gitschier J. Molecular analysis of hemophilia A mutations in the Finnish population. Am J Hum Genet. 1990;46(1):53.
52. Vidaud M, Chabret C, Gazengel C, Grunebaum L, Cazenave J, Goossens MA. de novo intragenic deletion of the potential EGF domain of the factor IX gene in a family with severe hemophilia B. Blood. 1986;68(4):961–3.
53. Cattaneo M. Inherited platelet-based bleeding disorders. J Thromb Haemost. 2003;1(7):1628–36.
54. Kern M, Blanchette V, Stain AM, Einarson TR, Feldman BM. Clinical and cost implications of target joints in Canadian boys with severe hemophilia A. J Pediatr. 2004;145(5):628–34.
55. Manco-Johnson MJ, Abshire TC, Shapiro AD, Riske B, Hacker MR, Kilcoyne R, et al. Prophylaxis versus episodic treatment to prevent joint disease in boys with severe hemophilia. N Engl J Med. 2007;357(6):535–44.
56. Castaman G, Goodeve A, Eikenboom J. Principles of care for the diagnosis and treatment of von Willebrand disease. Haematologica. 2013;98(5):667–74.
57. Castaman G, Rodeghiero F, Tosetto A, Cappelletti A, Baudo F, Eikenboom J, et al. Hemorrhagic symptoms and bleeding risk in obligatory carriers of type 3 von Willebrand disease: an international, multicenter study. J Thromb Haemost. 2006;4(10):2164–9.
58. Anwar R, Minford A, Gallivan L, Trinh CH, Markham AF. Delayed umbilical bleeding—a presenting feature for factor XIII deficiency: clinical features, genetics, and management. Pediatrics. 2002;109(2):e32.
59. Angles-Cano E, Mathonnet F, Dreyfus M, Claeyssens S, de Mazancourt P. A case of afibrinogenemia associated with A-alpha chain gene compound heterozygosity (HUMFIBRA c.[4110delA]+[3200+ 1G> T]). Blood Coagul Fibrinolysis. 2007;18(1):73–5.
60. Lebreton A, Casini A. Diagnosis of congenital fibrinogen disorders. Ann Biol Clin. 2016;74:405–12.
61. Dorgalaleh A, Kazemi A, Zaker F, Shamsizadeh M, Rashidpanah J, Mollaei M. Laboratory diagnosis of factor XIII deficiency, routine coagulation tests with quantitative and qualitative methods. Clin Lab. 2016;62(4):491–8.
62. Awasthy N, Aggarwal K, Gupta H, Saluja S. Congenital hypofibrinogenemia. Indian Pediatr. 2004;41(2):185–6.
63. Kihlberg K, Strandberg K, Rosén S, Ljung R, Astermark J. Discrepancies between the one-stage clotting assay and the chromogenic assay in haemophilia B. Haemophilia. 2017;23(4):620–7.
64. Barrowcliffe T. Monitoring haemophilia severity and treatment: new or old laboratory tests? Haemophilia. 2004;10(s4):109–14.
65. Castellone DD, Adcock DM. Factor VIII activity and inhibitor assays in the diagnosis and treatment of hemophilia A. Semin Thromb Hemost. 2017;43:320–30.
66. Verbruggen B, Meijer P, Novakova I, Van Heerde W. Diagnosis of factor VIII deficiency. Haemophilia. 2008;14(s3):76–82.

67. Cattaneo M, Hayward C, Moffat K, Pugliano M, Liu Y, Michelson AD. Results of a worldwide survey on the assessment of platelet function by light transmission aggregometry: a report from the platelet physiology subcommittee of the SSC of the ISTH. J Thromb Haemost. 2009;7(6):1029.
68. Cattaneo M, Cerletti C, Harrison P, Hayward C, Kenny D, Nugent D, et al. Recommendations for the standardization of light transmission aggregometry: a consensus of the working party from the platelet physiology subcommittee of SSC/ISTH. J Thromb Haemost. 2013;11(6):1183–9.
69. Nair S, Ghosh K, Kulkarni B, Shetty S, Mohanty D. Glanzmann's thrombasthenia: updated. Platelets. 2002;13(7):387–93.
70. Favaloro EJ, Pasalic L, Curnow J. Laboratory tests used to help diagnose von Willebrand disease: an update. Pathology. 2016;48(4):303–18.
71. Favaloro EJ, Soltani S, McDonald J, Grezchnik E, Easton L, Favaloro JW. Reassessment of ABO blood group, sex, and age on laboratory parameters used to diagnose von Willebrand disorder: potential influence on the diagnosis vs the potential association with risk of thrombosis. Am J Clin Pathol. 2005;124(6):910–7.
72. Royal S, Schramm W, Berntorp E, Giangrande P, Gringeri A, Ludlam C, et al. Quality-of-life differences between prophylactic and on-demand factor replacement therapy in European haemophilia patients. Haemophilia. 2002;8(1):44–50.
73. Valentino L, Mamonov V, Hellmann A, Quon D, Chybicka A, Schroth P, et al. A randomized comparison of two prophylaxis regimens and a paired comparison of on-demand and prophylaxis treatments in hemophilia A management. J Thromb Haemost. 2012;10(3):359–67.
74. De Moerloose P, Neerman-Arbez M. Treatment of congenital fibrinogen disorders. Expert Opin Biol Ther. 2008;8(7):979–92.
75. Federici A, Castaman G, Mannucci P. Guidelines for the diagnosis and management of von Willebrand disease in Italy. Haemophilia. 2002;8(5):607–21.
76. Mumford AD, Ackroyd S, Alikhan R, Bowles L, Chowdary P, Grainger J, et al. Guideline for the diagnosis and management of the rare coagulation disorders. Br J Haematol. 2014;167(3):304–26.
77. Mannucci PM. Treatment of von Willebrand's disease. N Engl J Med. 2004;351(7):683–94.
78. Bertolini J, Goss N, Curling J. Production of plasma proteins for therapeutic use. Hoboken: Wiley; 2012.

Part II

Common Bleeding Disorders

3 von Willebrand Disease

Akbar Dorgalaleh, Shadi Tabibian, Yavar Shiravand, and Emmanuel J. Favaloro

3.1 Introduction

von Willebrand disease (VWD) is the most common congenital bleeding disorder (CBD) and is inherited in an autosomal dominant or autosomal recessive manner [1]. The disorder is classified into quantitative deficiency (types 1 and 3) or qualitative defects (type 2) in von Willebrand factor (VWF) [2]. VWD represents a very heterogeneous bleeding disorder with variable bleeding tendency. The bleeding symptoms may be so mild as to not easily distinguish potential sufferers from a normal condition or else may be so severe that it is accompanied by life endangering bleeding (e.g., recurrent occurrence in central nervous system (CNS)). Generally, mucocutaneous bleeds such as epistaxis and menorrhagia are more typical presentations of the disorder, but other rare presentations also can be observed [1, 2]. In addition to the accepted ISTH SSC (International Society on Thrombosis and Hemostasis Scientific Standardization Committee) classification of the disorder, affected individuals are characterized according to clinical manifestations and laboratory findings [3]. In practice, VWD can be classified to mild (VWF:ristocetin cofactor (VWF:RCo): 30–50 U dL^{-1} and/or factor VIII (FVIII) coagulant activity (FVIII:C): 40–60 U dL^{-1}), moderate (VWF:RCo 10–30 U dL^{-1} and/or FVIII:C 20–40 U dL^{-1}), or severe (VWF:RCo <10 U dL^{-1} and/or FVIII:C <20 U dL^{-1}) [4]. Based on such a classification, type 3 VWD, as well as some cases of type 1, type

A. Dorgalaleh · S. Tabibian · Y. Shiravand
Department of Hematology and Blood Transfusion, School of Allied Medicine, Iran University of Medical Sciences, Tehran, Iran

E. J. Favaloro (✉)
Haematology, Institute of Clinical Pathology and Medical Research, NSW Health Pathology, Westmead Hospital, Westmead, NSW, Australia

Sydney Centres for Thrombosis and Haemostasis, Westmead, NSW, Australia
e-mail: Emmanuel.Favaloro@health.nsw.gov.au

A. Dorgalaleh (ed.), *Congenital Bleeding Disorders*,
https://doi.org/10.1007/978-3-319-76723-9_3

2A, type 2M, and type 2N VWD, can be classified to severe VWD [5]. Diagnosis of VWD is a challenge worldwide, and a precise laboratory approach and proper clinical assessment, although mandatory for timely diagnosis of disorder, is sometimes elusive [4]. Although significant progress has occurred in the laboratory diagnosis of VWD in recent years, proper diagnosis of most types of the disorder requires a sophisticated approach, and is thus challenging. This difficulty is due to several issues, including lack of a definitive cutoff between normal and abnormal levels of VWF reflecting normal individuals vs VWD, the effect of different molecular pathogenesis of VWD on VWF level and activity, other factors such as genetic modifiers and physiological factors that can reduce or increase plasma levels of VWF, overlap of bleeding symptomology in normal individuals and those with VWD, and difficulties with performance and interpretation of laboratory tests. Three foremost criteria are proposed for proper diagnosis of VWD: (1) presence of bleeding symptoms, (2) decreased VWF level and/or activity, and (3) the pattern of inheritance [6]. On-demand therapy is the current mainstay of treatment in VWD, but long-term prophylaxis can significantly improve the quality of life in patients with severe hemorrhages, such as hemarthrosis and GI bleeding, and even recurrent epistaxis. Desmopressin is the main therapeutic choice in patients with type 1 and a subset of patients with type 2 VWD, while replacement therapy with VWF/FVIII concentrates represents the main therapeutic option in type 3 and most patients with type 2 VWD, as well as those responsive to desmopressin but with long-term treatment needs [7, 8].

3.2 von Willebrand Factor Synthesis, Structure, and Function

3.2.1 von Willebrand Factor Biosynthesis

The biosynthesis of VWF consists of a series of sequential steps that ultimately leads to incorporation of the protein to storage organelles. These steps include protein production, removal of signal peptide, tail-to-tail dimerization, heat-to-head multimerization, N-linked glycosylation, maturation of N-glycan, O-linked glycosylation, formation of tubules, and incorporation to storage organelles [9].

3.2.2 von Willebrand Factor Structure

VWF is mapped to the tip of short arm of chromosome 12. The *VWF* gene spans 178 kb and consists of 52 exons [10], reflecting a unique gene structure consisting of different repeated sequences [11]. The intron 40 contains 14 Alu repeat and 670-bp repeat of TCTA. In addition the 5′ flanking region has AT repeat resemble to TATA element [12].

VWF is a multimeric protein with molecular weight of 350 kDa, which is coded by 9 kb mRNA and consists of 2813 amino acids, including 22 amino acid signal peptides, a 741 amino acid propeptide and a 2050 amino acid mature polypeptide [13]. VWF is synthesized as a precursor and processed in endoplasmic reticulum (ER) and Golgi apparatus in endothelial cells. After processing, this protein undergoes dimerization in the ER by disulfide bridging and cleavage into two components, the mature protein and a 97 kDa propeptide. The propeptide, also sometimes referred to as a von Willebrand antigen II, is secreted and circulates independently of the mature VWF and has unknown function [9].

VWF precursor consists of four distinct domains, each of them presenting with two to five tandem copies to arrange as D1-D2-D′-D3-A1-A2-A3-D4-B1-B2-B3-C1-C2-CK (Fig. 3.1a). The current domain organization recently proposed by Zhou et al. is different to the classical domain structure, with replacement of the B1–B3 and C1–C2 domain regions by six homologous C domains (C1–C6) (Fig. 3.1b) [14]. The D1 and D2 domains correspond to the propeptide, and the remainder represents the mature VWF subunit. The D domains consist of different distinct structures. D1, D2, and D3 domains contain VW domains (VW domain 1, 2, and 3), a C8 fold, a trypsin inhibitor-like (TIL) structure, and an E module. The D4 domain lacks the E module and contains a D4N subunit. In addition, the D′ domain only has TIL and an E module, and the VW and C8 fold are absent [14].

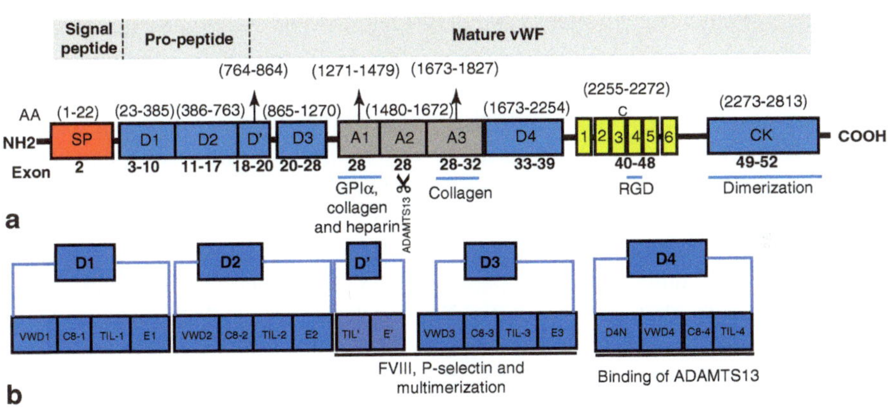

Fig. 3.1 von Willebrand factor (VWF) domain organization. (**a**) The classical structure of VWF. In this organization, VWF is arranged as D1-D2-D′-D3-A1-A2-A3-D4-B1-B2-B3-C1-C2-CK. The current revised structure of VWF. (**b**) In this structure, as proposed by Zhou et al. in 2012, the B1–B3 domains and C1–C2 domains are replaced by 6 homologous C domains (C1–C6). VWF contains 2813 amino acids and consists of a signal peptide (SP) comprising the first 22 residues, a propeptide comprising the subsequent 750 amino acids (the 23th to 763th amino acid), and a mature subunit (the 764th to 2813th amino acid). The signal sequence is cleaved in the endoplasmic reticulum and separated from VWF. Furin cleaves the propeptide to generate mature VWF. The propeptide consists of two domains (D1 and D2) while mature VWF consist of D′D3 complex, A domains, D4 complex, and stem complex. Stem complex has six domains comprising C1, C2, C3, C4, C5, and C6. Each D domain includes different subdomains. D1, D2, and D3 domains consist of VW domain, a C8 fold, a trypsin inhibitor-like (TIL) structure, and an E module. The D4 domain contains VWD, a C8 fold, TIL, and D4N subunit whereas D′ domain only has TIL and E module

3.2.3 Disulfide Bridging and Multimerization of von Willebrand Factor

About 8.3% of VWF is composed of the amino acid cysteine (234 of the 2813 residues), which if compared to most other human proteins is fourfold higher. In contrast to other domains, the triplicated domain A has only six cysteine residues. The cysteine residues are paired in disulfide bonds in the secreted protein. However, there exist several unpaired cysteines, which are essential for proper folding and secretion of VWF [15]. In ER, the subunits of pro-VWF undergo dimerization by disulfide bonds in C-terminal cysteine knot (CK) domains. This tail-to-tail dimerization needs only the sequence of the last 150 residues. Tail-to-tail pro-VWF is transported to Golgi and forms head-to-head dimerization by further disulfide bonding in D3 domain (Fig. 3.2b). The important point to consider here is the significant role of VWF propeptides (domain D1 and D2) and also D′ in multimerization. These domains are involved in the alignment of the pro-VWF dimer in order to facilitate the interdimeric cross-linking. Although the removal of the propeptide does not prevent the transportation to Golgi, it does inhibit the multimerization of VWF. The D1 and D2 domains contain CxxC sequence (Cys(c) 159-Gly-Leu-Cys(c) 162 and Cys(c) 521-GlyLeu-Cys(c) 524) which resembles the thiol disulfide functional sites and catalyzes disulfide binding in the D3 domain by its disulfide isomerase activity [16]. By adding any extra glycine to the sequences, the dimerization in ER occurs, but the dimers transported to the Golgi are secreted without the formation of multimers [17]. Therefore, D3 and D′ domains are necessary for multimer formation, and any deletion in these domains leads to expansion of only the dimeric form of VWF [18]. After multimerization, the multimers are organized into a helical structure that leads to 100-fold compaction of the protein. In this compacted structure, the D1 and D2 domains (propeptide) and also D′ and D3 domains form the wall of this helical structure, whereas other domains (A1-CK domains) protrudes outward and occupy the space between the tubules. VWF tubules assemble into ministacks that show the initial Weibel-Palade body (WPB)-like structure. In the trans-Golgi network, co-packaging of VWF that contains these ministacks results in maturation and formation of larger WPBs [9].

The regulation of the multimeric size of VWF is mediated by A Disintegrin and Metalloproteinase with ThromboSpondin type 1 motif, member 13 (ADAMTS13) which cleaves VWF at a single site (Tyr1605-Met1606) in the A2 domain [19, 20]. It appears that domain D4, at residues from 1874 to 2813, has a role in binding to ADAMTS13, and this acts as the initial step for proteolysis of VWF by ADAMTS13 (Fig. 3.3) [21].

3.2.4 Post-translational Modifications of von Willebrand Factor

During synthesis, VWF undergoes different post-translational modifications including the removal of the propeptide by the protease furin (Fig. 3.4), completion of N- and O-glycosylation, and sulfation of specific N-oligosaccharides [22]. In ER,

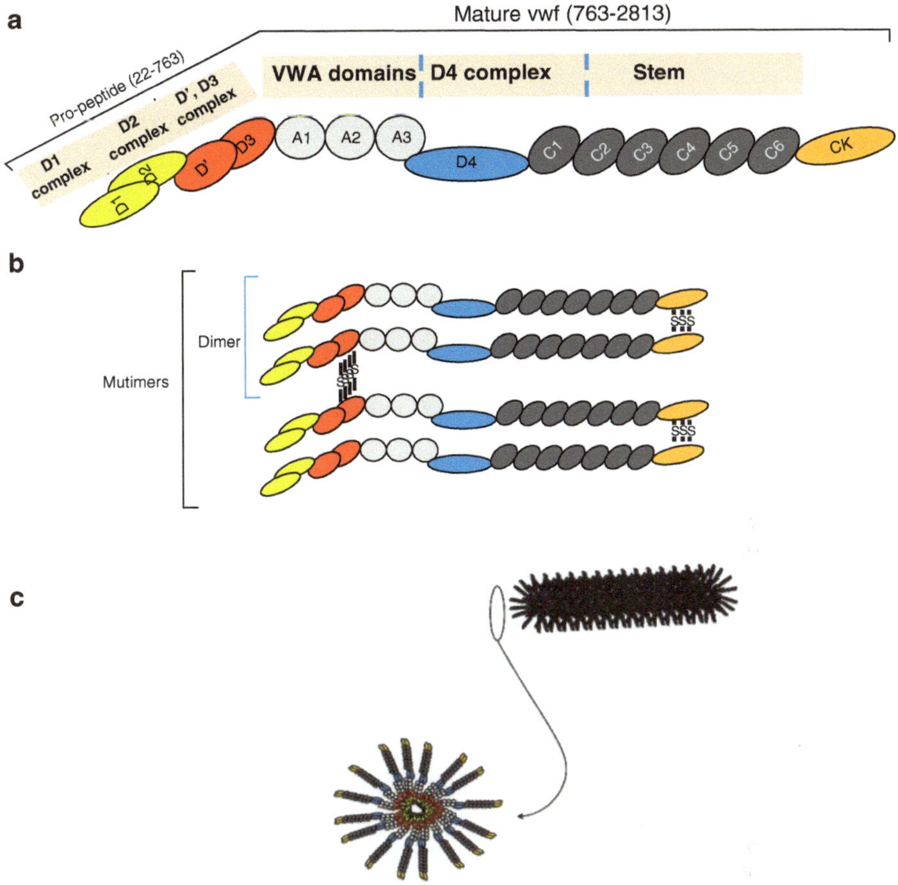

Fig. 3.2 (**a**) The structure of von Willebrand factor (VWF) including both the propeptide and mature VWF). (**b**) Dimer formation occurs via disulfide bonds in the C-terminal (CK) domain. This tail-to-tail dimerization occurs in ER. The tail-to-tail dimers are transported to the Golgi and the multimers formed via disulfide binding in D3 domain. (**c**). The multimers organize in a helical structure. In this right-handed helical structure (tubules), the D1–D2 and D′ and D3 form the wall, while other domains of VWF occupy the spaces of tubules. The tubules assemble in the form of ministacks that show the Weibel-Palade body (WPB)-like structures. Co-packaging of VWF that contains the ministacks leads to large WPB formation

oligosaccharyl tranferase is involved in attachment of 14 saccharide units to asparagine residues. Various studies have shown that pro-VWF has 17 N-linked carbohydrate structures with 4 of them located in the propeptide and 13 in the mature VWF. In addition, along with maturation of N-linked glycan in Golgi, 10 O-linked glycans are added. The N-linked oligosaccharides of this protein are different from other proteins because they contain ABO blood group oligosaccharides [23]. More than 90% of the glycans are capped by sialic acid. In N-linked glycan, there are five

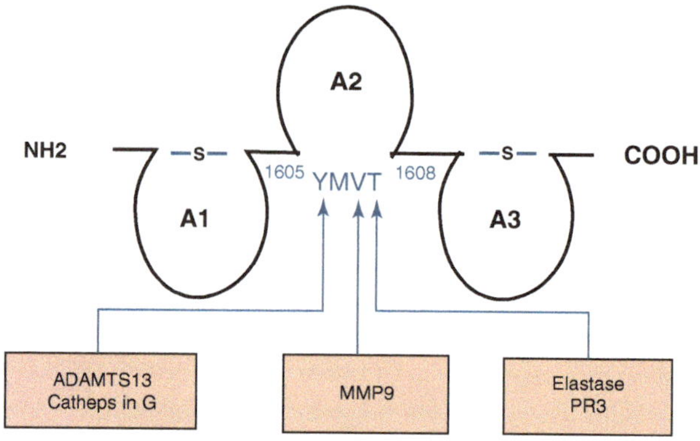

Fig. 3.3 The A domains are organized in loop structures. This structure is formed by disulfide bonds in the A1 and A3 domains. These bonds are between C1272 and C1458 in A1 and C1686 and C1872 in A3 domains. The multimeric size of VWF is regulated by cleavages that occur in the A2 domain. The site of this cleavage is located in Tyr1605-Met1606 and mediated by the metalloproteinase ADAMTS13. *MMP9* matrix metalloproteinase 9

sites for terminal sulfation [23]. The functional role of these sulfated residues remains under investigation [24]. Fig. 3.4 shows the sequential steps for biosynthesis of VWF.

3.2.5 Intracellular Storage and Secretion of VWF

Following synthesis, VWF is stored in α-granules of megakaryocytes/platelets or in Weibel-Palade bodies (WPBs) of endothelium (Fig. 3.4). α-Granules can still be formed in the absence of VWF, while the formation of WPBs depends on the presence of VWF [25]. About 95% of the VWF formed is constitutively secreted while the remainder is stored. In the WPBs, the VWF contained comprises large multimers, whereas the VWF that is constitutively secreted contains smaller multimers. The largest VWF multimers have a greater number of sites for interaction with platelets and vessel wall. Therefore, the thrombogenic risk of these larger molecules is high [26]. As mentioned, these large multimers are typically present in endothelial cells and platelets and are not normally present in plasma. Different studies suggest that size control of circulating VWF is for prevention of thrombosis [26, 27]. After synthesis and packaging of VWF in WPBs, a complex pathway is initiated that leads to secretion of VWF. The WPBs move in an undirected manner and are located to the cellular periphery. Following their fusion with the plasma membrane, their contents are released into the blood or the subendothelium [28]. Some studies assert that the fusion mechanism is random, whereas in some situations, release of WPB content including interlukin-8 and eotaxin-3 results in fusion of WPBs and plasma membrane. The secretion can occur in different ways. In basal secretion, single WPBs are fused with plasma membrane and

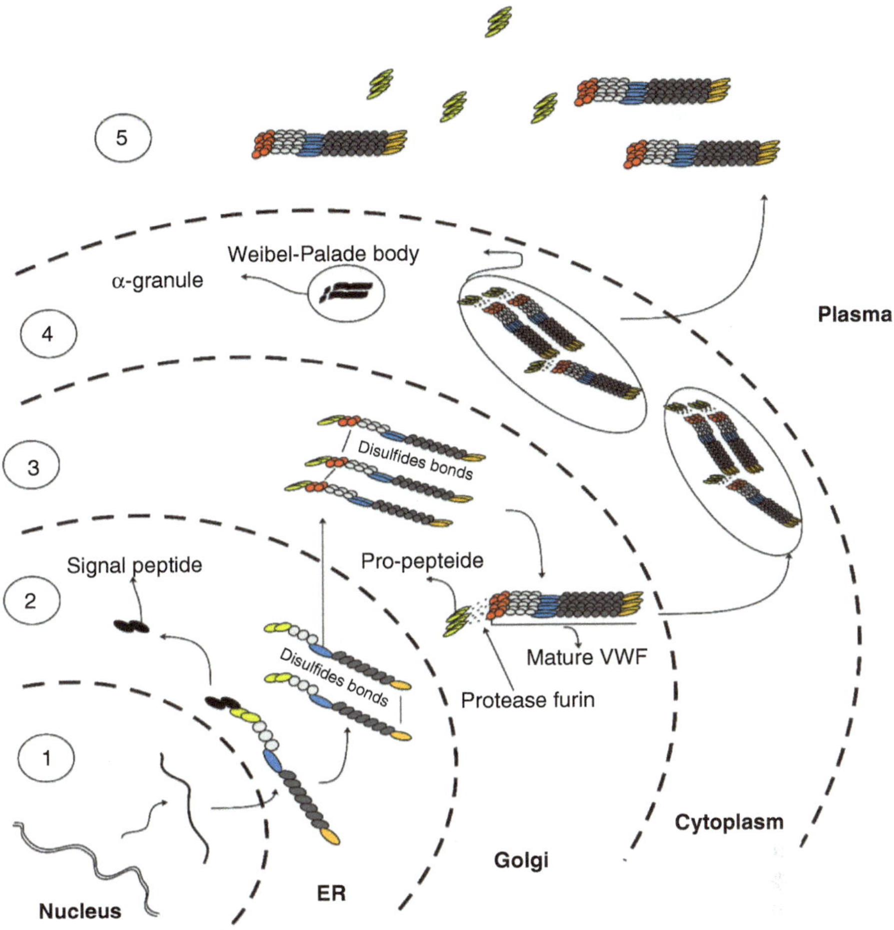

Fig. 3.4 The biosynthesis of von Willebrand factor (VWF). (*1*) The *VWF* gene encodes VWF mRNA which is translated to pre-propeptide VWF. (*2*) The synthesized VWF precursor is transported to the endoplasmic reticulum (ER) and undergoes several processes such as removal of signal peptide, tail-to-tail (C-terminal) dimerization, and addition of N-linked oligosaccharides. (*3*) VWF dimer is transported to Golgi apparatus and undergoes other processes including propeptide cleavage, N-terminal head-to-head multimerization, N-linked glycan maturation, and O-linked glycosylation. (*4*) The mature VWF is stored in storage organelles (Weibel-Palade bodies (WPBs) and α-granules of endothelial cells and megakaryocytes, respectively). (*5*) The contents of secretory granule storage are released into plasma, which thereby contributes to primary hemostasis

release all their contents, including VWF and other proteins. In massive secretion, multiple WPBs aggregate and are fused to secretory vesicles, which results in secretion of massive amounts of VWF multimers. This kind of secretion is potentially highly thrombogenic, therefore necessitating the presence of ADAMTS13 (Fig. 3.5) [9, 28].

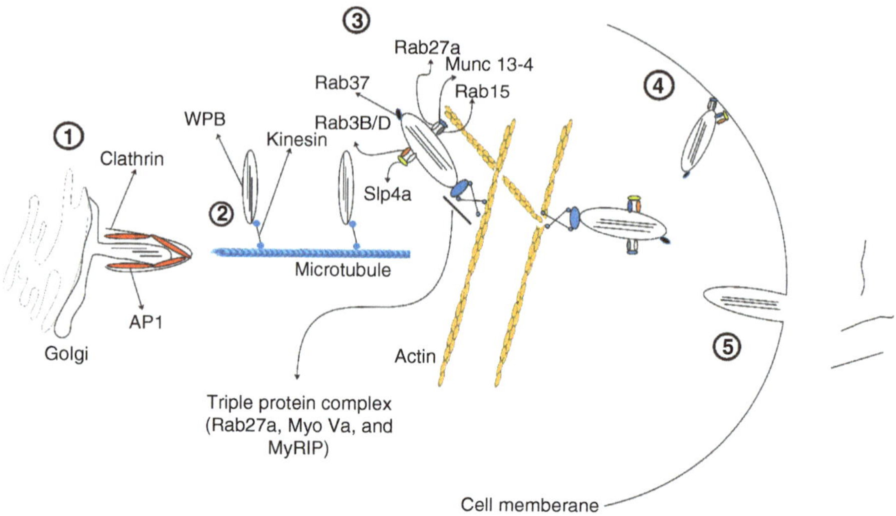

Fig. 3.5 A schematic presentation of VWF secretion. (*1*) The formation of WPBs begins at trans-Golgi network and involves AP1 and clathrin. (*2*) Within the endothelial cell, immature WPBs are transported along microtubules by the kinesin/dynein complex. (*3*) Following secretion, immature WPBs are adhered to the filamentous actin (F-actin) by the tripartite complex Rab27a, MyRIP, and MyoVa. Other proteins such as Rab3, 15, 27a, 37, Munc13-4, and Slp4a are attracted by WPBs. (*4*) Following secretion, F-actin adherence is lost, and three sequential steps tethering, docking, and priming occur, after which WPBs fuse with the cell membrane. A Rab27a and Slp4a-dependent docking step is necessary for the WPBs to release their contents. (*5*) WPBs fuse with the cell membrane and discharge their contents. *VWF* von Willebrand Factor, *WPBs* Weibel-Palade bodies, *AP1* adaptor protein complex 1, *MyRIP* myosin and Rab27a-interacting protein, *MyoVa* myosin Va

3.2.6 Biological Activities of von Willebrand Factor

The mature VWF consists of different functional sites that are capable of binding to other molecules and which exert various biological activities. These sites in each subunit act independent of multimer assembly; indeed, after proteolysis of the large native molecules, the isolated monomeric fragments still have substrate recognition specificity [27].

3.2.7 Stabilization and Transport of Coagulation Factor VIII

In patients affected by hemophilia A, due to defects in the *F8* gene, the FVIII level is decreased and the VWF level is normal. In contrast, in most of the patients with VWD, largely due to defects in the *VWF* gene, concomitant reduction of both FVIII and VWF occurs, because the survival of FVIII is dependent on its interaction with VWF [29]. The location of VWF that binds to FVIII is located with the first 272 amino acids of mature VWF, with the amino acids 78–96 having the substantive role

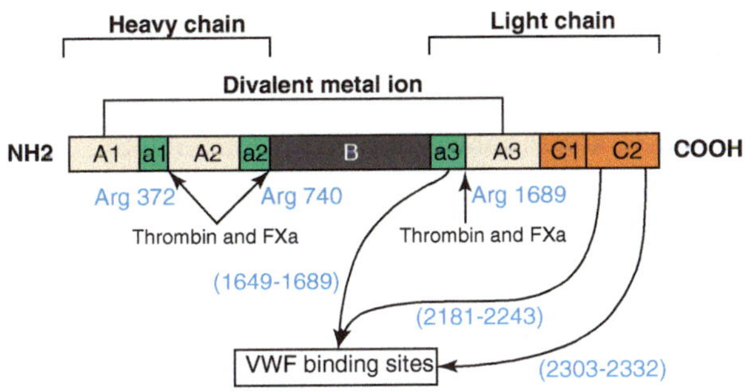

Fig. 3.6 Factor VIII (FVIII) structure and major binding sites for von Willebrand factor (VWF). FVIII consists of two chains including heavy and light chain. Heavy chain consists of A1, A2, and B domains while the light chain contains A3, C1, and C2 domains. Each A domain flanked by short segments (a1, a2, and a3) which have a high content of acidic amino acids. FVIII has different binding sites for different proteins. This factor is activated by thrombin and activated factor X (FXa) via proteolysis which occurs at Arg372, Arg740, and Arg1689 residues. This proteolysis leads to the release of B domain. FVIII has three binding sites for VWF, located at residues 1649–1689, 2181–2243, and 2303–2333. Following the activation of FVIII, thrombin cleaves FVIII at the Arg1689 residue and effectively destroys the binding site for VWF

in binding of VWF to FVIII [30]. In addition, the disulfide bond in the N-terminal of VWF has a crucial role in binding of FVIII. The respective binding sites in FVIII are located in the terminus of the light chain in the segment between 1669 and 1689 and also N-terminal and C-terminal of C2 domain including residues 2181–2243 and residues 2303–2332 [31, 32]. After transport of the FVIII to the location of hemostatic need, and the activation of FVIII, thrombin cleaves this coagulation factor at Arg1689. Thus, the binding site of VWF is destroyed and activated FVIII (FVIIIa) is released. In this way, VWF at the site of thrombus formation may deliver FVIIIa for coagulation reactions (Fig. 3.6) [9].

3.3 Platelet Adhesion

Following injury to the endothelium, VWF binds to different components of subendothelium as well as to platelets in order to sequester them to the injury site [33].

3.3.1 Interaction of von Willebrand Factor with Extracellular Protein

VWF is capable of binding to different types of collagen including type I, II, III, IV, V, and VI. Domains A1 and A3 are responsible for interaction with the main components of extracellular matrix (especially collagen). Each domain is capable of binding to different types of collagen [34] [35]. The A1 domain, which covers residues 497 to 716, binds to collagen type VI while the A3 domain, comprising residues 910 to 1111, binds to collagen types I and III [36, 37]. Collagen types I and III support VWF-dependent platelet adhesion in high shear rate, whereas collagen type IV mostly supports platelet adhesion at lower shear rates. The more important collagen binding site of VWF is therefore the A3 domain [38].

3.3.2 Interaction of von Willebrand Factor with Glycoprotein Ibα

The A1 domain has a site of interaction with glycoprotein (GP) Ibα, which in turn is a component of the platelet GPIb-V-IX receptor complex [39]. This interaction has a significant role in platelet activation, platelet adhesion, and finally platelet aggregation. In addition, binding of VWF to this receptor is crucial for the formation of thrombus. Initial platelet adhesion results from interaction between VWF and GpIbα under high fluid shear. In laboratory tests, the bacterial glycopeptide antibiotic ristocetin can bind to VWF and facilitate platelet GPIbα binding under low shear, and thereafter provokes platelet aggregation. This property of ristocetin is exploited in several VWF tests, including the ristocetin-induced platelet aggregation (RIPA) assay and VWF the ristocetin cofactor (VWF:RCo) assay, both of which permit laboratory estimation of the binding of VWF to GpIbα [40]. Botrocetin is a venom derived from viper *Bothrops jararaca* and can also activate platelets via GpIbα binding to cause VWF-dependent platelet aggregation [38]. The botrocetin-induced platelet aggregation (BIPA) is used more selectively in laboratory diagnostics [41].

The VWF binding site for GPIb is located in 293 residues of N-terminal and for optimal binding requires the sulfation of amino acid tyrosine at positions of 276, 278, and 279 [42]. Several studies have shown that the amino acids located in the boundary region between domain D3 and A1 (474 to 488 residues) and also the region in A1 domain (694–708 residues) are probably involved in this binding [43, 44]. Other studies have shown that another region in the A1 domain (residues 514 to 542) mediates the binding of VWF to GPIbα. In addition, carbohydrate chain has a role in binding of VWF to GPIbα. Although glycosylation of VWF is not necessarily needed for this binding, the O-linked sugars in each side of the A1 domain enhance this function [45–47].

3.3.3 Interaction of von Willebrand Factor with Integrin αIIbβ3 (GPIIb/IIIa)

Platelet GPIIb-IIIa, also known as the integrin αIIbβ3, is a surface receptor that, after platelet activation, can bind to different ligands, including fibrinogen, fibronectin, and VWF [48]. In domain C1 of VWF, the tetra peptide motif Arg-Gly-Asp-Ser (located in the C-terminal of the molecule) is a binding site for αIIbβ3 (GPIIb/IIIa). Although the major interaction for platelet adhesion is GbIb binding, inhibition of integrin αIIbβ3 (GPIIb/IIIa) also impairs platelet adhesion [38, 49]. In fact, VWF-integrin αIIbβ3 (GPIIb/IIIa) interaction leads to further platelet adhesion and facilitation of platelet aggregation initiated through the binding of GpIb to VWF [50].

3.4 von Willebrand Disease

VWD, with an estimated incidence of ~1%, is the most common CBD and is most often inherited in an autosomal dominant pattern. The disorder was first described by Erik von Willebrand in 1926, naming it "hereditary pseudohemophilia." VWD is caused by defects and/or deficiencies in VWF concentration, structure, or function. Patients with VWD present with variable bleeding episodes, mostly mucocutaneous bleeds. Epistaxis and bruising are the most common presentations in children, while menorrhagia and hematoma are common in adults, somewhat dependent on gender and type of VWD [2]. Generally, the severity and frequency of bleeding also depends on the type of disease, severity of defects, or deficiency in VWF and sometimes also the age and gender of the individual. Plasma levels of VWF gradually increase with age, and this may ameliorate the diagnosis of the disorder or its effect in some cases. VWD is classified into three main types: types 1 and 3 represent partial and complete deficiency of VWF, respectively, while type 2 reflects qualitative defects further characterized into four subgroups. These comprise (i) type 2A VWD, with loss of high- and sometimes intermediate-molecular-weight VWF multimers; (ii) type 2B VWD, with increased affinity of VWF for GPIb; (iii) type 2M VWD, with defects in VWF function such as platelet adhesion but a relatively normal pattern of (i.e., no substantial decrease in high molecular weight) VWF multimers; and (iv) type 2N, with markedly decreased VWF binding affinity to FVIII (Table 3.1) [1, 51].

Table 3.1 Classification of von Willebrand disease

Disorder		Definition	Prevalence	Inheritance
Type 1 VWD		Partial deficiency of VWF	1 in 1000 (40–80%)	AD
Type 2 VWD	2A	Qualitative defect with loss of high and sometimes intermediate-molecular-weight VWF multimers	~20%[a]	AD or AR
	2B	Qualitative defect with increased affinity to platelet GPIb	–	AD
	2M	Qualitative defect with decreased platelet adhesion property but relatively normal pattern of VWF multimers	–	AD
	2N	Qualitative defect with markedly decreased affinity of VWF to factor VIII	–	AR
Type 3 VWD		Complete deficiency of VWF	1 in 1 million (<1%)	AR

VWD von Willebrand disease, *VWF* von Willebrand factor, *AD* autosomal dominant, *AR* autosomal recessive

[a]Overall incidence of all type 2 VWD, with types 2A, 2M, 2B, and 2N each representing up to 25% or more of type 2 VWD cases, depending on the geography and the local study population

Table 3.2 Frequency of different types of von Willebrand disease

VWD type	London (*n*: 134)	German Democratic Republic (*n*: 111)	Swedish (*n*: 106)	UK (*n*: 116)	Jordan (*n*: 65)	Italy (*n*: 1286)
Type 1 VWD (%)	75	76	70	71	59	73
Type 2 VWD (%)[a]	19	12	10	23	29.5	21
Type 3 VWD (%)	6	12	20	6	11.5	6

VWD von Willebrand disease
[a]Overall incidence for type 2 VWD

Type 3 VWD, with an estimated incidence of 1 per 1 million in the general population in developed countries, is the rarest and the most severe form of disorder, while type 1 is the most commonly diagnosed form of VWD (Table 3.2). Relative frequency depends on the geographical location and the team making the diagnosis. For example, the diagnosis of type 3 VWD in some locations may include patients that would otherwise be identified as severe type 1 in other locations [52].

Types 1 and 2 VWD are highly heterogeneous disorders, and bleeding tendency is related to circulating level of functional VWF. Triad diagnostic criteria have been proposed for VWD: (1) bleeding symptoms, (2) decreased VWF activity measured (e.g., as measured by VWF:RCo), and (3) pattern of inheritance (autosomal dominant or recessive). Among these criteria, bleeding history is perhaps the most important criteria, although this is often elusive in young children due to lack of exposure to bleeding risk situations [53]. In respect to bleeding history, it is always important to determine whether the bleeding tendency is "lifelong" or of recent onset, the latter potentially indicating an acquired abnormality rather than an inherited one [53].

Diagnosis of VWD is a challenge worldwide, especially in the mildest form of the disease, as well as in complex types, and misdiagnosis is common and can occur due to use of the wrong methods or tests or ineffective test panels. Correct diagnosis and classification of VWD is crucial as it can influence patient management. However, in practice, typing of the disorder may be difficult because the patient's phenotype might vary over the time, the patient's genotype may not show a mutation or may show complex patterns, and some laboratory tests have low sensitivity and specificity. Moreover, the boundary between normal and abnormal phenotypes is not clearly defined [54].

3.4.1 Type 1 von Willebrand Disease

Type 1 VWD with an estimated incidence of 1 per 1000 is not only the most common form of VWD but also the most often diagnosed CBD. This disorder is inherited in autosomal dominant manner with variable penetrance and a highly variable phenotype. Type 1 VWD accounts for 40–80% of all cases with VWD, and based on molecular pathogenesis, VWF level is between 5 and 40%. A considerable number of factors are responsible for the highly variable clinical and laboratory phenotype in type 1 VWD. In about 30% of patients with type 1 VWD, a mutation cannot be detected in the *VWF* gene. Genetic modifiers and physiological factors are major factors that can reduce plasma level of VWF, with one well-known genetic modifier outside the *VWF* gene being ABO blood group [55].

Plasma VWF level is ~25% lower in individuals with O blood group than non-O blood group. Other genetic modifiers that can help explain the low level of VWF in type 1 VWD with undetectable mutation in *VWF* gene are CLEC4M (C-type lectin domain family 4, member M) and STXBP5 (syntaxin-binding protein 5), which are probably involved in clearance and exocytosis of VWF, respectively [56, 57]. The severity of bleeding episodes in type 1 VWD depends on severity of the VWF deficiency in plasma; therefore, risk of severe bleeds is higher in patients with lower plasma levels of VWF. Plasma FVIII level is also reduced in parallel with VWF but normally is at ~1.5× the level of VWF and is usually between 5 and 50% (5 to 50 IU/dL). Since type 1 VWD phenotypically defines an inherited bleeding disorder with partial quantitative VWF deficiency, both VWF antigen (VWF: Ag) and VWF activity fall in parallel, and functional abnormality can be excluded if all VWF activity/VWF:Ag ratios are around unity (generally >0.6) [58]. With use of sensitive assays, a considerable number of patients with historical diagnosis of type 1 VWD may have mild abnormalities of multimer structure or distribution; however, bleeding in this form of the disorder is generally attributed to the VWF concentration and not to any selective decrease in large VWF multimers or specific abnormalities in ligand binding sites [59]. Increased susceptibility of VWF to proteolytic cleavage may also contribute to the severity of type 1 VWD. The Tyr1584Cys mutation, for example, increases the susceptibility of VWF to cleavage by ADAMTS13. Desmopressin is generally suitable as the therapeutic choice in most patients with type 1 VWD, especially for short duration or minor treatments [59].

3.4.2 Type 2 von Willebrand Disease

Type 2 VWD is characterized by qualitative defects in structure and function of VWF and is classified in four types: 2A, 2B, 2M, and 2N. Classically, type 2A has been considered the most common form, while 2N and 2B represent the rarest forms. However, the relative frequency of type 2 VWD depends in part on the geography in which the diagnosis is made, as well as the diagnostic team. For example, type 2N VWD is relatively more frequent in some parts of France and Italy, and type 2B diagnosis requires performance of RIPA, which if omitted may lead to diagnosis of such patients as 2A VWD [60, 61]. Type 2 VWD is mostly transmitted in an autosomal dominant manner, except for type 2N, which has an autosomal recessive pattern of inheritance. Type 2 VWD is less common than type 1 VWD and represents ~20% of all cases of VWD. Type 2 VWD is usually attributable to mutations that either impair specific functional domains of VWF or which affect VWF multimer assembly or proteolysis. Generally, mutations responsible for type 2 VWD are highly penetrant, and bleeding episodes are highly reproducible in a given family. Type 2 VWD is diagnostically the most challenging form of VWD [62]. The hallmark of this type of disorder is low-functional VWF/VWF:Ag ratio (<0.7).

Functional VWF is usually assessed as VWF:RCo, although other assays such as collagen binding (VWF:CB) may be utilized. Lack of large multimers is evident in types 2A and 2B VWD, with loss of intermediate multimers also often seen in type 2A VWD. Impaired RIPA in platelet-rich plasma (PRP) or in whole blood is evident in types 2A and 2M VWD, whereas an increased RIPA responsiveness is seen in 2B VWD [41].

3.4.2.1 Type 2A von Willebrand Disease

Type 2A is classically considered the most frequent type 2 VWD, comprising up to 20% of all cases with VWD and typically >50% of all type 2 VWD. Impaired VWF multimerization or increased susceptibility of multimers to degradation with ADAMTS13 is the key impairment evident in this disorder, causing selective reduction of high-molecular-weight multimers (HMWM) and sometimes intermediate-molecular-weight multimers (IMWM), leading to diminished activity of the binding domains for GPIb and probably GPIIb/IIIa [61].

3.4.2.2 Type 2B von Willebrand Disease

In type 2B VWD, gain-of-function mutations, usually in the A2 domain of VWF, cause an increased affinity of VWF for platelet GpIb. This is often identified in laboratory testing by elevated RIPA responsiveness. In 2B VWD, the platelet-VWF complex is removed from the plasma circulation, often leading to loss of HMWM also (mild) thrombocytopenia. Although these features are seen with varying degree in the majority of patients, not all cases present with the "classic" 2B VWD presentation. Additional features of 2B VWD include slightly decreased to normal levels of VWF:Ag and FVIII and relatively decreased VWF:RCo and VWF:CB (ratios of VWF:RCo/Ag and VWF:CB/Ag both <0.7). VWF multimeric pattern is normal in some patients with ("atypical") type 2B, and in such patients, the functional VWF/VWF:Ag ratio may also be normal. In 2B VWD patients in their second and third trimester of pregnancy, the pregnancy associated with increased level of VWF may worsen the thrombocytopenia due to an increase of abnormal endogenous VWF and increased clearance. A similar situation can occur if desmopressin is administrated in patients with 2B VWD [63].

3.4.2.3 Type 2M von Willebrand Disease

Type 2M is mostly due to mutations in the A1 domain of VWF, leading to conformational changes in VWF protein and decreased affinity to GpIbα. VWF multimeric pattern is essentially normal, but platelet-dependent VWF activities are decreased. Rarely, these mutations can occur in the A3 domain, and thus also affect collagen binding. Generally, type 2M VWD cases are identified by low VWF:RCo/Ag ratios without lack of HMWM or low VWF:RCo/Ag ratio and normal VWF:CB/Ag ratio. Misdiagnosis is an important and largely under-recognized issue in type 2M VWD, and a considerable number of clinicians or laboratories identify this type "incorrectly" as type 1 or type 2A VWD. Patients with type 2M present with mild to moderate bleeding tendency but severe bleeds also may occur [64].

3.4.2.4 Type 2N von Willebrand Disease

Type 2N VWD (VWD "Normandy") was originally described in patients from the Normandy region of France, in 1989, as a variant of VWD caused by defects in the ability of VWF to bind FVIII. This defect causes decreased plasma level of FVIII, thereby resembling hemophilia A. However, the inheritance pattern of 2N VWD is autosomal recessive (whereas hemophilia A is sex-linked, being carried on the X chromosome), and the defect is present on VWF (whereas in hemophilia A, the defect is in FVIII). Symptoms of type 2N VWD are similar to that of (mild) hemophilia A [65]. Phenotypically, VWF:Ag, VWF:RCo, and multimeric pattern are normal in type 2N VWD, but the level of FVIII is decreased due to the increased clearance of FVIII (since the VWF does not bind FVIII, the FVIII is easily degraded in circulation). Sometimes 2N VWD may arise as a duplex defect. For example, patients with a 2N VWD mutation on one *VWF* gene and another defect in the other *VWF* gene may show more complex phenotypes and more severe/complex bleeding patterns. For example, if the second *VWF* gene carries a null mutation, essentially mimicking a "heterozygous type 3 VWD," then the resulting phenotype will express with lowered VWF levels. Although the majority of patients with type 2N VWD have normal multimeric patterns, occasional patients may show loss of HMWM should a complex genotype be evident [60].

3.4.3 Type 3 von Willebrand Disease

Type 3 VWD is the most severe form of the disorder, although fortunately also the rarest type of VWD (1 in 1 million in the general population); however, frequency is higher in developing countries due to high rates of consanguinity [66].

By definition, type 3 VWD is a severe bleeding disorder with undetectable plasma and platelet level of VWF and also a low level of FVIII:C (<20 U dL^{-1}). The clinical presentations and bleeding episodes are generally more severe than other types of VWD and are often similar to those of moderately severe hemophilia A. Due to concomitant decrease of VWF and FVIII, these patients not only present mucocutaneous hemorrhages but also with hemarthrosis and hematomas, as associated to decreased FVIII level [52].

3.5 Clinical Manifestations of von Willebrand Disease

Clinical manifestations and bleeding tendency among patients with VWD are highly variable and range from quite mild conditions to severe bleeding diathesis sufficient to require urgent medical intervention. Mucocutaneous bleeding such as epistaxis and menorrhagia is the typical presentation of VWD, and post-dental extraction bleeding is the most common post-surgical bleeding event. Since VWF also binds to FVIII and facilitates platelet function, VWD may cause bleeding symptoms that are typical of platelet function disorders or mild to moderately severe hemophilia A or both [3, 67].

In some patients, especially in males, surgery may be the first hemostatic challenge that leads to "abnormal bleeding" and therefore facilitates the diagnosis in previously unrecognized cases.

A wide overlap can be observed between the bleeding diathesis of patients with mild VWD and the normal population; therefore, a proper bleeding history is a critical and crucial component in the diagnosis of VWD and should be done carefully. Women with mild VWD are often more symptomatic than men, because they are subject to greater hemostatic challenges (menstruation and childbirth). In children with VWD, the pattern of hemorrhagic symptoms are different from children with more severe congenital bleeding disorders, with life-threatening bleeds such as intracranial hemorrhage (ICH) and umbilical cord bleeding being more rare among young VWD patients. In children with VWD, the most common clinical presentations are bruising and epistaxis, although these presentations are also frequent in normal healthy children, further challenging their diagnosis [68]. Some of standard clinical presentations in VWD, such as menorrhagia and post-surgical bleeding, are not clearly prevalent or evaluable in the pediatric population. Standard bleeding assessment tools (BATs) and scoring systems may be useful for correct assessment of bleeding episodes among these patients because significant bleeding diathesis may be overlooked while minimal bleeding symptoms may be over emphasized [69].

In adults, hematoma, menorrhagia, and bleeding from minor wounds are the most frequent symptoms, depending on VWD type, disease severity, and patient gender. Post-dental extraction and post-surgical bleeds are common and occur in about two-thirds of VWD patients. Gastrointestinal bleeding (GI) is also reported in VWD, predominantly among adults, and this can sometimes be severe [70]. In some patients, especially those with severe VWD, epistaxis can be so severe as to require medical intervention with clotting factor concentrates or blood transfusion. This diathesis can be life-threatening in some patients and may require long-time secondary prophylaxis [66].

Post-partum hemorrhage (PPH) can also be observed among women with VWD, but with lower frequency than may be expected because of increasing VWF levels during pregnancy. Delayed PPH can occur due to gradual decrease of VWF level to baseline level post-delivery. Prolonged vaginal bleeding following normal vaginal delivery is a common presentation of women with VWD. Menorrhagia (>80 mL of blood loss per menstrual period) is a common and important bleeding symptom of women with VWD and ~15% of women with menorrhagia have VWD. Therefore, menorrhagia is a sensitive but nonspecific presentation of VWD in women. This symptom can be accompanied by anemia and iron deficiency. Therefore, careful gynecological assessment of women with VWD is crucial [52, 69].

In general, bleeding symptoms are mild in type 1 VWD and more severe in type 2 and type 3 VWD. Since, FVIII level is only slightly reduced in most types of VWD, spontaneous hemarthrosis or hematoma are rare in type 1, 2A, and 2B VWD, while in type 3 VWD the severity of diathesis often resembles that of hemophilia.

Table 3.3 Clinical manifestations of patients with von Willebrand disease

	Scandinavian (*n*: 264)	Iranian (*n*: 385)	Italian		
Bleeding	VWD	Type 3	Type 1 (*n*: 671)	Type 2 (*n*: 497)	Type 3 (*n*: 66)
Epistaxis (%)	62	77	61	63	66
Menorrhagia (%)	60	69	32	32	56
Post-dental extraction bleeding (%)	51	–	31	39	53
Hematoma (%)	49	52	13	14	33
Bleeding from minor wounds (%)	36	–	36	40	50
Gum bleeding (%)	35	70[a]	31	35	56
Post-surgical bleeding (%)	28	41	20	23	41
Post-partum bleeding (%)	23	15	17	18	26
Gastrointestinal bleeding (%)	14	20	5	8	20
Hemarthrosis (%)	8	37	3	4	45
Hematuria (%)	7	1	2	5	12
CNS bleeding (%)	–	2	1	2	9

CNS central nervous system
[a]Oral cavity bleeding

Type 3 VWD mostly is accompanied with severe bleeds, while type 1 and type 2 VWD are very heterogeneous, and the severity of clinical presentations is associated with circulation level of functional VWF (e.g., as measured by VWF:RCo). Severe life-threatening bleeding can occur in type 3 VWD and sometimes in patients with type 2 VWD but is a rare presentation of type 1 VWD. ICH is a rare presentation of VWD that usually is only reported in type 3 VWD. An interesting recent finding is the reduced risk of cardiovascular disease and ischemic stroke among patients with VWD (Table 3.3).

3.5.1 Type 1 von Willebrand Disease

Although the bleeding symptoms are variable in type 1 VWD, bleeding tendency in these patients is usually mild, and major bleeds are rare. The heterogeneity in bleeding symptoms in Type 1 VWD may be partially explained by presence of genetic variations [71].

Due to the physiological rise in plasma VWF level throughout life, patients with type 1 VWD may have normal levels of VWD later in life; however, the severity and frequency of bleeding symptoms in older patients may still be significant, especially if there is an increase in hemostatic challenges (e.g., older patients more likely to be candidates for surgery). The most common clinical presentations in children with type 1 VWD are easy bruising and epistaxis, while menorrhagia, oral cavity bleeding, prolonged bleeding from minor lacerations, GI bleeding, and bleeding after tooth extractions or oral surgery are other presentations [72].

Clinical manifestations and bleeding episodes are an important part of the diagnosis of type 1 VWD. Out of three main criteria for diagnosis of VWD, clinical symptoms assessment is perhaps the most important part of the diagnosis [53]. A patient that meets all three diagnostic criteria may be diagnosed as type 1 VWD, while an asymptomatic patient with low level of VWF and positive family history of VWD without personal history of VWD and without personal history of clinical symptoms can be assigned to a category of "possible type 1 VWD." To fulfill this definition, an asymptomatic patient with low level of VWF should have at least two relatives with definitive VWD [58].

Based on a multicenter study on sensitivity and specificity of bleeding symptoms in the diagnosis of type 1 VWD, it was shown that menorrhagia and epistaxis are not good predictors of type 1 VWD, while cutaneous bleeding and post-dental extraction bleeding should be considered as the most sensitive symptoms. It was proposed that laboratory investigation for VWD should be done for those with at least three minor bleeds or those with at least two major bleeds if they include cutaneous bleeding or post-dental extraction bleeding [73].

3.5.2 Type 2 von Willebrand Disease

Patients with type 2 VWD have variable bleeding tendency with moderate to severe hemorrhagic tendency. The severity and incidence of hemorrhagic symptoms vary between different subtypes of type 2 VWD, often explainable by differences in levels of FVIII, VWF, and/or HMWM VWF. The bleeding tendency in type 2A VWD is generally greater that in type 2M; this cannot easily be explained by differences in residual FVIII or VWF levels but may be attributed to higher rate of GI bleeding in type 2A VWD. The higher relative risk of type 2A VWD can also be attributed to a lesser extent to a higher rate of menorrhagia. In type 2B VWD, thrombocytopenia is a contributory factor that can worsen the hemorrhage risk in affected patients. Intra-articular bleeding (hemarthrosis) is a common presentation of hemophilia that in addition to type 3 VWD can also be observed in type 2N. The risk of hemarthrosis is strongly dependent on residual plasma FVIII levels as well as the severity of VWD [60].

GI bleeding due to angiodysplasia is a well-known complication of VWD, notably in types 2A and 2B VWD. Two main reasons for the occurrence of this kind of bleeding are older age and lack of HMWM in plasma. It was shown in a long term prospective study that GI bleeding due to angiodysplasia was not observed in VWD Vicenza, which is accompanied by presence of ultra-large VWF multimers. The development of angiodysplasia in VWD is attributed to the role of VWF in regulation of angiogenesis, and enhanced angiogenesis is observed with reduced VWF level. It appears that some forms of type 2A VWD expressing the S1506L mutation are associated with higher risk of angiodysplasia [74]. GI bleeding due to angiodysplasia with an incidence of ~2–6 is a common cause of digestive tract bleeding in elderly people (Table 3.4).

Table 3.4 Clinical manifestations of patients with type 2 von Willebrand disease

Disorder	Clinical manifestations
Type 2A VWD	Gastrointestinal bleeding (36.9%)
	Post-surgical bleeding (80%)
	Post dental extraction bleeding (73%)
	Menorrhagia (50%)
	Epistaxis (34%)
	Prolonged bleeding from minor wounds (33%)
	Post-circumcision bleeding (32%)
	Bruising (24%)
	Cephalohematoma (~9%)
	Hematuria (4%)
	Central nervous system bleeding (3%)
	Umbilical stump bleeding (6%)
Type 2B VWD	Easy bruising (59%)
	Epistaxis (52%)
	Menorrhagia (25%)
	Oral cavity bleeding (23%)
	Prolonged bleeding from minor wounds (~27%)
	Gastrointestinal bleeding (14%)
	Umbilical stump bleeding (10%)
	Hemorrhage (~2%)
Type 2M VWD	Gastrointestinal bleeding (3.3%)
	Cephalohematoma (~9%)
	Bruising after birth (~7%)
	Prolonged bleeding from minor wounds (~32%)
Type 2N VWD	Cephalohematoma (~11%)
	Hemarthrosis
	Bruising after birth (~11%)
	Prolonged bleeding from minor wounds (~33%)

VWD von Willebrand disease

3.5.3 Type 3 von Willebrand Disease

Type 3 is the most severe form of VWD that from a clinical aspect is similar to some extent to hemophilia. Although hemophilia-like hemarthrosis or recurrent spontaneous mucosal bleeding is more frequent in type 3 VWD than in type 1 or 2 VWD, the rate of these bleeds is significantly lower than hemophilia A. The bleeding symptoms in type 3 are due to concomitant reduction of FVIII and VWF, leading to occurrence of both primary and secondary hemostasis presentations. Life-endangering hemorrhage in CNS is a rare presentation of VWD that is usually only reported in type 3 VWD [52]. Although the rate of GI bleeding is relatively high in type 3 VWD patients, the incidence of other life-threatening bleeds such as umbilical cord bleeding is relatively low in this disorder, and therefore the pattern of bleeding in type 3 VWD is different from other severe congenital bleeding disorders such as factor XIII deficiency. Since type 3 VWD represents an autosomal recessive congenital bleeding disorder, patients are homozygote or double heterozygotes. Carriers of type 3 VWD, with a single defective *VWF* gene, are typically asymptomatic, similar to most of other congenital bleeding disorders [66].

3.6 Diagnosis of von Willebrand Disease

VWD is diagnosed on clinical features, comprising personal and family history of bleeding or bruising, and confirmed by laboratory testing. As VWD is due to deficiencies or defects in the plasma protein VWF, a large adhesive protein with multiple activities, laboratory testing therefore centers on assessment of VWF by means of a panel of assays [6]. The more comprehensive the assay panel is, the more likely it is to achieve a correct diagnosis or exclusion of VWD. Vice versa, the less comprehensive the assay panel is, the more likely it is to achieve an incorrect diagnosis. The minimum recommended test panel comprises Factor VIII coagulant (FVIII:C), VWF antigen (VWF:Ag), and VWF "activity" using several other assays, generally including evaluation of platelet Glycoprotein (GP) Ib binding and collagen binding (VWF:CB), with factor VIII (FVIII) binding (VWF:FVIIIB) performed more selectively. Decreases in VWF:Ag and the various VWF activities, as well as the pattern of such changes, help define VWD and its type and the need (if any) for further testing. The most often used assay for measuring GPIb binding activity is the ristocetin cofactor assay (VWF:RCo), which historically measured the agglutination by VWF of fixed human platelets in the presence of ristocetin [75]. This assay is now often replaced or supplemented with other assays based on binding of VWF to recombinant GPIb, generally without the use of platelets and with or without ristocetin [75–77].

Because of the large number of different laboratory tests now available and the many different methodologies in use, associate terminology for tests involving "platelet-dependent" function has recently been updated by the International Society on Thrombosis and Haemostasis (ISTH) Scientific and Standardization Committee (SSC) [6, 77]. The main elements of the recommended nomenclature are summarized in Table 3.5.

Nevertheless, the assay group reflecting assays of GPIb binding (i.e., classical VWF:RCo, as well as methodologies now defined as "VWF:GPIbR" and "VWF:GPIbM") would be expected to broadly derive similar test results for VWD patients and are thus essentially recognized to be "interchangeable" in VWD diagnostics.

In respect to an "ideal" diagnostic test panel, then, (i) VWF:Ag assays quantify the level of VWF protein without reference to its functional activity; (ii) "GPIb-binding assays," as defined above, define platelet binding; (iii) VWF:CB assays quantify the activity of VWF binding to subendothelial matrix components (in this case collagen); (iv) FVIII coagulant function quantifies the activity of FVIII; (v)

Table 3.5 Recommended nomenclature of the ISTH VWF SSC for VWF test parameters

Abbreviation for assay	Description of assay	Comments
VWF:Ag	von Willebrand factor antigen	All assays that provide a quantitative level of VWF protein, be it by ELISA, LIA, or other methodology
VWF:CB	von Willebrand factor collagen-binding capacity	All assays that provide a quantitative level of VWF collagen-binding capacity, be it by ELISA or other methodology
VWF:RCo	von Willebrand factor ristocetin cofactor activity	Historically, this referred to assays that used ristocetin to facilitate VWF binding to GPIb, where the only such assay type available was that based on platelet agglutination. This has changed with the advent of non-platelet-based methods, which incorporated rGPIb. The updated recommendations place these new assays into new categories, namely, VWF:GPIbR
VWF:GPIbR	All assays that are based on the ristocetin-induced binding of von Willebrand factor to a recombinant wild-type GPIb fragment	Essentially, these are VWF:RCo assays that do not use platelets and which currently comprise several IL Werfen assays, as performed by either CLIA or LIA technology. These assays essentially generate test results that are very similar to those generated using "standard" VWF:RCo assays that utilize platelets
VWF:GPIbM	All assays that are based on the spontaneous binding of von Willebrand factor to a gain-of-function mutant GPIb fragment	Essentially a GPIb-binding assay that does not utilize platelets or ristocetin and which currently comprises the Siemens Innovance VWF Ac assay (by LIA), as well as non-commercialized ELISA-based assays. These assays essentially generate test results that are very similar to those generated using VWF:GPIbR or classical VWF:RCo assays, despite the lack of ristocetin in the assay
VWF:Ab	All assays that are based on the binding of a monoclonal antibody (MAB) to a von Willebrand factor A1 domain epitope	Essentially a VWF-binding assay that utilizes a monoclonal antibody; this currently comprises the IL Werfen "VWF Activity" assay (LIA), as well as ELISA-based assays. Like VWF:GPIbM assays, VWF:Ab assays do not use ristocetin. VWF:Ab assays provide results that may or may not match VWF:GPIbM, VWF:GPIbR, or classical VWF:RCo assays
VWF:FVIIIB	von Willebrand factor: factor VIII binding capacity	All assays that provide a quantitative level of VWF—factor VIII binding capacity, irrespective of specific methodology. Generally performed by ELISA

CLIA chemiluminescent immuno-assay, *ELISA* enzyme-linked immunosorbent assay, *GPIb* (platelet) glycoprotein Ib, *LIA* Latex immunoassay, *ISTH* International Society on Thrombosis and Haemostasis, *rGPIb* recombinant (platelet) glycoprotein Ib, *VWF* von Willebrand factor, *SSC* Scientific and Standardization Committee

VWF:FVIIIB (as required for 2N VWD) quantifies the activity of VWF binding to FVIII; and (v) VWF multimers (as selectively required) assess the multimeric profile or structure of VWF.

For the purpose of this section, the VWD classification scheme proposed by the ISTH SSC, and last updated in 2006, will be utilized [3], and provides the simplest and most clinically relevant classification scheme, separating VWD into six types, as summarized previously (Table 3.1).

The anticipated test patterns in different types of VWD are summarized in Table 3.6, with greater detail provided in Table 3.7. Type 1 VWD represents a partial quantitative deficiency of (functionally normal) VWF, so there is concordant decrease in VWF measured by any VWF assay (be it VWF:Ag, VWF:CB, or GPIb binding), and the ratio of any one VWF assay to any other is close to unity (in practice, >0.7). Type 3 VWD represents a total loss of VWF, and all VWF test results will be close to 0 U/dL, albeit recognizing that lower limit VWF sensitivity issues means that some assays cannot detect to these low levels.

In contrast, type 2 VWD represents qualitative VWF defects/deficiencies, such that VWF activity is proportionally decreased below that of VWF:Ag; furthermore, the VWD type can be defined by the type of activity reduced. In type 2A VWD, defining a loss of HMW VWF multimers, patients express a relative reduction of all VWF activities sensitive to this loss (this includes both GPIb binding and VWF:CB assays). In practice, this is expressed as the ratio of VWF activity/VWF:Ag assays being lower than ~0.7. Type 2B VWD defines an increased affinity of VWF for GPIb which often leads to loss of HMW VWF multimers and similar VWF test patterns to type 2A VWD. Type 2M VWD defines decreased VWF-dependent platelet adhesion without a selective deficiency of HMW VWF multimers. In type 2M VWD, there are specific changes in VWF function related to specific *VWF* mutations. In practice, most type 2M mutations affect GPIb binding, and less so collagen binding; thus, there is usually a low GPIb binding/VWF:Ag ratio, but the CB/Ag ratio may be normal. Type 2N VWD defines a decreased binding affinity for FVIII, as identified by the specific test VWF:FVIIIB. Phenotypically, however, these patients present similarly to those with hemophilia A, showing relatively lower FVIII:C to VWF:Ag ratios.

The impetus for testing of FVIII:C as part of a VWD diagnostic profile is manyfold. As VWF protects FVIII, lower levels of VWF (viz., VWD), in general, also mean lower levels of FVIII:C. In type 3 VWD, for example, levels of FVIII:C are generally <10 U/dL. In type 1 VWD, the FVIII:C is generally proportional to VWF:Ag. In type 2N VWD, FVIII:C is proportionally lower than VWF:Ag.

In summary, a recommended approach to diagnosis or exclusion of VWD is shown as an algorithm in Fig. 3.7. All patients being screened for VWD should be tested with the 4-test panel of VWF:Ag, VWF:CB, VWF GPIb binding, and FVIII:C. This recommendation is made based on decades of experience with this panel, and the issues arising with diagnostic errors when a different or smaller first line testing panel is employed [6, 78–82].Which tests within each category should be employed by laboratories is to some extent dependent on local instrumentation and test availability. For example, VWF:Ag by ELISA may be preferred if VWF:CB

Table 3.6 Classification scheme for von Willebrand disease

VWD type	Description	Phenotypic diagnosis	Incidence/comments
1	Partial quantitative deficiency of VWF	Low levels of VWF, with VWF functional concordance (i.e., ratio of functional VWF/ VWF:Ag approximates unity)	Most common presentation of "VWD" to most laboratories, with most patients presenting with mildly reduced levels of VWF
2A	Decreased VWF-dependent platelet adhesion and a selective deficiency of high-molecular-weight (HMW) VWF multimers	Loss of HMW VWF. Usually low levels of VWF, with VWF functional discordance (i.e., ratios of GPIb binding/Ag *and* CB/Ag typically <0.7)	Globally considered to be the most common presentation of type 2 VWD
2B	Increased affinity of VWF for platelet glycoprotein Ib	Low to normal levels of VWF, typically with VWF functional discordance (i.e., ratios of GPIb binding/Ag *and* CB/Ag generally <0.7), loss of HMW VWF and (mild) thrombocytopenia. Atypical cases may not show this pattern	Rare form (generally 10–20%) of type 2 VWD (= ~1–5 cases per million population). Defined by enhanced responsiveness in a RIPA assay
2M	Decreased VWF-dependent platelet adhesion without a selective deficiency of high-molecular-weight (HMW) VWF multimers	Low to normal levels of VWF, usually with VWF functional discordance detected by GPIb binding/Ag generally <0.7, but relatively normal CB/Ag ratio. HMW VWF present, but multimers may show other abnormalities	Under-recognized form of type 2 VWD. Probably as common as 2A VWD. Some (rare) 2M cases show low CB/Ag ratio, with normal GPIb binding/Ag. Some 2M cases show low CB/Ag ratio and low GPIb binding/Ag
2N	Markedly decreased binding affinity for factor VIII	Defined by VWF:FVIIIB assay, with low FVIIIB/VWF ratios (~0.5 for heterozygous mutations, and <0.3 for more severe genetic changes)	Rare form (generally <10%) of type 2 VWD (= ~1–5 cases per million population)
3	Virtually complete deficiency of VWF	Typically defined by VWF levels <2 U/dL and FVIII:C <10 U/dL	Rare form of VWD in developed countries (~1–5 cases per million population) but disproportionately more common in developing countries

testing is also being performed by ELISA. Alternatively, the availability of latex-based technology may drive the combined use of latex-based VWF:Ag and GPIb-binding assays, or availability of an AcuStar instrument may drive the utility of chemiluminescence test procedures [78]. Also, problems with classical VWF:RCo assays may drive usage of more modern GPIb binding assay alternatives such as VWF:GPIbR or VWF:GPIbM.

Table 3.7 Anticipated test patterns in different types of von Willebrand disease (VWD) and VWD type

VWD type	VWF:Ag	VWF:GPIb binding[a]	VWF:CB	FVIII:C	Multimers	GPIb binding / Ag[b]	CB/Ag[b]	FVIII/VWF[b]	Comments/additional testing
1	↓ to ↓↓	↓ to ↓↓	↓ to ↓↓	N to ↓↓	Normal pattern but reduced intensity	>(0.5–0.7)	>(0.5–0.7)	>(0.5–0.7)	VWF levels between ~30 and 50 U/dL will generally not be associated with *VWF* mutations and can be considered as representing "low" VWF as a risk factor for bleeding. VWF levels below ~30 U/dL will often be associated with *VWF* mutations and can be considered as representing "true" VWD
2A	N to ↓↓	↓↓ to ↓↓↓	↓↓ to ↓↓↓	↓ to ↓↓	Loss of HMW VWF	<(0.5–0.7)	<(0.5–0.7)	>(0.5–0.7)	2A and 2B VWD can only be distinguished by means of RIPA. Platelet-type (PT-) VWD phenotypically resembles 2B VWD; these can be distinguished by means of RIPA mixing studies, or by genetic analysis of *VWF* and/or platelet *GPIb* genes
2B	N to ↓↓	↓ to ↓↓↓	↓ to ↓↓↓	N to ↓↓	Loss of HMW VWF	<(0.5–0.7)	<(0.5–0.7)	>(0.5–0.7)	
2N	N to ↓↓	N to ↓↓	N to ↓↓	↓↓to ↓↓↓	Normal pattern	>(0.5–0.7)	>(0.5–0.7)	<(0.5–0.7)	Phenotypically similar to hemophilia A; distinguish using VWF:FVIII-binding assay or genetic analysis of *FVIII* and/or *VWF* genes

2M	N to ↓↓	(↓ to ↓↓↓)	(↓ to ↓↓↓)	↓ to ↓↓	No loss of HMW VWF; some multimer defects may however be observed	<(0.5–0.7) (platelet-binding defect) or >(0.5–0.7) (collagen-binding defect)	<(0.5–0.7) (collagen-binding defect) or >(0.5–0.7) (platelet-binding defect)	>(0.5–0.7)	2A and 2M VWD can only be distinguished by comprehensive or composite panel testing, including VWF:Ag, GPIb binding assay[a], *plus* VWF:CB or multimer analysis. Platelet binding dysfunction 2M VWD is far more common than collagen binding defect variants
3	↓↓↓ (absent)	↓↓↓ (absent)	↓↓↓ (absent)	↓↓↓	No VWF present	NA	NA	NA	Type 3 VWD can only be identified when VWF tests are performed, and these are sensitive to very low levels of VWF. The parents of affected patients should also be tested for VWF levels

Ag antigen, *CB* collagen binding, *FVIII* factor VIIII, *HMW* high-molecular-weight (VWF), *GPIb* glycoprotein Ib (the platelet VWF receptor), *N* normal, *NA* not applicable, *RCo* ristocetin cofactor, *RIPA* ristocetin-induced platelet aggregation, *VWF* von Willebrand factor, *VWD* von Willebrand disease

[a]For the purpose of this review, VWF GPIb-binding assays here include classical VWF:RCo assays plus “VWF:GPIbM” assays (such as the Siemens VWF Ac assay) and latex or CLIA-based “VWF:GPIbR” assays. Monoclonal antibody-based “activity” assays (“VWF:Ab” or “VWF:Act”) will also often match, but there will be some significant discrepancies

[b]Assay ratios used as cutoff for type 1 vs 2 VWD discrimination generally range in the region of 0.5–0.7 (viz., 0.5, 0.6, or 0.7). Different assays and different laboratories will use different cutoffs based on local evaluation. Type 2N VWD patients yield FVIIIB/VWF:Ag ratios around 0.5 (0.3–0.7) for heterozygous mutations and <0.3 for more severe genetic changes (including homozygous, double heterozygous, or combined heterozygous 2N mutation with second null allele)

Once the methodology has been selected by laboratories, the recommended basic VWD test panel should be able to diagnose or exclude VWD with additional investigations selected on a case-by-case basis, dependent on the results from the 4-test panel. The basic caveat always remains that diagnosis or exclusion of VWD requires, at the very least, repeat testing using a fresh sample, due to pre-analytical and also analytical limitations.

If all VWF tests are normal, confirmed on repeat testing, then either the patient does not have VWD, or else has a form of VWD that is not able to be defined with current testing. Additional assays to define the bleeding disorder, inclusive of platelet function, may be required. If all VWF tests are low, confirmed on repeat testing, but all VWF values are concordant (ratios of GPIb binding/Ag and CB/Ag both >0.7), then the patient has type 1 VWD. In this case, an assessment of severity based on absolute VWF level can ensure; however, unlike the case for hemophilia [83], there is no available consensus for cutoff values defining severity of VWD, and the values presented in Fig. 3.7 are only meant to provide a guide.

If there is a low ratio of GPIb binding/Ag and/or CB/Ag, and this pattern is confirmed on repeat testing with a fresh sample, then the patient may have type 2A, 2B, or 2M VWD (or even possibly platelet type VWD). Here further studies are also indicated. Generally, this means either ristocetin-induced platelet aggregation (RIPA) assessment and/or multimer assessment, depending on test findings and

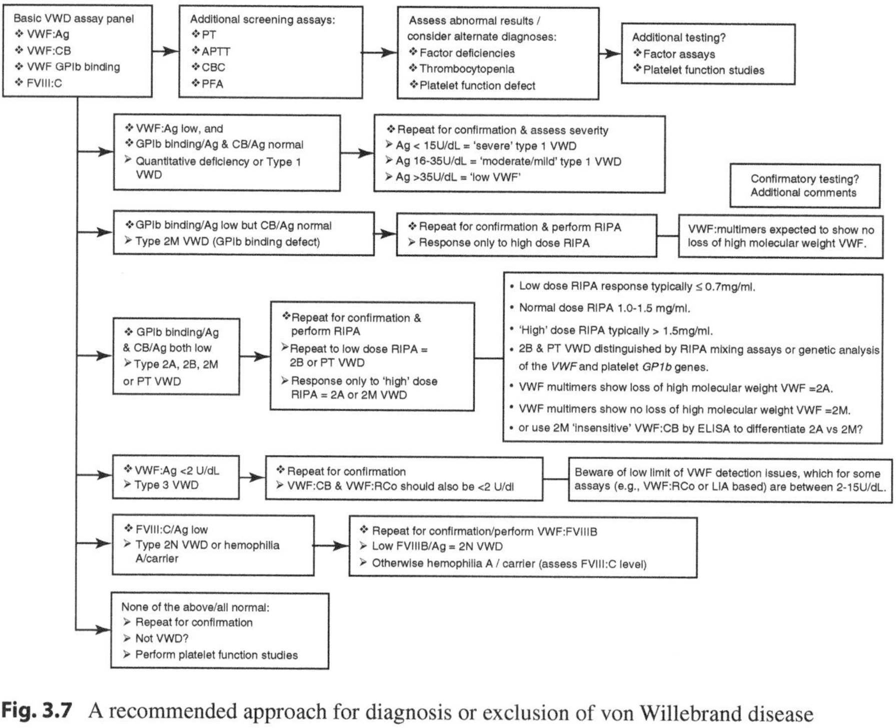

Fig. 3.7 A recommended approach for diagnosis or exclusion of von Willebrand disease

local availability. In our experience, RIPA analysis is usually more important than multimer analysis, and indeed, selection of the right test methodologies for VWF:Ag, VWF:CB, and GPIb-binding assays will often enable prediction of the mutimer pattern negating the need for its performance. Thus, a low ratio of GPIb binding/Ag plus a low ratio of CB/Ag usually points to a loss of HMW VWF, and thus likely 2A, 2B, or platelet-type VWD; instead, a low ratio of GPIb binding/Ag ***or*** CB/Ag (but not both) usually discounts a loss of HMW VWF and instead points to a type 2M VWD.

If all VWF test results are below the measuring range of the assays used, then this will create problems with clear diagnosis, but this usually means severe type 1 VWD or else type 3 VWD; therapy is similar in both cases, although clinical severity is often worse in type 3 VWD.

Finally, if the ratio of FVIII:C/VWF:Ag is low, this suggests either hemophilia A or 2N VWD. Hemophilia A is more common, and being sex-linked affects males more than females; however, misdiagnoses of both hemophilia A and 2N VWD, where the correct diagnosis was the other, do occur. Thus, testing by performance of a VWF:FVIIIB assay is recommended and, after repeat testing for confirmation, could include genetic analysis of *FVIII* and/or *VWF* for final definitive verification.

Genetic analysis may also be useful where patients have been defined to be type 2A, 2B, 2M, or platelet-type VWD and is also typically successful when performed on such patients. Genetic analysis is useful in some type 3 VWD investigations, but generally not useful in type 1 VWD [84].

3.7 Molecular Basis of von Willebrand Disease

VWD is an autosomal hemorrhagic disorder that is defined by dysfunction or deficiency of VWF, which has a critical role in the initiation of platelet adhesion at the site of vascular injury and which can also bind to and stabilize FVIII [85]. VWF is encoded by the *VWF* gene, which is located on the short arm of chromosome 12 (12p13.3), spans 180 kb, and consists of 52 exons, of which exon 50 (40 kb) and exon 28 (1/3 kb) are considered the longest and smallest exons, respectively. The intron 40 contains 14 Alu repeat and 670 bp repeat of TCTA. In addition, the 5′ flanking region has AT repeat resemble to TATA element. The *VWF pseudogene 1* (*VWFP1*), which is located on the long arm of chromosome 22 (22q11–13), spans ~21–29 kb and shows 97% homology with 23–34 exons of the *VWF* gene but encodes no functional transcript. The *VWF* gene is transcribed to an 8.8 kb mRNA which translates to a 2813-amino acid pre-pro-VWF protein. Pre-pro-VWF comprises of a signal peptide (pre) with 22 amino acids, a pro-peptide (pro) with 741 amino acids and a 2050-amino acid mature protein. Therefore, any mutation that leads to qualitative and/or quantitative abnormalities in VWF can be associated with VWD. Different biosynthetic events such as gene expression (transcription, translation), post-translational processing, dimerization/multimerization mechanisms, proteolytic processing, storage, secretion processing, structure, clearance, and function of VWF can be affected by these mutations. According to the ISTH-SSC VWF

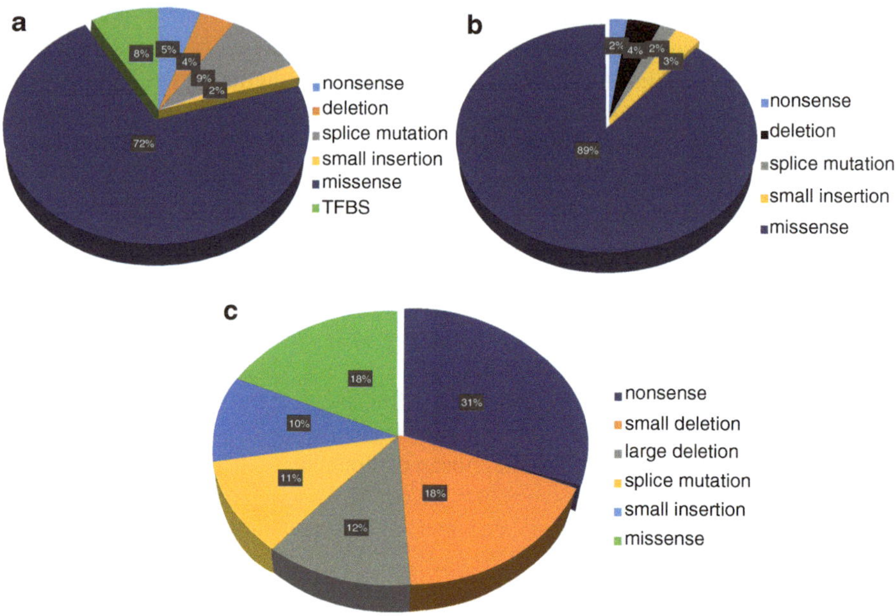

Fig. 3.8 Mutation distribution in patients with von Willebrand disease. (**a**) Patients with type 1 von Willebrand disease, (**b**) patients with type 2 von Willebrand disease, and (**c**) patients with type 3 von Willebrand disease. *TFBS* transcription factor binding sites

Online database (http://ragtimedesign.com/vwf/mutation/) and other studies, over 400 separate mutations have currently been reported in patients with VWD. VWD based on mutation locations and type of the nucleotides and protein abnormalities is divided into three hereditary types, comprising types 1, 2, and 3. Patients with acquired VWD do not have hereditary *VWF* mutations [85]. Different types of mutations associated with congenital VWD include (1) mutations that involve transcription factor binding sites (TFBS) and which lead to absent or reduced RNA transcription, (2) splice site mutations that disrupt the splice donor site (GT) and splice acceptor site (AG) of each intron and leading to exon skipping and production of shortened RNA and protein, (3) nonsense mutations, (4) small deletions, (5) insertions, (6) duplications, (7) large deletions, and (8) missense mutations (Fig. 3.8).

3.7.1 Type 1 von Willebrand Disease

Type 1 VWD is the most common type of VWD, is inherited in an autosomal dominant manner, and accounts for 40–80% of all VWD. Based on the ISTH-SSC VWF online database (http://ragtimedesign.com/vwf/mutation/), more than 130 different mutations have currently been identified in patients with type 1 VWD. About 65%

of these mutations occur within the splice site, promoter, or coding region of the *VWF* gene. In addition, about 70% of all mutations are missense substitutions, which may increase VWF clearance or interrupt the intracellular traffic, storage, and secretion of VWF. Approximately 15–20% of patients with type 1 VWD show more than one *VWF* mutation, and 30% of type 1 VWD patients show no evident mutations (Fig. 3.7). The Vicenza mutation (c.3614G>A, p.Arg1205His) in exon 27 of *VWF* gene is associated with VWD type 1C (clearance). The common laboratory findings of this variant includes decreased levels of VWF:Ag, VWF:RCo, and FVIII to ~0.15 U/mL, ~0.20 U/mL, and <0.30 U/mL of normal, respectively. The Vicenza variant often occurs with another variant of type 1 VWD (c. 2220G>A, p.Met740Leu). Another variant of type 1 VWD occurs following a c.4751A>G mutation in exon 28 of *VWF* gene leading to p.Tyr1584Cys and is associated with mild phenotype [86].

3.7.2 Type 2 von Willebrand Disease

Type 2 VWD is inherited in an autosomal dominant or recessive manner and is characterized by a qualitative deficiency that affects the function of VWF. Type 2 VWD accounts for ~20% of all VWD. Missense, frame shift mutations, duplications, and insertions are considered as the mutations mostly causing type 2 VWD. More than 160 different mutations have currently been identified in the *VWF* gene in type 2 VWD [85, 87, 88].

3.7.2.1 Type 2A von Willebrand Disease

Type 2A is an autosomal dominant or autosomal recessive disorder characterized by a qualitative defect of VWF and associated with an absence of large multimers VWF and reduction of VWF-mediated platelet adhesion. Mutations in the *VWF* gene encoding the A1 and A2 domains of VWF lead to two groups (I and II) of type 2A VWD. Misfolded VWF in group I leads to increased intracellular retention of VWF. The examples of this group are c.4513G>C and c.4820T>A mutations in exon 28 of *VWF* gene that lead to p.Gly1505Arg and p.Val1607Asp amino acid substitution (AAS), respectively. In group II, the biosynthesis, multimerization, and secretion of VWF is normal, but the sensitivity of synthesized VWF to ADAMTS13 cleavage is increased; the c.4789C>T mutation in exon 28 of *VWF* gene that leads to p.Arg1597Trp AAS is an example of group II. Multimerization of VWF can be affected by different mutations that involved D2 and D3 domains of VWF. Type 2A has been classified into the subtypes IIA, IIC, IID, and IIE. Subtype IIA is related to mutations affecting the A2 domain, which leads to enhanced proteolysis of the mutant VWF by ADAMTS13. Subtype IIC is associated with mutations affecting the D1 and D2 domains (pro-VWF), which leads to impaired multimerization in Golgi complex. The mutant VWF in subtype IID shows mutations affecting the CK domain and is associated with impaired dimerization in ER. Finally, subtype IIE is related to the mutations that impair disulfide bond formation of inter subunits in the Golgi complex [85, 89, 90].

3.7.2.2 Type 2B von Willebrand Disease

Type 2B is an autosomal dominant disorder that accounts for ~20% of all type 2 VWD. The GpIb-, heparin-, and collagen-binding sites are located within the A1 domain, and more than 20 different missense gain-of-function mutations that occur within *VWF* gene (exon 28) affecting this domain have been identified that lead to increased VWF affinity to GPIb. About 90% of type 2B VWD occur due to four mutations in exon 28 of *VWF* gene: (1) c.3916C>T mutation that leads to p.Arg1306Trp AAS, (2) c.4022G>A mutation that leads to p.Arg1341Gln AAS, (3) c.3946G>A mutation that leads to p.Val1316Met AAS, and (4) c.3922C>T mutation that leads to p.Arg1308Cys AAS [91, 92].

3.7.2.3 Type 2M von Willebrand Disease

Type 2M VWD, like type 2B, is an autosomal dominant disorder, but unlike type 2B, the disorder is due to loss-of-function mutations (missense, deletion, and frame shift) affecting the A1 domain (exon 28 of *VWF*), which prevent the interaction of VWF with GpIb. Type 2M VWD less frequently can occur following mutations that affect the A3 domain. Based on the ISTH-SSC VWF online database (http://ragtimedesign.com/vwf/mutation/) and other studies, about 30 different type 2M causing mutations have currently been identified. The c.5356C>G mutation in exon 31 of *VWF* gene leads to p.His1786Asp AAS with defective binding site for both types (I and III) of collagen [85, 91, 93].

3.7.2.4 Type 2N von Willebrand Disease

Type 2N VWD is a qualitative VWF abnormality that in contrast to other subtypes of type 2 VWD is inherited in an autosomal recessive manner and caused by defective VWF-FVIII interaction. The FVIII binding site spans the D′ and D3 domains and lies between amino acid Ser764 and Arg1035 of pre-pro-VWF, which is encoded by exons 18–28 of the *VWF* gene. Therefore, mutations within these domains can cause type 2N VWD. The majority of these mutations occur in exons 18–28, but some rare variants have been identified within exons 17 and 21–27. These mutations impair binding of VWF to FVIII, which leads to reduction of VWF-FVIII binding capacity and therefore causes a reduction in the level of plasma FVIII. About 30 different mutations have been reported to date, with the c.2561G>A mutation in exon 20 of *VWF* gene leading to p.Arg854Gln AAS being most frequent. Some of the mutations causing type 2N VWD are 1) c.2363G>A and c.2362T>C mutations in exon 18 of *VWF* gene that lead to p.Cys788Tyr and p.Cys788Arg AASs and 2) c.2635G>A and c.2573G>T mutations in exon 20 of *VWF* gene that lead to p.Asp879Asn and p.Cys858Phe AASs and which not only decrease the VWF-FVIII binding but also lead to reduction of HMWM VWF [89, 92, 94].

3.7.3 Type 3 von Willebrand Disease

Type 3 VWD is the most severe type of VWD and is inherited in an autosomal recessive manner. A wide range of mutations is detected in these patients including deletions, missense, frame shift, nonsense, and splice site. These mutations lead to absence or severe quantitative defects in VWF. Null mutations comprise ~80% of all mutation causing type 3 VWD. Some nonsense mutations such as p.Arg1659Stop and p.Arg2535Stop occur at CpG sequences. According to the ISTH-SSC VWF online database (http://ragtimedesign.com/vwf/mutation/), about 120 different mutations have been reported to date. Mutation distribution in patients with type 3 VWD is shown in Fig. 3.9.

3.8 Treatment of von Willebrand Disease

Management of patients with VWD includes prevention or treatment of bleeding diathesis by correction of dual hemostatic defects of primary hemostasis (due to lack or decrease of VWF) and secondary hemostasis (due to FVIII deficiency). These corrections can be performed by raising endogenous VWF (usually using desmopressin) or in unresponsive patients, by infusion of exogenous VWF/FVIII (typically as plasma concentrates) [7, 95, 96].

Several therapeutic choices are available for management of patients with VWD. Fresh frozen plasma (FFP) and cryoprecipitate represent older or traditional therapies. Cryoprecipitate was actually the main therapeutic choice for many years in the past, and even today it remains a major therapeutic option in a considerable number of developing countries where commercial VWF/FVIII concentrates may be unavailable or unaffordable; however, the risk of virus transmission and the need to transfuse a high volume of product reflect substantive obstacles for its continued use. More commonly, desmopressin, plasma-derived VWF/FVIII concentrates, purified plasma VWF, and recombinant VWF (rVWF) reflect the main therapeutic choices. In addition, adjuvant therapies can also be used for management of hemorrhagic symptoms in patients with VWD. Such agents include antifibrinolytic therapy with tranexamic acid or epsilon aminocaproic acid, which can improve hemostasis in patients without changing their plasma level of VWF [7, 96].

In summary, the different therapeutic choices that can be used for the management of patients with VWD are:

1. Desmopressin
2. Adjuvant agents
3. Cryoprecipitate
4. FFP
5. Intermediate purity factor VIII/VWF concentrate
6. High-purity factor VIII/VWF concentrate
7. Recombinant VWF
8. Platelet concentrate

Choice of treatment depends on several factors including type of VWD, severity of disorder, severity of bleeding episodes, and type and duration of surgery. In patients with less severe forms of VWD, such as type 1 VWD and some patients

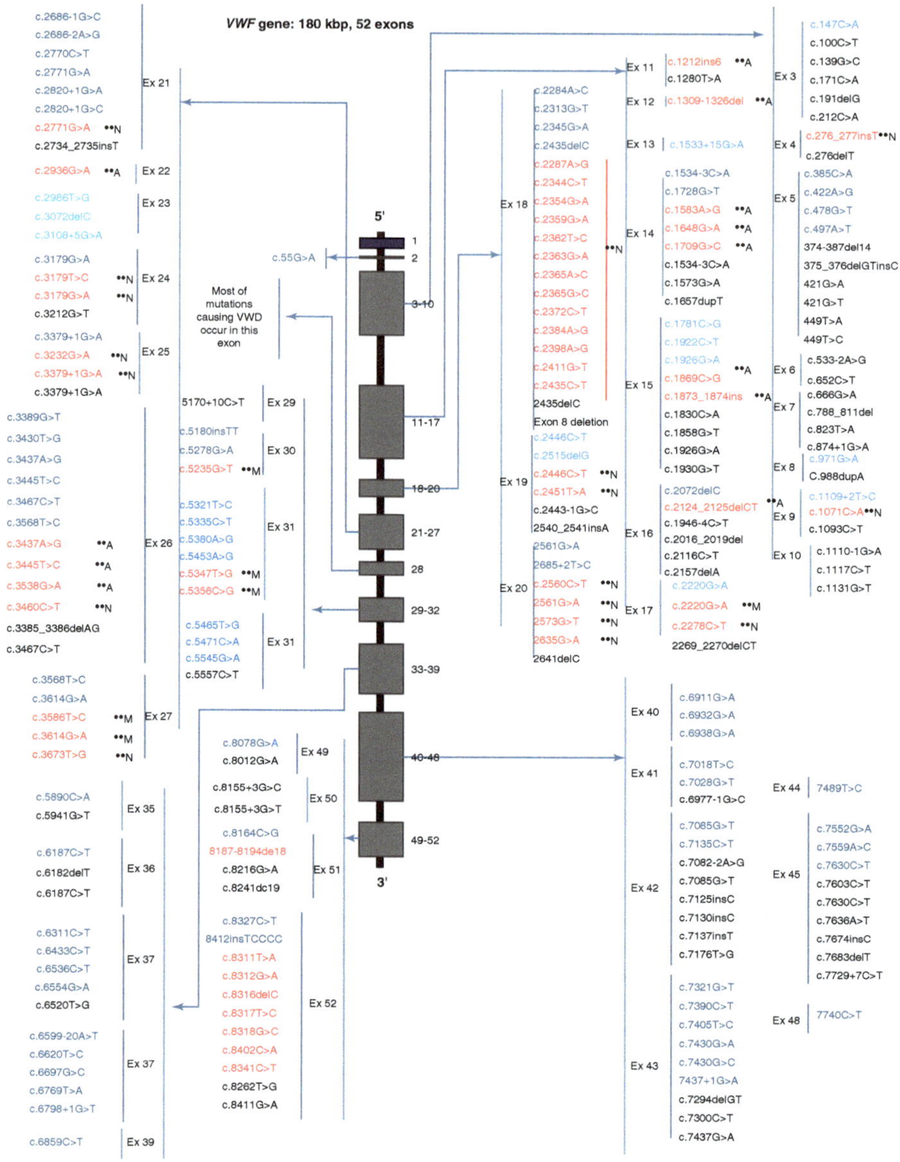

Fig. 3.9 The schematic presentation of *von Willebrand factor (vWF)* gene structure, which comprises of 52 exons with genetic abnormalities that lead to von Willebrand disease (VWD). Based on ISTH-SSC VWF online database (http://ragtimedesign.com/vwf/mutation/), approximately 400 different mutations have currently been reported and include mutations causing type 1 VWD (blue mutations), mutations causing type 2 VWD (red mutations), and mutations causing type 3 VWD (black mutations). *inv* inversion, *del* deletion, *ins* insertion, *dup* duplication

with type 2 VWD, desmopressin is a suitable choice, while in those patients with severe VWD (including type 3VWD and most of the patients with type 2 VWD), replacement therapy comprises the main therapeutic choice. Although on-demand therapy (meaning treatment of hemorrhage as soon as possible after onset of bleeding) is the mainstay of treatment of patients with VWD, long-term prophylaxis for those patients with severe hemorrhages (e.g., type 3 VWD) can significantly improve the quality of life [7].

3.8.1 Desmopressin

Desmopressin (1-deamino-8-D-arginine vasopressin (DDAVP)) is a synthetic analogue of vasopressin that (in a lower concentration) was primarily used for the treatment of diabetes insipidus. This synthetic drug causes an increase of endogenous FVIII and VWF by their release from storage sites into plasma. VWF is released from Weibel-Palade bodies of endothelial cells, while the source of FVIII is not well-known. However the exact cellular mechanism of DDAVP has not been fully elucidated. It seems that DDAVP activates the endothelial vasopressin V2 receptor (VR2), which results in the activation of cAMP-mediated signaling pathway. This leads to exocytosis of VWF and t-PA from WPB and also production of nitric oxide (NO) by NO synthase (NOS) activation in endothelial cells (Fig. 3.10) [7, 97].

Patients with baseline FVIII and functional VWF levels of 10–20 IU/dL or greater are more likely to show sufficient response to DDAVP to attain hemostasis. Therefore, this agent is useful in the management of patients with mild hemophilia or mild VWD, and if required, patients can receive repeated doses of drug in 12–24 h intervals. However, repeated doses of desmopressin cause less effective responses, and eventual depletion of FVIII and VWF stores, with this tachyphylaxis affecting patients with hemophilia more than those with VWD.

Desmopressin can be used for most patients with type 1 VWD, possible type 1 VWD, and some patients with type 2 VWD and can increase FVIII and VWF levels three to five times within 30 min (Table 3.8) [7, 95, 96].

Most patients with type 1 VWD with available ("releasable") VWF in storage sites are responsive to desmopressin, while those with low levels of releasable VWF are less responsive or their response is short-lasting. In the former group, FVIII, VWF, and bleeding time (BT) are usually corrected after administration of desmopressin. Although desmopressin is effective in some patients with type 2 VWD, mostly in types 2A and 2M, it's ineffective in the majority of patients, and in patients with type 2B, it is considered contradicted because it may lead to release of abnormal VWF that may worsen thrombocytopenia and may increase the risk of bleeding. Due to the lack of releasable stores of VWF in type 3 VWD, these patients are typically unresponsive to DDAVP [7, 98].

Desmopressin can be given intravenously, intranasally, or subcutaneously. Intravenous administration of DDAVP is preferred for acute hemorrhages and for surgical procedures. Stimate (CSL Behring, LLC, Kiel, Germany) nasal spray contains 1.5 mg/mL desmopressin acetate contains 150 μg DDAVP per puff [99].

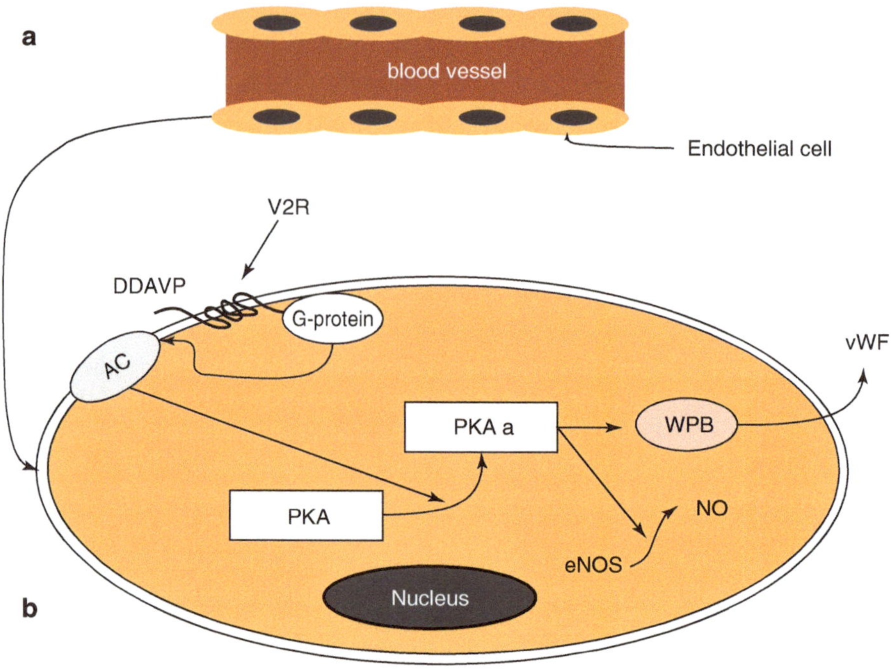

Fig. 3.10 Mechanism of DDAVP-induced VWF secretion. (a) the schematic presentation of a blood vessel. (b) DDAVP binds to V2 receptor on the endothelial cells and result in G-protein activation, adenylyl cyclase (AC) activation, cAMP production, and protein kinase A (PKA) activation. PKA stimulates the secretion of VWF from Weibel-Palade bodies (WPBs). In addition PKA phosphorylate the Ser1177 residue of nitric oxide synthase (NOS) and leads to NO production. *V2R* V2 receptor, *DDAVP* 1-deamino-8-D-arginine vasopressin (DDAVP) or desmopressin, *PKA* protein kinase A, *eNOS* endothelial nitric oxide synthase, *NO* nitric oxide

Table 3.8 Therapeutic response to desmopressin in von Willebrand disease

Disorder	Response
Possible type 1 VWD	Usually effective
Type 1 VWD	Usually effective
Type 2A VWD	Occasionally effective
Type 2B VWD	May be contraindicated
Type 2M VWD	Occasionally effective
Type 2N VWD	Rarely effective
Type 3 VWD	Ineffective

VWD von Willebrand disease

Desmopressin may have some side effects in some patients such as hypotension, cardiovascular complications, flushing, and hyponatremia. Hyponatremia can be prevented by limited fluid intake to 1500 mL for 24 h after desmopressin administration, while other side effects are mostly due to vasodilating effects of the DDAVP and can usually be attenuated by slowing the infusion rate. Since genotype and phenotype of VWD can affect the effectiveness of desmopressin response, a test dose is recommended before establishment of the magnitude and duration of the drug response. In fact, determination of desmopressin responsiveness in a non-bleeding state is a requirement in patients with moderate type 1, 2A, and 2M ahead of such treatment for bleeds [98].

For this purpose, 0.3 μg/kg in 50 mL is administrated intravenously over 30 min. FVIII:C, VWF:Ag, and functional VWF (e.g., VWF:RCo) should be assessed pre-infusion and at 1, 2, and/or 4 and 24 h post-infusion. Patients with sufficient response have a two to five times increase from baseline levels and have FVIII and VWF levels above 50 U/dL at 1 hour post-infusion. The levels remain above 30 U/dL at 4 h post-infusion but generally return to baseline levels by 24 h [56, 98, 100].

3.8.2 Concentrates

Transfusion therapy with human blood products containing FVIII/VWF is the main therapeutic choice in patients unresponsive to desmopressin, or for long-term therapy. Early studies revealed successfully the management of VWD patients with cryoprecipitate administration every 12–24 h, and subsequently cryoprecipitate was used for many years as the main treatment option in VWD. Although the risk of transmission of blood-borne diseases is the main concern for continued use of cryoprecipitate, this product may still reflect the main therapeutic choice in a considerable number of patients, especially in developing countries, due to low cost and easy production process [8, 56, 98, 100].

Virus-inactivated VWF/FVIII concentrates that were initially developed for the management of hemophilia are considered safer and more suitable therapeutic option for patients unresponsive to desmopressin. VWF/FVIII concentrates can be used for on-demand therapy (to stop bleeding when they occur) and to prevent bleeding in surgery or for long-term secondary prophylaxis [101].

In patients with type 3, most patients with type 2 VWD, and a number of patients with type 1 VWD, this treatment type reflects the current treatment of choice (Table 3.9) [8, 56].

The three main requirements for VWF/FVIII concentrates are as follows: (1) they should contain enough biologically active VWF to correct the platelet adhesion defect otherwise due to the low level of plasma VWF and enable stabilization of endogenous FVIII; (2) their efficacy and pharmacokinetics should be assessed in clinical trials prior to clinical use; and (3) they should be efficacy-virus inactivated [102].

A number of concentrates have been used for the treatment of VWD. These concentrates were primarily produced as "FVIII concentrates" for the treatment of hemophilia, but since they also contained VWF, they also were then also used for the treatment of VWD. The amount of HMWM of these products differs, and those without HMWM are less effective in the management of mucosal hemorrhages. Today, most "FVIII concentrates" actually lack VWF, and only those with high amounts of functional VWF are useful for the treatment of VWD. Although many concentrates are now available for this purpose, there is considerable difference

Table 3.9 Therapeutic options for management of patients with von Willebrand disease

Disorder	Therapeutic choice	Additional treatment
Type 1 VWD	Desmopressin: (1) Intravenously: 0.3 μg/kg or (2) Subcutaneously: 0.3 μg/kg or (3) Intranasally: 300 μg (150 μg per nostril)[a]	Tranexamic acid: 3 or 4 times daily
Type 2 VWD	(1) Desmopressin: (1) Intravenously: 0.3 μg/kg[a] or (2) Subcutaneously: 0.3 μg/kg or (3) Intranasally: 300 μg (150 μg per nostril)[b] or (2) VWF-FVIII concentrate or (3) VWF concentrate	Tranexamic acid: 3 or 4 times daily
Type 3 VWD	(1) VWF-FVIII concentrate or (2) VWF concentrate	Tranexamic acid: 3 or 4 times daily

VWD von Willebrand disease, *VWF* von Willebrand factor, *FVIII* Factor VIII
[a]For indication of desmopressin use, refer to Table 3.1
[b]For those with body weight <50 kg, only one dose of 150 μg is sufficient

among concentrates in the amount and activity of VWF and FVIII. Specific activity is crucial to determine the degree of relative purity of FVIII/VWF concentrates. VWF:RCo/Ag ratio can be used as a surrogate marker for determination of VWF activity while VWF:RCo/FVIII:C ratio gives data on the amount of FVIII:C protein associated with VWF in the VWF/FVIII concentrate. It is important to avoid excessive concentrations of FVIII:C with injection of repeated doses in patients with VWD [56, 100].

In patients with VWD, a VWF:RCo/VWF:Ag ratio <0.7 is considered as representative of dysfunctional VWF (and thus a type 2 VWD). In a study of six concentrates, only three had a ratio of >0.7, with Immunate (Baxter Bioscience, Austria) having the lowest ratio. Immunate is therefore not approved for treatment of VWD in some countries, including Sweden. HMWM VWF was largely preserved in Haemate-P/Humate-P (Aventis Behring, Marburg, Germany), Innobrand and Facteur Willebrand (LFB, Lille, France) concentrates, with well-preserved multimeric composition being preferred for management of mucosal bleeding (Table 3.10) [56, 98, 100, 103].

For proper management of VWD, the correct dose of concentrate should be used. Several factors should be considered in defining a correct dose, including type and severity of bleeding episodes, type of concentrate, baseline FVIII and VWF levels and VWD type, as well as bleeding history and therapeutic response. The type of hemorrhage is an important issue and this should receive particular attention. Some bleeding, such as mucosal hemorrhage (especially GI bleeding), is difficult to stop, while management of post-traumatic hemorrhage and post-surgical bleeding from soft tissues can be managed more easily. For estimation of VWF

Table 3.10 Main characteristics of VWF-FVIII concentrates and recombinant VWF

Concentrate	Company	Country	Purity	Virus inactivation	Contents	VWF:RCo/ FVIII:C	VWF:RCo/ VWF:Ag
Immunate	Baxter Bioscience, Vienna	Austria	IEX	S/D + vapor heat	FVIII:C 1000 IU 10 mL^{-1}	0.67	0.15
Alphanate	Grifols, Los Angeles	USA	HLCT	S/D + dry heat		0.9	0.47
Fanhdi	Grifols, Cambridgeshire	UK	Precipitation, HLCT	S/D + dry heat		1	0.47
Wilate	Octapharma Hoboken, NJ	USA	Affinity CT, size exclusion	S/D + dry heat		0.9	0.9
Biostate	CSL Behring, Melbourne	Australia	Precipitation, HLCT	S/D + dry heat		2	0.8
Facteur Willebrand	LFB, Lille	France		Solvent/detergent	VWF:RCo 1000 IU 20 mL^{-1}		0.72
Wilfactin	LFB, Les Ulis	France	Ion exchange, affinity CTs	S/D + nanofiltration + dry heat		>10	0.95
Innobrand	LFB	France	Ion exchange CT	S/D	VWF:RCo 1100 IU 20 mL^{-1}		0.89
Haemate-P[a] Humate-P[b]	Aventis Behring	Germany	Polyelectrolyte precipitation	Pasteurization	FVIII:C 250 IU 10 mL^{-1}	2	0.91
Factor 8Y	Bio Products Laboratory, Hertfordshire	UK	Heparin/glycine precipitation	Dry heat	FVIII:C 315 IU 10 mL^{-1}	0.81	0.29
Koate-DVI	Bayer Corp	USA	Precipitation, size exclusion	S/D + dry heat	FVIII:C 1050 IU 10 mL^{-1}		0.48
Vonicog alfa (Vonvendi)[c]	Baxalta, Bannockburn	USA	–	S/D		No FVIII:C	

[a]In Europe
[b]In the USA, *IEX* ion-exchange chromatography, *HLCT* heparin ligand chromatography
[c]Recombinant VWF, *S/D* Solvent/detergent

loading dose, it should be considered that 1 IU/kg of FVIII usually increases plasma FVIII:C 2 U/dL, whereas 1 IU/kg VWF:RCo usually increases the VWF:RCo 1.5 U/dL; therefore the following formulas can be used for the determination of proper dose [56, 95].

$$\text{Factor VIII}:\text{C}:1\,\text{U}/\text{kg}=2\%\text{rise in plasma dose}=$$
$$\%\text{desired FVIII rise}\times\text{wt}(\text{kg})\times0.5$$

$$\text{VWF}:\text{RCo}:1\,\text{U}/\text{kg}=1.5\%\text{rise in plasma dose}=$$
$$\%\text{desired VWF}:\text{RCo rise}\times\text{wt}(\text{kg})\times0.67$$

Different VWF/FVIII concentrate doses are recommended for different situations in patients with VWD (Table 3.11).

A high plasma level of FVIII is a risk factor for venous thromboembolism (VTE), and patients with VWD who received repeated dose of concentrates containing both FVIII and VWF may experience VTE. When a patient with VWD receives repeated dose of these concentrates, plasma FVIII:C should be monitored. With use of pure VWF, this risk can be avoided, but plasma level of FVIII increases very slowly, and therefore in acute situations, these concentrates should be used in combination with FVIII concentrate [56, 95].

Table 3.11 Recommended dose of factor VIII/von Willebrand factor concentrate for management of patients with von Willebrand disease (VWD) unresponsive to desmopressin

	Dose (IU/kg)		Number of infusion		Objective	
Bleeding type	Italian	Netherlands	Italian	Netherlands	Italian	Netherlands
Major surgery	50	50	Once a day (days 1–3), then every other day	Twice daily 25 IU FVIII/kg, based on FVIII:C levels	Maintain FVIII:C >50 U/dL for at least 7–14 days	FVIII:C 50 IU/dL for 7–10 days
Minor surgery	30	30–50	Once a day (days 1–3), then every other day	Twice daily 15–25 IU FVIII/kg, based on FVIII:C levels	Maintain FVIII:C >30 U/dL for at least 5–7 days	FVIII:C >50 IU/dL for 3 days and 30 IU/dL for additional 4–7 days
Dental extraction	20–40	20–40	Single	Single dose + tranexamic acid	Maintain FVIII:C >30 U/dL for up to 6 h	FVIII:C and VWF:RCo >50 IU/dL
Spontaneous or post-traumatic bleeding	20–40	20–40	Single	Usually single	Maintain FVIII >30 U/dL	–

3.8.3 Recombinant von Willebrand Factor

RVWF (Vonicog alfa (Vonvend)) is a new product for the management of VWD that is synthesized within genetically engineered Chinese hamster ovary (CHO) cell lines. This engineered cell line co-expresses both *VWF* and *FVIII* genes. The produced VWF is purified by immune-affinity chromatography that yields a rVWF with 99% purity. Since the product is not exposed to ADAMTS13, it retains all sizes of VWF multimers including HMWM and ultra-large multimers. In USA, rVWF is licensed for on-demand treatment of patients with VWD. This product should be given under supervision, and the proper dose of product should be used (Table 3.12) [104].

3.8.4 Prophylaxis

Since the bleeding tendency is less severe in VWD, prophylaxis treatment is not as common as in hemophilia A and B. Prophylaxis should be considered for patients with type 3 VWD and recurrent hemarthrosis. Patients with recurrent GI bleeding and those with frequent epistaxis can also benefit from prophylaxis treatment. Therefore, in such patients with frequent bleeding, long-term secondary prophylaxis should be considered. In fact, hemarthrosis, GI bleeding, menorrhagia, and recurrent epistaxis are the most common indications for long-term secondary prophylaxis. Although overall use of prophylaxis in VWD is low and is around 1.5%, this percentage is higher in type 3 VWD, and about one-fifth of patients undergo prophylaxis. Regular prophylaxis decreases the number of bleeds, decreases the severity of hemorrhages, prevents arthropathy, and improves the quality of life in

Table 3.12 Recommended dose of intravenous recombinant von Willebrand factor (Vonvendi) for the management of patients with von Willebrand disease in the USA

Bleeding type	Initial dose	Subsequent doses
Minor bleeding	40–50 IU/kg (adjust dose based on the extent and location of bleeding; should achieve VWF levels >60%, based on VWF:RCo >0.6 IU/mL)	40–50 IU/kg every 8–24 h (as clinically required)
Major bleeding	50–80 IU/kg (adjust dose based on the extent and location of bleeding; should achieve VWF levels >60%, based on VWF:RCo >0.6 IU/mL)	40–60 IU/kg every 8–24 h for ~2–3 days (as clinically required; maintain trough VWF:RCo levels >50% as long as deemed necessary)
When a rapid increase in FVIII is needed and baseline FVIII values are <40% of normal activity or unknown	Administer the first dose of rVWF with an approved rFVIII (one that does not contain VWF) within 10 min of completing rVWF infusion at a ratio of 1.3:1 (i.e., 30% more rVWF than rFVIII; calculate by dividing rVWF dose by 1.3)	

patients with VWD. It should be noted that all patients with VWD are candidates for regular long-term prophylaxis; however, most patients with type 3 VWD, and some other entities of VWD, including type 2A and type 2B with GI bleeding, are candidates of long-term prophylaxis [102, 105].

Different therapeutic doses are used for long-term prophylaxis, and 50 IU of VWF:RCo/kg two or three times a week reflects a commonly used dose [56, 95].

3.8.5 Surgery

Surgical procedures represent an important hemostatic challenge in patients with VWD, and the majority of patients with major surgery should be managed by replacement therapy, as therapy with DDAVP is precarious owing to the frequent onset of poor responsiveness following repeated doses. For successful management of these patients, a strict cooperation between the patient's surgeon and hematologist is mandatory [56, 106].

Strategies for preoperative management of patients with VWD depends on several important factors including the type of VWD, kind of surgery, baseline levels of VWF and FVIII, and therapeutic response to desmopressin. The type of hemorrhagic problem, including mucosal or soft-tissue bleeding, also can affect treatment strategies. A strict follow-up is recommended for the first 10–15 days post-surgery, especially in those patients who undergo major surgery, since delayed hemorrhage may occur until complete wound healing is achieved. Although FVIII is the main determinant of post-surgical hemorrhage in patients with VWD, it is not sufficient to only substitute FVIII in these patients, because the half-life of FVIII is very low in the absence of VWF. Since the ability of infused VWF in raising and maintaining plasma FVIII is not dependent on VWF multimeric composition of concentrates, those concentrates with loss of HMWM may be effective in some surgeries. However, when surgery involves mucous membranes, then concentrates that contain HMWM VWF should be used [56].

A characteristic of VWF concentrates that are almost devoid of FVIII:C is delay in the plasma increase in FVIII:C. This is an important issue especially in patients with type 3 VWD who undergo emergency surgical procedures representing acute life-threatening bleeds. In patients with scheduled surgical procedure, FVIII should be administrated 12 h before surgery. In elective surgery, a pure VWF should be given 12–24 h prior to the surgical procedure in order to increase FVIII levels sufficiently [106].

3.8.6 Pregnancy

VWF and FVIII levels increase two- to threefold during the second and third trimesters in patients with types 1 and 2 VWD and fall to baseline by 7–21 days postpartum; however, this increase is not observed in type 3 VWD, and thus, management of pregnant women with VWF/FVIII is required. A rapid decrease in plasma VWF and FVIII can occur post-partum, and subsequently PPH, including delayed PPH with a risk of 30%, can occur [107].

In type 2B VWD, this increase in VWF reflects an "abnormal VWF" which can worsen thrombocytopenia. Generally, patients VWD should be monitored for functional VWF (e.g., VWF:RCo) and FVIII:C once during the third trimester and within 10 days of expected date of delivery. In pregnant women with VWD, the risk of hemorrhage is minimum when the VWF:RCo and FVIII levels are >30 U/dL. In women with type 1 VWD with FVIII:C level <30 U/dL, it may be necessary to administer desmopressin at parturition and for 3–4 days thereafter. To prevent late hemorrhage, VWF:RCo and FVIII:C levels should be monitored for at least 2 weeks post-partum [56, 108].

References

1. Robertson J, Lillicrap D, James PD. von Willebrand disease. Pediatr Clin N Am. 2008;55(2):377–92.
2. James PD, Goodeve AC. von Willebrand disease. Genet Med. 2011;13(5):365–76.
3. Sadler J, Budde U, Eikenboom J, Favaloro E, Hill F, Holmberg L, et al. Update on the pathophysiology and classification of von Willebrand disease: a report of the Subcommittee on von Willebrand Factor. J Thromb Haemost. 2006;4(10):2103–14.
4. Federici A. Clinical diagnosis of von Willebrand disease. Haemophilia. 2004;10(s4):169–76.
5. Federici AB. Diagnosis of inherited von Willebrand disease: a clinical perspective. Semin Thromb Hemost. 2006;124:S1.
6. Favaloro EJ, Pasalic L, Curnow J. Laboratory tests used to help diagnose von Willebrand disease: an update. Pathology. 2016;48(4):303–18.
7. Sadler J, Mannucci P, Berntorp E, Bochkov N, Boulyjenkov V, Ginsburg D, et al. Impact, diagnosis and treatment of von Willebrand disease. Thromb Haemost. 2000;84(2):160–74.
8. Mannucci PM, Chediak J, Hanna W, Byrnes J, Ledford M, Ewenstein BM, et al. Treatment of von Willebrand disease with a high-purity factor VIII/von Willebrand factor concentrate: a prospective, multicenter study. Blood. 2002;99(2):450–6.
9. Lenting PJ, Christophe OD, Denis CV. von Willebrand factor biosynthesis, secretion, and clearance: connecting the far ends. Blood. 2015;125(13):2019–28.
10. Ginsburg D, Handin RI, Bonthron DT, Donlon TA, Bruns GA, Latt SA, et al. Human von Willebrand factor (vWF): isolation of complementary DNA (cDNA) clones and chromosomal localization. Science. 1985;228:1401–7.
11. Mancuso D, Tuley E, Westfield L, Worrall N, Shelton-Inloes B, Sorace J, et al. Structure of the gene for human von Willebrand factor. J Biol Chem. 1989;264(33):19514–27.
12. Collins CJ, Underdahl JP, Levene RB, Ravera CP, Morin MJ, Dombalagian MJ, et al. Molecular cloning of the human gene for von Willebrand factor and identification of the transcription initiation site. Proc Natl Acad Sci. 1987;84(13):4393–7.
13. Federici AB, Lee CA, Berntorp EE, Lillicrap D, Montgomery RR. Von Willebrand disease: basic and clinical aspects. Hoboken: Wiley; 2011.
14. Zhou Y-F, Eng ET, Zhu J, Lu C, Walz T, Springer TA. Sequence and structure relationships within von Willebrand factor. Blood. 2012;120(2):449–58.
15. Shapiro S, Nowak A, Wooding C, Birdsey G, Laffan M, McKinnon T. The von Willebrand factor predicted unpaired cysteines are essential for secretion. J Thromb Haemost. 2014;12(2):246–54.
16. Tjernberg P, Vos HL, Castaman G, Bertina RM, Eikenboom JC. Dimerization and multimerization defects of von Willebrand factor due to mutated cysteine residues. J Thromb Haemost. 2004;2(2):257–65.

17. Hommais A, Stépanian A, Fressinaud E, Mazurier C, Pouymayou K, Meyer D, et al. Impaired dimerization of von Willebrand factor subunit due to mutation A2801D in the CK domain results in a recessive type 2A subtype IID von Willebrand disease. Thromb Haemost. 2006;95(5):776–81.
18. Voorberg J, Fontijn R, Van Mourik J, Pannekoek H. Domains involved in multimer assembly of von Willebrand factor (vWF): multimerization is independent of dimerization. EMBO J. 1990;9(3):797.
19. Sadler JE. Von Willebrand factor, ADAMTS13, and thrombotic thrombocytopenic purpura. Blood. 2008;112(1):11–8.
20. Zanardelli S, Crawley JT, Chion CKCK, Lam JK, Preston RJ, Lane DA. ADAMTS13 substrate recognition of von Willebrand factor A2 domain. J Biol Chem. 2006;281(3):1555–63.
21. Zanardelli S, Chion AC, Groot E, Lenting PJ, McKinnon TA, Laffan MA, et al. A novel binding site for ADAMTS13 constitutively exposed on the surface of globular VWF. Blood. 2009;114(13):2819–28.
22. Samor B, Michalski JC, Debray H, Mazurier C, Goudemand M, Halbeek H, et al. Primary structure of a new tetraantennary glycan of the N-acetyllactosaminic type isolated from human factor VIII/von Willebrand factor. FEBS J. 1986;158(2):295–8.
23. Canis K, McKinnon TA, Nowak A, Haslam SM, Panico M, Morris HR, et al. Mapping the N-glycome of human von Willebrand factor. Biochem J. 2012;447(2):217–28.
24. Carew JA, Browning PJ, Lynch DC. Sulfation of von Willebrand factor. Blood. 1990;76(12):2530–9.
25. Haberichter SL, Merricks EP, Fahs SA, Christopherson PA, Nichols TC, Montgomery RR. Re-establishment of VWF-dependent Weibel-Palade bodies in VWD endothelial cells. Blood. 2005;105(1):145–52.
26. Sporn LA, Marder VJ, Wagner DD. Inducible secretion of large, biologically potent von Willebrand factor multimers. Cell. 1986;46(2):185–90.
27. Ruggeri ZM. Structure of von Willebrand factor and its function in platelet adhesion and thrombus formation. Best Pract Res Clin Haematol. 2001;14(2):257–79.
28. Nightingale T, Cutler D. The secretion of von Willebrand factor from endothelial cells; an increasingly complicated story. J Thromb Haemost. 2013;11(s1):192–201.
29. Skipwith CG, Cao W, Zheng XL. Factor VIII and platelets synergistically accelerate cleavage of von Willebrand factor by ADAMTS13 under fluid shear stress. J Biol Chem. 2010;285(37):28596–603.
30. Foster PA, Fulcher CA, Marti T, Titani K, Zimmerman TA. major factor VIII binding domain resides within the amino-terminal 272 amino acid residues of von Willebrand factor. J Biol Chem. 1987;262(18):8443–6.
31. Bahou W, Ginsburg D, Sikkink R, Litwiller R, Fass D. A monoclonal antibody to von Willebrand factor (vWF) inhibits factor VIII binding. Localization of its antigenic determinant to a nonadecapeptide at the amino terminus of the mature vWF polypeptide. J Clin Investig. 1989;84(1):56.
32. Ginsburg D, Bockenstedt P, Allen E, Fox D, Foster P, Ruggeri Z, et al. Fine mapping of monoclonal antibody epitopes on human von Willebrand factor using a recombinant peptide library. Thromb Haemost. 1992;67(1):166–71.
33. Ruggeri ZM, Mendolicchio G. Interaction of von Willebrand factor with platelets and the vessel wall. Hämostaseologie. 2015;35(3):211–24.
34. Roth GJ, Titani K, Hoyer LW, Hickey MJ. Localization of binding sites within human von Willebrand factor for monomeric type III collagen. Biochemistry. 1986;25(26):8357–61.
35. Cruz MA, Yuan H, Lee JR, Wise RJ, Handin RI. Interaction of the von Willebrand factor (vWF) with collagen Localization of the primary collagen-binding site by analysis of recombinant vWF a domain polypeptides. J Biol Chem. 1995;270(18):10822–7.
36. Pareti FI, Niiya K, McPherson J, Ruggeri Z. Isolation and characterization of two domains of human von Willebrand factor that interact with fibrillar collagen types I and III. J Biol Chem. 1987;262(28):13835–41.
37. Hoylaerts MF, Yamamoto H, Nuyts K, Vreys I, Deckmyn H, Vermylen J. von Willebrand factor binds to native collagen VI primarily via its A1 domain. Biochem J. 1997;324(1):185–91.

38. Sadler JE. Biochemistry and genetics of von Willebrand factor. Annu Rev Biochem. 1998;67(1):395–424.
39. Fujimura Y, Titani K, Holland L, Russell S, Roberts J, Elder J, et al. von Willebrand factor. A reduced and alkylated 52/48-kDa fragment beginning at amino acid residue 449 contains the domain interacting with platelet glycoprotein Ib. J Biol Chem. 1986;261(1):381–5.
40. Scott J, Montgomery R, Retzinger G. Dimeric ristocetin flocculates proteins, binds to platelets, and mediates von Willebrand factor-dependent agglutination of platelets. J Biol Chem. 1991;266(13):8149–55.
41. Wohner N, Legendre P, Casari C, Christophe O, Lenting P, Denis C. Shear stress-independent binding of von Willebrand factor-type 2B mutants p. R1306Q & p. V1316M to LRP1 explains their increased clearance. J Thromb Haemost. 2015;13(5):815–20.
42. Andrews RK, López J, Berndt MC. Molecular mechanisms of platelet adhesion and activation. Int J Biochem Cell Biol. 1997;29(1):91–105.
43. Shelton-Inloes BB, Titani K, Sadler JE. cDNA sequences for human von Willebrand factor reveal five types of repeated domains and five possible protein sequence polymorphisms. Biochemistry. 1986;25(11):3164–71.
44. Mohri H, Fujimura Y, Shima M, Yoshioka A, Houghten R, Ruggeri Z, et al. Structure of the von Willebrand factor domain interacting with glycoprotein Ib. J Biol Chem. 1988;263(34):17901–4.
45. Titani K, Kumar S, Takio K, Ericsson LH, Wade RD, Ashida K, et al. Amino acid sequence of human von Willebrand factor. Biochemistry. 1986;25(11):3171–84.
46. Berndt MC, Ward CM, Booth WJ, Castaldi PA, Mazurov AV, Andrews RK. Identification of aspartic acid 514 through glutamic acid 542 as a glycoprotein Ib-IX complex receptor recognition sequence in von Willebrand factor. Mechanism of modulation of von Willebrand factor by ristocetin and botrocetin. Biochemistry. 1992;31(45):11144–51.
47. Knott HM, Berndt MC, Kralicek AV, O'Donoghue SI, King GF. Determination of the solution structure of a platelet-adhesion peptide of von Willebrand factor. Biochemistry. 1992;31(45):11152–8.
48. Plow EF, Pierschbacher MD, Ruoslahti E, Marguerie GA, Ginsberg MH. The effect of Arg-Gly-Asp-containing peptides on fibrinogen and von Willebrand factor binding to platelets. Proc Natl Acad Sci. 1985;82(23):8057–61.
49. Fressinaud E, Baruch D, Girma J-P, Sakariassen KS, Baumgartner HR, von Meyer D. Willebrand factor-mediated platelet adhesion to collagen involves platelet membrane glycoprotein IIb-IIIa as well as glycoprotein Ib. Transl Res. 1988;112(1):58–67.
50. Aoki T, Tomiyama Y, Honda S, Mihara K, Yamanaka T, Okubo M, et al. Association of the antagonism of von Willebrand factor but not fibrinogen by platelet αIIbβ3 antagonists with prolongation of bleeding time. J Thromb Haemost. 2005;3(10):2307–14.
51. von Ginsburg D. Willebrand disease. In: Williams hematology. 6th ed. Philadelphia: McGraw-Hill; 2001. p. 1813–28.
52. Eikenboom JC. Congenital von Willebrand disease type 3: clinical manifestations, pathophysiology and molecular biology. Best Pract Res Clin Haematol. 2001;14(2):365–79.
53. Goodeve A, Eikenboom J, Castaman G, Rodeghiero F, Federici AB, Batlle J, et al. Phenotype and genotype of a cohort of families historically diagnosed with type 1 von Willebrand disease in the European study, Molecular and Clinical Markers for the Diagnosis and Management of Type 1 von Willebrand Disease (MCMDM-1VWD). Blood. 2007;109(1):112–21.
54. Laffan M, Brown S, Collins PW, Cumming A, Hill F, Keeling D, et al. The diagnosis of von Willebrand disease: a guideline from the UK Haemophilia Centre Doctors' Organization. Haemophilia. 2004;10(3):199–217.
55. Peake I, Goodeve A. Type 1 von Willebrand disease. J Thromb Haemost. 2007;5(s1):7–11.
56. Laffan MA, Lester W, O'donnell JS, Will A, Tait RC, Goodeve A, et al. The diagnosis and management of von Willebrand disease: a United Kingdom Haemophilia Centre Doctors Organization guideline approved by the British Committee for Standards in Haematology. Br J Haematol. 2014;167(4):453–65.
57. Gill JC, Endres-Brooks J, Bauer PJ, Marks WJ, Montgomery RR. The effect of ABO blood group on the diagnosis of von Willebrand disease. Blood. 1987;69(6):1691–5.

58. Quiroga T, Goycoolea M, Belmont S, Panes O, Aranda E, Zuniga P, et al. Quantitative impact of using different criteria for the laboratory diagnosis of type 1 von Willebrand disease. J Thromb Haemost. 2014;12(8):1238–43.
59. Sadler JE. Von Willebrand disease type 1: a diagnosis in search of a disease. Blood. 2003;101(6):2089–93.
60. Mazurier C, Goudemand J, Hilbert L, Caron C, Fressinaud E, Meyer D. Type 2N von Willebrand disease: clinical manifestations, pathophysiology, laboratory diagnosis and molecular biology. Best Pract Res Clin Haematol. 2001;14(2):337–47.
61. Sutherland JJ, O'Brien LA, Lillicrap D, Weaver DF. Molecular modeling of the von Willebrand factor A2 Domain and the effects of associated type 2A von Willebrand disease mutations. J Mol Model. 2004;10(4):259–70.
62. Woods AI, Kempfer AC, Paiva J, Sanchez-Luceros A, Bermejo E, Chuit R, et al. Phenotypic parameters in genotypically selected type 2B von Willebrand disease patients: a large, single-center experience including a new novel mutation. Semin Thromb Hemost. 2017;43: 92–100.
63. Leebeek FW, Eikenboom JC. Von Willebrand's disease. N Engl J Med. 2016;375(21):2067–80.
64. Patzke J, Favaloro EJ. Laboratory testing for von Willebrand factor activity by glycoprotein Ib binding assays (VWF:GPIb). Methods Mol Biol. 1646;2017:453–60.
65. Perez Botero J, Pruthi RK, Nichols WL, Ashrani AA, Patnaik MM. von Willebrand disease type1/type 2N compound heterozygotes: diagnostic and management challenges. Br J Haematol. 2017;176(6):994–7.
66. Lak M, Peyvandi F, Mannucci P. Clinical manifestations and complications of childbirth and replacement therapy in 385 Iranian patients with type 3 von Willebrand disease. Br J Haematol. 2000;111(4):1236–9.
67. Federici A, Castaman G, Mannucci P. Guidelines for the diagnosis and management of von Willebrand disease in Italy. Haemophilia. 2002;8(5):607–21.
68. Federici AB, Bucciarelli P, Castaman G, Mazzucconi MG, Morfini M, Rocino A, et al. The bleeding score predicts clinical outcomes and replacement therapy in adults with von Willebrand disease. Blood. 2014;123(26):4037–44.
69. Rodeghiero F, Tosetto A, Abshire T, Arnold D, Coller B, James P, et al. ISTH/SSC bleeding assessment tool: a standardized questionnaire and a proposal for a new bleeding score for inherited bleeding disorders. J Thromb Haemost. 2010;8(9):2063–5.
70. Makris M. Gastrointestinal bleeding in von Willebrand disease. Thromb Res. 2006;118:S13–S7.
71. Tosetto A, Rodeghiero F, Castaman G, Goodeve A, Federici A, Batlle J, et al. A quantitative analysis of bleeding symptoms in type 1 von Willebrand disease: results from a multicenter European study (MCMDM-1 VWD). J Thromb Haemost. 2006;4(4):766–73.
72. Hyatt SA, Wang W, Kerlin BA, O'brien SH. Applying diagnostic criteria for type 1 von Willebrand disease to a pediatric population. Pediatr Blood cancer. 2009;52(1):102–7.
73. Castaman G, Tosetto A, Cappelletti A. Clinical presentation of type 1 von Willebrand disease in obligatory carriers: final results from a collaborative, international, multicentre study. J Thromb Haemost. 2003; Suppl. 1: Abstract OC078.
74. Castaman G, Federici A, Tosetto A, La Marca S, Stufano F, Mannucci P, et al. Different bleeding risk in type 2A and 2M von Willebrand disease: a 2-year prospective study in 107 patients. J Thromb Haemost. 2012;10(4):632–8.
75. Favaloro EJ. Diagnosing von Willebrand disease: a short history of laboratory milestones and innovations, plus current status, challenges, and solutions. Semin Thromb Hemost. 2014;40(5):551–70.
76. Just S. Laboratory testing for von Willebrand disease: the past, present, and future state of play for von Willebrand factor assays that measure platelet binding activity, with or without Ristocetin. Semin Thromb Hemost. 2017;43(1):75–91.
77. Bodo I, Eikenboom J, Montgomery R, Patzke J, Schneppenheim R, Di Paola J. Platelet-dependent von Willebrand factor activity. Nomenclature and methodology: communication from the SSC of the ISTH. J Thromb Haemost. 2015;13(7):1345–50.

78. Favaloro EJ, Bonar RA, Meiring M, Duncan E, Mohammed S, Sioufi J, et al. Evaluating errors in the laboratory identification of von Willebrand disease in the real world. Thromb Res. 2014;134(2):393–403.
79. Favaloro E, Bonar R, Mohammed S, Arbelaez A, Niemann J, Freney R, et al. Type 2M von Willebrand disease–more often misidentified than correctly identified. Haemophilia. 2016;22(3):e145–55.
80. Favaloro EJ, Bonar R, Kershaw G, Sioufi J, Baker R, Hertzberg M, et al. Reducing errors in identification of von Willebrand disease: the experience of the Royal College of Pathologists of Australasia Quality Assurance Program. Semin thromb hemost. 2006;32:505–13.
81. Favaloro EJ, Mohammed S. Towards improved diagnosis of von Willebrand disease: comparative evaluations of several automated von Willebrand factor antigen and activity assays. Thromb Res. 2014;134(6):1292–300.
82. Favaloro EJ, Mohammed S. Evaluation of a von Willebrand factor three test panel and chemiluminescent-based assay system for identification of, and therapy monitoring in, von Willebrand disease. Thromb Res. 2016;141:202–11.
83. Blanchette VS, Srivastava A. Definitions in hemophilia: resolved and unresolved issues. Semin Thromb Hemost. 2015. https://doi.org/10.1055/s-0035-1564800
84. Favaloro E. Genetic testing for von Willebrand disease: the case against. J Thromb Haemost. 2010;8(1):6–12.
85. Lillicrap D. The molecular genetics of von Willebrand disease. Haematol Rep. 2005;1: 3–8.
86. Pruss CM, Golder M, Bryant A, Hegadorn CA, Burnett E, Laverty K, et al. Pathologic mechanisms of type 1 VWD mutations R1205H and Y1584C through in vitro and in vivo mouse models. Blood. 2011;117(16):4358–66.
87. Goodeve AC. The genetic basis of von Willebrand disease. Blood Rev. 2010;24(3):123–34.
88. Mannucci PM. Treatment of von Willebrand's Disease. N Engl J Med. 2004;351(7):683–94.
89. Zimmerman TS, Dent JA, Ruggeri ZM, Nannini LH. Subunit composition of plasma von Willebrand factor. Cleavage is present in normal individuals, increased in IIA and IIB von Willebrand disease, but minimal in variants with aberrant structure of individual oligomers (types IIC, IID, and IIE). J Clin Invest. 1986;77(3):947.
90. Shen M-C, Chen M, Ma G-C, Chang S-P, Lin C-Y, Lin B-D, et al. De novo mutation and somatic mosaicism of gene mutation in type 2A, 2B and 2M VWD. Thromb J. 2016;14(1):36.
91. Fressinaud E, Mazurier C, Meyer D. Molecular genetics of type 2 von Willebrand disease. Int J Hematol. 2002;75(1):9–18.
92. Ahmad F, Jan R, Kannan M, Obser T, Hassan MI, Oyen F, et al. Characterisation of mutations and molecular studies of type 2 von Willebrand disease. Thromb Haemost. 2013;109(1):39–46.
93. Hillery CA, Mancuso DJ, Sadler JE, Ponder JW, Jozwiak MA, Christopherson PA, et al. Type 2M von Willebrand disease: F606I and I662F mutations in the glycoprotein Ib binding domain selectively impair ristocetin-but not botrocetin-mediated binding of von Willebrand factor to platelets. Blood. 1998;91(5):1572–81.
94. Ginsburg D, Bowie E. Molecular genetics of von Willebrand disease. Blood. 1992;79(10):2507–19.
95. Mannucci PM. How I treat patients with von Willebrand disease. Blood. 2001;97(7):1915–9.
96. Rodeghiero F, Castaman G, Tosetto A. How I treat von Willebrand disease. Blood. 2009;114(6):1158–65.
97. Federici AB, Mazurier C, Berntorp E, Lee CA, Scharrer I, Goudemand J, et al. Biologic response to desmopressin in patients with severe type 1 and type 2 von Willebrand disease: results of a multicenter European study. Blood. 2004;103(6):2032–8.
98. Castaman G, Goodeve A, Eikenboom J. Principles of care for the diagnosis and treatment of von Willebrand disease. Haematologica. 2013;98(5):667–74.
99. Amesse LS, Pfaff-Amesse T, Leonardi R, Uddin D, French JA. Oral contraceptives and DDAVP nasal spray: patterns of use in managing vWD-associated menorrhagia: a single-institution study. J Pediatr Hematol/Oncol. 2005;27(7):357–63.
100. Curnow J, Pasalic L, Favaloro EJ. Treatment of von Willebrand disease. Semin Thromb Hemost. 2016 Mar;42(2):133–46.

101. Thompson AR, Gill JC, Ewenstein B, Mueller-Velten G, Schwartz B. Successful treatment for patients with von Willebrand disease undergoing urgent surgery using factor VIII/VWF concentrate (Humate-P®). Haemophilia. 2004;10(1):42–51.
102. Federici A, Barillari G, Zanon E, Mazzucconi M, Musso R, Targhetta R, et al. Efficacy and safety of highly purified, doubly virus-inactivated VWF/FVIII concentrates in inherited von Willebrand's disease: results of an Italian cohort study on 120 patients characterized by bleeding severity score. Haemophilia. 2010;16(1):101–10.
103. Lethagen S, Kyrle P, Castaman G, Haertel S, Mannucci P. von Willebrand factor/factor VIII concentrate (Haemate® P) dosing based on pharmacokinetics: a prospective multicenter trial in elective surgery. J Thromb Haemost. 2007;5(7):1420–30.
104. Gill JC, Castaman G, Windyga J, Kouides P, Ragni M, Leebeek FW, et al. Hemostatic efficacy, safety, and pharmacokinetics of a recombinant von Willebrand factor in severe von Willebrand disease. Blood. 2015;126(17):2038–46.
105. Schinco P, Dorina C, Valeri F, Borchiellini A, Teruzzi C, Mantuano M. Long-Term Prophylaxis in Patients with Von Willebrand Disease and Recurrent Bleeding in Italy. Blood. 2014;124(21):50–6.
106. Mannucci P, Franchini M. Laboratory monitoring of replacement therapy for major surgery in von Willebrand disease. Haemophilia. 2017;23:182–7.
107. James A, Konkle B, Kouides P, Ragni M, Thames B, Gupta S, et al. Postpartum von Willebrand factor levels in women with and without von Willebrand disease and implications for prophylaxis. Haemophilia. 2015;21(1):81–7.
108. Simionescu AA, Buinoiu NF, Berbec N. Von Willebrand disease type 2 in pregnancy—a critical clinical association. Transfus Apher Sci. 2017;56:269–71.

Hemophilia A

4

Mohammad Saeed Gholami, Mohsen Valikhani,
Akbar Dorgalaleh, Sayed Hamid Mousavi,
and Behnaz Pezeshkpoor

4.1 Introduction

The word "hemophilia" was first used by Hopff in 1828 [1]. Hemophilia (either A or B) is a bleeding disorder which is inherited in an X-linked recessive manner. The most common type of hemophilia is hemophilia A caused by defect or deficiency in coagulation factor VIII (FVIII) [2]. Hemophilia A or classical hemophilia is the most common severe bleeding disorder comprised of ~80% of all types of hemophilia [2]. The main feature of the hemophilia A is prolonged and abnormal bleeding, especially into joints and soft tissues.

The precise incidence of the disorder is not clear, but the estimated incidence is estimated between ~5 and ~20 per 100,000 males, but the majority of the patients remains underdiagnosed [3]. Approximately 40–60% of people with hemophilia A

M. S. Gholami
Student Research Committee, School of Allied Medicine,
Iran University of Medical Sciences, Tehran, Iran

Department of Hematology and Blood Transfusion, School of Allied Medicine,
Iran University of Medical Sciences, Tehran, Iran

M. Valikhani · A. Dorgalaleh
Department of Hematology and Blood Transfusion, School of Allied Medicine,
Iran University of Medical Sciences, Tehran, Iran

S. H. Mousavi
Department of the Clinical Biochemistry, Faculty of Medical Sciences, Kateb University,
Kabul, Afghanistan

Afghanistan National Charity Organization for Special Diseases (ANCOSD),
Kabul, Afghanistan

B. Pezeshkpoor (✉)
Institute of Experimental Hematology and Transfusion Medicine, University of Bonn,
Bonn, Germany
e-mail: Behnaz.Pezeshkpoor@ukbonn.de

A. Dorgalaleh (ed.), *Congenital Bleeding Disorders*,
https://doi.org/10.1007/978-3-319-76723-9_4

have the severe form of the disease, and they are at risk of post-dental extraction, post-surgical and post-trauma hemorrhages, as well as internal hemorrhage. They also exhibit spontaneous bleeding without trauma or injury. Intra-articular joint hemorrhage is the most common spontaneous bleeding that can lead to chronic physical disability due to arthropathy. In fact, the majority of people with hemophilia develops chronic disability, typically in the form of hemophilic arthropathy, because of repeated joint bleeds [4].

Hemarthrosis is the main cause of functional disability and even psychological depression of patients with hemophilia [4]. Hemorrhage into the central nervous system (CNS) is the leading cause of death in hemophilia, accounts for ~20% of non-infective deaths, as reported in developed countries [5].

Based on FVIII activity, hemophilia A is classified into mild (>5% to <40%), moderate (1–5%), and severe (<1%) deficiency. FVIII coagulant activity (FVIII:C) can be measured by either one-stage or chromogenic assays, but chromogenic assay is recommended for FVIII:C assay in plasma and concentrate [6, 7]. Primary prophylaxis is the treatment of choice in patients with severe hemophilia A. Several therapeutic choices are available including fresh frozen plasma (FFP) and cryoprecipitate as traditional options, and FVIII concentrate and recombinant FVIII (rFVIII) as more advanced choices, but the most promising therapeutic strategy is gene therapy [8].

4.2 Factor VIII Structure and Function

The mature FVIII protein consists of three homologous A domains, two homologous C domains, and a unique B domain, which are arranged in the order of A1-A2-B-A3-C1-C2 from the N-terminus to the C-terminal end of protein (Fig. 4.1) [9, 10].

The A1 and A2 domains have about 30% homology with each other. A1-A2-B domains compose the heavy chain of FVIII, while the A3-C1-C2 domains form light chain of FVIII protein. The two chains non-covalently bind together and require a metal ion-dependent linkage, with the responsible residues, which are located within the A1 and A3 domains. Each domain contains a copper atom [11, 12]. Two main antibody epitopes have been detected in the A2 domain. One of them is located in amino acid 484–508, while another one is placed between amino acids 558 and 565. Immunization against these epitopes affects its interaction with activated FIX (FIXa) [13, 14]. There are three acidic peptides named a1, a2, and a3 which are clusters of aspartic and glutamic residues and surround the A domains. The C domains of FVIII and FV are structurally related domains. The C domains are structurally discoid and belong to the phospholipid-binding domains families [15]. The B domain is unique without significant homology with any other known

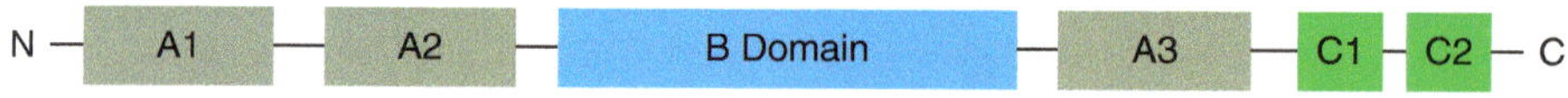

Fig. 4.1 Structure of factor VIII protein; human factor VIII is a single chain protein with a molecular weight of 300 kDa, consists of six domains including A1-A2-B-A3-C1-C2. The mature factor VIII protein consists of three homologous A domains, two homologous C domains, and a B domain

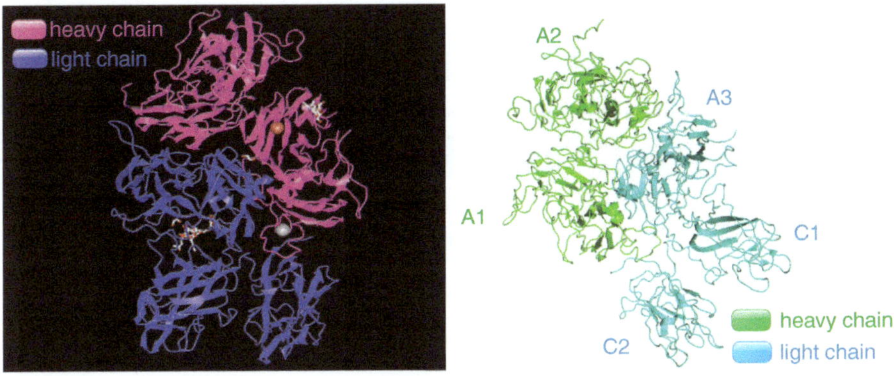

Fig. 4.2 Three-dimensional crystalloid structure of B-domain deleted factor VIII protein. There are three A domains, A1, A2, and A3, and two C domains, C1 and C2 (www.pdb.org)

protein [16]. This domain does not affect FVIII activity in the process of blood coagulation. When the B domain is cleaved and released, FVIII is converted to the active form (FVIIIa). The protein in active form consists of a heavy chain and a light chain. This process requires two cleavages by thrombin (Fig. 4.2).

Different domains of FVIII protein have different functions. An acidic peptide, which spans from amino acid 337 to 374 and called a1, separates A1 from A2 domain. Second acidic peptide, a2, links A2 to B domain. The next short acidic peptide termed a3 is connected with A3 domain. There is a pair of homologous C domains (C1 and C2) at the C-terminal of FVIII protein. A region of the C2 domain contains a membrane-binding site and the site for interaction with von Willebrand factor (VWF) [17]. The 2303 to 2332 sequence of the C2 domain has been suggested to form an interactive site for both VWF and phospholipids. The organization of the FVIII domains and linker peptides can thus be ordinated as A1.a1.A2.a2.B.a3. A3.C1.C2. Notably, there are seven disulfide bonds within the FVIII molecule: two in each A domain and one within the C1 domain [18]. In the A1 domain, Cys310, Met320, His267, and His315 create a copper-binding site, and Cys2000, His1954, and His2005 constitute another copper-binding site in the A3 domain [12, 19].

First cleavage by thrombin at Arg1689 (at the B-a3) position generates a heavy chain with variable size (90–210 kDa) and consists of A1 and A2 domains and heterogeneous fragments of the partially proteolyzed B domain; during this process, a 40-amino-acid acidic peptide (a3) is released from the C-terminal product to form a 73 kDa product that includes A3-C1-C2 domains which is called the light chain. Further cleavage by thrombin cleaves the protein between the A1 and A2 domains and removes most of the B domain: cleavage at Arg372 (between the A1 and A2 domains) and at Arg740 (between the A2 and B domains) generates a 54 kDa A1 and a 44 kDa A2 domain (Fig. 4.3) [20, 21].

Both chains form a non-covalently linked complex in a calcium-dependent manner. This complex is the procoagulant FVIIIa [22]. Next step in coagulation cascade is activation of FX by tenase complex, which consists of FVIIIa, and FIXa, platelet surface phospholipids and calcium cation (Table 4.1) [23].

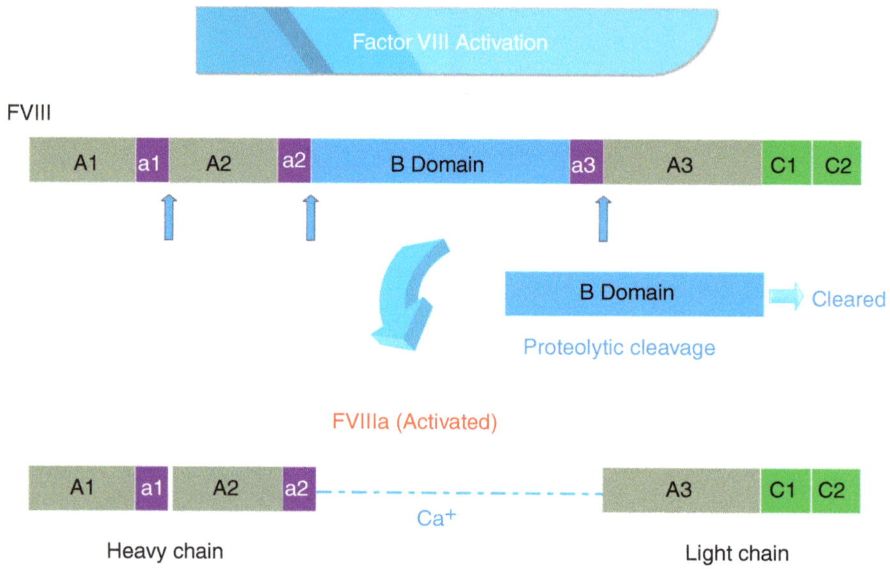

Fig. 4.3 Activation of factor VIII. Cleavage by thrombin removes the B domain and divides factor VIII to two chains: the heavy and light chains. Then the calcium cations link them together. Factor VIII in its nonactivated form circulates in plasma in a complex with von Willebrand factor (VWF). Upon activation by thrombin or factor X-mediated site-specific proteolysis, activated factor VIII serves as a cofactor for factor IXa

Table 4.1 Characteristics of factor VIII domains

Domain	Number of amino acids	Function	Molecular manifestation of the defected domain
A	FVIII A domains consist of A1(336 aa), A2 (337 aa), and A3 (329 aa)	Coagulation FVIII A domains are homologous with coagulation FV domains and ceruloplasmin 40% amino acid identity with each other and to the A domains of FV	–
A1	336	Creates the heavy chain (200 kDa) (A1-A2) Contains single copper atom	Reduced stability of the FVIIIa Impaired thrombin activation

Table 4.1 (continued)

A2	337	Creates the heavy chain (200 kDa) (A1-A2) The main antibody epitope is present in the A2 domain in amino acid 484–508 sites	Alter FVIII intracellular trafficking and/or secretion Alter interaction with FIXa Impaired thrombin activation
A3	329	Creates the light chain (80 kDa) (A3-C1-C2) linked by metal ions Contain single copper atom	Alter interaction with FIXa Reduce stability of the FVIIIa
B[a]	907	Creates the heavy chain (200 kDa) (A1-A2) Intracellular synthesis quality control: Enables interaction of FVIII with chaperone proteins that distinguish properly folded tertiary structure of proteins; stabilizes folded domains, prevents aggregation Secretion: Interacts with cargo-specific sorting receptor complex that enables endoplasmic reticulum to Golgi transport; increases secretion efficiency Plasma activation: Possibly shields thrombin activation site from premature proteolysis Platelet binding: Decreases affinity of inactivated FVIII for activated platelets, thus preserving circulating FVIII Inactivation: Reduces proteolysis by activated protein C and FXa Clearance: May play a role in FVIII quality control through interaction with asialoglycoprotein receptor	–
C1	153	C1 domain an impact on VWF and C2 domain linkage strengthening Creates the light chain (80 kDa) (A3-C1-C2) linked by metal ions	Reduction of FVIII binding to VWF FVIII intracellular trafficking and/or secretion Misfolded protein Defect at phospholipid-binding surface

(continued)

Table 4.1 (continued)

C2	160	C2 domain surface responsible for phospholipid linkage to coagulation FVIII Creates the light chain (80 kDa) (A3-C1-C2) linked by metal ions	Reduce the FVIII secretion rate Misfolded protein Reduction of FVIII binding to VWF Defect at phospholipid-binding surface
a1	37	–	Impaired thrombin activation
a2	31	–	Impaired thrombin activation
a3	42	–	Impaired thrombin activation Reduction of FVIII binding to VWF

aa amino acids, *FVIII* factor VIII, *FVIIIa* activated factor VIII, *FV* factor V, *FIXa* activated factor IX, *FXa* activated factor X, *VWF* von Willebrand factor
[a]Comprising 40% of FVIII mass

4.3 Hemophilia A

The word hemophilia comes from two Greek words: the haima, which means blood, and the philia meaning affection. Hemophilia A or classic hemophilia is an X-linked recessive bleeding disorder characterized by dysfunctional blood clotting, due to a mutation in the gene for the clotting component, FVIII. This problem may transport everyone to the second century AD, when the Talmud, a collection of Jewish rabbinical writings, stated that male newborns should not be circumcised if their two brothers had already died from this procedure. During the twentieth century, this problem had been estimated that it has affected 1 in 5032 live male births in the United States [24, 25].

Clinical presentations of patients with hemophilia A vary from mild condition to severe bleeding tendency. Approximately 50% of people with hemophilia A have the severe form of the disease. Patients with hemophilia A are at higher risk of post-traumatic bleeding such as post-dental hemorrhage and post-surgical bleeding; spontaneous bleeding is relatively common in patients with hemophilia A. The intra-articular joint hemorrhage is the most common spontaneous bleeding and can lead to chronic disability as a result of arthropathy. This issue may result in loss of a range of motion and severe pain. In fact, the majority of people with severe hemophilia A develops chronic disability, typically in the form of hemophilic arthropathy, because of repeated joint bleeds [4]. Furthermore, people with severe hemophilia have

Table 4.2 Classification of hemophilia A and severity of clinical presentations

Severity of disease	Factor level % activity (IU/mL)	Sign and symptoms	Relative incidence (%)	Age at diagnosis
Severe	<1% (<0.01)	Spontaneous bleeding, predominantly in the joints, muscles, and internal organs	50	First year of life
Moderate	1–5% (0.01–0.05)	Occasional spontaneous bleeding, severe bleeding after trauma or surgery	30	Up to age 5–6 years
Mild	>5–40% (0.05–0.40)	Severe bleeding with major trauma or surgery	20	Often later in life

less than 1% of the normal level of FVIII in their blood. They can experience repeated spontaneous bleedings per month. People with moderate hemophilia usually bleed less than severely affected patients and post-minor traumatic hemorrhages can occur. Finally, people with mild hemophilia A have even fewer hemorrhages. Sometimes they are not aware of their bleeding problem, and an invasive procedure such as surgery or tooth extraction can make them aware (Table 4.2) [26].

Diagnosis of disorder can be made based on clinical presentations, appropriate laboratory assessment, and familial history. Because hemophilia A is an X-linked disease, females can be carriers. Carriers have one normal and one abnormal gene. They have a 50% chance of giving the hemophilia gene to each child. Boys who receive the abnormal gene will have hemophilia; girls who inherit it will become carriers. Therefore, if the father of a family has hemophilia and the mother has a hemophilic gene, their daughter can have hemophilia. With regard to phenotype, carriers are usually unaffected or only mildly affected with some bleeding symptoms. Carriers who have >50% of clotting FVIII levels can control bleeding [27]. But half of them have < 50% FVIII and therefore manifest a bleeding tendency proportional to how low the level is in their blood.

Carriers are divided into two groups: mandatory carriers, who necessarily carry the affected X chromosome, and possible carriers [27].

Mandatory Carriers Are:

- All female offspring of a man with hemophilia
- Mothers who have a boy with hemophilia and at least one other family member with hemophilia (brother, grandparent, uncle, nephew, or cousin)
- Mothers who have a boy with hemophilia and a family member carrying the hemophilia gene (mother, sister, mother's grandmother, aunt, or uncle)
- Mothers of two or more boys with hemophilia

Possible Carriers Are:

- All girls born of a carrier
- Mothers of one boy with hemophilia who have no other family members have hemophilia or are carriers of hemophilia
- Sisters, mothers, maternal grandmothers, aunts, nieces, and female cousins of carriers (Fig. 4.4)

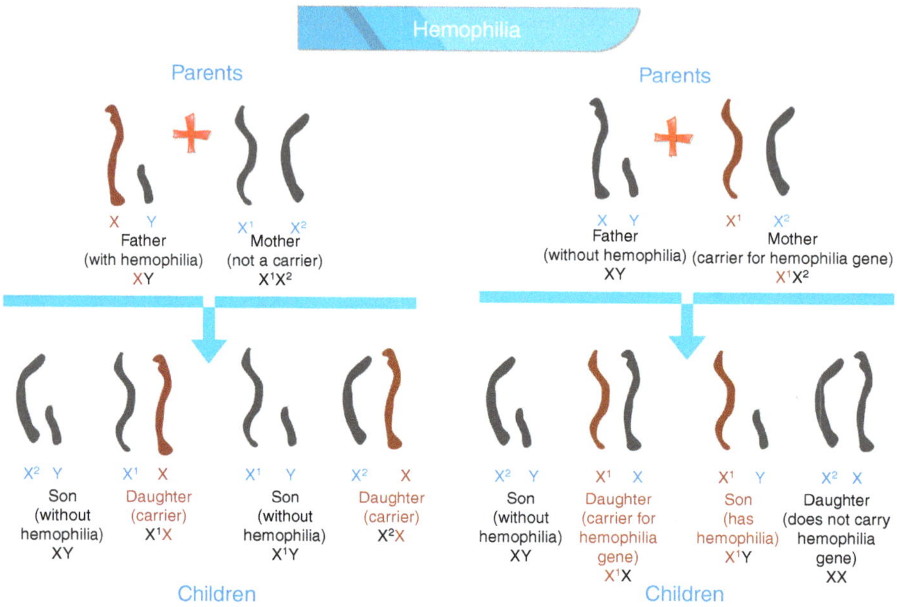

Fig. 4.4 Hereditary chance of giving the hemophilia gene in each child: left; when the father is affected, right; when the mother is a carrier

4.4 Clinical Manifestations

Hemophilia A is the most common severe congenital bleeding disorder, and patients present variable clinical presentations. There is a direct correlation between FVIII:C and severity of clinical presentations. Based on residual FVIII:C level, the disorder is classified into severe (<0.01 IU/dL (<1% of normal)), moderate (0.01–0.05 IU/dL (1–5% of normal)), and mild (>0.05 to <0.40% IU/dL (>5 to <40% of normal) deficiency [7].

Mild, moderate, and severe forms comprise 20%, 30%, and 50% of all cases with hemophilia, respectively [28]. Individuals with FVIII:C higher than 30% are usually asymptomatic, but a mild bleeding tendency presents in hemophilia A carrier females with low to low-normal FVIII:C level [29].

Severely affected individuals present severe bruising and joint hemorrhage during their first 2 years of life [30].

Phenotypically, hemarthrosis (particularly in the knee, ankle, and elbow joints), soft tissue hematoma, easy bruising, retroperitoneal bleeding, intracranial hemorrhage (ICH), and post-surgical bleeding are the most concerning problems in hemophilia A that may present at any age [31]. ICH is the main concern at time of birth that can occur immediately after birth or within the birth. Severity of disorder and type of delivery can affect the rate of ICH in neonates with hemophilia. Neonates with forceps delivery and Cesarean section delivery are at higher risk of ICH, while non-traumatic normal vaginal delivery imposes less risk. Overlay incidence of ICH in hemophilia is variable, but 3.5–4% is the more acceptable rate of ICH (Table 4.3).

Table 4.3 Clinical manifestations of congenital factor VIII deficiency

Prevalence (%)	Bleeding episodes	Iran% (*N*: 885)[a]	Northeastern Iran% (*N*: 287)	India% (*N*: 56)[b]	Pakistan% (*N*: 229)	Iran% (*N*: 100)	Iran% Severe/moderate (*N*: 50)	Iran% Mild (*N*: 50)
~20–100	Ecchymosis	13.2	71	–	–	–	–	–
	Hemarthrosis	8.7	72.6	73.2	–	86	86	6
	Oral cavity bleeding	–	–	–	–	64	64	30
	Post-partum bleeding	–	–	–	–	36	–	–
	Post-operative bleeding	–	–	–	18.4	–	76	30
	Post-dental extraction bleeding	6.8	89	–	0.9	–	–	–
	Epistaxis	–	55.9	26.7		20	20	12
~5–20	Post-circumcision bleeding	14.5	–	–	62	–	–	–
	Gastrointestinal bleeding	0.4	21	3.5	–	10	10	0
	Hematuria	–	32.3	1.78	–	12	12	0
	Hematoma	1.2	4.2	–	0.9	93	82	8
	Skin bleeding	–	–	80.3	–	–	–	–
	Muscle bleeding			46.4	–	–	–	–
~<5	Central nervous system bleeding	–	2.4	–	–	4	4	0
	Umbilical cord bleeding	0.5	1.8	–	5.2	–	–	–
	Menorrhagia	0.3	–	–	–	–	–	–
	Iliopsoas muscle	–	–	1.7	–	–	–	–

[a]First clinical presentations
[b]Fifty one cases had hemophilia A, while five cases had hemophilia B

In early childhood, large hematomas might also be observed following intramuscular injections (e.g., immunizations) and should persuade the physician to rule out a bleeding disorder [2, 32].

Bleeding symptoms also may appear later when the teeth erupt. Prolonged severe oral bleeding can lead to anemia [33].

As the child's activity increases with age, the presentation of bleeding episodes is changed. During the toddler age, bumps and falls can cause prolonged oral bleeding from the frenula, superficial hematoma, and intramuscular hemorrhages. Physicians must thoroughly examine the patients who have such symptoms to differentiate hemophilia from child abuse. The family history of bleeding disorders can be helpful [2, 34].

Spontaneous hematuria may occur in children and adults but usually disappears in a few days [35, 36]. Large intramuscular hematoma is also a major bleeding problem in childhood and adulthood periods and should immediately be treated by clotting factor concentrate. Bleeding into a muscle causes it to be swollen hard and tender. Hemorrhages in large muscles may cause anemia and severe pain [2, 37]. Bleeding in the iliopsoas may present as an acute abdominal pain and could be mistaken as appendicitis or other intra-abdominal surgical emergencies [38]. On the other hand, some mouth problems can occur during infancy, when teeth's roots of infant are mobile. Bleeding also occurs when a tooth falls out or is extracted by a dentist. The teenage years sometimes need for orthodontic braces. The orthodontist must be aware of the child's disorder and should consider the necessary considerations. Another problem is gum diseases. Chronic periodontitis (pyorrhoea), which is typically seen in adults, and gingivitis are both painless but may lead to gum bleeding, particularly during brushing [39].

Moreover, gastrocnemius, quadriceps, and forearm bleedings may increase pressure on neurovascular bundles, causing a situation that is known as compartment syndrome. It can lead to ischemia, fibrosis, neuropathy, and atrophy and even may require amputation [40].

The major bleeding problem throughout the patient's life is hemarthrosis that requires immediate treatment. Bleeding into the joint leads to synovitis, causing increased proliferation and vascularization. Repeated bleeding episodes, causing a hot swollen joint, which resulted from the synovial hypertrophy and, with further bleeding, muscle weakness and loss of joint stability. This cycle of bleeding leads to erosion of the joint cartilage, resulting in arthritis and the paralyzed, disfigured limb of patients with hemophilia [2, 41, 42].

4.5 Molecular Basis

F8 gene that encodes FVIII protein is one of the largest genes located on the long arm of chromosome X (Xq28 position). *F8* gene contains high GC content and, within the 9.1 kb coding region, includes 25 introns and 26 exons organized in several domains, A1, A2, A3, B, and C1-C2 [43]. Exons are ranged from 69 bp (exon 5) to 3.1 kb (exon 14) in size. The FVIII precursor protein of 2351 amino acids is encoded by FVIII mRNA which is 9.1 kb in size [44].

4.5.1 Factor VIII Gene Mutations

The sequence of the *F8* gene was published in 1984, and since that time, a large number of mutations that cause hemophilia A have been identified [45].

FVIII deficiency is caused by a wide spectrum of mutations, which occur along the entire length of the *F8* gene. The mutations can cause quantitative or qualitative defects. In quantitative defects the level of transcription or translation and in qualitative defects changes of individual amino acids in FVIII protein occurred. Severe hemophilia is typically caused by inversions, deletions, insertions, missense mutations, and by nonsense mutations. Milder forms of hemophilia are usually caused by missense mutations, while single nucleotide deletions or splicing errors also may occur [21]. There are about 70 CpG dinucleotides within *F8* gene. This results in to hypermutation status, and approximately 30% of variants are usually novel [43]. Human gene mutation database (HGMD) has reported 2320 mutations within the *F8* gene [46]. The most frequent gene defect is the intron 22 inversion which leads to hemophilia A with a frequency of 52% among individuals with severe hemophilia A [28]. The second most frequent mutation is the intron 1 inversion with a prevalence of about 1–5% among hemophilia A patients (Table 4.4) [47–49].

The remaining cases are caused by numerous mutations spread all over the gene. As outlined in the FVIII HAMSTeRS (homology, mutation, structure, testing, and site resources) mutation database, there are over 1200 mutations in *F8* coding and untranslated regions. Most of these mutations are point mutations or small rearrangement [50]. Most of the missense mutations which are detected in mild to moderately severe hemophilia A are located within the exons coding for the three A domains or the two C domains.

4.5.2 Intron 22 Inversion

About 40–50% of patient with severe hemophilia A show intron 22 inversion of *F8* gene, the most frequent inversion mutation in severe hemophilia A [51]. The intron 22 of the *F8* gene contains a 9.5 kb region, which is present outside of the gene, near the telomere of the X chromosome in two additional copies; these are

Table 4.4 Frequency of *F8* gene mutation

Type of mutation	Frequency percentage (%)	Most reported relevant type of disease
Intron 22 inversions	52	Severe
Intron 1 inversions	2	Severe
Large deletions	1	Severe
Small deletions	10	Severe
Nonsense mutations	9	Severe
Splice site mutation	4	Severe
Missense mutations	68	Moderate

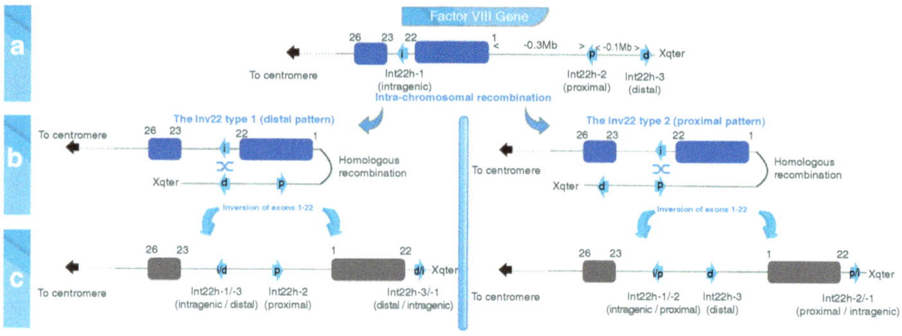

Fig. 4.5 The intron 22 inversion of the *F8* gene. Intrachromosomal homologous recombination between inverted repeats on the X chromosome accounts for about half of severe hemophilia A cases. Identification of a third rearrangement at Xq28 that causes severe hemophilia A as a result of homologous recombination between inverted repeats. (**a**) shows normal alleles, (**b**) shows the intrachromosomal homologous recombination, (**c**) shows the Inv22 type 1 (distal pattern) and type 2 (proximal pattern). Functional *F8* is indicated by blue arrows, while nonfunctional *F8* sequences are indicated by gray arrows. *Xqter* the end of the long arm of the X chromosome, *Int* intron, *F8*, coagulation factor VIII, *i* Int22h-1 (intragenic), *P* Int22h-2 (proximal), *d* Int22h-3 (distal)

termed *int22h2* and *int22h3*. *int22h1* is the sequence in intron 22 that include the *F8* gene [52, 53]. The sequence identity of the three regions is 99.9%. An inversion of the *F8* gene can be caused by an intrachromosomal homologous recombination between *int22h1* and one of its two telomeric copies. This inversion occurs almost particularly in the male germ cells because the proposed intrachromosomal recombination would be probably inhibited by pairing Xq with its homologous in female meiosis (Fig. 4.5) [54].

4.5.3 Insertions and Deletions in the *F8* Gene

Insertions and deletions that cause severe hemophilia can be large (more than 50 bp) or small, usually one or more nucleotides. Insertions and deletions of a single nucleotide lead to a shift of the reading frame and, thus, cause severe form of the disease. Several types of repetitive sequences, including SINES and LINES, which are present in the *F8* gene, may be mutated. Hemophilia in such patients is somewhere on the border between the severe and moderate forms. In severe hemophilia A, gross gene alterations (including large deletions or insertions, frameshift and splice junction changes, and nonsense and missense mutations) of FVIII account for approximately 50% of mutations detected. The most recent update of the HAMSTeRS database listed more than 200 small deletions (50 nucleotides or less than) and more than 80 insertions in hemophilia A [55–57].

Genetic defects can affect the interaction sites of FVIII with other clotting factors such as FIX or VWF and cause hemophilia A [9, 10].

4.6 Diagnosis

Diagnosis and management of hemophilia A is required precise laboratory assessment of patients, especially precise determination of FVIII:C level. FVIII:C assay can be used for precise classification of disease, determination of the dose of replacement therapy, and pre-operative management and therapeutic response in patients with hemophilia A. Based on FVIII activity, hemophilia A is classified to mild (> 5% to 40%), moderate (1–5%), and severe (< 1%) deficiency. Since FVIII is not an enzyme, FVIII assay is an indirect method performed by clot bases or chromogenic assays. A high variation is observed in FVIII assays in different laboratories. This variation is sometime more profound with use of new recombinant modified FVIII products. Different methods are available for FVIII assay based on one-stage assay and chromogenic assay. Each of these methods has its own advantages and disadvantages.

4.6.1 Chromogenic Assay

The chromogenic assay has similar principle with two-stage assay and including two stages: at first stage, activated FX (FXa) is generated, and subsequently, at second stage, amount of FXa is determined. In the first stage, patient's plasma is incubated with FIXa, excess FX and thrombin, calcium, and phospholipids. In this step, FVIIIa accompanied with FIXa generates intrinsic tenase (FIXa–FVIIIa) and converts FX to FXa. In the second step, FXa cleaves the chromogenic substrate, and the intensity of generated color is directly proportional to amount of FXa and therefore amount of FVIII in patient's plasma (Fig. 4.6).

This mixture consists of purified FIXa, purified FX, phospholipids (PL), calcium, and chromogenic substrate. This mixture also consists of highly diluted patient's plasma or reference plasma as a source of FVIIIa. FX is converse to FXa, and this activated coagulation factor, hydrolyze FX-specific chromogenic substrate, leads to release of chromophoric group *para*-nitroaniline (pNA). The extinction can be read on 405 nm.

This method was recommended by FVIII and FIX subcommittee of International Society of Thrombosis and Hemostasis (ISTH) as a reference method for FVIII:C assay in plasma and in concentrate. Chromogenic assay has lower variation between laboratories than one-stage assay (Table 4.5).

The advantages of chromogenic assay over one-stage assay are the precision and sensitivity to low amounts of factor, but the complexity of procedure and operator burden may increase the risk of inaccuracy and errors.

Advantages:

1. FVIIIa cannot affect the chromogenic assay as it is seen in two-stage assay.
2. Additionally, direct thrombin inhibitors (DTI) or heparin can affect chromogenic assay less than the one-stage assay.

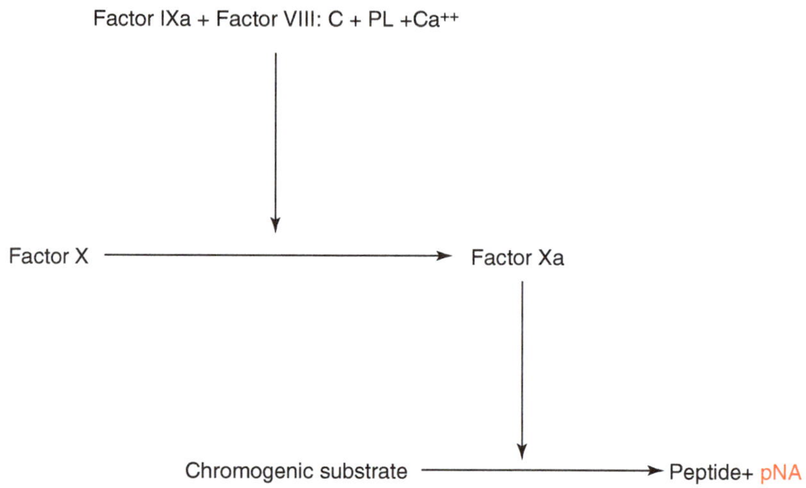

Fig. 4.6 Principle of chromogenic assay: At the first, patient's plasma is incubated with FIXa, FVIII, excess FX and thrombin, CA^{2+}, and PL. Then intrinsic tenase (FIXa–FVIIIa) generates and converts FX to FXa. Finally, FXa cleaves the chromogenic substrate to peptide and pNA. *pNA* para-nitroaniline, *CA^{2+}* calcium, *PL* phospholipids, *FVIII* factor VIII, *FVIIIa* activated factor VIII, *FIXa* activated factor IX, *FXa* activated factor X

3. In comparing with the one-stage assay, variability of the chromogenic assay is much lower.
4. The chromogenic assay is not dependent on FVIII deficient plasma.

Disadvantages:
1. However, falsely reduced FVIII activity may be measured when a direct FXa inhibitor is present.
2. Generally, chromogenic FVIII assay is more expensive than clot-based FVIII activity assays such as one-stage assay [6, 58, 59].

4.6.2 One-Stage Assay

The most common method to measure FVIII activity is the one-stage assay which is based on partial thromboplastin time (PTT) or activated partial thromboplastin time (aPTT).

For such assay, standard plasma and FVIII-deficient plasma are required. Standard plasma can be made in laboratory or can be a commercial one. In any case, standard plasma should be calibrated against international standard for FVIII, and it is not acceptable to assume polled plasma to has 100 U/dL FVIII:C. FVIII-deficient plasma can be commercially available or can be obtained from patients with FVIII level <1 U/dL without inhibitor and with normal liver function tests. Although both methods can be used, today, the former is the predominant method.

Table 4.5 Characteristics of chromogenic factor VIII assay kits

Kit	Vendor	Intended use	FXa substrate	Thrombin inhibitor	Detection limit (%)	Total CV	Advantages/ Disadvantages	Measuring range (%)
Coatest® SP4[a]	Chromogenix, Milan, Italy	Plasma and concentrate	S-2765: N-a-Z-D-Arg-Gly-Arg-pNA	I-2581	<1	Range 1–20%: 5.6 ($n = 80$) Range 20–150%: 5.3 ($n = 80$)	Rapid applications for a wide range of automated instruments	1. 1–20 2. 20–150
Coatest® SP[a]	Chromogenix, Milan, Italy	Plasma and concentrate	S-2765: N-a-Z-D-Arg-Gly-Arg-pNA	I-2581	<1	Range 1–20%: 5.6 ($n = 80$) Range 20–150%: 5.3 ($n = 80$)	1) No drug interference 2) Heparin concentrations 0.2 IU/mL do not interfere 3) 0.5 IU/mL gives 5% inhibition 4) Due to the high dilutions used, there is no underestimation of FVIII activity in samples containing lupus anticoagulant	1. 1–20 2. 20–150
Coamatic®	Chromogenix, Milan, Italy	Plasma and concentrate	S-2765: N-a-Z-D-Arg-Gly-Arg-pNA	I-2581	<1	Range 1–20%: 5.6 ($n = 80$) Range 20–150%	Applications for a wide range of automated instruments	20–150 (0.2–1.5 IU/mL) • 1–20 (0.01–0.2 IU/mL)

(continued)

Table 4.5 (continued)

Kit	Vendor	Intended use	FXa substrate	Thrombin inhibitor	Detection limit (%)	Total CV	Advantages/ Disadvantages	Measuring range (%)
Technochrom® FVIII:C	Technoclone, Vienna, Austria	Plasma	FXa-1 (pNA)	α-NAPAP	<1	–	1) Stability on board 24 h Reagents may be capped and refroze 2 weeks at −20 °C after opening 2) Excellent accuracy and precision 3) Economical use For plasma samples and concentrates 4) Adaptation sheets for common autoanalyzers are available	0.6–1.5 IU F VIII (60–150 of normal)
DG-Chrom FVIII	Grifols, Barcelona, Spain	Plasma	FXa-1 (pNA)	α-NAPAP		4.06%	Rapid	1 to130
FVIII chromogenic assay	(Siemens, Marburg, Germany)	Plasma	CH3OCO-D-CHG-Gly-Arg-pNA. AcOH	α-NAPAP		–	Extended on board reagent stability	–
Biophen	Hyphen biomed, Neuville-sur-Oise, France	Plasma and concentrate	SXa-11 (pNA)	Thombin inhibitor	High range) ~10 Low range ~2	FVIII deficient plasma is not required Insensitive to lupus anticoagulant	1) More expensive than one stage 2) More sophisticated than one stage 3) Difficult for automation	Low: 0 to 25 and high: 0 to 200

[a]The formulation of the two kits is same; they are optimized for different test volumes, *FVIII* factor VIII

In this assay, FVIII-deficient plasma is added to patient's plasma and aPTT reagent and incubated for appropriate time (most often 3 to 5 min). Then calcium is added to this mixture and clotting time is recorded. In fact, patient's plasma is diluted in buffer and is mixed with equal amount of deficient plasma. For determination of FVIII activity in patient's plasma, clotting time of patients sample is compared with standard curve. Standard curve is constructed by plotting the clotting time of serial dilution of standard plasma vs FVIII activity on logarithmic/linear scale graph paper. An important issue with this assay is parallelism between standard dilutions and patients plasma dilutions. Therefore, FVIII activity assay should be performed at least on three different dilutions to check parallelism. Non-parallelism FVIII activity should be considered as incorrect. It is generally accepted that the main reasons for non-parallelism results are presence of specific FVIII inhibitor, lupus anticoagulants, or other non-specific inhibitors.

Benefits of the One-Stage Methodology Include:

1. Simplicity and readily automation.
2. As it is shown by CV (%), the one-stage assay may be more suitable to detect a normal or decreased FVIII level when the plasma has low FVIII activity.

Limitations of the One-Stage Assay Include:

1. Lipemia more likely affects the one-stage assay than chromogenic assay.
2. In addition, this method can also be influenced by anticoagulant drugs, specifically heparin, direct thrombin inhibitors, or direct FXa inhibitors.
3. When FVIII is converted to the FVIIIa during sample collection, the one-stage assay shows a false increase of FVIII activity.
4. The one-stage assay may be nonoptimal for detecting an increased level of FVIII as it shown by CV%.
5. Finally, due to the presence of different reagents of aPTT, various instrumentations, calibration standards, and factor deficient plasmas, there is a significant difference between one-step FVIII tests performed in different laboratories [58].

4.6.3 Discrepancy Between Chromogenic and One-Stage Assays

One-stage and chromogenic assays give comparable results, but discrepancies can occur between two types of assay in a number of circumstances including some hemophilia A phenotypes and some specific mutations. In 30% of patients with mild hemophilia A, discrepancy between one-stage assay and chromogenic assay can be observed. In approximately 5–10% of patients with mild hemophilia A, FVIII activity assay is placed within normal range, while lower FVIII activity assay with other methods. In these patients, if only one assay is used, diagnosis may be missed; thus simultaneous use of one-stage and chromogenic assays is recommended for diagnosis of mild hemophilia A.

When missense mutations occur in A1, A2, and A3 domain interfaces, the result of FVIII activity is lower by chromogenic assay than one-stage assay. This difference can be as much as twofold or higher. It seems that such mutations can decrease FVIII heterodimer and FVIIIa heterotrimer stability. These changes have minimum effect on one-stage assay, while in chromogenic assay, this effect is more profound because incubation in first stage of this assay increases A2 dissociation and subsequently decreases FVIII activity in this assay.

In the other hand, mutations around thrombin cleavage site, FXa binding site, and VWF binding site cause lower FVIII activity in one-stage assay in comparison with chromogenic assay. These mutations cause impaired FVIII activation by thrombin and its binding to VWF and FXa. In one-stage assay, physiological concentration of thrombin is affected by mutations around thrombin cleavage site, while in chromogenic stage, high concentration of thrombin and time of incubation help to appropriate activation of FVIII, and therefore this assay is less sensitive to these kinds of mutations.

4.6.4 Determination of Factor VIII Concentrates Potency

FVIII activity assay is important for monitoring of patients' response to replacement therapy and for potency labeling of different FVIII products. Discrepancies were observed between FVIII activity assay by one-stage assay and chromogenic assay in laboratory assessment of some long-acting rFVIII products and in diagnosis of some patients with different genotypes. Although long-acting products have several advantages including decreased number of injection and improved quality of life, their FVIII assay required specific considerations. One-stage assays are more sensitive to PEGylation than chromogenic assay; for example, in N8-GP (Novo Nordisk A/S, Bagsværd, Denmark) as a PEGylated rFVIII, PEG moiety of this product interferes with one-stage aPTT assay, and therefore when some particular aPTT reagents especially silica-based aPTT reagents are used, this effect is more profund. Although it seems that ellagic acid and polyphenol aPTT reagents are not sensitive to PEGylated products and can be used for potency measurement of PEGylated rFVIII, chromogenic is certified for potency testing of this product. Although one-stage assay can accurately determine FVIII activity in plasma-derived FVIII products, they give 20–50% lower FVIII activity than chromogenic assay in B-domain deletion (BDD) rFVIII products. For full-length rFVIII, chromogenic assay gives higher FVIII activity than one-stage assay, and there is 8–20% discrepancy that is clinically significant [60–67] (Table 4.6).

For labeling of a FVIII product, both methods are acceptable when the results agree, but when a significant discrepancy was observed between one-stage and chromogenic assays, the proper method should be used for this purpose. Although one-stage assay is the most commonly used method in clinical use, the ability of chromogenic assay in accurate assay of new modified products will increase its role in potency assignment and probably also in clinical monitoring in the future.

Table 4.6 Comparison the potency of factor VIII replacement products

Product	Nature of product	Company	The certified potency of	Half-life
N8-GP	A PEGylated, B-domain truncated derivative of rFVIII, turoctocog alfa pegol	Novo Nordisk A/S, Bagsværd, Denmark	Chromogenic assay	19 h
Novoeight (turoctocog alfa)	rFVIII B-domain truncation	Novoeight, Novo Nordisk A/S, Bagsværd, Denmark	One-stage clotting assay or the chromogenic substrate assay	10.8 h (in children is about 29% shorter than in adults)
Advate®	Full-length rFVIII	rFVIII, Advate, Baxter bioscience, Deerfield, IL, USA	One-stage clotting assay	8.7–25.2 h
BAY 94–9027	K1804C directed PEGylation	Bayer, Leverkusen, Germany	One-stage FVIII assays, with ellagic acid aPTT reagents	19 h
ReFacto	rFVIII-BDD	Pfizer, Sandwich, UK	One-stage clotting assay	14.8 ± 5.6 h (range 7.6–28.5 h)
Efmoroctocog alfa	rFVIII-Fc fusion protein	Eloctate®; Biogen Idec Inc., Cambridge, MA, USA	One-stage clotting or chromogenic assays	1.48 to 1.56-fold greater than that of rFVIII
BAX 855	PEGylated full-length rFVII	Baxter, Deerfield, IL, USA	Chromogenic FVIII assay	1.4- to 1.5-fold increased half-life compared to Advate
CSL627	Single-chain variant of FVIII-BDD	CSL Behring, King of Prussia, PA, USA	Chromogenic assay	13 h

FVIII: factor VIII; rFVIII: recombinant factor VIII; aPTT: activated partital thromboplastin time; BDD: B-domain deleted

4.7 Treatment of Patients with Hemophilia A

In the 1960s and 1970s, the advent of concentrates, self-infusion, and treatment centers improved the quality of life in patients with hemophilia. Today, as a result of advances in eradication of infectious agents in clotting factor concentrates, almost all patients with 30 years old or younger with hemophilia are HIV negative and hepatitis C negative. Although hepatitis C infection remained as a complication, to reach the goal "best quality of life" in a patients with hemophilia, several strategies should be taken: first, preventive therapy, such as therapeutic abortion or vaccination against hepatitis in prenatal and postnatal, respectively; second, aggressive new treatment such as prophylaxis; third, improved surgical techniques such as arthroscopic synovectomy; and finally better rehabilitation techniques [2].

4.7.1 Replacement Therapy

The traditional and common way to treat this genetic disorder is regular supplementation with intravenous recombinant or plasma derived FVIII concentrates in severe cases. However, some people with severe hemophilia and more often those with moderate and mild hemophilia treat only as needed. In children, to minimize frequent traumatic intravenous cannulation, an easily accessible intravenous port (port-a-cath) may have to be used [68]. These devices eliminate problems of finding a vein for infusion, which may be required, several times in a week. Therefore, this devise make the prophylaxis program in hemophilia easier. There are other studies that showed risk of clot formation at the tip of the catheter [69]. But a number of patients with severe hemophilia and most with moderate and mild hemophilia only receive on-demand therapy [70]. Individuals with mild hemophilia often are managed with desmopressin, which releases stored FVIII from blood vessel walls [71].

4.7.2 Treatment of Arthritis

Briefly, symptom relief, prevention of the progression of the joint damage, and maintenance of function are the physician goals in hemophilic arthritis. These are similar to inflammatory arthropathy. In hemophilic arthritis, in an early stage, these goals can be achieved by limiting the effects of chronic synovitis and more importantly by early treatment of hemarthrosis. In the subject with degenerative changes, function would be corrected by surgical/physical methods with adequate hemostatic cover [4].

4.7.3 Management of Bleeding

The first choice for treatment of joint disease in patients with hemophilia is the prophylaxis with factor concentrates which is recommended by the World Health Organization (WHO) and the World Federation of Hemophilia (WFH). The level of the factor must be greater than 1% for the maximum profit. This can usually be achieved by giving 25–50 IU/kg of FVIII three times per week [72].

4.7.4 Adjunctive Management

Analgesics like paracetamol/acetaminophen or aspirin-containing drugs can be used to relieve the arthritis pain, but aspirin-containing drugs sometimes exacerbate bleeding. So milder opioid painkillers are more common.

4.7.5 Anti-inflammatory Treatment

To treat chronic synovitis, some experts have recommended the intra-articular corticosteroid infusion.

4.7.6 Rest, Ice, Compression, and Elevation (RICE)

This strategy may be useful to relieve the pain of the patients with minor pain, but prolonged rest may cause motion limitation and muscle atrophy [73].

4.7.7 Physiotherapy

Physiotherapy is an important way to preserve or return movement and function to the joints. It also reduces swelling and pain, prevents injury, and maintains muscle strength [74].

4.7.8 Joint Aspiration

In hip hemarthrosis and other major and painful hemarthrosis, aspiration can be prescribed and should be performed immediately after a bleeding episode (<12 h) [74].

4.7.9 Surgical Treatment

When conservative therapies fail, open surgical procedures are often the best or even the only way to cure patients with severe joint disease. The advantages of surgery must be more than the potential risks, particularly in patients with severe hemophilia and/or inhibitors.

4.7.10 Synovectomy

If a patient suffers from synovitis that is refractory to treatment, synovectomy is recommended. However, the first step to treat incurable synovitis and to relieve its pain is the use of nonsurgical synovectomies (synoviortheses), which involve the percutaneous injection of radioisotopes or chemical agents. This treatment can generate fibrosis of the hypertrophied synovium [75, 76]. However, sometimes inevitably synovectomy is the best way to prevent not only the progression of hemophilic arthropathy but also the development of end-stage arthropathy. Severe cartilage damage is a limiting factor to use this method.

4.7.11 Joint Debridement

Joint debridement is a surgical procedure that removes synovitis in young patients to prevent or delay articular arthroplasty [77].

4.7.12 Joint Arthroplasty

To reach the normal quality of life in patients with severely annoying joint pain, replacement surgery, which also is known as arthroplasty, could be considered. Results from the most commonly replaced joints are generally good or excellent [78].

4.7.13 Fusion (Arthrodesis)

Fusion is also known as arthrodesis. It comprises joint removal and fusion of the bones. Ankle arthrodesis is carried out today. Other joints in the foot can move normally. So the patient can have a close-to-normal walk [78].

4.7.14 Treatment in Carriers

Most carriers are asymptomatic, but, if they are subject to trauma or surgical intervention, they may show prolonged bleeding. In these instances, carriers must be treated, in the same way, as patients with hemophilia. Pre-existing clotting factor level and the cause and severity of the bleed determine the dosage and duration of treatment [27].

4.8 Problems Related to Treatment of Hemophilia

Virus infections and immunization against FVIII are the most reported problems related to treatment of patient with hemophilia. The main issue with factor replacement therapy is the development of inhibitor antibodies against FVIII. In fact as the patient's body does not have its own copy, recognizes the "normal form" FVIII as foreign. The consequence is that in these cases, FVIII infusions are ineffective. Recently FVIII a has become available as a treatment for hemorrhage in patient with hemophilia and FVIII inhibitors [70, 79]. An inhibitor may be suspected when unexpected bleeding in the response to treatment is not stopped by factor substitution as quickly as it should. After suspicion, the inhibitor may be discovered during routine screening as it defines later, and after detection, its titer must be determined. Inhibitor titer is important for the physician's decision to select a suitable treatment based on patient's inhibitor titer.

4.8.1 Inhibitor

An inhibitor is a polyclonal high-affinity immunoglobulin G (IgG) that is directed against the FVIII protein [80]. IgG4 antibodies are the predominant antibodies that do not fix complement [80, 81]. The domains A2, A3, and C2 are the main domains that inhibitory antibodies are directed against them [82].

The most dangerous complication of the hemophilia A management is development of inhibitor against FVIII. Based on data reported worldwide, the frequency of inhibitor is 5–10% patients with hemophilia without consideration the severity of disorder, and 10–15% in severe patients [83, 84].

Based on different studies from around the world, prevalence of inhibitor in hemophilia A is more in compare with hemophilia B [85]. For instant, in Saudi Arabia, patients with FVIII inhibitor were observed in 43 (29.3%) out of the 147 patients, and only 1 out of the 54 patients developed FIX inhibitor [86].

4.8.2 Inhibitor Generation Risk Factors

The following risk factors were mentioned as the main risk factors for inhibitor development [82, 87].

1. Number of exposures to clotting factor concentrates
2. Increased dosage of clotting factor concentration
3. Spanish ethnicity or black race
4. The positive history of inhibitors in family
5. High-risk mutation such as multiple exon deletion or stop codon

4.8.3 Inhibitor Evaluation

Bethesda assay for several mixtures of patient plasma with normal pool plasma (NPP) by different, distinctive dilutions and also several control mixtures containing buffer and NPP with different, distinctive dilutions are incubated. Then remaining FVIII activity in the test tube is compared with those in control tube. Therefore, the percent of residual FVIII activity in the patient mix is converted to Bethesda units (BU). One BU is defined as the amount of inhibitor producing a residual activity of 50% [88]. In Nijmegen assay, modified method NPP that is used in patient and control mixtures are buffered with imidazole, and control tube contains FVIII-deficient plasma instead of buffer [88, 89].

4.8.4 Treatment in Patient with Inhibitor

The healthcare costs associated with inhibitor formation can be worrying because of the amount and type of treatment products required to stop bleeding in such patients. In addition, these patients are much likely to be hospitalized for a bleeding complications, and they are at increased risk of lethal hemorrhges [90–92].

4.8.5 Virus Infections

Adults with hemophilia have one of the highest prevalence of hepatitis C virus (HCV) infectious among all populations at risk of HCV infection. Prior to 1987, approximately all patients treated for hemophilia with plasma products were exposed to HCV, and more than 80% had chronic infections. On the other hand, ribavirin, an essential component of HCV therapy, typically induces hemolysis [93]. In a study on the 350 patients with hemophilia A and B, 232 individuals (about 66%) had been infected with HCV. There was no independent risk factor based on multivariate logistic regression analysis [94]. The prevalence of HCV infection serologically among HCV-infected patient with hemophilia was evaluated. It is reported that the prevalence of anti-HCV antibodies is 66%. Out of 31 patients with HCV/HIV, 21 persons (67.7%) had no history of transfusion. The authors noted that contaminated FVIII (clotting factor) could be responsible for disease acquisition [95].

4.8.6 Treatment of Bleeding in Patients with Inhibitor

In persons with low-responding inhibitors and low Bethesda titers (less than 5 units), therapy with further FVIII replacement products is usually possible. In these cases, higher doses of the factor and/or more frequent (or continuous) factor infusions may be useful to overcome the effect of antibody. However, when there is a high titer antibody (at least five Bethesda units) in the body, higher dose of therapeutic FVIII or FIX is usually not effective because the inhibitor can neutralize even the large factor doses. Plasmapheresis or immune absorption may be useful in eliminating inhibitors, especially when a life-threatening bleeding is treated with an excess factor but a high level of inhibitor exists. However, as soon as the patient receives the factor, he makes large amounts of new antibody within several days. The further approach is bypass therapy, which includes various therapeutic products. These include prothrombin complex concentrate (PCC), activated PCC (APCC), and rFVIIa. Therapeutic choice is based on several circumstances such as inhibitor characteristics, nature, and severity of the bleeding, age, and treatment response pattern of the individual (Table 4.7) [85].

High-Dose Clotting Factor Concentrates People with low titer inhibitor (<5 BU) may be treated with higher amount or more frequent factor concentrate.

Table 4.7 Treatment of bleeding in patients with hemophilia A and inhibitor

Inhibitor titer	Approach	Advantages	Disadvantages
<5 Bethesda units	Higher doses of the factor and/or more frequent, or continuous factor infusion	May be useful to overcome the antibody	It may trigger stronger immune response and increases inhibitor titer
≥5 Bethesda units with life-threatening bleeding	Plasmapheresis or immune adsorption, then factor replacement	Eliminate the risk of bleeding or lethal episodes	After the patient receives, the factor provokes formation of a large amounts of new antibody within few days
≥5 Bethesda units without life-threatening bleeding	Bypass therapy with PCC	Bypasses the requirement for factor	1) Short-acting 2) Paradoxically causes either more bleeding or exces clotting 3) Worsens problem if antifibrinolytic drugs are used along with PCC 4) Contains small amounts of FVIII and stimulates new antibody production
	APCC with doses of 50–100 units/kg every 8–24 h, depending on the severity of the bleeding	Effective for 60–90% of musculoskeletal bleeds, major and minor surgery prophylaxis	Same with PCC
	rFVIIa multiple doses of 90 units/kg or more every 2–6 h	1) Bypasses the requirement for factor 2) Effective in the prevention and treatment of joint hemorrhage, life-threatening bleeding, and surgical bleeding 3) Contains no FVIII, therefore doesn't restimulate antibody production	1) Short-acting 2) Excess blood clotting
	Immune tolerance induction (ITI) infusions of variable doses of FVIII or FIX administered for a period of weeks to years in an effort to tolerize the immune system	Accept treatment with the missing clotting factor without producing further antibodies	Time-consuming and expensive

Consequently factor VII (rFVIIa) is frequently the bypass therapy of choice for patient with hemophilia *FVIII* factor VIII, *rFVII* recombinant factor VII, *PCC* prothrombin complex concentrate, *APCC* activated prothrombin complex concentrate

Bypassing Agents Bypassing agents, which can proceed the coagulation cascade without the requirement for the desired factor are used to treat bleeding complications in people with high titer inhibitors (>5 BU).

Immune Tolerance Induction (ITI) Therapy The purpose of ITI therapy is to halt the inhibitor production by the immune system of individuals with hemophilia. This method teaches the body to accept factor as a normal part of blood. In this way, patients receive more frequent, low dose factor [96].

4.8.7 Bypassing Therapy Products

Factor eight inhibitor bypass activity (FEIBA) is an anti-inhibitor coagulant complex, which is indicated in patients with hemophilia A or hemophilia B and inhibitors for [97]:

- Control and prevention of bleeding episodes
- Peri-operative management
- Prophylaxis to prevent or decrease the rate of acute bleeding

4.8.8 Autoplex

Autoplex is an APCC. Despite the unknown mechanism of action for bypassing FVIII, Autoplex appears to be a useful and needed interim product and is safe and effective in management of bleeding. To avoid possible thrombosis, simultaneous use of fibrinolytic inhibitors must be avoided [98].

4.8.9 Mouth Care in Hemophilia

For patients with severe hemophilia, factor replacement therapy is necessary before surgery or regional block injections. Some studies proposed a dose of 50 IU/kg FVIII before a tooth extraction in patients with hemophilia. The safe and cost-effective method to control bleeding due to teeth extraction is the use of fibrin glue and antifibrinolytic agents such as tranexamic acid.

Lifestyle is significantly responsible for gum diseases. Smoking and tobacco use may contribute to periodontal disease and oral cancer. Oral hygiene is the best way to prevent gum diseases such as chronic periodontitis gingivitis [39, 99].

4.8.10 Following Rules Might Be Useful

Reducing the frequency and amount of sugars in the diet, avoiding smoking, and using fluoride, mouth protection, and soft plastic mouth guards may be needed to prevent damage from trauma, tooth grinding (bruxism), and acid erosion in individuals with hemophilia [39, 100].

4.9 Gene Therapy

The most promising curative strategy in hemophilia is gene therapy. Theoretically, this process includes identifying the missing or defective clotting factor gene in a patient, replaces it by a normal gene fragment and inserts the normal gene in the genetic material of cells of the hematopoietic system, liver, skin, muscle, or blood vessels. Because the *F9* gene is very large and difficult to insert compared with the *F9* gene, hemophilia B was the first candidate to be treated by gene therapy. Several studies have reported that gene therapy will be effective by using the test tube and animal studies. Recently, the *F9* gene was successfully administered in dogs with FIX deficiency [101]. A clinical trial that began in 2010 has reported long-lasting conversion of severe hemophilia B to mild status by elevating FIX levels above 5% [102]. Subsequently five other trials in hemophilia B have started using similar vectors based on adeno-associated virus (AAV).

The goal of treatment of gene-deficient diseases is the elimination of disease for the lifetime of the patient. Gene therapy is the best and only way to achieve this goal, which contains the replacement of the faulty gene sequence with the correct one. Continuous delivery of FVIII in a patient with hemophilia by gene therapy would result in a higher clinical development than nonpersistent FVIII administration. First clinical trials attempting to treat hemophilia with gene transfer primarily demonstrate good safety but without good efficacy. The next efforts, which reengineered the vector plasmids and delivery systems, resulted in markedly improved outcomes in animal models. Retroviral vectors that can permanently insert the *F8* gene into the DNA of the host cell appear as the most suitable things for this specific purpose (Fig. 4.7) [103].

Gene therapy strategies can be divided in two groups:

1. Gene replacement by an ex vivo or in vivo approach
2. Other proposed approaches

4.9.1 The Gene Replacement by an Ex Vivo or In Vivo Approach

Ex vivo and in vivo treatments for hemophilia gene therapy have been proposed. Ex vivo gene therapy involves isolating the cells from the patient, expanding and genetically modifying them in the culture medium with vectors which express FVIII, then transferring the transfected cells to the patient's liver, skin, etc. Different cell types such as skin fibroblasts, endothelial cells, epithelial cells, myoblasts, hematopoietic stem/progenitor cells, and bone marrow (BM) stromal cells have been considered as potential targets for hemophilia gene therapy [104].

Another particular creative target is megakaryocytes. An ex vivo hemophilic treatment gene that uses megakaryocytes has shown an effective homeostatic

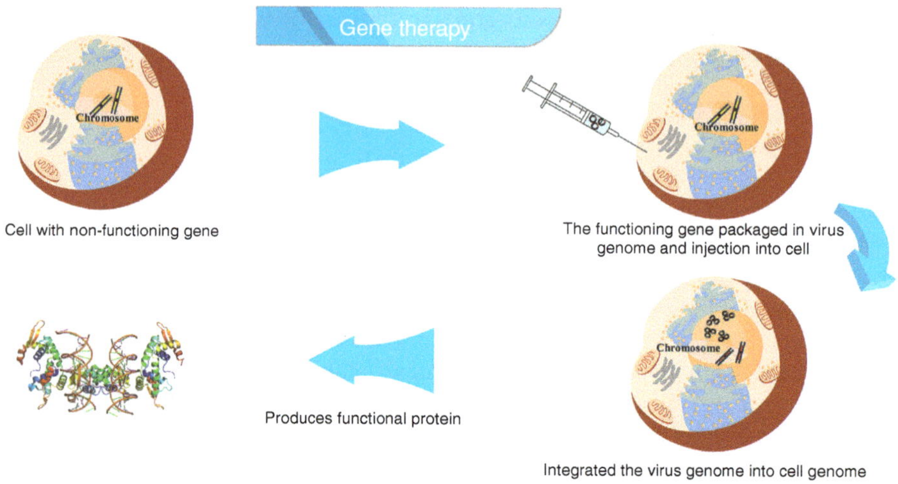

Fig. 4.7 The in vivo approach of gene therapy. The target gene packaged in virus genome and then delivered in the body organ such as the liver. The virus genome is integrated into cell genome and produces functional protein. *ITR* long terminal repeats, *PA* palindromic repeat

response in standard hemophilia [75, 105]. The initial cell capacity for transferring FVIII to the bloodstream is highly dependent on the site of implantation. The liver appears to be a suitable target for hemophilia gene therapy. FVIII produced in the transduced hepatocyte should have readily access to the circulation. In addition, the stability of FVIII increases when it is secreted in the environment in which it has access to circulation VWF or to VWF produced in sinusoidal endothelial. In contrast, coagulation factors produced in non-hepatic tissues might not be properly processed due to differences in post-translational modification. Ex vivo gene therapy is based on the use of viral vectors (especially retrovirus) and sometimes in non-viral transfer systems [76].

The in vivo gene therapy is more affordable than ex vivo. However, the host immune response toward the viral vector is the major drawback of in vivo gene therapy. The gene delivery system in the gene therapy of hemophilia should be efficient, safe, and non-immunogenic and allows for long-term gene expression. Most importantly, the compare between gene therapies for hemophilia A with existing protein replacement therapies must be in favor of gene therapy [106]. Retroviral, lentiviral, adenoviral, and AAV vectors, each with their own benefits and limitations, are the most commonly used vectors in hemophilia gene therapy. Moloney murine leukemia virus (MoMLV)-based retroviral vectors are the first and the most commonly used vectors for clinical trials [107]. Although non-viral vectors are less immunogenic than viral vectors, the viral vectors are the most chosen method (Table 4.8) [106]. If the immune system is stimulated, the treatment strategy can be combined with immune-modulating drugs. For instance, inhibition of poly (ADP-ribose) polymerase-1 (PARP-1) and nuclear factor kappa B (NF-κB) signaling

Table 4.8 Viral-based vectors used for gene therapy of factors VIII deficiency

Vector	Nucleic acid	Advantages	Disadvantages
Retroviral	RNA	Efficient transduction Genomic integration Persistent expression	Oncogene derivation Random insertion Cell division-dependent (except for lentiviral)
Adenoviral	DNA	Transduces nondividing cells Accommodates large cDNAs don't have chronic toxicity	Immune responses to AV Episomal (no integration) Transient expression
Adeno-associated viral	DNA	Integration (partial) Persistent expression Different serotypes	Limited size of cDNA Possible rearrangements Pre-existing anti-AAV antibody able to prevent successful transduction Liver disease in patient especially HCV positives Immune response to the capsid

AV adenoviral, *AAV* adeno-associated viral, *HCV* hepatitis C virus

synergistically downregulates immune response against recombinant AAV vectors. A combination of non-viral vector systems with some viral components can combine the benefits of both systems. The *F9* gene is cloned, but this is too large to be packaged efficiently into any commonly used gene therapy vectors. However, there is a full-length recombinant PEGylated FVIII [108]. FVIII-BDD cDNA had been shown to express a higher level of FVIII protein as compared to the full-length FVIII cDNA and is suitable to lie in restricted packaging limits of vectors [106]. The packaging capacity of AAV is about 5 kb, but the FVIII expression cassette is about 7 kb. The use of a FVIII-BDD (4.37 kb in size) overcomes this challenge but constrains a tight constraint on the size of the regulatory elements that control FVIII expressions [109]. Several FVIII-BDD products by different trade names are available including BAY94-9027, Novoeight, Eloctate, and others [108]. Studies in hemophilia A dogs that had developed inhibitors have demonstrated that inhibitors would be eradicated following AAV-mediated liver-directed gene therapy [110]. Proprotein convertases are a family of proteins that activate other proteins by proteolytic activity. One member of this family is furin [111]. When furin processes FVIII-BDD, its procoagulant activity is degraded. This process also reduces its secretion. Therefore, inhibition of furin leads to secretion of FVIII-BDD in mammalian cells [112]. Now the challenges include ensuring long-term stable protein expression, vector immunogenicity, and the potential risk of insertional mutagenesis and hepatic toxicity (Table 4.8) [113].

Advantages of Lentivirus (LV) Transduction:

1. A long-term therapeutic effect can result.
2. There are some evidences, which say that a single treatment of LV-mediated gene therapy will be sufficient for lifelong effect.

3. LV can transduce both nondividing and dividing cells, and this is the most important advantage of LV in comparison with traditional retroviral vectors. This leads to a considerable increase in LV efficacy in the targeting of primitive stem cells.
4. An addition to SIN LTR elements in self-inactivating (SIN)-LVs provided improved safety by reducing transactivation capacity [114].

4.9.2 Adeno-Associated Virus Gene Therapy for Hemophilia A

Recently a trial has reported that patients with severe hemophilia A treated by peripheral vein infusion of a single dose of vector achieved and have maintained normal level of FVIII for more than a year (Biomarin study).

4.9.3 Other Proposed Approaches

1. Aminoglycoside antibiotics such as gentamycin can transiently suppress the nonsense mutations at the ribosomal level in a patient with hemophilia. This could potentially convert severe hemophilia to a moderately severe phenotype, however, failed to show a clinically significant effect [115].
2. At the RNA level, trans-splicing could potentially be feasible and effective to inversions in mice [116].
3. Some prokaryotes such as bacteria and even archaea use the clustered regularly interspaced short palindromic repeats or Regularly Interspaced Short Palindromic Repeats (CRISPR) and CRISPR-associated (Cas) system in their immune system. This provides the CRISPR/Cas9 genome editing technology that allows for permanent changes in the genes of organisms [117]. This process leads to the creation of a double-strand break (DSB) at a distinctive region of the genome. Then the DSB(s) are typically repaired by an error-prone path which is named nonhomologous end joining (NHEJ) or error-free path which is known as homology-directed repair (HDR). Thus, the HDR pathway could be used to correct the monogenetic diseases including hemophilia after CRISPR-induced DSB. However, it has been reported that gene correction with NHEJ is also possible [118].

Acknowledgment We appreciate Professor Edward Tuddenham for his valuable comments that significantly improved the quality of this chapter.

References

1. Gitschier J, Wood WI, Goralka TM, Wion KL, Chen EY, Eaton DH, et al. Characterization of the human factor VIII gene. Nature. 1984;312:326–30.
2. Bell B, Canty D, Audet M. Hemophilia: an updated review. Pediatrics in review. Am Acad Pediatr. 1995;16(8):290–8.

3. Anwarul M, Yakub C. A review on hemophilia in children. Bangladesh J Child Health. 2013;37:27–40.
4. Madhok R, York J, Sturrock RD. Haemophilic arthritis. Ann Rheum Dis. 1991;50(8):588.
5. Luck Jr JV, Silva M, Rodriguez-Merchan CE, Ghalambor N, Zahiri CA, Finn RS. Hemophilic arthropathy. J Am Acad Orthop Surg. 2004;12(4):234–45.
6. Moser KA. Chromogenic factor VIII activity assay. Am J Hematol. 2014;89(7):781–4.
7. White G, Rosendaal F, Aledort L, Lusher J, Rothschild C, Ingerslev J. Recommendation of the scientific subcommittee on factor VIII and factor IX of the scientific and standardization committee of the International Society on Thrombosis and Haemostasis. Thromb Haemost. 2001;85(3):560.
8. Srivastava A, Brewer A, Mauser-Bunschoten E, Key N, Kitchen S, Llinas A, et al. Guidelines for the management of hemophilia. Haemophilia. 2013;19(1). https://doi.org/10.1111/j.1365-2516.2012.02909.x.
9. Bowen D. Haemophilia A and haemophilia B: molecular insights. J Clin Pathol. 2002;55(2):127.
10. Keeney S, Mitchell M, Goodeve A. The molecular analysis of haemophilia A: a guideline from the UK haemophilia centre doctors' organization haemophilia genetics laboratory network. Haemophilia. 2005;11(4):387–97.
11. Bihoreau N, Pin S, Kersabiec AM, Vidot F, Fontaine-Aupart MP. Copper-atom identification in the active and inactive forms of plasma-derived FVIII and recombinant FVIII-ΔII. Eur J Biochem. 1994;222(1):41–8.
12. Tagliavacca L, Moon N, Dunham WR, Kaufman RJ. Identification and functional requirement of Cu (I) and its ligands within coagulation factor VIII. J Biol Chem. 1997;272(43):27428–34.
13. O'brien S, Mayewski P, Meeker L, Meese D, Twickler M, Whitlow S. Complexity of Holocene climate as reconstructed from a Greenland ice core. Science. 1995;270(5244):1962–4.
14. Bajaj MS, Birktoft JJ, Steer SA, Bajaj SP. Structure and biology of tissue factor pathway inhibitor. Thromb Haemost. 2001;86(4):959–72.
15. Macedo-Ribeiro S, Bode W, Huber R, Quinn-Allen MA, Kim SW, Ortel TL, et al. Crystal structures of the membrane-binding C2 domain of human coagulation factor V. Nature. 1999;402(6760):434–9.
16. Church WR, Jernigan RL, Toole J, Hewick RM, Knopf J, Knutson GJ, et al. Coagulation factors V and VIII and ceruloplasmin constitute a family of structurally related proteins. Proc Natl Acad Sci. 1984;81(22):6934–7.
17. Pratt KP, Shen BW, Takeshima K, Davie EW, Fujikawa K, Stoddard BL. Structure of the C2 domain of human factor VIII at 1.5 Å resolution. Nature. 1999;402(6760):439–42.
18. McMullen BA, Fujikawa K, Davie EW, Hedner U, Ezban M. Locations of disulfide bonds and free cysteines in the heavy and light chains of recombinant human factor VIII (antihemophilic factor A). Protein Sci. 1995;4(4):740–6.
19. Saenko EL, Shima M, Rajalakshmi K, Scandella D. A role for the C2 domain of factor VIII in binding to von Willebrand factor. J Biol Chem. 1994;269(15):11601–5.
20. Watzka SB, Steiner M, Samorapoompichit P, Gross K, Coles JG, Wolner E, et al. Establishment of vessel-like structures in long-term three-dimensional tissue culture of myocardium: an electron microscopy study. Tissue Eng. 2004;10(11–12):1684–94.
21. Faridi NJ, Kumar P, Husain N, Siddiqi MI. Factor VIII genetic mutations and protein alterations in hemophilia A: a review. Clin Rev Opin. 2014;6(1):1–10.
22. Thorelli E, Kaufman RJ, Dahlbäck B. The C-terminal region of the factor V B-domain is crucial for the anticoagulant activity of factor V. J Biol Chem. 1998;273(26):16140–5.
23. Swieringa F, Kuijpers MJ, Lamers MM, Van der Meijden PE, Heemskerk JW. Rate-limiting roles of the tenase complex of factors VIII and IX in platelet procoagulant activity and formation of platelet-fibrin thrombi under flow. Haematologica. 2015;100(6):748–56.
24. Grillberger L, Kreil TR, Nasr S, Reiter M. Emerging trends in plasma-free manufacturing of recombinant protein therapeutics expressed in mammalian cells. Biotechnol J. 2009;4(2):186–201.
25. Soucie JM, Evatt B, Jackson D. Occurrence of hemophilia in the United States. Am J Hematol. 1998;59(4):288–94.

26. Manno CS. Difficult pediatric diagnoses: bruising and bleeding. Pediatr Clin N Am. 1991;38(3):637–55.
27. Mauser-Bunschoten EP. Symptomatic carriers of hemophilia, vol. 46. Montreal: World Federation of Hemophilia; 2008. p. 2–3.
28. Antonarakis SE, Rossiter J, Young M, Horst J, De Moerloose P, Sommer S, et al. Factor VIII gene inversions in severe hemophilia A: results of an international consortium study. Blood. 1995;86(6):2206–12.
29. Plug I, Mauser-Bunschoten EP, Bröcker-Vriends AH, van Amstel HKP, van der Bom JG, van Diemen-Homan JE, et al. Bleeding in carriers of hemophilia. Blood. 2006;108(1):52–6.
30. Khair K, Liesner R. Bruising and bleeding in infants and children–a practical approach. Br J Haematol. 2006;133(3):221–31.
31. Kasper CK. Hereditary plasma clotting factor disorders and their management. Haemophilia. 2000;6:13–27.
32. Sahu S, Lata I, Singh S, Kumar M. Revisiting hemophilia management in acute medicine. J Emerg Trauma Shock. 2011;4(2):292.
33. Shastry SP, Kaul R, Baroudi K, Umar D. Hemophilia A: dental considerations and management. J Int Soc Prev Community Dent. 2014;4(Suppl 3):S147.
34. Hardisty RM, Ingram GIC. Bleeding disorders: investigation and management. Hoboken: Blackwell Scientific Publications; 1965.
35. Holme PA, Tait RC, Combescure C, Berntorp E, Tagliaferri A, Staritz P, et al. Renal status and hematuria in older patients with hemophilia. Blood. 2015;126(23):2290.
36. Kulkarni R, Soucie JM, Evatt B. Renal disease among males with haemophilia. Haemophilia. 2003;9(6):703–10.
37. Sørensen B, Benson G, Bladen M, Classey S, Keeling D, McLaughlin P, et al. Management of muscle haematomas in patients with severe haemophilia in an evidence-poor world. Haemophilia. 2012;18(4):598–606.
38. Balkan C, Kavakli K, Karapinar D. Iliopsoas haemorrhage in patients with haemophilia: results from one Centre. Haemophilia. 2005;11(5):463–7.
39. Jover Cerveró A, Poveda Roda R, Bagán JV, Jiménez Soriano Y. Dental treatment of patients with coagulation factor alterations: an update. Med Oral Patol Oral Cir Bucal. 2007;12(5):380–7.
40. Rodriguez-Merchan EC. Acute compartment syndrome in haemophilia. Blood Coagul Fibrinolysis. 2013;24(7):677–82.
41. Leslie R, Catherine M. Modern management of haemophilic arthropathy. Br J Haematol. 2007;136(6):777–87.
42. Ghosh K, Ghosh K. Management of chronic synovitis in patients with hemophilia: with special reference to developing countries. Indian J Hematol Blood Transfusion. 2008;24(4):151–4.
43. Nair PS, Shetty SD, Chandrakala S, Ghosh K. Mutations in intron 1 and intron 22 inversion negative haemophilia A patients from western India. PLoS One. 2014;9(5):e97337.
44. Vehar GA, Keyt B, Eaton D, Rodriguez H, O'Brien DP, Rotblat F, et al. Structure of human factor VIII. Nature. 1984;312(5992):337–42.
45. Margaglione M, Castaman G, Morfini M, Rocino A, Santagostino E, Tagariello G, et al. The Italian AICE-genetics hemophilia A database: results and correlation with clinical phenotype. Haematologica. 2008;93(5):722–8.
46. Stenson PD, Mort M, Ball EV, Howells K, Phillips AD, Thomas NS, et al. The human gene mutation database: 2008 update. Genome Med. 2009;1(1):13.
47. Salviato R, Belvini D, Radossi P, Tagariello G. Factor VIII gene intron 1 inversion: lower than expected prevalence in Italian haemophiliac severe patients. Haemophilia. 2004;10(2):194–6.
48. Schröder J, EL-MAARRI O, Schwaab R, Müller C, Oldenburg J, Factor VIII. Intron-1 inversion: frequency and inhibitor prevalence. J Thromb Haemost. 2006;4(5):1141–3.
49. Tantawy AA. Molecular genetics of hemophilia A: clinical perspectives. Egyptian J Med Human Genet. 2010;11(2):105–14.
50. Chen YC, Hu SH, Cheng SN, Chao TY. Genetic analysis of haemophilia A in Taiwan. Haemophilia. 2010;16(3):538–44.

51. Lakich D, Kazazian HH, Antonarakis SE, Gitschier J. Inversions disrupting the factor VIII gene are a common cause of severe haemophilia A. Nat Genet. 1993;5(3):236–41.
52. Levinson B, Kenwrick S, Lakich D, Hammonds G, Gitschier J. A transcribed gene in an intron of the human factor VIII gene. Genomics. 1990;7(1):1–11.
53. Naylor JA, Buck D, Green P, Williamson H, Bentley D, Gianneill F. Investigation of the factor VIII intron 22 repeated region (int22h) and the associated inversion junctions. Hum Mol Genet. 1995;4(7):1217–24.
54. Gitschier J. Molecular genetics of hemophilia A. Schweiz Med Wochenschr. 1989;119(39):1329–31.
55. Kemball-Cook G, Tuddenham EG. The factor VIII mutation database on the world wide web: the haemophilia a mutation, search, test and resource site HAMSTeRS update (version 3.0). Nucleic Acids Res. 1997;25(1):128–32.
56. Goodeve AC, Peake IR. The molecular basis of hemophilia A: genotype-phenotype relationships and inhibitor development. Semin Thromb Hemost. 2003;29:23–30.
57. El-Maarri O, Herbiniaux U, Graw J, Schröder J, Terzic A, Watzka M, et al. Analysis of mRNA in hemophilia A patients with undetectable mutations reveals normal splicing in the factor VIII gene. J Thromb Haemost. 2005;3(2):332–9.
58. Chandler WL, Ferrell C, Lee J, Tun T, Kha H. Comparison of three methods for measuring factor VIII levels in plasma. Am J Clin Pathol. 2003;120(1):34–9.
59. Kitchen S, McCraw A, Echenagucia M. Diagnosis of hemophilia and other bleeding disorders. A laboratory manual. Montreal: World Federation of Hemophilia; 2000.
60. Hillarp A, Bowyer A, Ezban M, Persson P, Kitchen S. Measuring FVIII activity of glycopegylated recombinant factor VIII, N8-GP, with commercially available one-stage clotting and chromogenic assay kits: a two-centre study. Haemophilia. 2017;23(3):458–65.
61. Di Paola J, Smith M, Klamroth R, Mannucci P, Kollmer C, Feingold J, et al. ReFacto® and Advate®: a single-dose, randomized, two-period crossover pharmacokinetics study in subjects with haemophilia A. Haemophilia. 2007;13(2):124–30.
62. Mei B, Pan C, Jiang H, Tjandra H, Strauss J, Chen Y, et al. Rational design of a fully active, long-acting PEGylated factor VIII for hemophilia A treatment. Blood. 2010;116(2):270–9.
63. Peyvandi F, Oldenburg J, Friedman K. A critical appraisal of one-stage and chromogenic assays of factor VIII activity. J Thromb Haemost. 2016;14(2):248–61.
64. Reding M, Ng H, Poulsen LH, Eyster M, Pabinger I, Shin HJ, et al. Safety and efficacy of BAY 94-9027, a prolonged-half-life factor VIII. J Thromb Haemost. 2017;15(3):411–9.
65. Powell JS, Josephson NC, Quon D, Ragni MV, Cheng G, Li E, et al. Safety and prolonged activity of recombinant factor VIII fc fusion protein in hemophilia A patients. Blood. 2012;119(13):3031–7.
66. Turecek P, Bossard M, Graninger M, Gritsch H, Höllriegl W, Kaliwoda M, et al. BAX 855, a PEGylated rFVIII product with prolonged half-life. Hamostaseologie. 2012;32(1):S29–38.
67. Zhang Y, Limsakun T, Bensen-Kennedy DM, Veldman A, Yao Z. Population pharmacokinetic modeling and simulation of recombinant single-chain factor VIII (r VIII-SingleChain) in patients with hemophilia A. J Thromb Haemost. 2017;15(6):1106–14.
68. Ma AD, Roberts HR, Escobar MA. Hemophilia and hemostasis: a case-based approach to management. Hoboken: Wiley; 2012.
69. O'grady NP, Alexander M, Burns LA, Dellinger EP, Garland J, Heard SO, et al. Guidelines for the prevention of intravascular catheter-related infections. Clin Infect Dis. 2011;52(9):e162-e93.
70. Ljung R. The risk associated with indwelling catheters in children with haemophilia. Br J Haematol. 2007;138(5):580–6.
71. Franchini M, Lippi G. The use of desmopressin in acquired haemophilia A: a systematic review. Blood Transfus. 2011;9(4):377.
72. Aledort L, Haschmeyer RH, Pettersson H. A longitudinal study of orthopaedic outcomes for severe factor-VIII-deficient haemophiliacs. J Intern Med. 1994;236(4):391–9.
73. Knobe K, Berntorp E. Haemophilia and joint disease: pathophysiology, evaluation and management. J Comorb. 2011;1(1):51–9.

74. Rodriguez-Merchan E. Articular bleeding (hemarthrosis) in hemophilia. In: Schulman S, editor. An orthopedist's point of view. 2nd ed. Montréal: The World Federation of Hemophilia; 2008. p. 1–5.
75. Shi Q, Fahs SA, Wilcox DA, Kuether EL, Morateck PA, Mareno N, et al. Syngeneic transplantation of hematopoietic stem cells that are genetically modified to express factor VIII in platelets restores hemostasis to hemophilia A mice with preexisting FVIII immunity. Blood. 2008;112(7):2713–21.
76. Rea CJ, Aledort L, Rangarajan S. Haemophilia: a race for cure. Hematol Transfus Int J. 2017;4(5):00094.
77. Rodriguez-Merchan E. Ankle surgery in haemophilia with special emphasis on arthroscopic debridement. Haemophilia. 2008;14(5):913–9.
78. Rodriguez-Merchan E. Orthopaedic surgery in persons with haemophilia. Thromb Haemost. 2003;89(1):34–42.
79. Pagon R, Adam M, Ardinger H, Wallace S, Amemiya A, Bean L, et al. Hemophilia A, GeneReviews®. Seattle: University of Washington; 2000.
80. Fulcher CA, de Graaf Mahoney S, Zimmerman TSFVIII. Inhibitor IgG subclass and FVIII polypeptide specificity determined by immunoblotting. Blood. 1987;69(5):1475–80.
81. Lollar P. Pathogenic antibodies to coagulation factors. Part one: factor VIII and factor IX. J Thromb Haemost. 2004;2(7):1082–95.
82. Witmer C, Young G. Factor VIII inhibitors in hemophilia A: rationale and latest evidence. Ther Adv Hematol. 2013;4(1):59–72.
83. Wintrobe MM. Wintrobe's clinical hematology/clinical hematology: Wolters Kluwer Health/ Lippincott Williams & Wilkins; 2009.
84. Astermark J. Overview of inhibitors. Semin Hematol. 2006;43:S3–7.
85. DiMichele DM. Inhibitors in haemophilia: a primer. Haemophilia. 2000;6:38–40.
86. Owaidah T, Al Momen A, Alzahrani H, Almusa A, Alkasim F, Tarawah A, et al. The prevalence of factor VIII and IX inhibitors among Saudi patients with hemophilia: results from the Saudi national hemophilia screening program. Medicine. 2017;96(2):e5456.
87. Hoots W, Shapiro A. Factor VIII and factor IX inhibitors in patients with hemophilia. Waltham, MA: UpToDate; 2016.
88. Miller C, Platt S, Rice A, Kelly F, Soucie J. Validation of Nijmegen–Bethesda assay modifications to allow inhibitor measurement during replacement therapy and facilitate inhibitor surveillance. J Thromb Haemost. 2012;10(6):1055–61.
89. Duncan E, Collecutt M, Street A. Nijmegen-Bethesda assay to measure factor VIII inhibitors. Methods Mol Biol. 2013;992:321–33.
90. Guh S, Grosse S, McAlister S, Kessler C, Soucie J. Healthcare expenditures for males with haemophilia and employer-sponsored insurance in the United States, 2008. Haemophilia. 2012;18(2):268–75.
91. Guh S, Grosse S, McAlister S, Kessler C, Soucie J. Health care expenditures for medicaid-covered males with haemophilia in the United States, 2008. Haemophilia. 2012;18(2):276–83.
92. Walsh CE, Soucie JM, Miller CH. Impact of inhibitors on hemophilia A mortality in the United States. Am J Hematol. 2015;90(5):400–5.
93. Orman ES, Fried MW. Hepatitis C viral infection in patients with hemophilia and hemolytic disorders. Clin Liver Dis. 2012;1(3):95–7.
94. Reza Yazdani M, Kassaian N, Ataei B, Nokhodian Z, Adibi P. Hepatitis C virus infection in patients with hemophilia in Isfahan, Iran. Int J Prev Med. 2012;3(Suppl 1):S89–93.
95. Al-Kubaisy W, Al-Naib K, Habib M. Prevalence of HCV/HIV co-infection among haemophilia patients in Baghdad. East Mediterr Health J. 2006;12(3/4):264.
96. Berntorp E, Shapiro A, Astermark J, Blanchette V, Collins P, Dimichele D, et al. Inhibitor treatment in haemophilias A and B: summary statement for the 2006 international consensus conference. Haemophilia. 2006;12(s6):1–7.
97. Tjonnfjord G, Holme PA. Factor eight inhibitor bypass activity (FEIBA) in the management of bleeds in hemophilia patients with high-titer inhibitors. Vasc Health Risk Manag. 2007;3(4):527.

98. Abildgaard CF, Penner JA, Watson-Williams EJ. Anti-inhibitor coagulant complex (Autoplex) for treatment of factor VIII inhibitors in hemophilia. Blood. 1980;56(6):978–84.
99. Scully C, Dios PD, Kumar N. Special care in dentistry: handbook of oral healthcare. London: Elsevier Health Sciences; 2006.
100. Scully C, Dios PD, Giangrandc P. Oral care for people with hemophilia or a hereditary bleeding tendency, Treatment of hemophilia monograph series. Montreal: The World Federation of Hemophilia; 2008. p. 10–1.
101. Wang L, Zoppè M, Hackeng TM, Griffin JH, Lee K-F, Verma IM. A factor IX-deficient mouse model for hemophilia B gene therapy. Proc Natl Acad Sci. 1997;94(21):11563–6.
102. Nathwani AC, Reiss UM, Tuddenham EGD, Rosales C, Chowdary P, McIntosh J, Peruta MD, Lheriteau E, Patel N, Raj D, Riddell A, Pie J, Rangarajan S, Bevan D, Recht M, Shen Y-M, Halka KG, Basner-Tschakarjan E, Mingozzi F, High KA, Allay J, Kay MA, Ng CYC, Zhou J, Cancio M, Morton CL, Gray JT, Srivastava D, Nienhuis AW, Davidoff AM. Long-term safety and efficacy of factor IX gene therapy in hemophilia B. N Engl J Med. 2014;371(21):1994–2004.
103. Murphy SL, High KA. Gene therapy for haemophilia. Br J Haematol. 2008;140(5):479–87.
104. Hao Q-L, Malik P, Salazar R, Tang H, Gordon EM, Kohn DB. Expression of biologically active human factor IX in human hematopoietic cells after retroviral vector-mediated gene transduction. Hum Gene Ther. 1995;6(7):873–80.
105. Swystun LL, Lillicrap D. Gene therapy for coagulation disorders. Circ Res. 2016;118(9):1443–52.
106. Ponder KP. Gene therapy for hemophilia. Curr Opin Hematol. 2006;13(5):301–7.
107. Chuah MK, Collen D, VandenDriessche T. Gene therapy for hemophilia: hopes and hurdles. Crit Rev Oncol Hematol. 1998;28(3):153–71.
108. Morfini M. A new era in the Hemophilia treatment: lights and shadows. J Hematol Transfus. 2016;4(3):1051.
109. High KA, Anguela XM. Adeno-associated viral vectors for the treatment of hemophilia. Human Mol Genet. 2015:ddv475.
110. Finn JD, Ozelo MC, Sabatino DE, Franck HW, Merricks EP, Crudele JM, et al. Eradication of neutralizing antibodies to factor VIII in canine hemophilia A after liver gene therapy. Blood. 2010;116(26):5842–8.
111. Artenstein AW, Opal SM. Proprotein convertases in health and disease. N Engl J Med. 2011;365(26):2507–18.
112. Siner JI, Samelson-Jones BJ, Crudele JM, French RA, Lee BJ, Zhou S, et al. Circumventing furin enhances factor VIII biological activity and ameliorates bleeding phenotypes in hemophilia models. JCI Insight. 2016;1(16):e89371.
113. Powell JS, Ragni MV, White GC, Lusher JM, Hillman-Wiseman C, Moon TE, et al. Phase 1 trial of FVIII gene transfer for severe hemophilia A using a retroviral construct administered by peripheral intravenous infusion. Blood. 2003;102(6):2038–45.
114. Miao CH. Hemophilia A: gene therapy via intraosseous delivery of factor VIII-lentiviral vectors. Thromb J. 2016;14(1):41–e89371.
115. James PD, Raut S, Rivard GE, Poon M-C, Warner M, McKenna S, et al. Aminoglycoside suppression of nonsense mutations in severe hemophilia. Blood. 2005;106(9):3043–8.
116. Chao H, Mansfield SG, Bartel RC, Hiriyanna S, Mitchell LG, Garcia-Blanco MA, et al. Phenotype correction of hemophilia A mice by spliceosome-mediated RNA trans-splicing. Nat Med. 2003;9(8):1015–9.
117. Zhang F, Wen Y, Guo X. CRISPR/Cas9 for genome editing: progress, implications and challenges. Hum Mol Genet. 2014;23(R1):R40–6.
118. Nguyen TH, Anegon I. Successful correction of hemophilia by CRISPR/Cas9 genome editing in vivo: delivery vector and immune responses are the key to success. EMBO Mol Med. 2016;8(5):439–41.

Hemophilia B

5

Hoda Motlagh, Behnaz Pezeshkpoor,
and Akbar Dorgalaleh

5.1 Introduction

Blood coagulation factor IX (FIX) is a vitamin K-dependent glycoprotein which consists of 415 amino acid residues with a molecular weight of 57 kDa [1]. This coagulation factor has a vital role in coagulation cascade. FIX is mainly activated to FIXa by tissue factor-FVII (TF-FVII) complex and also by FXIa. FIXa with FVIIIa, phospholipid and calcium, makes an activating complex, called tenase, which converts FX to FXa. This reaction has a crucial role in the propagation phase of the coagulation cascade (please refer to Chap. 1) [2].

Hemophilia B is a congenital bleeding disorder caused by mutation in the *F9* gene, which is located in chromosome Xq27.1 [3]. Although hemophilia B is an inherited sex-linked recessive disorder, in ~30% of patients, mutations are sporadic, with no preceding family history of the disease [1]. In addition to genetically determined defect, FIX deficiency can be an acquired deficiency due to vitamin K deficiency, in which all vitamin K-dependent coagulation factors including FII, FVII, FIX, and FX and proteins C, S, and Z are decreased [4].

There is a strong correlation between severity of the disorder and residual FIX activity in the bloodstream in hemophilia B. Hemophilia B is classified according to residual plasma FIX activity into severe (<1%), moderate (1–5%), and mild (>5–30%) deficiency [1]. Hemarthrosis, ecchymosis, epistaxis, and dental-related bleeding are common clinical presentations of patients with hemophilia B. Rarely,

H. Motlagh · A. Dorgalaleh (✉)
Department of Hematology and Blood Transfusion, School of Allied Medicine,
Iran University of Medical Sciences, Tehran, Iran
e-mail: motlagh.h@tak.iums.ac.ir

B. Pezeshkpoor
Institute of Experimental Hematology and Transfusion Medicine, University of Bonn,
Bonn, Germany
e-mail: behnaz.pezeshkpoor@ukbonn.de

A. Dorgalaleh (ed.), *Congenital Bleeding Disorders*,
https://doi.org/10.1007/978-3-319-76723-9_5

patients with severe deficiency may present with life-threatening bleeds such as intracranial hemorrhage (ICH) [5].

In initial laboratory examination, patients with hemophilia B have prolonged activated partial thromboplastin time (aPTT) and normal prothrombin time (PT), thrombin time (TT), and platelet count. Factor assay should be performed to confirm the diagnosis. In addition, molecular studies can contribute to detection of underling mutation, carrier detection, and prenatal diagnosis (PND) [5].

Fresh frozen plasma (FFP) and prothrombin complex concentrate (PCC) were therapeutic choices, but these possessed risks of blood-borne disease transmission [2]. Todays, plasma-derived FIX (pdFIX) and recombinant FIX (rFIX) are treatments of choice. With timely diagnosis and appropriate management, burden of the disorder can be decreased, and the patients' quality of life can be improved [6].

5.2 Factor IX Structure and Function

FIX is a vitamin K-dependent single-chain glycoprotein which contains 17% carbohydrates and is produced by hepatocytes in the liver. Plasma half-life of FIX is ~18 h, and its average plasma concentrate is 2.5–5 μg/ml [7].

The complete sequence of *F9* gene was determined in 1985 [7]. The gene is located in the long arm of the X chromosome in the chromosomal location Xq27.1 and spans 33 kb. *F9* gene has eight exons that transcribe to a 2.8 kb mRNA. Of this, 1.4 kb mRNA translate to a precursor protein with 461 amino acids, from which the signal peptide (28 amino acid residues) and propeptide (18 amino acid residues) are removed by proteolytic cleavage. As a result, mature FIX zymogen of 415 amino acids and 57 kDa of molecular weight are released to bloodstream (Fig. 5.1) [8].

Blood coagulation FIXa glycoprotein has several domains including γ-carboxylation domain (Gla domain), short hydrophobic stack, epidermal growth factor-1 (EGF-1)-like domain, EGF-2, activation peptide (AP), and serine protease (SP) domain (Fig. 5.2) [9, 10].

Gla domain has 11 glutamic acids which post-translationally is modified to γ-carboxy-glutamate. These modified residues are necessary for binding to calcium ions. These calciums with positive charge make feasible binding of Gla domain to membrane phospholipids with negative charge. Regions with high affinity for connecting to calcium were reported in SP and EGF-1 domains [8].

Both EGF domains are related to EGF superfamily and have six cysteine residues, which form disulfide bridges. AP is removed to convert FIX zymogen to FIXa. The catalytic activity of FIXa results from a catalytic triad of Ser411, Asp315, and His267 in SP domain [1].

However, crystal structure of full-length human FIX has not been determined, but a structure model could be constructed by considering porcine FIXa (because of 84% identity) and determined three partial structures of human FIXa, Gla, EGF-1, and EGF2-SP domains (Fig. 5.3). According to these findings, FIXa comprises of a light chain with three domains (Gla, EGF-1, and EFG-2) and a heavy chain with one domain (SP domain), which linked together by a single disulfide

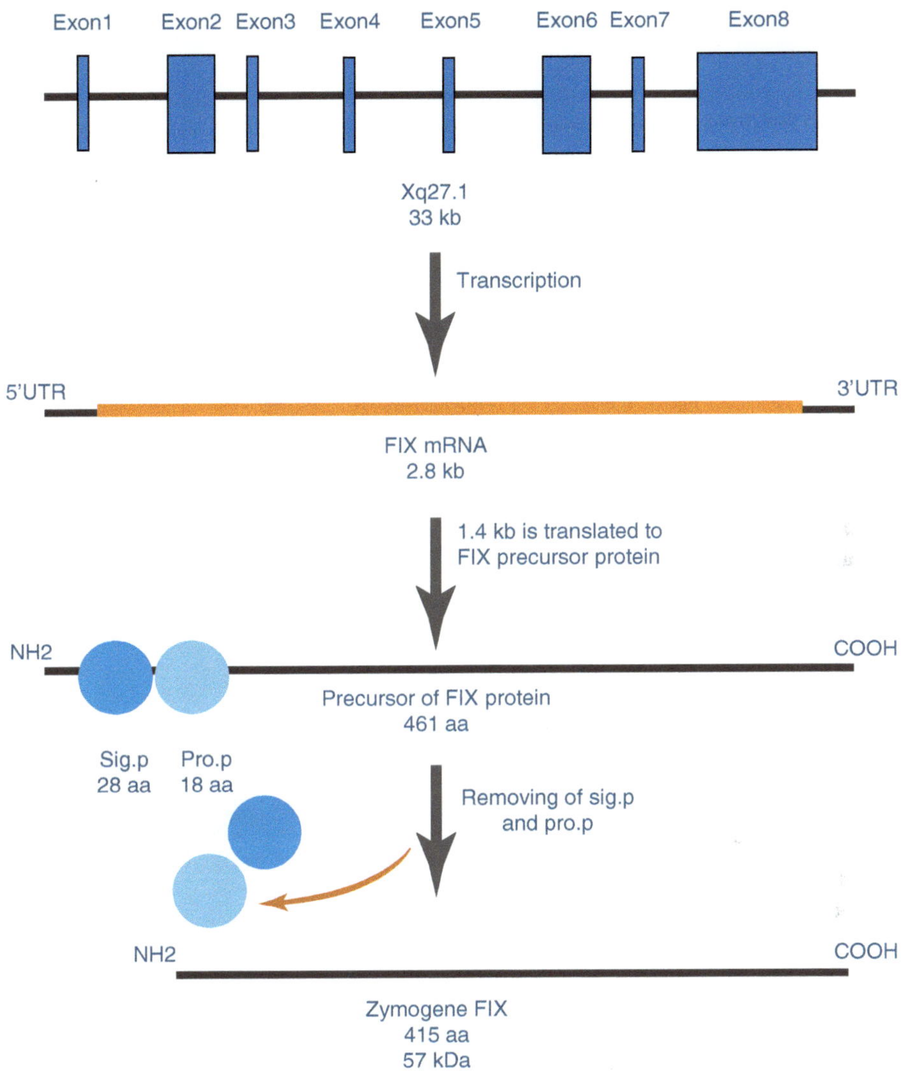

Fig. 5.1 *F9* gene located in Xq27.1. It has eight exons and spans 33 kilobase (kb) pairs . *F9* gene transcribed to an mRNA with 2.8 kb, from which 1.4 kb translated to a precursor FIX with 461 amino acids. Then two domains of FIX, including signal peptide and propeptide domains, are removed by proteolytic cleavage. The remained zymogene FIX has 415 amino acids with 57 kDa molecular weight. *UTR* untranslated region, *aa* amino acid, *FIX* factor IX, *sig.p* signal peptide, *pro.p* propeptide

bond (Cys178-Cys335) [10]. Light chain of FIX which includes Gla, EGF-1, and EGF-2 domains creates a stalk so that Gla domain connects to the phospholipid membrane. Serine protease which is catalytic domain places above the structure [8, 10]. FVIIIa as cofactor of FIX, in order to playing its important cofactor role, makes interaction with catalytic domain and critical residues in EGF-1 and EGF-2 domains either [11, 12].

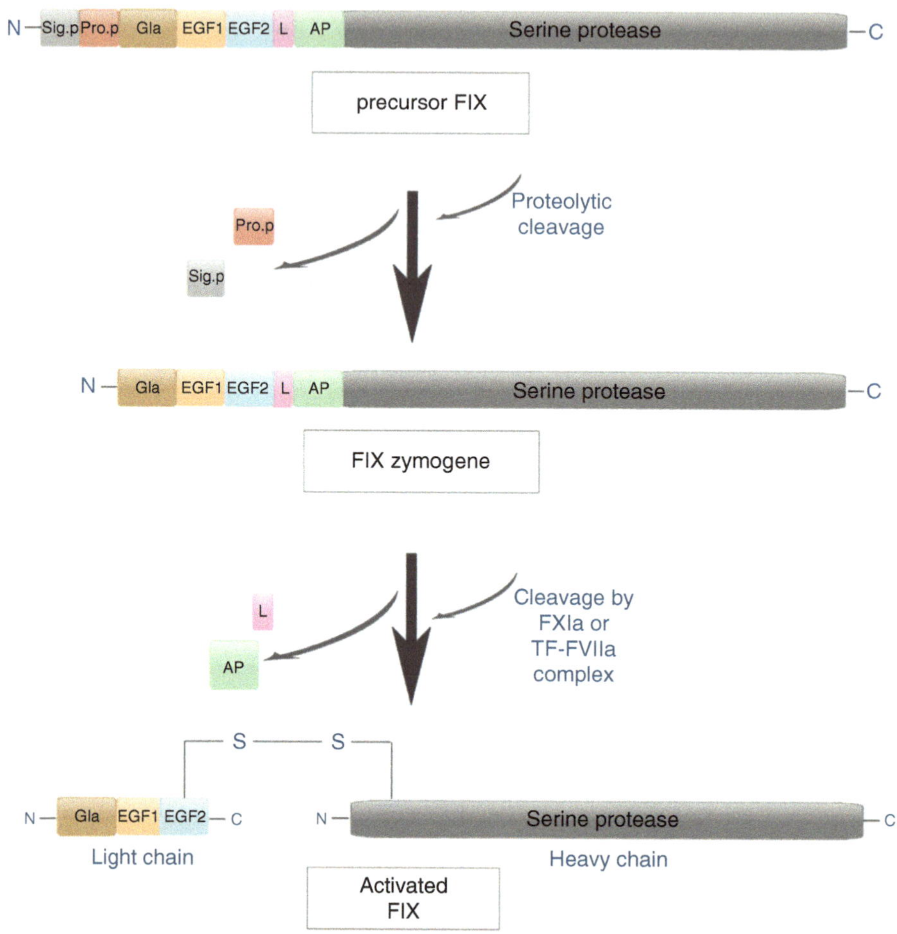

Fig. 5.2 Precursor FIX which synthesized in the liver has several domains including Gla domain, EGF1 and EGF2 domains, activation peptide, and serine protease domain. Proteolytic cleavages remove signal peptide and propeptide domains. Thus initial FIX converts to FIX zymogene. Then FIX zymogene is released to blood circulation. Cleavage of activated peptide by activated FXI (FXIa) or tissue factor-FVII (TF-FVII) complex leads to conversion of FIX to activated FIX (FIXa). FIXa comprises of a light chain (Gla, EGF-1, EGF-2) and a heavy chain (serine protease domain) which bonded together by a single disulfide bridge. *L* linker, *Gla* glutamic acid, *EGF* epidermal grow factor, *FIX* factor IX, *AP* activated peptide, *sig.p* signal peptide, *Pro.p* propeptide, *TF-FVIIa*, tissue factor-activated factor VII

Activation of FIX either via extrinsic pathway by TF-FVII complex, or via intrinsic pathway by FXI, occurs upon double cleavages of peptide bonds after Arg192 and Arg226 residues. This phenomenon leads to removal of AP and release of FIXa to the plasma [13]. When FIXa binds to FVIIIa as its cofactor, its function is dramatically increased by 50,000 fold. In addition, its binding to membrane phospholipid increases its catalytic activity. FIXa as a component of intrinsic complex which includes FVIIIa, calcium, and phospholipid cleaves an arginine-isoleucine

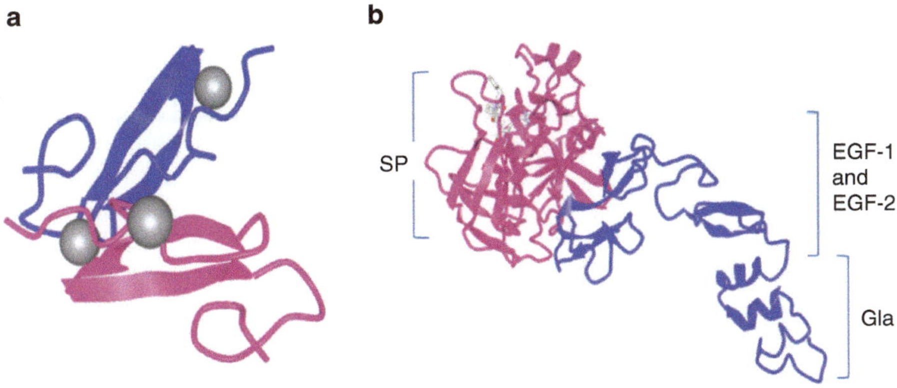

Fig. 5.3 (**a**) Epidermal growth factor (EGF)-like domain from human factor IX. B chain and C chain are shown in purple and blue, respectively. Calcium ions are illustrated in gray residues. (**b**) Porcine FIX domains. The blue color shows light chain which includes Gla domain and EGF-1 and EGF-2 domains. The serine protease (SP) domain which is the catalytic region of the coagulation factor is shown in purple color

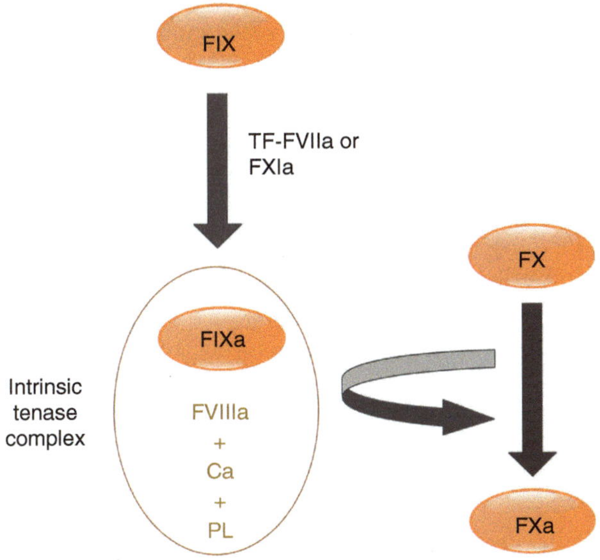

Fig. 5.4 Factor IX (FIX) which activated by tissue factor-activated FVIIa (FVIIa) complex or factor FXIa leads to formation of intrinsic tenase complex that converts FX to FXa. *Ca* calcium, *PL* phospholipid, *TF* tissue factor, *FIX* factor IX, *FIXa* activated factor IX, *FVIIIa* activated factor VIII, *FX* factor X

bond to convert FX to FXa (Fig. 5.4). Then, FXa initiates prothrombin to thrombin conversion and ultimately results in clot formation. Therefore, FIX has a vital role in the coagulation cascade. Hence mutations in *F9* gene causing FIX quantitative deficiencies (type I) or/and qualitative defects (type II) lead to hemophilia B—a bleeding disease [10].

5.3 Hemophilia B

Hemophilia B or Christmas disease is a congenital X chromosome-linked bleeding disorder, which arises from different mutations in *F9* gene located in Xq27.1 [13, 14]. The overall incidence of hemophilia B is 1 per 30,000 male live births, whereas hemophilia A has a prevalence of 1 per 5000 male infants [15]. Although most cases of hemophilia B are hereditary, 30% of cases are due to sporadic mutations. In the case of hereditary deficiency, because of X-linked recessive manner of inheritance, a male with one mutant X chromosome and a female with two mutants X chromosome (although scarce) have hemophilia. Females by one mutant X chromosome are carriers of this genetic abnormality. In the case of a hemophilic father and a normal mother, all sons would be non-hemophilic, while daughters would be carriers of hemophilia B. On the other hand, when father has none mutant X chromosome and mother is carrier, 50% of sons would have mutant allele, and 50% of their daughters would be carrier (Fig. 5.5) [1].

The most prevalent genetic abnormalities in patients with hemophilia B with a frequency of 64% are point mutations. Overall, mutations are categorized in two main groups: type I mutations which cause quantitative deficiency of FIX and type II mutations which manifest as functional defects [1, 10]. In rare cases, hemophilia B can be an acquired phenomenon due to antibody against FIX [16].

Patients with hemophilia B present with recurrent joint bleeding, soft tissue hematoma, and rarely in severely affected cases, life-threatening manifestations

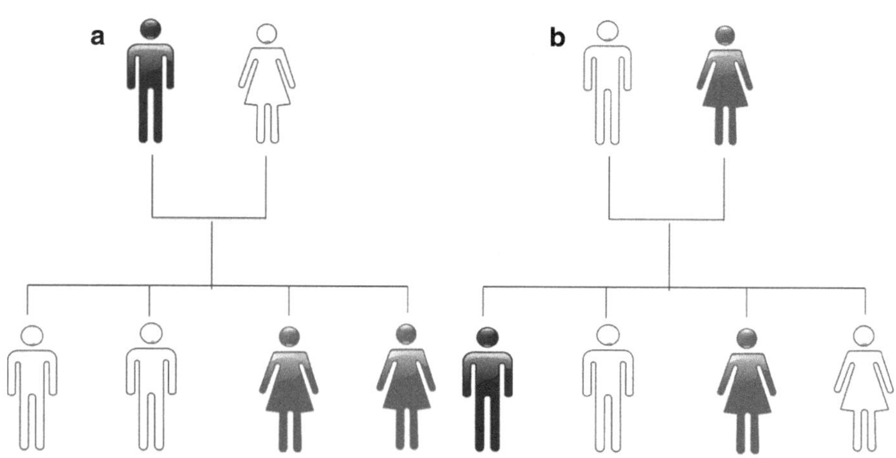

Fig. 5.5 Inheritance pattern in hemophilia B. (**a**) In a family with hemophilic father and non-hemophilic mother, all daughters are genetic carrier, and all sons are non-hemophilic. (**b**) In the case of a non-hemophilic father and carrier mother with one mutant X chromosome, 50% of sons are hemophilic, and 50% of daughters are hemophilic carrier. Black, hemophilia patient; white, nonhemophilia; gray, carrier

such as ICH. Recurrent joint bleeding may lead to disabling arthropathy [5]. Diagnosis of disorder can be made based on clinical presentations, family history, and appropriate laboratory approach. Routine coagulation tests such as PT and aPTT accompany with FIX activity assay, and in well-equipped laboratories, molecular analysis can be used for diagnosis of the disorder [5]. The main drawback with replacement therapy via injection of plasma-derived protein and rFIX is producing of inhibitors against exogenous factor [17].

5.4 Molecular Basis

F9 gene is located on Xq27.1 and comprises of eight exons. Approximately 1000 distinct mutations have been reported in *F9* gene, up to now [3]. The miscellaneous genetic abnormalities were observed within *F9* gene including missense/nonsense mutations (64%), small insertion/deletion (indels) (18%), splicing (9%), large indels (6%), regulatory (2%), and complex rearrangement (1%) (Fig. 5.6) [1]. Therefore, unlike hemophilia A, the most common abnormalities in hemophilia B are missense mutations which most of them are combined with normal FIX antigen level (type II mutations) [15].

There are some mutational hotspots within *F9* gene that are more prone to occurrence of mutation. For instance, the high rate of mutations in regions with high frequency of guanine and cytosine, typically near the initiation transcript region, revealed that they are mutational hotspots. The loci of mutation can affect

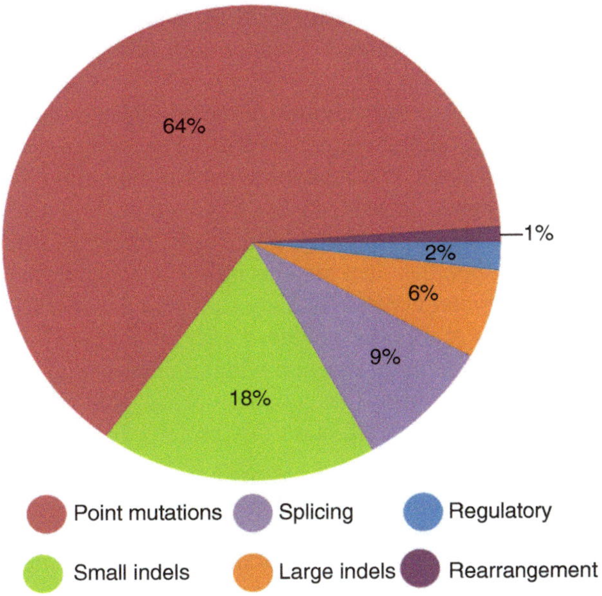

Fig. 5.6 This pie illustrates percentage of genetic abnormalities in patients with hemophilia B. The most prevalent genetic abnormalities are point mutations (64%). Prevalence of other abnormalities reported within *F9* gene are small indels (insertion and deletion) (18%), splicing (9%), large indels (6%), regulatory (2%), and rearrangement (1%)

production and function of coagulation FIX and therefore can influence disease severity. Point mutations can manifest as missense, premature stop codon, or splice site mutations. *F9* gene mutations are classified in two main types, type I and type II, which lead to quantitative deficiencies and qualitative defects, respectively. Type I mutations often result in reduced transcription and FIX secretion to the bloodstream and can cause severe hemophilia B [1].

A signal peptide (residues 1–28) directs intracellular trafficking of the protein and has no effect on the protein function; its mutations lead to impaired FIX secretion and therefore lead to type I mutation. An example of functional deficit in *F9* gene is mutation in triad residues of serine protease domain which produces protein defective in catalytic activity. This results in severe hemophilia B and associated with increased susceptibility to inhibitor formation. In addition, mutations in propeptide (residues 29–46) which mediates interaction with the vitamin K-dependent γ-carboxylase lead to impaired phospholipid-binding capacity that presents as mild or moderate phenotype [10].

Generally, nonsense mutations are associated with severe type I defect, without any protein production. Nevertheless, when a nonsense mutation occurs in coding gene of C-terminal region of protein, results in producing nonfunctional FIX and type II defect. However a splicing defect creates a variable range of disease severity; a single point mutation that impairs a splice donor site or occurs in the sequence of an intron which creates an alternative splice acceptor site results in a nonsense mRNA and severe hemophilia B. In north America, England, and Ireland, some recurrent mutations due to founder effect were reported. Founder effect illustrates how certain genetic abnormalities occur more frequently in a specific geographically restricted hemophilia B population due to identity by descent. These are usually mild or moderate disease causing mutations for the reason that a severe defect reduces reproductive fitness of affected males (please refer to Chap. 2) [1].

There are some mutations in the *F9* gene promoter that cause permanent low level of FIX throughout patient's life. However in hemophilia B Leyden with more than 20 different identified mutations in proximal *F9* gene promoter, a severe FIX deficiency presents at birth. The FIX level starts to increase in the second decade of life at the onset of puberty, and finally reaches to near normal level in the third decade of life, that then remains stable throughout life. It is apparent that the defect in the promoter makes FIX transcription dependent on testosterone level, and hence the severity of disease is reduced after puberty [18].

Small insertion or deletion with a prevalence of 18%, generally occurs in association with runs of dinucleotide repeats. This abnormality usually occurs within introns without any effect on FIX protein. However, occasionally these indels can occur in regulatory regions or lead to frameshifts which result in a severe hemophilia B. As inhibitor formation is influenced by genetic abnormalities, a null allele which means complete deletion of *F9* gene has the most probability for inhibitor formation [19]. Although the overall prevalence of inhibitor formation against therapeutic products is 1–3%, this rate is increased to nearly 20% in cases with complete deletion of the *F9* gene [10].

5.5 Factor IX Propeptide Mutation-Associated Hypersensitivity to Coumarin Therapy

There are two missense mutations in FIX propeptide which lead to major bleeding after coumarin therapy. These mutations occur in Ala-10 locus which is a high protected site in vitamin K-dependent clotting factors (FII, FVII, FIX, and FX). These two point mutations, Ala-10(GCC) → Val(GTC) and Ala-10(GCC) → Thr(ACC) in exon 2 of *F9* gene result in a propeptide to which carboxylase enzyme has low affinity and therefore exhibit extremely low FIX coagulant activity (FIX:C) after coumarin therapy. It is considered that these patients have normal phenotype and coagulation screening test without any bleeding episodes in their life. They only show a defect once they undergo oral anticoagulation therapy with warfarin. Upon receipt of anticoagulant, they would show extreme fall in FIX:C to <1–3% and subsequently abnormal increase in aPTT in therapeutic range of PT and INR. In other people usually after coumarin therapy FIX:C decreases to 15–30% as do other vitamin K-dependent factors [20–22].

Prothrombin complex factors (FII, FVII, FIX and FX) for connection to membrane phospholipid need γ-carboxylation in NH2 terminal of mature protein. The propeptide is a carboxylase recognition site, and their junction together is a key step of the reaction (Fig. 5.7). In cases with propeptide mutations, although the affinity of hydroxylase enzyme is reduced, its activity is normal in absence of coumarin therapy. So it could be the probable cause of normal FIX:C and lack of bleeding before treatment with oral anticoagulants as warfarin. After coumarin therapy, in addition of low affinity, the activity of enzyme falls down because of inhibition of vitamin K reductase and lack of KH2 as cofactor (Table 5.1). Therefore, the result

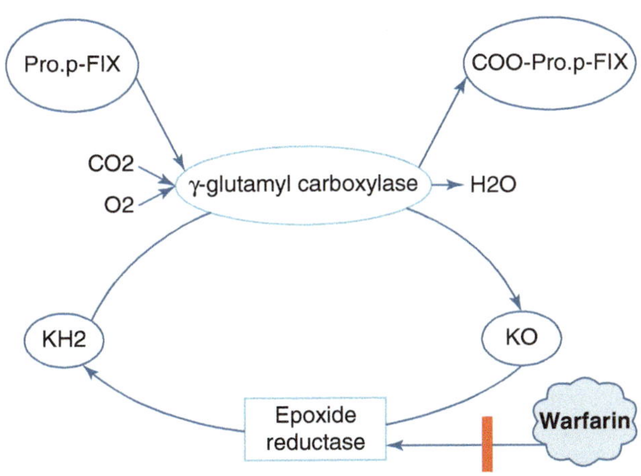

Fig. 5.7 The mechanism of vitamin K-dependent clotting factor carboxylation. The propeptide is carboxylase recognition site, and after connection, KH2 is used as enzyme cofactor. Generated KO coverts to KH2 through epoxide reductase function. It is goal enzyme for inhibition by warfarin. *Pro.p* propeptide, *FIX* factor IX, *KH2* dihydro vitamin K, *KO* epoxide vitamin K

Table 5.1 Activity and affinity of carboxylase enzyme in wild-type factor IX propeptide and mutant factor IX propeptide in the presence and absence of coumarin

	Wild-type FIX propeptide		Mutant FIX propeptide	
Enzyme characteristics[a]	Activity	Affinity	Activity	Affinity
Absence of coumarin	N	N	N	L
Coumarin therapy	L	N	L	L

In absence of coumarin, although enzyme activity and affinity are normal in wild-type factor IX propeptide, affinity of enzyme is reduced in mutant propetide. In wild-type, enzyme activity is reduced after coumarin therapy. Low activity and low affinity after coumarin therapy in mutant factor IX propeptide are the main causes of bleeding complications

N normal, *L* low, *FIX* factor IX

[a]Enzyme is referred to γ-glutamyl carboxylase

is FIX:C less than 1–3%, abnormally increased aPTT, and severe bleeding in these patients after treatment with coumarin [20–22].

Propeptide mutations in other vitamin K-dependent clotting factors show less coumarin sensitivity due to their autosomal recessive inheritance (unlike to *F9* gene which is located on X chromosome). Consequently, the effect of these mutations should be observed greatly in males [21, 22]. In conclusion, in cases with unusual bleeding pattern after treatment with oral anticoagulant which are vitamin K antagonist, aPTT and FIX:C should be evaluated, even in therapeutic range of PT and INR [22].

5.6 Clinical Manifestations

Patients with hemophilia B present various clinical symptoms including hemarthrosis, epistaxis, ecchymosis, and post-dental extraction bleeding. The most common site of spontaneous bleeding is the joints [5]. Life-threatening symptoms such as central nervous system (CNS) bleeding and umbilical cord bleeding are rare and usually only seen in severely affected individuals [5]. Over the long period, the main complications of recurrent joint bleeding and soft tissue hematomas are extensive arthropathy, muscle contractures, and pseudotumors that result in disability and chronic pain [15].

According to FIX:C, hemophilia B is classified into three types: severe (FIX:C <1% or <0/01 IU ml^{-1}), moderate (FIX:C of 1–5% or 0/01–0/05 IU ml^{-1}), and mild (FIX:C of 5–30% or >0/05–<0/30 IU ml^{-1}) deficiency. The main presentation of patients with severe hemophilia B is spontaneous bleeding, while patients with moderat FIX deficiency has seldom spontaneous bleeding and patient with mild FIX deficiency is lack of this clinical feature. Most commen clinical presentations in patients with moderate hemophilia B is post-traumatic hemorrhage, while post-surgical bleeding, post-dental extraction hemorrhage and bleeding after major injories are more common in patients with mild phenotype (Table 5.2) [3, 10, 14].

In overall, severity of disease influenced by type of mutation and some of mutations lead to severe hemophilia B. Frameshifts, nonsense mutations, large deletions, and splicing mutations are the most common genetic abnormalities that lead to severe hemophilia B. However, small deletions and missense mutations cause severe, moderate, or mild deficiency, depending on their location on genome (Table 5.3) [23].

Table 5.2 Classification and characteristics of hemophilia B according to residual plasma factor IX activity

Factor IX activity (%)	Disease severity	Prevalence (%)	Clinical symptoms	Bleeding frequency	Mean age at diagnosis
<1	Severe	60	Spontaneous joint or deep muscle bleeding	Up to 2–5 per month	<2 years
1–5	Moderate	15	Seldom spontaneous bleeding, usually after minor trauma	Vary from 1 per month to 1 per year	2–5 years
>5–30	Mild	25	No spontaneous bleeding, usually bleeding after severe trauma, surgery and tooth extraction	Vary from 1 per year to 1 every 10 years	Often later in the life

Table 5.3 Genotype-phenotype correlation in hemophilia B

Genetic abnormality	Severity of disease
Frameshifts	Severe (95%)[a]
Nonsense mutations	Severe (84%)[a]
Large deletions	Severe (100%)[a]
Splicing mutations	Severe (100%)[a]
Missense mutations	Severe, moderate, or mild deficiency, depending on the genetic abnormality location

[a]The percentage refer to phenotype that causes by the mentioned genetic abnormality

Generally, hemophilia B is a less severe bleeding disease with lower bleeding frequency and better long-term outcomes than hemophilia A [14]. Approximately one-third of heterozygous women are classified as symptomatic carriers because their FIX activity is between 40% and 60%. Their clinical manifestations are similar to mild hemophilia B. In addition, they often have more prolonged menstrual bleedings [1].

5.7 Diagnosis

The usual age of patients with hemophilia B at diagnosis relies on the severity of disorder. In the case of severe hemophilia, usual age at diagnosis is ≤2 years. Moderate hemophilia typically is diagnosed at age of 2–5 years, while mild deficiency is often diagnosed later in the life. In the cases with sporadic mutations or in the cases without family history, the time of diagnosis is related to outward symptoms of patients [1].

Generally, diagnosis of disorder is based on clinical presentations, family history, and appropriate laboratory approach. As recurrent bleeding episodes are relatively similar in various coagulopathies, proper laboratory assessment is necessary for correct and timely diagnosis of the disorder [5]. Complete blood count (CBC) is normal in hemophilia B; however a reduction in hemoglobin and RBC might be seen due to prolonged hemorrhages. In screening coagulation tests, aPTT is prolonged up to 2.5 times, while PT is normal [1].

Diagnosis of hemophilia B should be differentiated from vitamin K deficiency, heparin consumption, von Willebrand disease (VWD), and hemophilia A which all presented with increased aPTT (Table 5.4) [24].

Factor assay could be used for determining each factor activity level. In hemophilia B, FIX level is decreased [5]. There are two methods for FIX activity assay including one-stage clot assay which is based on aPTT and chromogenic assay. The former is traditional common method, whereas the later rarely is used for hemophilia B. Chromogenic assay is used more commonly in hemophilia A than hemophilia B. According to recent reports from seven countries, chromogenic assay is used in 68% of laboratories for hemophilia A, while only 11% of laboratories used this method for hemophilia B [25].

For FIX:C, blood should be collected in citrated tube and immediately be centrifuged in 2000*g* for 20 min. Then plasma should be separated and be freezed in −70 °C [25]. After melting, FIX:C could be performed with one of two methods: one-stage assay or chromogenic assay [26]. The one-stage assay is an aPTT-based method and the most routinely used method. Patient plasma and FIX-deficient plasma preincubate with aPTT reagent for 3–5 min. Then, after addition of calcium, the clotting time should be recorded. The result of patient's plasma clotting time is compared with a standard curve that is generated from plasma samples with determined FIX activity. Each patient's plasma at least should be measured in three different dilutions for analyzing of parallelism between standard dilutions and patient plasma dilutions. Two lines should be parallel, unless there is an inhibitor [24].

Chromogenic assay include two stages: at first stage, a reactive mixture consisting of FXIa, thrombin, phospholipid, and calcium chloride adding to patient's plasma with unknown FIX activity. It is assumed that amount of generated FXa is proportional with the amount of residual plasma FIX. In the second stage, a specific peptide of FXa, nitroanilin substrate, is measured through a peptide cleavage. Generated *p*-nitroaniline is analyzed photometrically in absorbance of 405 nm. The created color is directly proportional with the amount of functional FIX in plasma according to a standard curve (Fig. 5.8) [24, 25].

According to a study on patients with hemophilia B, discrepancy between two activities assay methods is not observed in patients with severe hemophilia B, while in non-severe hemophilia B, discrepancy between one-stage assay and chromogenic assay is observed. This study illustrated that those patients with non-severe hemophilia B and mutation in N-terminal site of activation peptide and propeptide domains of FIX have twofold more differentiate between results of one-stage and chromogenic stage assays (higher activity in chromogenic assay) [25].

Different aPTT reagents don't have any impact on discrepancy between these assays. In fact, each method has some advantages and disadvantages (Table 5.5). Furthermore, the use of both assays is contributory for favorable diagnosis and classification of hemophilia B (Table 5.6) [25].

To assess inhibitor development in response to factor replacement therapy or when presence of inhibitor is suspected, a mixing test is used, in which normal

Table 5.4 Differential diagnosis of hemophilia B

Disease	PT	aPTT	Cause of disease	Differentiation
Bleeding disorders with low factor IX activity level				
Combined vitamin K-dependent factors deficiency	↑	↑	Genetic abnormalities in *GGCX* and *VCORC1* genes	Increased PT, multiple coagulation factor deficiencies (factor II, VII, IX, X), autosomal recessive inheritance
Acquired vitamin K-dependent factor deficiency	↑↑	↑	Warfarin treatment, liver disease	Increased PT, multiple coagulation factor deficiencies (factor II, VII, IX, X)
Bleeding disorders with prolonged aPTT and normal factor IX activity level				
Hemophilia A	N	↑	Genetic abnormalities in the *F9* gene	It is undistinguishable clinically from hemophilia B. A decreased FVIII activity level (<30%) with normal VWF level
VWD	N	↑ or N	Genetic abnormalities in *VWF* gene	VWD type 1: Multimers—normal pattern but reduced intensity GPIb binding/Ag: >(0.5–0.7) CB/Ag: >(0.5–0.7) FVIII/VWF: >(0.5–0.7) VWD type 2 variable VWD type 3: Multimers—no VWF present GPIb binding/Ag: NA CB/Ag: NA FVIII/VWF: NA
FXI deficiency	N	↑	Genetic abnormalities in *F11* gene	A specific FXI activity assay which is normal in HB
FXII, prekallikrein, or HMWK deficiencies	N	↑	Genetic abnormalities in underling gene	Don't cause any clinical bleeding
Prothrombin (FII), FV, or FX deficiencies	↑	↑	Genetic abnormalities in underling gene	A specific coagulation factor assay
FVII deficiency	↑	N	Genetic abnormality in *F7* gene	Prolonged PT with normal aPTT
Inherited fibrinogen disorders	↑	↑	Genetic abnormality in *FGA, FGB, or FGG* genes	Usually prolonged PT, aPTT, TT, RT
FXIII deficiency	N	N	Genetic abnormality in *F13A1*or *F13B* genes	All routine coagulation test are normal, joint bleeding is rare, a specific FXIII assay should be used
Inherited platelet function disorders	N	N	Underling gene defect	Joint, muscle, and intracranial bleeding are rare. Platelet aggregation assays, flow cytometry, and platelet electron microscopy could be used for differential diagnosis

FIX factor IX, *PT* prothrombin time, *aPTT* activated partial thromboplastin time, *GGCX* Gamma-Glutamyl Carboxylase, *VKORC1* vitamin K epoxide reductase complex, subunit 1, *N* normal, *VWF* von Willebrand factor, *VWD* von Willebrand disease, *HMWK* high molecular weight kinase

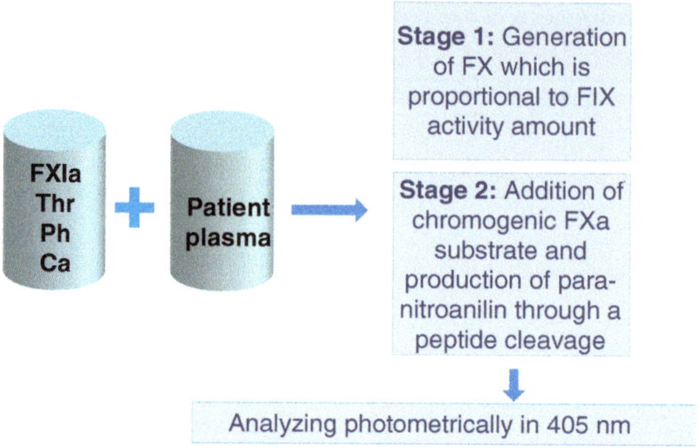

Fig. 5.8 Principle of factor IX (FIX) chromogenic assay. A reactive mixture (FXIa, Thr, Ph, and Ca) adding to patient plasma with unknown FIX activity. In the first stage, generated FX is directly proportional to FIX activity in patient's plasma. In the second stage, a peptide cleavage of chromogenic FXa substrate leading to generation of *p*-nitroaniline and therefore analyzing of this color in absorbance of 405 nm. *FXIa* activated factor XI, *Thr* thrombin, *Ph* phospholipid, *Ca* calcium, *FX* factor X, *FXa* activated factor X, *FIX* factor IX

Table 5.5 Advantages and disadvantages of one-stage assay and chromogenic assay

	One-stage assay	Chromogenic assay
Advantages	Simple, readily automated	Added thrombin allows unlimited FIX activation. High dilution of coagulation factors leading to reduction of interferences of heparin, anticoagulants, lupus anticoagulant. The limited number of their kits leads to reduction of variability in results
Disadvantages	Influenced by lipemia, heparin, direct thrombin inhibitors, direct FXa inhibitors. Differences between laboratories in results owing to using of different aPTT reagents, instruments, and FIX deficiency plasma	More expensive, influenced by direct FXa inhibitors which cause false reduction

FIX factor IX, *FXa* activated factor X, *aPTT* activated partial thromboplastin time

Table 5.6 Chromogenic assay reagents for factor IX assay

Company	Kit	Country
Diagnostica Stago	STA-R FIX kit	France
Diagnostica Stago	Asserachrom IX:AG	France
Aniara	BIOPHEN Chromogenic Factor FIX: C kit	USA
Siemens Healthcare	Unsp	Germany
Rossix	Unsp	Sweden

Unsp, unspecified

pooled plasma as a source of FIX is mixed with equal parts of patient's plasma. The assay is based on incubation of this mixture for 1 h at 37° followed by aPTT assay. A prolonged repeated aPTT should be followed by Nijmegen assay to determine the inhibitor titer. One unit of inhibitor is the amount of inhibitor that will inactivate 50% or 0.5 unit of FIX activity over 10 min at 37°. This assessment helps to make a correct decision for management of patients with hemophilia B with inhibitor [5, 24].

In the case of a known carrier mother, chorionic villus sampling (CVS) and amniocentesis can be performed for screening of the fetus. After birth, coagulation tests for identifying clotting factor level should be performed for such cases. It is considerable that although low level of FVIII is pointing to hemophilia A, results for FIX are not so decisive. FIX takes approximately 6 months after age to reach normal level, so in interpretation of FIX assay at birth, this issue should be considered. On the other hand, if there is mild decrease in FIX level at birth, it is not representative of hemophilia B, while an extensive reduction of FIX level is suggestive of the disorder [1].

Molecular analysis can be used for confirmation of the disorder and can assist to achieving valuable data about carrier detection, prenatal diagnosis (PND), and prediction of inhibitor formation and therefore management of disorder [5]. Additionally determination of eligibility for gene therapy in future will benefit from molecular analysis. Since there is no common reported mutation within *F9* gene, for molecular diagnosis full *F9* gene sequencing is required. The DNA amplification by polymerase chain reaction (PCR) and then direct sequencing is a well-standardized manner for molecular analysis; however large deletions or other gross abnormalities due to the existence of other normal allele could not be detectable by this method. Multiplex ligation-dependent probe amplification (MLPA) and multiplex amplification and probe hybridization (MAPH) could be used to reduce percent of *F9* gene mutations in patients with hemophilia B [27, 28].

5.8 Treatment

In the past, initial treatment of patients with hemophilia B was injection of fresh frozen plasma (FFP) or prothrombin complex concentrate (PCC) which, in addition to FIX, contains additional coagulation factors. The problems associated with these products were extreme activation of coagulation cascade, volume enhancement, and risk of blood-borne diseases especially in using of FFP [1, 2].

Next achievement for hemophilia treatment was advent of plasma-derived FIX (pdFIX) products and recombinant FIX (rFIX) concentrates. pdFIX and FVIII are available since 1970 which lead to self-infusion and home therapy. rFIX which are available since 1999 eradicate risk of animal and human infectious agent transmission. In addition, rFIX is safe and effective and with lower rate of allergic and thrombosis reactions and inhibitor formation [29].

The purpose of replacement therapy is achievement of plasma FIX level to 60–80% and 20–40% for major and minor bleeding, respectively. There are several plasma-derived and recombinant FIX products for treatment of hemophilia B

(Table 5.7) [30]. Over past years, the safety and purity of these products were improved, so the current treatment of choice for hemophilia B is intravenous injection of these products. However, the fear, pain, and annoyance related to needle-based injection of these products are causes of low patient requisition [5].

In 2014, for the first time, Food and Drug Administration (FDA) confirmed a long-lasting rFIX Fc fusion protein (rFIXFc) which required a lower frequency of injections to maintain hemostasis. This product meets the current goal of producing a FIX with extended circulation time which can decrease injection frequency and

Table 5.7 Factor IX products for hemophilia B treatment

Product	Company	Country	Explanation
Plasma-derived factor IX			
Aimafix	Kedrion	Italy	
AlphaNine SD	Grifols	Spain	FDA approval in 1996
Mononine/ Berinin-P	CSL Behring	Australia	FDA approval in 1992
Betafact	LFB	Several countries	
Factor IX Grifols	Grifols	Spain	
Haemonine	Biotest	Germany	
Hemo-B-RAAS	Shanghai RAAS	China	
Immunine	Baxter BioScience	America	
Nanotiv	Octapharma	Switzerland	
Nonafact	Sanquin	Amsterdam	
Octanine F	Octapharma	Switzerland	
Replenine	BPL	England	
TBSF FIX	CSL Biotherapies	Australia	
Recombinant factor IX			
Rixubus	Baxter/Baxalta	America	FDA approval in June 2013, with a normal half life
Alprolix (rFIXFc)	Biogen Idec	America	FDA approval in March 2014, long-lasting recombinant Fc fusion. Phase II/III trials showed a 2.5 times increase in half-life
Ixinity (trenonacog alfa)	Emergent BioSolutions (previously Cangene)	Maryland	FDA approval in May 2015, with a normal half-life
Idelvion	CSL Behring	Australia	FDA approval in March 2016, long-lasting recombinant albumin fusion, a five times increase in half-life
NN79 (N9-GP)	Novo Nordisk	Denmark	PEGylated recombinant FIX, five times increase in half-life
BeneFIX	Pfizer	America	FDA approval in 1997

FDA food and drug administration, *FIX* factor IX

improve quality of life. rFIXFc has an extended half-life up to 48 h, compared to standard rFIX with half-life of approximately 18 h, in animal models of hemophilia B. Alprolix which is a rFIXFc comprises of a single-chain FIX that is recombinantly connected to constant region (Fc) of immunoglobulin IgG. Fc domain protects protein from catabolism via binding to Fc receptors (FcRn). These receptors protect IgG from degradation [30].

GlycoPEGylated rFIX is another rFIX concentrate which has twofolds recovery time and fivefolds longer half-life than standard FIX. PEG covalently connects to activation peptide, so PEGylation of rFIX in this special site, saves its biological activation and increases its circulation time Therefore patients requier lower frequency of injections. Once per week administration of 40 IU/kg of PEG-rFIX is required for hemophilia B treatment [30–32].

Another type of fusion protein is albumin-rFIX which has five times increased half-life compared with standard rFIX. However, more studies are required for establishing safety and efficacy of newer rFIX products [30, 33].

Replacement therapy could be administrated as prophylaxis or on-demand regimens [30]. Primary prophylaxis therapy is replacement protein injection in absence of bleeding as a protective procedure. This trend has improved life expectancy and quality of life in patients with hemophilia B. On-demand therapy is treatment when bleeding is occurred [29]. Recommended dosage of FIX concentrate for hemophilia B treatment is shown in Table 5.8 [30, 34]. Prophylaxis is recommended care for patients with severe hemophilia B; it prevents joint bleeding and hemophilic arthropathy and improves patient's quality of life [30]. Common prophylaxis is injection of FIX concentrate twice per week, but emergence of extended half-life of

Table 5.8 Recommended dosage of factor IX concentrate for treatment of hemophilia B

Factor IX dose (IU/kg)	Kind of hemorrhage
20–40	Mild or moderate hemarthrosis or hematoma
40–60	Severe hemarthrosis or hematoma External bleeding with anemia Moderate post-traumatic bleeding
50–100	Cranial trauma Cerebral hemorrhage Surgery prophylaxis
30–40	Primary prophylaxes
	Site of hemorrhage
30–40	Muscle
50–80	Joint
40–60	Gastrointestinal tract
30–40	Oral mucosa
30–50	Epistaxis
70–100	Hematuria
100	Retroperitoneal
100	CNS bleeding
100	Trauma or surgery

CNS central nervous system

FIX products leads to once per week injection. In a study, it has been shown that 100 IU/kg injection of rFIX nonacog alfa once per week is as effective as 50 IU/kg injection of it twice per week in 50 patients [35].

5.9 Inhibitor Formation a Challenge of Replacement Therapy

The most important complication of replacement therapy in hemophilia B is inhibitor development which leads to increasing risk of bleeding-related morbidity such as nephrosis and mortality [36]. The FIX inhibitor is commonly IgG4 subclass with affinity to Gla domain and SP domain in light and heavy chains, respectively. This phenomenon not only reduces efficacy of replacement therapy but also uses lots of economic resources [17, 37]. Although the prevalence of inhibitor in hemophilia B is less than 5%, in severely affected patients with major gene defects, this increases to 9–23% (Fig. 5.9) [19, 29, 36].

Approximately 50% of patients with FIX inhibitor might experience life-threatening anaphylactic reactions. The inhibitor development results from genetic and non-genetic reasons which the mutation type is the major risk factor. In HB, null mutations in which the genetic abnormality such as large deletions and nonsense mutations prevents synthesizes of coagulation factor result in inhibitor development. In contrast, in milder molecular defects such as small deletions, insertions, splice site, and missense mutations which result in synthesis of coagulation factor but loss of function, inhibitory development risk is less [5, 17, 36, 37]. Since the missense mutations are the most common molecular defects in hemophilia B, it

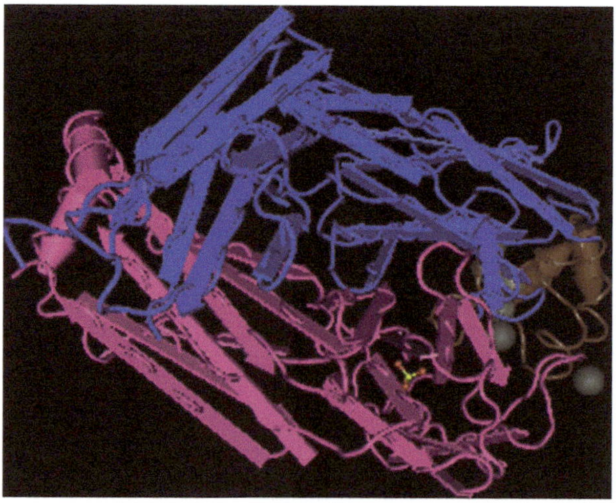

Fig. 5.9 Crystal structure of human factor IX GLA domain in complex with an inhibitory antibody. Heavy chain and light chain of inhibitory antibody are shown in blue and purple, respectively. Gla domain is shown in brown color. The grey residues are calcium ions. *Ab* antibody

might be the reason of low prevalence of inhibitor antibody in these patients than hemophilia A [5, 36]. The other risk factors, for instance, non-genetic reasons, are less studied and analyzed in hemophilia B because of rarity of inhibitor development in these patients [19].

The treatment strategy for these patients depends on the inhibitor levels. When the inhibitor titer is low (<5 Bethesda unit (BU)), the treatment approach is injection of FIX in high level of standard dose. In contrast, the high titer of inhibitor (>5 BU) requires more rigorous therapeutic options. In these cases, management of patients is divided into two parts: prevention of further hemorrhage and eradication of inhibitor. Bypassing agents, recombinant activated FVII (rFVIIa), and activated prothrombin complex concentrate (APCC) are main options for management of bleeding episodes. Immune tolerance induction (ITI), requiring high-dose injection of FIX for months to years, is used for inhibitor eradication. In cases of ITI-resistant, immunosuppressive drugs such as rituximab are the alternative choice for inhibitor elimination (Fig. 5.10). ITI is less effective in patients with hemophilia B in comparison with cases with hemophilia A (<50% and 60–80% for hemophilia B and hemophilia A, respectively) [17, 36]. Since rFVIIa as a bypassing agent doesn't include FIX, it's a suitable choice for hemophilia B patients who developed the inhibitor and manifest anaphylactic reactions to FIX injections [38].

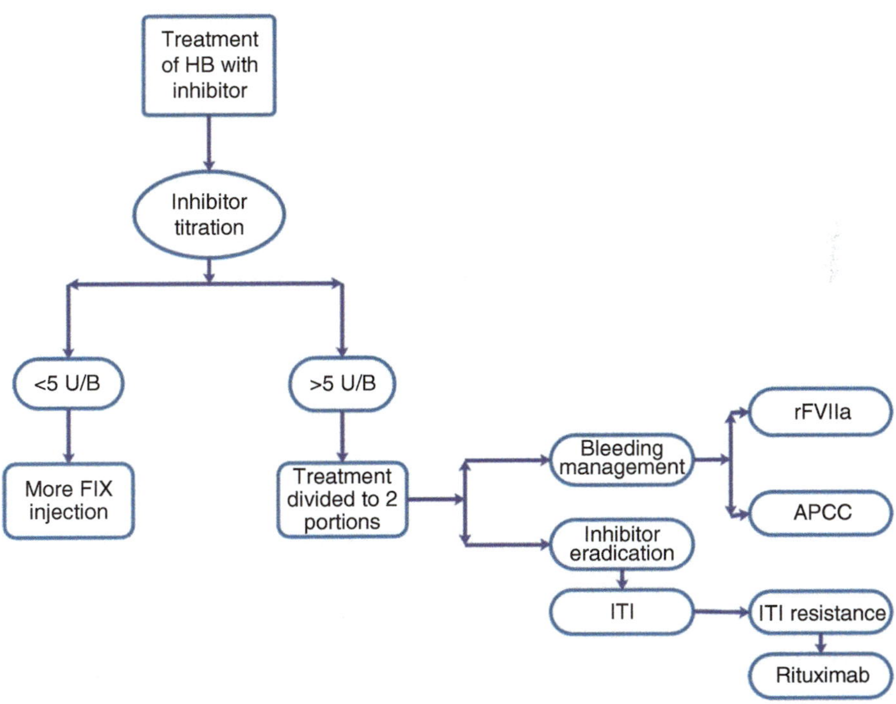

Fig. 5.10 The treatment approach for patients with hemophilia B and inhibitor antibody. *HB* hemophilia B, *U/B* unite/Bethesda, *FIX* factor IX, *ITI* immune tolerance induction, *rFVIIa* recombinant activated factor VII, *APCC* activated prothrombin complex concentrate

5.10 Gene Therapy

Gene therapy is one of the curative options for hemophilia B. It can lead to long-stay synthesis of FIX. Additionally, it can eliminate spontaneous bleeding and requiring for frequently injections. In fact gene therapy treats hemophilia completely. Adeno-associated virus (AAV)-mediated gene therapy is full of promise because this vector could induce long term FIX level [39, 40].

Current therapy using pdFIX products and rFIX concentrates has increased life expectancy and quality of life in patients with hemophilia B. However, these treatments require high-cost and lifelong factor injection [41, 42].

A promising strategy for effective treatment of patients with hemophilia disease is gene therapy. This approach is especially effevtive for severe untreated patients with less than 1% factor activity accompanied with arthropathy and life-threatening bleeds. Gene therapy is a conclusive treatment using AAV vectors to transfer *F9* gene through intramuscular injections or liver-targeting delivery [40]. According to a study on ten patients with severe hemophilia B, a single AAV8 vector dose injection causes long-term expression of FIX and clinical improvement [41].

AAV is a nonpathogenic virus with a single-strand genome which is 4.7 kb in length. Results of gene transferring through the AAV vector are reduction of prophylactic costs and bleeding episodes. Among various serotypes of AAV, AAV serotype 8 is more effective because it is lack of abiliy to cross react with antibodies produced against other AAV serotypes [40, 43]. Nevertheless the main complication of gene therapy is liver toxicity and aminotransferase elevation 7–10 weeks after gene transfer [41]. This phenomenon is a result of T cell-mediated immune responses to conducted hepatocytes. It can be simply resolved by using glucocorticoid therapy like prednisolone without loss of transgene expression. The level of increase of FIX is dose-dependent. In high-dose vector injection, FIX level reaches to 8–12% of normal levels [39].

In conclusion, gene therapy is the potential curative option for hemophilia because it induces long-term endogenous production of FIX. A small enhancement in factor level at least 1% of normal, ameliorates bleeding episodes [44]. So, despite increase in aminotransferase levels which could return to basic level through glucocorticoid therapy, without loss of gene expression, gene therapy could convert severe hemophilia to mild form or reverse it completely [39]. In fact, the future of gene therapy for management and treatment of hemophilia patients looks bright [40].

Acknowledgment We appreciate Professor Edward Tuddenham for his valuable comments that significantly improved the quality of this chapter.

References

1. Horava SD, Peppas NA. Recent advances in hemophilia B therapy. Drug Deliv Transl Res. 2017;7:359–71.
2. DeLoughery TG. Basics of coagulation. In: Hemostasis and thrombosis. Cham: Springer; 2015. p. 1–7.

3. Wang Q-Y, et al. A genetic analysis of 23 Chinese patients with hemophilia B. Sci Rep. 2016;6:25024.
4. Eby CS. Bleeding and vitamin K deficiency. In: Management of bleeding patients. Cham: Springer; 2016. p. 145–50.
5. Dorgalaleh A, Dadashizadeh G, Bamedi T. Hemophilia in Iran. Hematology. 2016;21(5):300–10.
6. Berntorp E, Shapiro AD. Modern haemophilia care. Lancet. 2012;379(9824):1447–56.
7. Yoshitake S, et al. Complete nucleotide sequences of the gene for human factor IX (antihemophilic factor B). Biochemistry. 1985;24(14):3736–50.
8. Lee C, Berntorp E, Hoots K. Textbook of hemophilia. Chichester, West Sussex, UK. Hoboken, NJ: Wiley-Blackwell; 2010.
9. Schmidt AE, Bajaj SP. Structure–function relationships in factor IX and factor IXa. Trends Cardiovasc Med. 2003;13(1):39–45.
10. Rallapalli P, et al. An interactive mutation database for human coagulation factor IX provides novel insights into the phenotypes and genetics of hemophilia B. J Thromb Haemost. 2013;11(7):1329–40.
11. Ngo JCK, et al. Crystal structure of human factor VIII: implications for the formation of the factor IXa-factor VIIIa complex. Structure. 2008;16(4):597–606.
12. Autin L, et al. Molecular models of the procoagulant factor VIIIa–factor IXa complex. J Thromb Haemost. 2005;3(9):2044–56.
13. Li T, et al. The CDC Hemophilia B mutation project mutation list: a new online resource. Mol Genet Genomic Med. 2013;1(4):238–45.
14. Li T, et al. Mutation analysis of a cohort of US patients with hemophilia B. Am J Hematol. 2014;89(4):375–9.
15. Mannucci P, Franchini M. Is haemophilia B less severe than haemophilia A? Haemophilia. 2013;19(4):499–502.
16. Jedidi I, et al. Acquired haemophilia B: a case report and literature review. Ann Biol Clin. 2011;69:685–8.
17. Franchini M, Mannucci PM. Inhibitors of propagation of coagulation (factors VIII, IX and XI): a review of current therapeutic practice. Br J Clin Pharmacol. 2011;72(4):553–62.
18. Crossley M, et al. Recovery from hemophilia B Leyden: an androgen-responsive element in the factor IX promoter. Science. 1992;257(5068):377–9.
19. DiMichele D. Inhibitor development in haemophilia B: an orphan disease in need of attention. Br J Haematol. 2007;138(3):305–15.
20. Ulrich S, et al. Congenital hypersensitivity to vitamin K antagonists due to FIX propeptide mutation at locus-10: a (not so) rare cause of bleeding under oral anticoagulant therapy in Switzerland. Swiss Med Wkly. 2008;138(7–8):100–7.
21. Chu K, et al. A mutation in the propeptide of Factor IX leads to warfarin sensitivity by a novel mechanism. J Clin Investig. 1996;98(7):1619.
22. Oldenburg J, et al. Missense mutations at ALA-10 in the factor IX propeptide: an insignificant variant in normal life but a decisive cause of bleeding during oral anticoagulant therapy. Br J Haematol. 1997;98(1):240–4.
23. Surin V, et al. Mutational analysis of hemophilia B in Russia: molecular-genetic study. Russ J Genet. 2016;52(4):409–15.
24. Kitchen S, McCraw A, Echenagucia M. Diagnosis of hemophilia and other bleeding disorders. A laboratory manual. Montreal: World Federation of Hemophilia; 2000.
25. Kihlberg K, et al. Discrepancies between the one-stage clotting assay and the chromogenic assay in haemophilia B. Haemophilia. 2017;23(4):620–7.
26. Kitchen S, Signer-Romero K, Key N. Current laboratory practices in the diagnosis and management of haemophilia: a global assessment. Haemophilia. 2015;21(4):550–7.
27. Sellner LN, Taylor GR. MLPA and MAPH: new techniques for detection of gene deletions. Hum Mutat. 2004;23(5):413–9.
28. KWON MJ, et al. Identification of mutations in the F9 gene including exon deletion by multiplex ligation-dependent probe amplification in 33 unrelated Korean patients with haemophilia B. Haemophilia. 2008;14(5):1069–75.

29. Bolton-Maggs PH, Pasi KJ. Haemophilias a and b. Lancet. 2003;361(9371):1801–9.
30. Franchini M, et al. Treatment of hemophilia B: focus on recombinant factor IX. Biol Targets Ther. 2013;7:33.
31. Elm T, Oestergaard H, Tranholm M. Dose response and prolonged effect of 40K PEG-FIX on bleeding in hemophilia B mice. J Thromb Haemost. 2009;7:134.
32. Carcao M, et al. Insight into health-related quality of life of young children with haemophilia B treated with long-acting nonacog beta pegol recombinant factor IX. Haemophilia. 2017;23(3):e222–4.
33. Metzner HJ, et al. Genetic fusion to albumin improves the pharmacokinetic properties of factor IX. Thromb Haemost. 2009;102(4):634–44.
34. Brown DL. Congenital bleeding disorders. Curr Probl Pediatr Adolesc Health Care. 2005;35(2):38–62.
35. Nummi V, Jouppila A, Lassila R. Monitoring once-weekly recombinant factor IX prophylaxis in hemophilia B with thrombin generation assay and factor IX activity. Int J Lab Hematol. 2017;39:359–68.
36. Dolan G, et al. Haemophilia B: Where are we now and what does the future hold? Blood Rev. 2017;32:52–60.
37. Key NS. Inhibitors in congenital coagulation disorders. Br J Haematol. 2004;127(4):379–91.
38. White G, et al. Recommendation of the scientific subcommittee on factor VIII and factor IX of the scientific and standardization committee of the International Society on Thrombosis and Haemostasis. Thromb Haemost. 2001;85(3):560.
39. Nathwani AC, et al. Adenovirus-associated virus vector–mediated gene transfer in hemophilia B. N Engl J Med. 2011;365(25):2357–65.
40. Nienhuis AW, Nathwani AC, Davidoff AM. Gene therapy for hemophilia. Mol Ther. 2017;25:1163–7.
41. Nathwani AC, et al. Long-term safety and efficacy of factor IX gene therapy in hemophilia B. N Engl J Med. 2014;2014(371):1994–2004.
42. Park C-Y, et al. Genome-editing technologies for gene correction of hemophilia. Hum Genet. 2016;135(9):977–81.
43. Kay MA, et al. Evidence for gene transfer and expression of factor IX in haemophilia B patients treated with an AAV vector. Nat Genet. 2000;24(3):257.
44. Herzog RW, et al. Long-term correction of canine hemophilia B by gene transfer of blood coagulation factor IX mediated by adeno-associated viral vector. Nat Med. 1999;5(1):56.

Part III

Rare Bleeding Disorders

Congenital Fibrinogen Disorders

6

Akbar Dorgalaleh, Alessandro Casini, and Parvin Rahmani

6.1 Introduction

Congenital fibrinogen disorders (CFD) are rare coagulation disorders inherited as autosomal dominant or recessive manner. CFD include four subtypes of disorders: afibrinogenemia (undetectable functional and antigenic levels of fibrinogen), hypofibrinogenemia (concomitant decrease of functional and antigenic levels of fibrinogen), dysfibrinogenemia (decreased fibrinogen activity with normal antigen levels), and hypodysfibrinogenemia (decreased level of dysfunction fibrinogen) [1]. Epidemiology of CFD is not known. Based on recent international databases, CFD represent 8% of rare coagulation disorders, although asymptomatic patients are underreported in such collections. The prevalence of afibrinogenemia is estimated to be 1 for 1,000,000 of person and more frequent in countries with consanguinity [2–4]. The prevalence of other subtypes is probably higher due to the number of asymptomatic patients [5]. Clinical features of CFD depend on the subtype and the level of fibrinogen [6]. Diagnosis is based on routine laboratory tests and confirmed by genotype [3]. Additional functional analysis can be performed in highly specialized centers to better define the patient's phenotype [7]. Management is often challenging and mainly based on personal and experts' recommendations due to the lack of randomized clinical trials or large

A. Dorgalaleh
Department of Hematology and Blood Transfusion, School of Allied Medicine, Iran University of Medical Sciences, Tehran, Iran

A. Casini (✉)
Division of Angiology and Haemostasis, Faculty of Medicine, University Hospitals of Geneva, Geneva, Switzerland
e-mail: alessandro.casini@hcuge.ch

P. Rahmani
Department of Hematology and Blood Transfusion, School of Allied Medicine, Tehran University of Medical Sciences, Tehran, Iran

A. Dorgalaleh (ed.), *Congenital Bleeding Disorders*,
https://doi.org/10.1007/978-3-319-76723-9_6

observational studies [3, 8]. In this chapter, after an overview of the structure, synthesis, and assembly of fibrinogen, we describe the clinical features of CFD as well as the diagnosis strategies and the management.

6.2 Fibrinogen Structure and Function

Fibrinogen is a high molecular weight protein (340 kD) with half-life of about 2–4 days, mostly synthetized in the liver although non-hepatocyte synthesis has also been reported in the epithelial cells of the intestine [9], cervix [10], and lungs [11]. A small amount of circulating fibrinogen is absorbed by megakaryocyte and platelets α-granules and is released into blood stream after platelet degranulation [12, 13]. Fibrinogen is an acute-phase protein which increased in pregnancy, inflammation, infection, and malignancies. Fibrinogen molecule is organized as a disulfide-linked hexamer comprised of two identical subunits, each of which formed by one Aα, one Bβ, and one γ chain with molecular weight of 64 (610 residues), 57 (461 residues), and 47 (411 residues) kDa, respectively [14–16]. These chains are encoded by three separated genes, *FGA*, *FGB*, and *FGG*, ordered from centromere to telomere and clustered in a 50 kb region on chromosome 4q32. *FGA* and *FGG* are transcribed from the reverse strand, in the opposite direction to *FGB*. Fibrinogen gene expression is controlled by the activity of proximal promoters and enhancers [17]. The *FGA*, *FGB*, and *FGG* genes consist of six exons (7.5 kb), eight exons (8 kb), and ten exons (8.5 kb), respectively [18–20]. Alternative splicing results in two isoforms for the fibrinogen α-chain and the γ-chain. The common Aα-chain is encoded by exons 1–5 and the Aα-E isoform, which represents only 1–2% of transcripts, is encoded by exons 1–6. Two mRNA transcripts arise from alternative splicing of *FGG* gene: the main one consists of ten exons which encode the common γA chain and the minor isoform (γ′) codes for 20 unique amino acids at the terminal end of the γ′-chain, which substitutes the 4 γA amino acids of exon 10 [21]. *FGB* gene encodes a unique 1.9 kb mRNA transcript [22–24]. Fibrinogen underwent posttranslational modifications including hydroxylation, oxidation, deamination, *N*-glycosylation, sulfation, sialylation, and phosphorylation [25, 26]. Post mRNA translation, disulfide bonds are formed by chaperone molecules in the rough endoplasmic reticulum.

Fibrinogen has a three-nodular structure with a central E region and two terminal D regions, each with several structural domains [27] (Fig. 6.1). The NH_2-terminal portion of all six chains composes the central nodule of the E region [15, 16, 28]. The D region is formed by the COOH-terminal portion of the Bβ and γ chains. The COOH-terminal portion of Aα-chain (αC) is flexible and tends to be developed at proximity of the E region. The soluble fibrinogen converts into insoluble fibrin in the presence of calcium and thrombin. First, the cleavage of fibrinopeptides A (FPA) and B (FPB) by thrombin at the AαArg16-Gly17 and BβArg14-Gly15 residues results in fibrin monomer (fragment X) formation [29–31]. FPA release happens earlier and faster than FPB and is sufficient to fibrin polymerization. After the conversion of insoluble fibrinogen to soluble fibrin, clot stabilization occurs by the

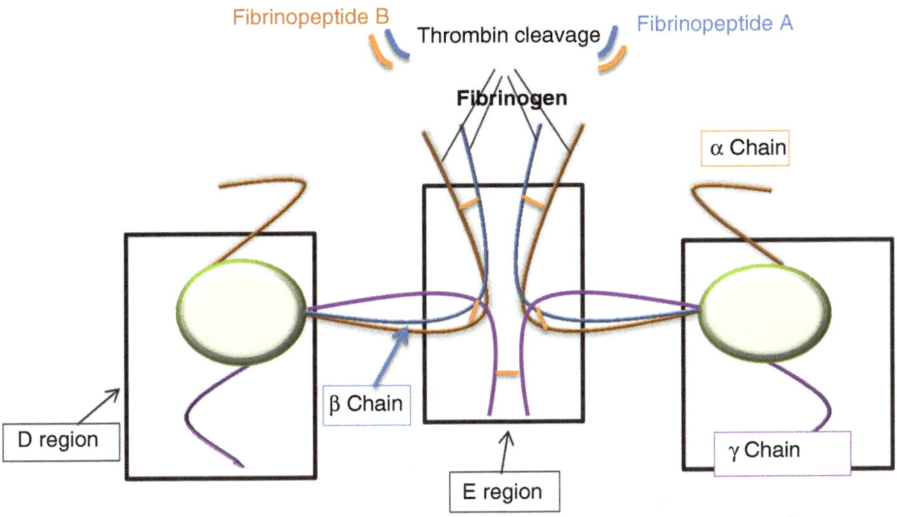

Fig. 6.1 Fibrinogen molecule structure; fibrinogen comprises of three polypeptide chains; Aα, Bβ, γ chains organize a symmetrical dimer structure which is joined together by disulfide bonds. The NH2-terminal part of the three chains forms the central E region. Fibrinopeptide A and fibrinopeptide B are cleaved and released by thrombin during fibrinogen to fibrin conversion. D region consists of the Bβ and γ chains COOH-terminal residues

transglutaminase activity of the factor XIII in presence of calcium. Factor XIII covalently link between D and E regions of adjacent fibrin monomers and give rise to protofibril which the glutamic acid of D or E domain links to lysine of an adjacent domain. Both the Aα and the γ chains participate in this reaction [32–34].

In addition to the well-known role in hemostasis supporting the platelet aggregation and the fibrin formation, fibrin(ogen) takes part in several additional processes including wound healing, angiogenesis, tumor development, cell proliferation and migration, cell matrix interactions by adhering to fibronectin, cell adhesion, and maintenance of pregnancy [35–41].

6.3 Congenital Fibrinogen Disorders

CFD are rare coagulation disorders, affecting either the quantity (type I) (afibrinogenemia and hypofibrinogenemia) or the quality (type II) (dysfibrinogenemia) or both (hypodysfibrinogenemia) of fibrinogen molecule. The precise prevalence of these disorders is not known due to the considerable number of asymptomatic patients. Afibrinogenemia is inherited in an autosomal recessive manner while hypofibrinogenemia and dysfibrinogenemia mainly in an autosomal dominant pattern [3, 42, 43] (Table 6.1). In addition to the subtype classification, sometimes CFD are classified according to the fibrinogen levels as mild (>1 g/L), moderate (0.5–1 g/L), and severe (undetectable) [44, 45]. Clinical features depend on the

Table 6.1 Congenital fibrinogen disorders

	Afibrinogenemia	Hypofibrinogenemia	Dysfibrinogenemia	Hypodysfibrinogenemia
Prevalence	1 per 1 million	Undetermined	Undetermined	Undetermined
Inheritance	Autosomal recessive	Mainly autosomal dominant	Mainly autosomal dominant	Mainly autosomal dominant
Fibrinogen activity	Undetectable	<1.5 g/L	<1.5 g/L	<1.5 g/L
Fibrinogen antigen	Undetectable	<1.5 g/L	>1.5 g/L	<1.5 g/L
Clinical features	Bleeding thrombosis Bone cysts Spontaneous spleen rupture Defective wound healing Miscarriages Postpartum hemorrhage	Mainly asymptomatic (bleeding according to the fibrinogen level) Fibrinogen storage disease Placenta abruption Miscarriages Postpartum hemorrhage	Mainly asymptomatic Thrombosis Bleeding Amyloidosis Pulmonary hypertension Miscarriage Postpartum hemorrhage	Thrombosis Bleeding Miscarriage Postpartum hemorrhage

fibrinogen levels as well as on the subtype. Furthermore, each subtype of CFD has some specific symptoms as indicated in Table 6.1.

CFD account for 8% of all rare bleeding disorders (RBDs) and are the third most common RBDs [2]. Diagnosis of disorder can be made based on clinical presentations and appropriate laboratory assessment but even in well-equipped coagulation laboratory, sometime diagnosis of these disorders can be a sophisticated process especially for dysfibrinogenemia and hypodysfibrinogenemia (Table 6.1) [46–48].

6.4 Clinical Manifestations

6.4.1 Afibrinogenemia

Bleeding, which can be life-threatening, is the main symptom of afibrinogenemia (Table 6.2). Umbilical cord bleeding, gingival bleeding, and epistaxis are common [4, 5, 49]. Muscular bleeding and hemarthroses are also frequent but less severe and invalidating than in patients with hemophilia. Although intracerebral hemorrhage is rare in afibrinogenemia, it's an important cause of morbidity and mortality [50–52]. A characteristic complication observed in afibrinogenemic patients are the painful bone cysts. They are described especially in long bones with histological features different from those reported in hemophiliac pseudotumor [53]. Another specific complication of afibrinogenemia is the spontaneous splenic rupture. Spontaneous splenic rupture is associated with an increased rate of mortality and sometimes leads to development of splanchnic thrombosis [54]. The physiopathology of these two afibrinogenemia-related disorders is not known; it could result either from a primary bleeding event or from a thrombotic event.

Table 6.2 Bleeding symptoms in afibrinogenemic and dysfibrinogenemic patients

Disorder	Clinical presentations
Afibrinogenemia	UCB (85%)
	Epistaxis (80%)
	Menorrhagia (70%)
	Hemarthrosis (54%)
	Gingival bleeding (70%)
	Postoperative bleeding (40%)
	CNS bleeding (5%)
Dysfibrinogenemia	Easy bruising (22%)
	Menorrhagia (27%)
	Gingival bleeding (6%)
	Epistaxis (5%)
	Cerebral hemorrhage (1%)

UCB umbilical cord bleeding, *CNS* central nervous system

Menorrhagia and obstetrical adverse outcomes are frequent in afibrinogenemic women. In a large series of patients, menorrhagia occurred in about half of woman. Hemorrhagic ovarian cyst rupture is a typical presentation at the menarche. As for women with factor XIII deficiency, replacement of the deficient factor is mandatory to maintain pregnancy to term. Insufficient fibrinogen replacement leads to metrorrhagia, placenta abruption, and miscarriage [5, 40, 55–57].

Paradoxically, afibrinogenemic patients are also at risk of thrombotic events, both in venous and arterial territories [58]. The mechanism has not been elucidated, although several hypotheses have been postulated [59]. One possibility is that in the absence of fibrin, there is an increased level of circulating thrombin due to the decreased antithrombin physiologic role of fibrin. Arterial thromboses could be correlated to an increase activation of platelets in response to damaged endothelium due to repeated intimal bleeding [60]. Thrombotic events are frequently recurrent, especially in the arterial peripheral territory, sometimes despite an accurate antithrombotic regimen.

6.4.2 Hypofibrinogenemia

Patients with hypofibrinogenemia are usually asymptomatic according to the fibrinogen levels. The bleeding phenotype in severe hypofibrinogenemic patients is sometimes similar to that of afibrinogenemic ones. Spontaneous bleeding can be observed among patients with fibrinogen levels lower than <0.5 g/L or post-surgery [3]. Usually, the fibrinogen level is sufficient to maintain pregnancy to term. However, recurrent pregnancy losses and placenta abruption have been reported, especially in severe hypofibrinogenemia with insufficient fibrinogen replacement. Postpartum hemorrhage can also be a complication of severe hypofibrinogenemia [51, 61–64].

Rarely, accumulation of fibrin aggregate occurs due to the impaired release of abnormal fibrinogen, resulting in chronic liver disease [65]. This “fibrinogen storage disease" is characterized by liver inflammation and hypofibrinogenemia [66–69]. It has been postulated that autophagy-induced agents can be efficient to decrease the progression of the liver disease [70].

6.4.3 Dysfibrinogenemia

The clinical presentation of dysfibrinogenemia is highly variable ranging from asymptomatic condition to severe bleeding and thrombotic complications [71]. Generally bleeding is mild in patients with dysfibrinogenemia, most often characterized by easy bruising and epistaxis. Major bleeding is usually related to trauma or injury, and spontaneous major bleeds are rare. In a large series of patients with a mean follow-up of 8.8 years, the incidence of major bleeding was 2.5 per 1000 patient-years, and the cumulative incidence at an age of 50 years was of 19.2% [72]. Most of these events occurred in child-bearing ages women. Indeed, in addition of menorrhagia, dysfibrinogenemic women can suffer from severe postpartum hemorrhage [73]. On the other hand, dysfibrinogenemia is associated with an increased risk of thrombotic events. In the aforementioned study, the incidence of venous and arterial thromboses was 18.7 per 1000 patient-years, and the cumulative incidence at an age of 50 years was of 30.1% [72]. To explain the dysfibrinogenemia-related hypercoagulability, several mechanisms have been reported. First, a defective binding of thrombin to fibrinogen can result in an increased level of circulating thrombin. Second, the abnormal fibrin network composed of thin and dense fibrin fiber decreased the overall permeability of the fibrin clot [74, 75]. Finally, fibrinolysis is impaired due to imperfect binding of tissue plasminogen activator and antiplasmin on the abnormal fibrin surface [7]. Even if most of fibrinogen variants participate only partially to this imbalance of the hemostasis system, some are clearly associated with a very strong risk of thrombotic event.

A few fibrinogen mutations lead to hereditary fibrinogen Aα-chain amyloidosis. In fibrinogen Aα-chain amyloidosis, fibrinogen molecules are fully functional (i.e., normal fibrinogen levels) but undergo an abnormal extravascular proteolysis resulting in deposit of amyloid fibrils [7, 76].

6.4.4 Hypodysfibrinogenemia

Patients with hypodysfibrinogenemia present various clinical presentations varying from mild to life-threatening bleeding such as central nervous system bleeding. About half of patients with these disorders present with at least one bleeding at time of diagnosis, while about one-fourth of them are asymptomatic at time of diagnosis. In comparison with dysfibrinogenemia, this disorder is more severe with higher rate of thrombotic events and has less asymptomatic patients [1, 77]. Bleeding is frequent in child-bearing women including postpartum hemorrhage and menorrhagia. One-fourth of women with this disorder experience at least one miscarriage. About half of these patients experience thrombotic complications, mostly in the arterial territory. The mean age of first thrombotic event is 30 years, while the mean age of diagnosis of hypodysfibrinogenemia is 32 years. In half of patients, thrombotic event occurred recurrently even with sufficient anticoagulant therapy [77–82].

6.5 Molecular Basis of Congenital Fibrinogen Disorders

In CFD, mutations are scattered throughout the three fibrinogen genes (i.e., *FGA*, *FGB*, *FGG*). Some hotspot mutations have been identified, but a number of new fibrinogen variants are still reported to date. For more details and an updated exhaustive list of causative mutations in CFD, we refer lectors to recent reviews on this topic and free online database. As example, in Fig. 6.2 are indicated selected causative mutations of quantitative fibrinogen disorders [7, 20, 77, 83–87].

6.5.1 Quantitative Fibrinogen Disorders

In quantitative disorders, null mutations (e.g., large deletions, frameshift mutations, early truncating nonsense mutations, splice-site mutations) are common. Overall, these molecular anomalies affect the fibrinogen assembly, stability, or secretion [20, 83, 88–90].

Although traditionally afibrinogenemia and hypofibrinogenemia were considered as two completely separated clinical entities, in fact they are the phenotypic expression of the heterozygote and homozygote allelic status for a given fibrinogen mutation. Afibrinogenemia is caused by homozygosity or compound heterozygosity, while hypofibrinogenemia is mostly due to heterozygosity. In most patients with afibrinogenemia and hypofibrinogenemia, amplification of coding sequences and exon-intron junctions of *FGA*, *FGB*, and *FGG* genes leads to identification of the causative mutation, but large deletions or deep intronic deletions required additional analyses [1, 20, 85, 87–89, 91]. Two recurrent mutations have been identified in quantitative fibrinogen disorders, both localize in *FGA*. The IVS4+1G>T splice-site mutation results in an early α-chain truncation. The 11-kb deletion leads to the absence of the Aα-chain.

A rare presentation of hypofibrinogenemia is the fibrinogen storage disease characterized by endoplasmic reticulum fibrinogen inclusions in the hepatocytes. Only six mutations, clustered in exon 8 and exon 9 of *FGG*, have been identified (Fig. 6.3). In patients with hypofibrinogenemia associated with a familial history of idiopathic liver disease, molecular analysis should be started with screening of these two exons [68, 69, 88, 92, 93].

6.5.2 Qualitative Fibrinogen Disorders

In qualitative fibrinogen disorders, non-null mutations are more frequent [7, 20, 94, 95]. Most dysfibrinogenemia cases are inherited in an autosomal dominant manner

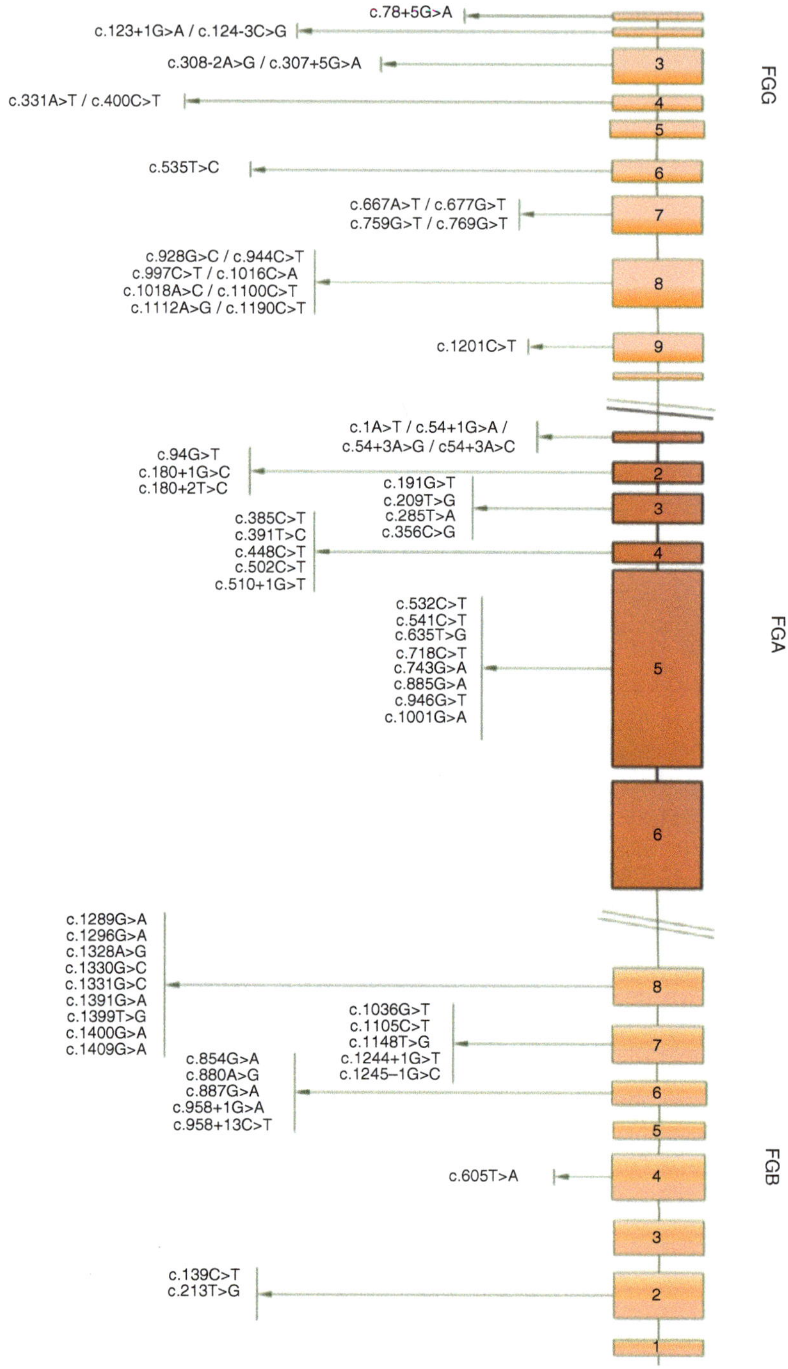

Fig. 6.2 Selected causatives mutations leading to quantitative fibrinogen disorders among the fibrinogen genes (*FGA, FGB, FGG*)

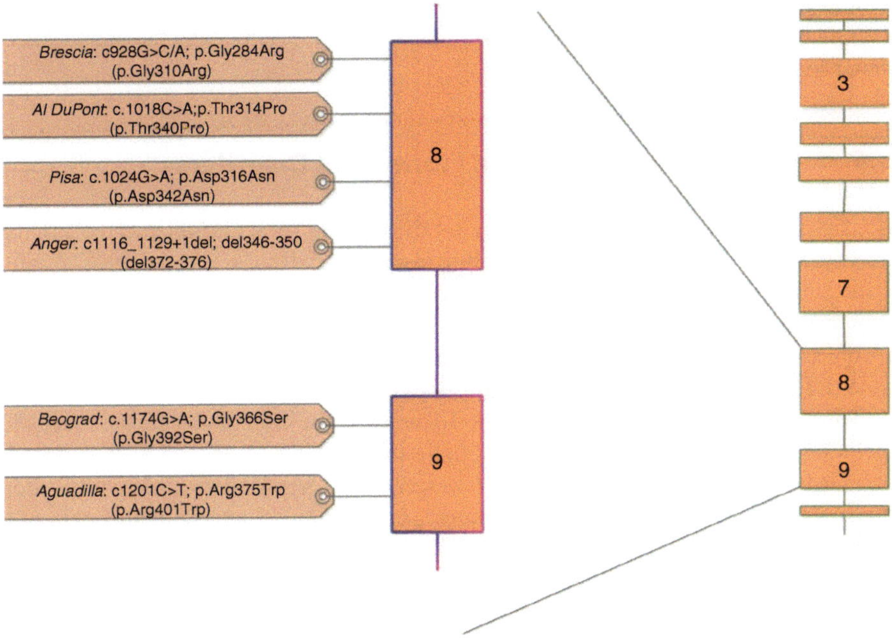

Fig. 6.3 Causative mutations of the fibrinogen storage disease

caused by heterozygote missense mutation in one of the three fibrinogen genes, although rarely homozygotes or compound heterozygote have been reported. In addition, deletion/insertion and frameshift mutations have also been identified [96, 97]. Overall, molecular anomalies leading to qualitative fibrinogen disorder affect the structure and the function of the fibrinogen molecule, including defects in fibrinopeptide cleavage and release, fibrin polymerization, and fibrin cross-linking. Two missense mutations (i.e., hotspot mutations) are frequent. The residue Arg35 of exon 2 of *FGA* (c.103C>T or c.104G>A) can be mutated in histidine or cysteine resulting in a defective thrombin binding and an abnormal release of FpA [8, 72, 87, 98]. The residue Arg301 of exon 8 of *FGG* (c.901C>T or c.902G>A) can also be mutated in histidine or cysteine affecting the D:D interactions, causing a defect in the early stage of fibrin polymerization [1, 5, 20, 88]. Considering hotspot mutations and the surrounding residues in exon 2 of *FGA* and exon 8 of *FGG*, about 85% of dysfibrinogenemia can be identified. During genetic exploration, these exons should be screened firstly [1, 7, 29, 47, 99].

In hypodysfibrinogenemia, a total of 32 causative mutations, mainly missense, nonsense, and frameshift, have been identified [77, 97]. The "hypo" phenotype of hypodysfibrinogenemia is due to impaired assembly of fibrinogen molecule, decreased secretion, or increased fibrinogen clearance, while the "dysf" phenotype is often due to defective fibrin polymerization or abnormal binding of calcium or tissue plasminogen activator [46, 77, 100, 101]. Several molecular mechanisms explain these phenotypes. On one hand, a single mutation can lead to production of an abnormal fibrinogen chain that is less effectively secreted. On other hand, two distinct heterozygous mutations can cause the qualitative defect and the quantitative one, respectively [77, 97, 102–104].

6.6 Diagnosis of Congenital Fibrinogen Disorders

A CFD should be suspected depending on the clinical presentation and the family history. For example, a prolonged umbilical cord bleeding in a relative of an afibrinogenemic family is highly suggestive. All relatives of a known CFD family should be screened [1, 4, 22, 46].

Initial investigation of CFD should include the thrombin time (TT), the reptilase time (RT), and functional and antigen fibrinogen assays (Table 6.3).

The sensitivity and the specificity of TT and RT are affected by several factors, including reagent and instrument. Although sensitivity of TT has not been properly assessed in this setting, it's broadly used as screening tests for detection of CFD. For the TT measurement, a standard amount of thrombin is added to the patient's citrated plasma and then clotting time is measured. Thrombin cleaves both molecules of FpA and FpB to mediate fibrin formation. For the RT, reptilase is used instead of thrombin to initiate the fibrin formation. In contrast to thrombin, reptilase induces fibrin formation only by cleavage of FpA. TT is prolonged in the presence of unfractionated heparin or direct thrombin inhibitors in patient's plasma, while RT is not affected in this situation [100].

A wide range of methods are available for the functional and antigen assessment of fibrinogen. Functional assays include the Clauss and the prothrombin time-derived method. The Clauss method is a modification of the thrombin time, in which citrated plasma is diluted and then excess thrombin, usually 100 U/ml (range 35–200 U/ml), is added and time of clotting is measured. High concentration of thrombin is used to ensure that clotting time is independent of thrombin concentration [1, 46, 105–107]. The clotting time is inversely proportional to the amount of fibrinogen in the sample. For determination of the plasma fibrinogen level, a calibration curve with a serial dilution of reference plasma with known concentration of fibrinogen is provided. Another method is PT-derived method [48]. As the Clauss assay, the PT-derived method is not a direct measure of the fibrinogen activity. The main advantage of PT-derived method is the limited additional cost to laboratory. In this method the PT is performed on plasma dilutions with known amount of fibrinogen, and a curve is drawn based on optical changes against different fibrinogen concentrations [1, 100, 107]. By this graph, an optical change in plasma with known amount of fibrinogen is converted to fibrinogen level. Limitations of the PT-derived method are the high rate of variability according to the reagent and the instrument. Moreover, it overestimates fibrinogen level in dysfibrinogenemia (Table 6.3) [1, 5, 46, 48, 100]. Fibrinogen antigen level can be determined by immunological (enzyme-linked immunosorbent assay, radial immunodiffusion), precipitation (heat, sulfite), and thrombin clotting methods. Fibrinogen degradation products can falsely increase fibrinogen antigen level in radial immunodiffusion, heat and sulfite precipitation, and thrombin clotting methods [1, 46, 47, 100, 108, 109].

Table 6.3 Coagulation tests in congenital bleeding disorders

	Afibrinogenemia	Hypofibrinogenemia	Dysfibrinogenemia	Hypodysfibrinogenemia	Limitations
Prothrombin time	↑↑↑	↑**	↑↑*	↑**	Low sensitivity
Activated partial thromboplastin time	↑↑↑	↑**	↑↑*	↑**	Low sensitivity
Thrombin time	↑↑↑	↑**	↑↑*	↑↑*	Low specificity and can be prolonged by: 1. Presence of heparin 2. Presence of direct thrombin inhibitors 3. Presence of paraproteins
Reptilase time	↑↑↑	↑**	↑↑*	↑↑*	Can be prolonged by: 1. High amount of FDP 2. Presence of paraproteins
Functional assay	↓↓↓	↓↓	↓↓	↓↓	In photo-optical analyzers, lipemia and high bilirubin can interfere with assay
Antigen assay	↓↓↓	↓↓	→	↓↓	Results required correlation with other assays
Activity/antigen ratio	–	>0.7	<0.7	<0.7	The sensitivity and specificity of this ratio have not been validated

*depending on the method and reagents used as well as on the fibrinogen variant
**depending on the fibrinogen level

6.6.1 Quantitative Fibrinogen Disorders

In afibrinogenemia all tests based on fibrin clot as end point are infinitely prolonged. Fibrinogen functional and antigen are undetectable (Table 6.3) [46, 100].

In hypofibrinogenemia, a proportional reduction of activity and antigen fibrinogen level (<1.5 g/L) is observed. The prolongation of PT, PTT, TT, and RT depends on the fibrinogen levels. Acquired hypofibrinogenemia can be seen in a considerable number of situations including liver disease, but they can be distinguished from congenital form based on the clinical features [110]. Distinguishing severe hypofibrinogenemia from afibrinogenemia can be difficult and depend on the limit detection of the fibrinogen assay. In such cases additional methods, such as mass spectrometry, can be useful. Finally, the genotype will confirm the diagnosis [111].

6.6.2 Qualitative Fibrinogen Disorders

Although patients with dysfibrinogenemia can be discovered due to bleeding or thrombotic phenotype, most patients are incidentally diagnosed. Initially, a similar approach to the quantitative fibrinogen disorder is performed (Table 6.3) [47, 62, 112]. Dysfibrinogenemia is suspected in case of discrepancy between functional and antigenic fibrinogen levels. A ratio activity/antigen below 0.7 is historically used to diagnose dysfibrinogenemia, although this cutoff has never been validated [46]. It should be noted that in dysfibrinogenemia the sensitivity of routine coagulation tests depends on the causative mutation, the reagents, and the instruments [112]. Shorten TT can be observed in a rare fibrinogen variants (e.g., fibrinogen Oslo I) [11, 113]. In a large series of patients with dysfibrinogenemia, TT and RT were prolonged in 87.6% and 89.7%, respectively [7]. Use of appropriate methods for activity and antigen fibrinogen assessment is crucial to minimize overestimation and misdiagnosis. In patients with dysfibrinogenemia, the PT-derived method overestimated fibrinogen level, five to six times compared with Clauss method [46–48, 100].

Hypodysfibrinogenemia is defined by low level of dysfunctional fibrinogen. It is suspected in case of discrepancy between decreased activity and decreased antigen fibrinogen levels. Since hypodysfibrinogenemia shares some features with both hypofibrinogenemia and dysfibrinogenemia, misdiagnosis is an important issue in this disorder. Distinguish it from hypofibrinogenemia is difficult especially in case with very low fibrinogen levels [46, 77, 100]. In a recent systematic review of literature, the functional/antigenic fibrinogen ratio of <0.7 showed a poor sensitivity (86%) with a mean functional/antigenic fibrinogen ratio of 0.46 (0.07–1.25) observed in 32 cases [77]. Overall, further assessments including fibrinogen functional and structural assays, performed in highly specialized research laboratories, can provide a better assessment of the patient's phenotype [1, 46, 47, 77, 100].

6.7 Treatment of Patients with Congenital Fibrinogen Disorders

Traditionally, CFD patients were treated with fresh frozen plasma (FFP) and/or cryoprecipitate, but use of these blood components has been restricted due to risk of blood-borne disease transmission. Virus-inactivated fibrinogen concentrates are nowadays the treatment of choice. However, they are still inaccessible in many areas of the world. Different plasma-derived fibrinogen concentrates are available, with minimal risk of blood-borne diseases (Table 6.4) [9, 114]. Three additional fibrinogen concentrates are at different phases of clinical trials [22].

6.7.1 Quantitative Fibrinogen Disorders

Conventionally, patients with quantitative fibrinogen disorders are treated "on-demand," although secondary prophylaxis regimens should be proposed after life-threatening bleeding. In case of primary or secondary prophylaxis, the target trough fibrinogen level should be more than 0.5 g/L. The long half-life of fibrinogen allows usually an administration every 7–14 days. Due to intraindividual differences, a pharmacokinetic profile should be proposed to each patient. In case of bleeding, the target peak fibrinogen level depends on the type and the severity of hemorrhage [115]. For surgical prophylaxis, fibrinogen level is recommended to be above 1 g/L and maintained above 0.5 g/L until complete wound healing. There is some concern on the fibrinogen-related risk of thrombosis in case of replacement. This risk should be kept in mind, and the physician should try to not over-increase the fibrinogen level. To determine required dose in patient with congenital fibrinogen disorders, below formula can be used:

$$\text{Amount of fibrinogen to be administered} = \left[\text{target fibrinogen level}\left(\text{g L\_1}\right) - \text{basal fibrinogen level}\right] \times 1/\text{R} \times \text{weight}\left(\text{kg}\right)$$

Antifibrinolytic agents, such as tranexamic acid, can be used for mucosal bleeding and to prevent postdental extraction bleeding. This therapeutic option may be increase the risk of thrombosis and should be used with caution in patients with previous personal or familial history of thrombosis and high risk of thrombosis. Another potential therapeutic choice for patients with afibrinogenemia is liver

Table 6.4 Available fibrinogen concentrates

Product	Company	Country
Clottafact/Clottagen®	LFB, les Ulis	France
Fibrinogen HT®	Benesis	Japan
Haemocomplettan/ RiaSTAP®	CSL Behring	Germany

transplantation [24, 115, 116]. Treatment of thrombosis in congenital fibrinogen disorders is difficult. This condition required both fibrinogen concentrate and anti-thrombosis agents [3, 8, 116]. Oral direct anticoagulants, especially with direct anti-thrombin activity, are promising agents. Women with quantitative fibrinogen disorder may benefit from introduction of contraceptive pills to decrease the risk of severe menorrhagia and hemorrhagic ovarian cyst rupture. In case of pregnancy, afibrinogenemic and severe hypofibrinogenemic women should receive a fibrinogen replacement. The fibrinogen requirement increases throughout the pregnancy.

6.7.2 Qualitative Fibrinogen Disorders

The overall management of patients with qualitative fibrinogen disorders should always consider the personal and familial history of bleeding and thrombosis as well as the genotype [7, 42]. In case of bleeding, the same recommendations for quantitative fibrinogen disorder are valuable [117]. Fibrinogen replacement prophylaxis before surgery is necessary only in case of a strong bleeding phenotype or in case of major surgery. Most often, the fibrinogen replacement is required only in case of complications [116]. Patients should receive an accurate thromboprophylaxis in high thrombotic risk situation. In case of thrombosis, low molecular weight heparin and direct oral anticoagulant are the molecules of choice. Length of thrombosis is dependent on the type of thrombosis (localization, recurrence), the genotype (some mutations correlate with the thrombotic risk), and the familial history [3]. Most often dysfibrinogenemic women do not require a fibrinogen replacement during the pregnancy but should carefully followed during the postpartum due to the risk of postpartum hemorrhage [72].

References

1. Neerman-Arbez M, De Moerloose P, Casini A. Laboratory and genetic investigation of mutations accounting for congenital fibrinogen disorders. Semin Thromb Hemost. 2016;42:356–65.
2. Palla R, Peyvandi F, Shapiro AD. Rare bleeding disorders: diagnosis and treatment. Blood. 2015;125(13):2052–61.
3. Casini A, De Moerloose P, Neerman-Arbez M. Clinical features and management of congenital fibrinogen deficiencies. Semin Thromb Hemost. 2016;42:366–74.
4. Dorgalaleh A, Alavi SER, Tabibian S, Soori S, Moradi EH, Bamedi T, et al. Diagnosis, clinical manifestations and management of rare bleeding disorders in Iran. Hematology. 2017;22(4):224–30.
5. De Moerloose P, Casini A, Neerman-Arbez M. Congenital fibrinogen disorders: an update. Semin Thromb Hemost. 2013;39:585–95.
6. Menache D. Congenital fibrinogen abnormalities. Ann N Y Acad Sci. 1983;408(1):121–30.
7. Casini A, Neerman-Arbez M, Ariens R, Moerloose P. Dysfibrinogenemia: from molecular anomalies to clinical manifestations and management. J Thromb Haemost. 2015;13(6):909–19.
8. De Moerloose P, Neerman-Arbez M. Treatment of congenital fibrinogen disorders. Expert Opin Biol Ther. 2008;8(7):979–92.
9. Molmenti EP, Ziambaras T, Perlmutter DH. Evidence for an acute phase response in human intestinal epithelial cells. J Biol Chem. 1993;268:14116–24.

10. Lee SY, Lee KP, Lim JW. Identification and biosynthesis of fibrinogen in human uterine cervix carcinoma cells. Thromb Haemost. 1996;75:466–70.
11. Simpson-Haidaris PJ. Induction of fibrinogen biosynthesis and secretion from cultured pulmonary epithelial cells. Blood. 1997;89:873–82.
12. Francis CW, Nachman RL, Marder VJ. Plasma and platelet fibrinogen differ in gamma chain content. Thromb Haemost. 1984;51(1):84–8.
13. Soria J, Soria C, Samama M, Poirot E, Kling C. Human platelet fibrinogen: a protein different from plasma fibrinogen. Pathol Biol. 1976;24:15–7.
14. Blombäck B. Fibrinogen structure, activation, polymerization and fibrin gel structure. Thromb Res. 1994;75(3):327–8.
15. Mosesson MW. Fibrinogen structure and fibrin clot assembly. Semin Thromb Hemost. 1998;24:169–74.
16. Söderqvist T, Blombäck B. Fibrinogen structure and evolution. Naturwissenschaften. 1971;58(1):16–23.
17. Fish RJ, Neerman-Arbez M. Fibrinogen gene regulation. Thromb Haemost. 2012;108(3):419–26.
18. Crabtree GR, Comeau CM, Fowlkes DM, Fornace AJ, Malley JD, Kant JA. Evolution and structure of the fibrinogen genes: random insertion of introns or selective loss? J Mol Biol. 1985;185(1):1–19.
19. Henry I, Uzan G, Weil D, Nicolas H, Kaplan J, Marguerie C, et al. The genes coding for A alpha-, B beta-, and gamma-chains of fibrinogen map to 4q2. Am J Hum Genet. 1984;36(4):760.
20. Asselta R, Duga S, Tenchini M. The molecular basis of quantitative fibrinogen disorders. J Thromb Haemost. 2006;4(10):2115–29.
21. Macrae FL, Domingues MM, Casini A, Ariëns RA. The (Patho)physiology of fibrinogen γ′. Semin Thromb Hemost. 2016;42(4):344–55.
22. De Moerloose P, Neerman-Arbez M. Congenital fibrinogen disorders. Semin Thromb Hemost. 2009;35:356–66.
23. Neerman-Arbez M, Tirefort Y, de Moerloose P. Can mutations identified in congenital fibrinogen disorders explain the clinical manifestations. J Coagul Disord. 2010;2(2):1–9.
24. Stanciakova L, Kubisz P, Dobrotova M, Stasko J. Congenital afibrinogenemia: from etiopathogenesis to challenging clinical management. Expert Rev Hematol. 2016;9(7):639–48.
25. Ogata Y, Hepplmann CJ, Charlesworth MC, Madden BJ, Miller MN, Kalli KR, et al. Elevated levels of phosphorylated fibrinogen-α-isoforms and differential expression of other post-translationally modified proteins in the plasma of ovarian cancer patients. J Proteome Res. 2006;5(12):3318–25.
26. Parastatidis I, Thomson L, Burke A, Chernysh I, Nagaswami C, Visser J, et al. Fibrinogen β-chain tyrosine nitration is a prothrombotic risk factor. J Biol Chem. 2008;283(49):33846–53.
27. Medved L, Weisel JW, Fibrinogen and Factor XIII Subcommittee of Scientific Standardization Committee of International Society on Thrombosis and Haemostasis. Recommendations for nomenclature on fibrinogen and fibrin. J Thromb Haemost. 2009;7(2):355–9.
28. Mosesson M. Fibrinogen and fibrin structure and functions. J Thromb Haemost. 2005;3(8):1894–904.
29. Olexa SA, Budzynski AZ. Evidence for four different polymerization sites involved in human fibrin formation. Proc Natl Acad Sci. 1980;77(3):1374–8.
30. Gorkun OV, Veklich YI, Medved LV, Henschen AH, Weisel JW. Role of the alpha C domains of fibrin in clot formation. Biochemistry. 1994;33(22):6986–97.
31. Li X, Galanakis D, Gabriel DA. Transient intermediates in the thrombin activation of fibrinogen evidence for only the desAA species. J Biol Chem. 1996;271(20):11767–71.
32. Dorgalaleh A, Rashidpanah J. Blood coagulation factor XIII and factor XIII deficiency. Blood Rev. 2016;30(6):461–75.
33. Muszbek L, Yee VC, Hevessy Z. Blood coagulation factor XIII: structure and function. Thromb Res. 1999;94(5):271–305.
34. Muszbek L, Adany R, Mikkola H. Novel aspects of blood coagulation factor XIII. I. Structure, distribution, activation, and function. Crit Rev Clin Lab Sci. 1996;33(5):357–421.

35. Drew AF, Liu H, Davidson JM, Daugherty CC, Degen JL. Wound-healing defects in mice lacking fibrinogen. Blood. 2001;97(12):3691–8.
36. Clark RA. Fibrin and wound healing. Ann N Y Acad Sci. 2001;936(1):355–67.
37. Ikeda Y, Handa M, Kawano K, Kamata T, Murata M, Araki Y, et al. The role of von Willebrand factor and fibrinogen in platelet aggregation under varying shear stress. J Clin Investig. 1991;87(4):1234.
38. Staton CA, Brown NJ, Lewis CE. The role of fibrinogen and related fragments in tumour angiogenesis and metastasis. Expert Opin Biol Ther. 2003;3(7):1105–20.
39. Rybarczyk BJ, Lawrence SO, Simpson-Haidaris PJ. Matrix-fibrinogen enhances wound closure by increasing both cell proliferation and migration. Blood. 2003;102(12):4035–43.
40. Suh TT, Holmbäck K, Jensen NJ, Daugherty CC, Small K, Simon DI, et al. Resolution of spontaneous bleeding events but failure of pregnancy in fibrinogen-deficient mice. Genes Dev. 1995;9(16):2020–33.
41. Cheresh DA, Berliner SA, Vicente V, Ruggeri ZM. Recognition of distinct adhesive sites on fibrinogen by related integrins on platelets and endothelial cells. Cell. 1989;58(5):945–53.
42. Peyvandi F. Epidemiology and treatment of congenital fibrinogen deficiency. Thromb Res. 2012;130:S7–S11.
43. El Boussaadni Y, Benajiba N, El Ouali A, Amrani R, Rkain M. Congenital afibrinogenemia: a case report. Archives de pediatrie: organe officiel de la Societe francaise de. Pediatrie. 2015;22(1):50–2.
44. Peyvandi F, Palla R, Menegatti M, Siboni S, Halimeh S, Faeser B, et al. Coagulation factor activity and clinical bleeding severity in rare bleeding disorders: results from the European Network of Rare Bleeding Disorders. J Thromb Haemost. 2012;10(4):615–21.
45. Peyvandi F, Di Michele D, Bolton-Maggs P, Lee C, Tripodi A, Srivastava A. Classification of rare bleeding disorders (RBDs) based on the association between coagulant factor activity and clinical bleeding severity. J Thromb Haemost. 2012;10(9):1938–43.
46. Lebreton A, Casini A. Diagnosis of congenital fibrinogen disorders. Ann Biol Clin. 2016;74:405–12.
47. Cunningham MT, Brandt JT, Laposata M, Olson JD. Laboratory diagnosis of dysfibrinogenemia. Arch Pathol Lab Med. 2002;126(4):499–505.
48. Miesbach W, Schenk J, Alesci S, Lindhoff-Last E. Comparison of the fibrinogen Clauss assay and the fibrinogen PT derived method in patients with dysfibrinogenemia. Thromb Res. 2010;126(6):e428–e33.
49. Al-Mondhiry H, Ehmann WC. Congenital afibrinogenemia. Am J Hematol. 1994;46(4):343–7.
50. Henselmans J, Meijer K, Haaxma R, Hew J, van Der Meer J. Recurrent spontaneous intracerebral hemorrhage in a congenitally afibrinogenemic patient. Stroke. 1999;30(11):2479–82.
51. Taslimi R, Golshani K. Thrombotic and hemorrhagic presentation of congenital hypo/afibrinogenemia. Am J Emerg Med. 2011;29(5):573.e3–5.
52. Paolini R, Sartori MT, Fiorin F, Gorinati M, Boeri G, Girolami A. Perinatal intracranial hemorrhage as first manifestation of congenital hypofibrinogenemia. Clin Appl Thromb Hemost. 1996;2(1):60–3.
53. Fettah A, Gökçebay DG, Çulha V, Yaralı N, Tunç B, Özbek N. A rare complication of congenital afibrinogenemia: bone cysts. Turk J Haematol. 2017;34(2):183.
54. Ehmann WC, Al-Mondhiry H. Congenital afibrinogenemia and splenic rupture. Am J Med. 1994;96(1):92–4.
55. Dorgalaleh A, Naderi M, Shamsizadeh M. Morbidity and mortality in a large number of Iranian patients with severe congenital factor XIII deficiency. Ann Hematol. 2016;95(3):451–5.
56. Trehan A, Fergusson I. Congenital afibrinogenaemia and successful pregnancy outcome. Case report. Br J Obstet Gynaecol. 1991;98(7):722–4.
57. Zdziarska J, Undas A, Basa J, Iwaniec T, Skotnicki AB, De Moerloose P, et al. Severe bleeding and miscarriages in a hypofibrinogenemic woman heterozygous for the γAla82Gly mutation. Blood Coagul Fibrinolysis. 2009;20(5):374–6.
58. Santoro C, Massaro F, Venosi S, Capria S, Baldacci E, Foà R, Mazzucconi MG. Severe thrombotic complications in congenital afibrinogenemia: a pathophysiological and management dilemma. Semin Thromb Hemost. 2016;42(5):577–82.

59. Rottenstreich A, Lask A, Schliamser L, Zivelin A, Seligsohn U, Kalish Y. Thromboembolic events in patients with severe inherited fibrinogen deficiency. J Thromb Thrombolysis. 2016;42(2):261–6.
60. Sartori MT, Milan M, de Bon E, Fadin M, Pesavento R, Zanon E. Thrombosis of abdominal aorta in congenital afibrinogenemia: case report and review of literature. Haemophilia. 2015;21(1):88–94.
61. Frenkel E, Duksin C, Herman A, Sherman DJ. Congenital hypofibrinogenemia in pregnancy: report of two cases and review of the literature. Obstet Gynecol Surv. 2004;59(11):775–9.
62. Awasthy N, Aggarwal K, Gupta H, Saluja S. Congenital hypofibrinogenemia. Indian Pediatr. 2004;41(2):185–6.
63. Hasselback R, Marion RB, Thomas J. Congenital hypofibrinogenemia in five members of a family. Can Med Assoc J. 1963;88(1):19.
64. Bay A, Coskun E, Leblebisatan G, Sivasli E. Epidural hematoma and cephalohematoma with congenital hypofibrinogenemia. Blood Coagul Fibrinolysis. 2012;23(3):229–31.
65. Rubbia-Brandt L, Neerman-Arbez M, Rougemont A-L, Malé P-J, Spahr L. Fibrinogen gamma375 arg→ trp mutation (fibrinogen aguadilla) causes hereditary hypofibrinogenemia, hepatic endoplasmic reticulum storage disease and cirrhosis. Am J Surg Pathol. 2006;30(7):906–11.
66. Wehinger H, Klinge O, Alexandrakis E, Schürmann J, Witt J, Seydewitz H. Hereditary hypofibrinogenemia with fibrinogen storage in the liver. Eur J Pediatr. 1983;141(2):109–12.
67. Pfeifer U, Ormanns W, Klinge O. Hepatocellular fibrinogen storage in familial hypofibrinogenemia. Virchows Arch B. 1981;36(1):247–55.
68. Casini A, Sokollik C, Lukowski S, Lurz E, Rieubland C, Moerloose P, et al. Hypofibrinogenemia and liver disease: a new case of Aguadilla fibrinogen and review of the literature. Haemophilia. 2015;21(6):820–7.
69. Asselta R, Robusto M, Braidotti P, Peyvandi F, Nastasio S, D'antiga L, et al. Hepatic fibrinogen storage disease: identification of two novel mutations (p. Asp316Asn, fibrinogen Pisa and p. Gly366Ser, fibrinogen Beograd) impacting on the fibrinogen γ-module. J Thromb Haemost. 2015;13(8):1459–67.
70. Puls F, Goldschmidt I, Bantel H, Agne C, Bröcker V, Dämmrich M, et al. Autophagy-enhancing drug carbamazepine diminishes hepatocellular death in fibrinogen storage disease. J Hepatol. 2013;59(3):626–30.
71. Casini A, Duval C, Pan X, Tintillier V, Biron-Andreani C, Ariëns R. Fibrin clot structure in patients with congenital dysfibrinogenaemia. Thromb Res. 2016;137:189–95.
72. Casini A, Blondon M, Lebreton A, Koegel J, Tintillier V, de Maistre E, et al. Natural history of patients with congenital dysfibrinogenemia. Blood. 2015;125(3):553–61.
73. Miesbach W, Galanakis D, Scharrer I. Treatment of patients with dysfibrinogenemia and a history of abortions during pregnancy. Blood Coagul Fibrinolysis. 2009;20(5):366–70.
74. Miesbach W, Scharrer I, Henschen A, Neerman-Arbez M, Spitzer S, Galanakis D. Inherited dysfibrinogenemia: clinical phenotypes associated with five different fibrinogen structure defects. Blood Coagul Fibrinolysis. 2010;21(1):35–40.
75. Hayes T. Dysfibrinogenemia and thrombosis. Arch Pathol Lab Med. 2002;126(11):1387–90.
76. Rowczenio D, Stensland M, de Souza GA, Strøm EH, Gilbertson JA, Taylor G, et al. Renal amyloidosis associated with five novel variants in the fibrinogen A alpha chain protein. Kidney Int Rep. 2017;2:461–9.
77. Casini A, Brungs T, Lavenu-Bombled C, Vilar R, Neerman-Arbez M, Moerloose P. Genetics, diagnosis and clinical features of congenital hypodysfibrinogenemia: a systematic literature review and report of a novel mutation. J Thromb Haemost. 2017;15(5):876–88.
78. Deering SH, Landy HJ, Tchabo N, Kessler C. Hypodysfibrinogenemia during pregnancy, labor, and delivery. Obstet Gynecol. 2003;101(5, Part 2):1092–4.
79. Cheah CY, Brennan SO, Kennedy H, Januszewicz EH, Maxwell E, Burbury K. Fibrinogen Melbourne: a novel congenital hypodysfibrinogenemia caused by γ326Cys-Phe in the fibrinogen γ chain, presenting as massive splanchnic venous thrombosis. Blood Coagul Fibrinolysis. 2012;23(6):563–5.

80. Ebert RF, Bell WR. Fibrinogen Baltimore II: congenital hypodysfibrinogenemia with delayed release of fibrinopeptide B and decreased rate of fibrinogen synthesis. Proc Natl Acad Sci. 1983;80(23):7318–22.
81. Lefebvre P, Velasco PT, Dear A, Lounes KC, Lord ST, Brennan SO, et al. Severe hypodysfibrinogenemia in compound heterozygotes of the fibrinogen AαIVS4+ 1G> T mutation and an AαGln328 truncation (fibrinogen Keokuk). Blood. 2004;103(7):2571–6.
82. Jayo A, Arnold E, González-Manchón C, Green D, Lord ST. Hypodysfibrinogenemia causing mild bleeding and thrombotic complications in a compound heterozygote of AαIVS4+ 1G> T mutation and Aα4841delC truncation (AαPerth). Thromb Haemost. 2009;101(4):770.
83. Duga S, Asselta R, Santagostino E, Zeinali S, Simonic T, Malcovati M, et al. Missense mutations in the human β fibrinogen gene cause congenital afibrinogenemia by impairing fibrinogen secretion. Blood. 2000;95(4):1336–41.
84. Neerman-Arbez M, De Moerloose P, Bridel C, Honsberger A, Schönbörner A, Rossier C, et al. Mutations in the fibrinogen Aα gene account for the majority of cases of congenital afibrinogenemia. Blood. 2000;96(1):149–52.
85. Neerman-Arbez M. The molecular basis of inherited afibrinogenaemia. Thromb Haemost. 2001;86(1):154–63.
86. Uzan G, Courtois G, Besmond C, Frain M, Sala-Trepat J, Kahn A, et al. Analysis of fibrinogen genes in patients with congenital afibrinogenemia. Biochem Biophys Res Commun. 1984;120(2):376–83.
87. Neerman-Arbez M, De Moerloose P. Mutations in the fibrinogen gene cluster accounting for congenital afibrinogenemia: an update and report of 10 novel mutations. Hum Mutat. 2007;28(6):540.
88. Brennan SO, Fellowes AP, George PM. Molecular mechanisms of hypo-and afibrinogenemia. Ann N Y Acad Sci. 2001;936(1):91–100.
89. Neerman-Arbez M, De Moerloose P, Honsberger A, Parlier G, Arnuti B, Biron C, et al. Molecular analysis of the fibrinogen gene cluster in 16 patients with congenital afibrinogenemia: novel truncating mutations in the FGA and FGG genes. Hum Genet. 2001;108(3):237–40.
90. Neerman-Arbez M, Vu D, Abu-Libdeh B, Bouchardy I, Morris MA. Prenatal diagnosis for congenital afibrinogenemia caused by a novel nonsense mutation in the FGB gene in a Palestinian family. Blood. 2003;101(9):3492–4.
91. Asselta R, Spena S, Duga S, Peyvandi F, Malcovati M, Mannucci PM, et al. Analysis of Iranian patients allowed the identification of the first truncating mutation in the fibrinogen Bbeta-chain gene causing afibrinogenemia. Haematologica. 2002;87(8):855–9.
92. Brennan SO, Davis RL, Conard K, Savo A, Furuya KN. Novel fibrinogen mutation γ314Thr→ Pro (fibrinogen AI duPont) associated with hepatic fibrinogen storage disease and hypofibrinogenaemia. Liver Int. 2010;30(10):1541–7.
93. Lee MJ, Venick R, Bhuta S, Li X, Wang HL. Hepatic fibrinogen storage disease in a patient with hypofibrinogenemia: report of a case with a missense mutation of the FGA gene. Semin Liver Dis. 2015;35:439–43.
94. Asselta R, Platè M, Robusto M, Borhany M, Guella I, Soldà G, et al. Clinical and molecular characterisation of 21 patients affected by quantitative fibrinogen deficiency. Thromb Haemost. 2015;113(3):567–76.
95. Sumitha E, Jayandharan G, Arora N, Abraham A, David S, Devi G, et al. Molecular basis of quantitative fibrinogen disorders in 27 patients from India. Haemophilia. 2013;19(4):611–8.
96. Koopman J, Haverkate F, Grimbergen J, Egbring R, Lord S. Fibrinogen Marburg: a homozygous case of dysfibrinogenemia, lacking amino acids A alpha 461-610 (Lys 461 AAA--> stop TAA). Blood. 1992;80(8):1972–9.
97. Vu D, Neerman-Arbez M. Molecular mechanisms accounting for fibrinogen deficiency: from large deletions to intracellular retention of misfolded proteins. J Thromb Haemost. 2007;5(s1):125–31.
98. Zhou J, Ding Q, Chen Y, Ouyang Q, Jiang L, Dai J, et al. Clinical features and molecular basis of 102 Chinese patients with congenital dysfibrinogenemia. Blood Cell Mol Dis. 2015;55(4):308–15.

99. Hill M, Dolan G. Diagnosis, clinical features and molecular assessment of the dysfibrinogenaemias. Haemophilia. 2008;14(5):889–97.
100. Verhovsek M, Moffat KA, Hayward CP. Laboratory testing for fibrinogen abnormalities. Am J Hematol. 2008;83(12):928–31.
101. Sadeghian MH, Keramati MR, Badiei Z, Ravarian M, Ayatollahi H, Rafatpanah H, et al. Alloimmunization among transfusion-dependent thalassemia patients. Asian J Transfus Sci. 2009;3(2):95.
102. Ridgway HJ, Brennan SO, Faed JM, George PM. Fibrinogen Otago: a major α chain truncation associated with severe hypofibrinogenaemia and recurrent miscarriage. Br J Haematol. 1997;98(3):632–9.
103. Martinez J, Holburn R, Shapiro S, Erslev A. Fibrinogen Philadelphia. A hereditary hypodysfibrinogenemia characterized by fibrinogen hypercatabolism. J Clin Investig. 1974;53(2):600.
104. Mukai S, Nagata K, Ikeda M, Arai S, Sugano M, Honda T, et al. Genetic analyses of novel compound heterozygous hypodysfibrinogenemia, Tsukuba I: FGG c. 1129+ 62_65 del AATA and FGG c. 1299+ 4 del A. Thromb Res. 2016;148:111–7.
105. Harr JN, Moore EE, Ghasabyan A, Chin TL, Sauaia A, Banerjee A, et al. Functional fibrinogen assay indicates that fibrinogen is critical in correcting abnormal clot strength following trauma. Shock. 2013;39(1):45.
106. Mackie I, Lawrie A, Kitchen S, Gaffney P, Howarth D, Lowe G, et al. A performance evaluation of commercial fibrinogen reference preparations and assays for Clauss and PT-derived fibrinogen. Thromb Haemost. 2002;87(6):997–1005.
107. Mackie IJ, Kitchen S, Machin SJ, Lowe G. Guidelines on fibrinogen assays. Br J Haematol. 2003;121(3):396–404.
108. Exner T, Burridge J, Power P, Rickard KA. An evaluation of currently available methods for plasma fibrinogen. Am J Clin Pathol. 1979;71(5):521–7.
109. Desvignes P, Bonnet P. Direct determination of plasma fibrinogen levels by heat precipitation. A comparison of the technique against thrombin clottable fibrinogen with spectrophotometry and radial immuno-diffusion. Clin Chim Acta. 1981;110(1):9–17.
110. Besser MW, MacDonald SG. Acquired hypofibrinogenemia: current perspectives. J Blood Med. 2016;7:217.
111. Casini A, de Moerloose P. Can the phenotype of inherited fibrinogen disorders be predicted? Haemophilia. 2016;22(5):667–75.
112. Shapiro SE, Phillips E, Manning RA, Morse CV, Murden SL, Laffan MA, et al. Clinical phenotype, laboratory features and genotype of 35 patients with heritable dysfibrinogenaemia. Br J Haematol. 2013;160(2):220–7.
113. Godal H, Brosstad F, Kierulf P. Three new cases of an inborn qualitative fibrinogen defect (Fibrinogen Oslo II). Eur J Haematol. 1978;20(1):57–62.
114. Acharya S, Coughlin A, Dimichele DM. Rare Bleeding Disorder Registry: deficiencies of factors II, V, VII, X, XIII, fibrinogen and dysfibrinogenemias. J Thromb Haemost. 2004;2(2):248–56.
115. Casini A, de Moerloose P, Congenital Fibrinogen Disorders Group. Management of congenital quantitative fibrinogen disorders: a Delphi consensus. Haemophilia. 2016;22(6):898–905.
116. Mumford AD, Ackroyd S, Alikhan R, Bowles L, Chowdary P, Grainger J, et al. Guideline for the diagnosis and management of the rare coagulation disorders. Br J Haematol. 2014;167(3):304–26.
117. Bolton-Maggs PH, Perry DJ, Chalmers EA, Parapia LA, Wilde JT, Williams MD, Collins PW, Kitchen S, Dolan G, Mumford AD. The rare coagulation disorders – review with guidelines for management from the United Kingdom Haemophilia Centre Doctors' Organisation. Haemophilia. 2004;10(5):593–628.

7 Congenital Factor II Deficiency

Yadollah Farshi, Akbar Dorgalaleh, and Shadi Tabibian

7.1 Introduction

Coagulation factor (F) II (prothrombin) is a vitamin K-dependent coagulation factor which plays a pivotal role in blood coagulation cascade. Prothrombin is a 72-kDa glycoprotein that synthesized as an inactive zymogen by hepatocytes [1]. Prothrombin is activated to thrombin by prothrombinase complex which consists of the activated FX (FXa), FVa, and calcium [2] (please refer to Chap. 1). Thrombin is a multifunctional enzyme which converts fibrinogen to fibrin in the blood coagulation cascade. In addition, this protein has different roles including platelet, FXIII, FV, FVIII, and protein C activation [3, 4]. Congenital FII deficiency which was first reported by Quick in 1947 is the rarest autosomal recessive coagulation disorder (similar to FXIII deficiency, please refer to Chap. 13) with incidence of 1:2 million in the general population. This disorder mostly presents in regions which parental consanguinity is commonly practiced [5]. Based on the FII activity level, prothrombin deficiency is classified into three groups including mild, moderate, and severe forms with >10%, <10%, and undetectable level of FII activity, respectively [6]. Moreover, this disorder can be classified into four main phenotypes including hypoprothrombinemia (type I deficiency) with concomitant decrease of both FII activity and antigen levels, dysprothrombinemia (type II deficiency) with normal or slightly decreased level of FII antigen, but low level of activity, hypo–dys or dys–dys forms, and combined deficiency of prothrombin and other γ-carboxylated coagulation factors [6, 7]. The most common clinical manifestations of this disorder are mucosal

Y. Farshi
Department of Hematology and Blood Transfusion, School of Allied Medicine, Tehran University of Medical Sciences, Tehran, Iran

A. Dorgalaleh · S. Tabibian (✉)
Department of Hematology and Blood Transfusion, School of Allied Medicine, Iran University of Medical Sciences, Tehran, Iran

A. Dorgalaleh (ed.), *Congenital Bleeding Disorders*,
https://doi.org/10.1007/978-3-319-76723-9_7

bleeding, hematoma, and post-surgical bleeding [3]. Life-threatening bleedings including central nervous system (CNS) bleeding, gastrointestinal (GI) bleeding, and umbilical cord (UC) bleeding are rarely presentations in affected patients [3, 8]. About 60 causing mutations in *F2* gene are identified; 80% of them are missense. Other mutations are insertion/deletion (10%), nonsense (6%), and splice site mutations (4%) [9]. FII deficiency is diagnosed based on family history, clinical manifestations, and routine and specific coagulation laboratory tests. FII deficiency is suspected through prolonged prothrombin time (PT) and activated thromboplastin time (aPTT) and confirmed by FII assays. The one-stage PT-based assay is the most commonly used FII activity assay technique [3]. Since there is no specific available prothrombin concentrates, prothrombin complex concentrate (PCC) and fresh frozen plasma (FFP) are the treatments of choice [10].

7.2 Coagulation Factor II (Prothrombin) Structure

Coagulation FII (prothrombin) is a vitamin K-dependent glycoprotein which plays a pivotal role in blood coagulation system. Prothrombin is a 72-KDa glycoprotein and synthesized in the liver and needs posttranslational carboxylation to become active. This protein circulates in blood stream at the concentration of 0.1 mg/mL with half-life of 60 h [6].

Prothrombin mapped to centromeric region of 11p11-q12 with length about 21 kb and composed of 14 exons and 13 introns (Fig. 7.1). This protein consists of 4 fragments and 579 amino acid residues including gamma carboxyglutamic (Gla) domain (residues 1–46), kringle-1 (residues 65–143), kringle-2 (residues 170–248), and protease domain (residues 285–579). Protease domain includes chain A (residues 285–320) and chain B (residues 321–579) [1].

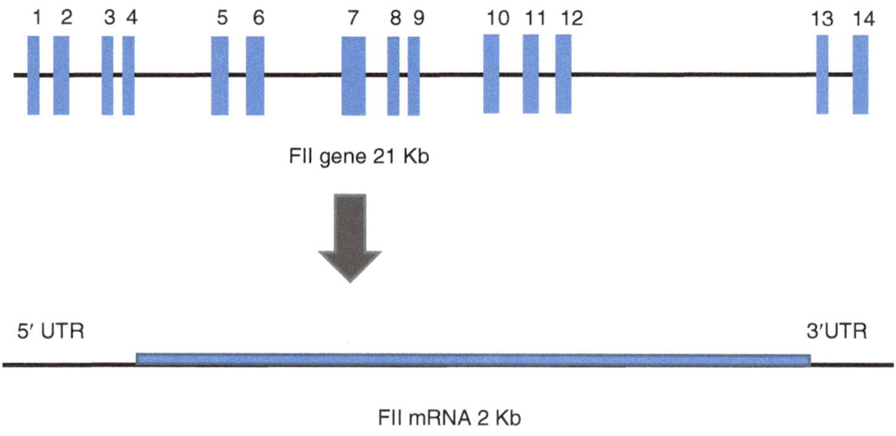

Fig. 7.1 Factor (F) II structure. The schematic presentation of *F2* gene. The *F2* gene composed of 14 exons and 13 introns covering a 21 kb region. This protein is mapped on short arm of chromosome 11 (11p11-q12)

Thrombin is highly homologous with serine proteinases including chymotrypsin. Crystal structure of thrombin shows that this protein consists of the active site, exosites I and II, and different loops including γ-loop, 60-loop, and loop which contains Na^+ binding site [11]. Thrombin-like chymotrypsin has serine residue (Ser195) which in conjugation with other residues including His57 and Asp189 forms the active site that is necessary for target peptide bond's nucleophilic attack [12]. In addition, surface of this thrombin is exposed to loops and is charged patched which has known as exosites around various residues in the active site. Thrombin contains two exosites including I and II which centered different residues including Lys36, His71, Arg73, Arg75, Tyr76, Arg77a, Lys109/110 and Arg93, Lys236, Lys 240, Arg101, Arg233, respectively. The roles of exosites are interaction with thrombin's cofactor and substrates [13, 14].

Moreover, thrombin contains different loops such as γ-loop and 60-loop that surround the active site. The 60-loop, which causes structural rigidity, interacts with residues in substrate's amino-terminal side, while the γ-loop which is more mobile interacts with substrate's residues in the carboxyl-terminal side. In addition, thrombin has another loop which contains Na^+ binding sites. This loop influences thrombin function allosterically by promoting the binding and hydrolysis of its substrates. These substrates include fibrinogen, FV, FVIII, and PAR1 [11, 15].

7.3 Synthesis of Prothrombin

Initially prothrombin is produced in the liver as a prepro-prothrombin which consists of signal peptide. Following the removal of signal peptide by signal peptidase, pro-prothrombin is generated. Pro-prothrombin has a Gla domain which contains ten glutamic acid residues in the N-terminal region [16]. Vitamin K-dependent carboxylase catalyzes the conversion of all ten glutamic acid residues of pro-prothrombin to Gla (γ-carboxylation) and produces the prothrombin (Fig. 7.2). Gla domain is involved in binding of prothrombin to the anionic phospholipid surfaces on the activated platelets and also on vascular injuries in the presence of Ca^{++} [1, 17, 18]. Following the γ-carboxylation, the propeptide is removed and the mature zymogen is generated. Then three N-linked carbohydrates were added which are located in kringle-1 and serine protease domain [16, 19].

7.4 Thrombin Generation

Prothrombin activation which leads to α-thrombin generation is a critical step in coagulation cascade. α-thrombin generation is mediated by prothrombinase complex which is composed of FXa and its cofactor FVa that are assembled in negatively charge surface provided by activated platelet in the presence of Ca^{++} ions (please refer to Chap. 1) [2].

Although FXa is capable to catalyze this process, the rate of prothrombin activation is markedly low. When prothrombinase complex is formed, the rate of prothrombin activation is raised about 10^5-fold [20]. Prothrombin activation occurs by cleavages in two sites. The first cleavage occurs in Arg271 residue (between kringle-2 and A chain) and generates inactive intermediate fragment 1.2 and prothrombin-2. The second cleavage occurs at Arg320 residue and leads to conversion of prothrombin-2 to α-thrombin. In an alternative pathway, the first cleavage occurs in Arg320 residue which leads to generation of active intermediate meizothrombin (mIIa) followed by cleavage at Arg271 and generation of α-thrombin [1, 21]. The rate of prothrombin activation is controlled through cofactor Va and phospholipids. In the absence of FVa, prothrombin activates via prothrombin-2 pathway, while in the presence of FVa, the preferred pathway is meizothrombin intermediate (Fig. 7.2) [22].

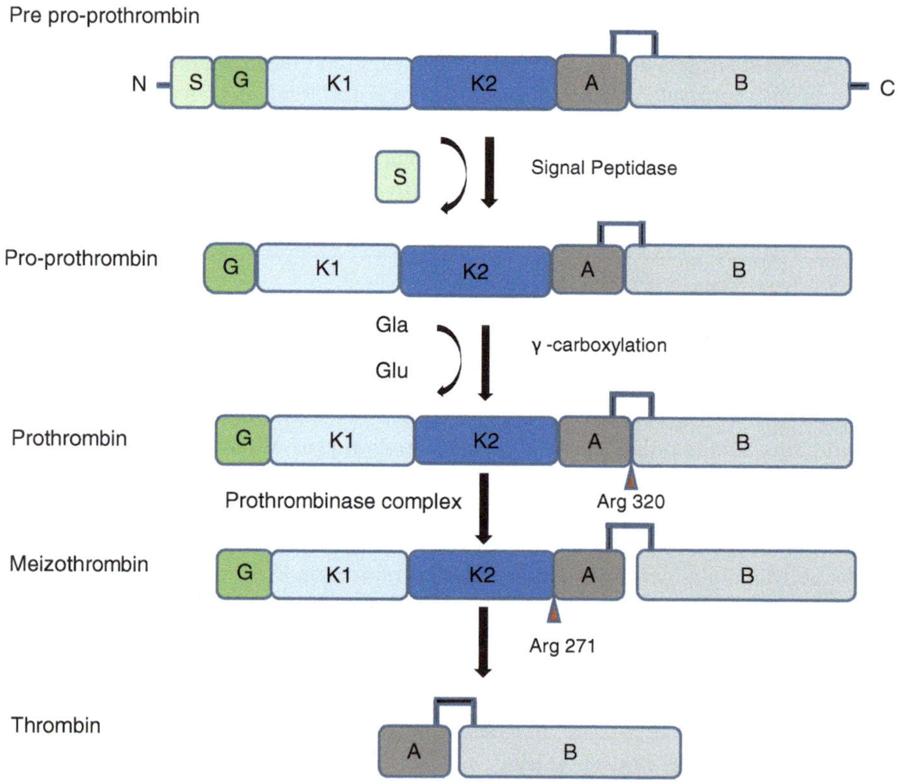

Fig. 7.2 Prothrombin synthesis and thrombin generation. Prepro-prothrombin is a precursor of prothrombin which synthesized in the liver. Following the removal of signal peptide by signal peptidase, the pro-prothrombin which consists of Gla domain is generated. The vitamin K-dependent carboxylase catalyzes the conversion of glutamic acid residues of pro-prothrombin to Gla (γ-carboxylation), and prothrombin is produced. Prothrombinase complex which consists of FXa and its cofactor (FVa) cleaves prothrombin and thrombin is produced. In an alternative pathway, prothrombinase complex cleaves prothrombin in two sites; the first cleavage occurs at Arg320 residue, and active intermediate meizothrombin is generated and the second cleavage occurs at Arg271 residue that results in conversion of meizothrombin to α-thrombin. *S* signal peptide, *G* gamma-carboxyglutamic acid-rich domain, *K1* kringle-1 domain, *K2* kringle-2 domain

The proteolytically active thrombin comprised of two polypeptides, the A-chain (36 residues) and the B-chain (259 residues) which are covalently linked by single disulfide bond through the Cys^{1}-Cys^{122} [23]. Autoproteolysis of thrombin in the A-chain at position of Arg284-Thr285 leads to removal of 13-residue N-terminal peptide of A-chain and generation of α-thrombin. In solution, α-thrombin automatically undergoes cleavage of the Arg62-Ile and Arg73-Asn bonds in B-chain and subsequently in the Arg123-Glu and Lys154-Gly bonds, giving rise to formation of β-thrombin and γ-thrombin, respectively. These forms of thrombin are much less active in comparison with α-thrombin [12, 16, 24].

7.5 Hemostatic Roles of Thrombin

Thrombin is a multifunctional serine protease which is involved in regulation of numerous pathophysiological coagulation and inflammation processes [4].

7.5.1 Fibrin Formation

The primary role of thrombin is conversion of soluble fibrinogen into insoluble fibrin. During this reaction, thrombin binds to the central E nodule of fibrinogen and cleaves four specific Arg-Gly bonds at the N-terminal of both Aα and Bβ chains, leading to the release of fibrinopeptide A (FPA) and B (FPB), respectively (Fig. 7.3). Following the cleavage of FPA, a fibrin monomer which is also termed as fibrin I is formed. Then fibrin I spontaneously polymerizes to protofibrils. Cleavage of FPB results in generation of fibrin II protofibrils. The deposition of fibrin leads to formation of extensive meshwork which by surrounding the platelet forms the stabilized clot [25, 26].

7.5.2 Factor XIII Activation

In the final stage of blood coagulation, thrombin activates FXIII by cleavage of an activating peptide on the A subunit of FXIII (FXIII-A) after Arg37 (Fig. 7.4). Following the cleavage, the activation peptide is released and the active site is exposed. Therefore, the transglutaminase cross-linked fibrin fibrils and increases clot's mechanical strength (please refer to Chap. 13) [27].

7.5.3 Factor V and Factor VIII Activation

A small amount of thrombin which is generated on the tissue factor-bearing cell acts as a positive feedback of coagulation cascade via activation of FV and FVIII. Following the activation of these two factors, the function of FXa and FIXa is enhanced and therefore leads to increased and more sustained thrombin generation and FXa formation. Thrombin activates these two factors by cleavage of them which is followed by removal of B domain [28]. The

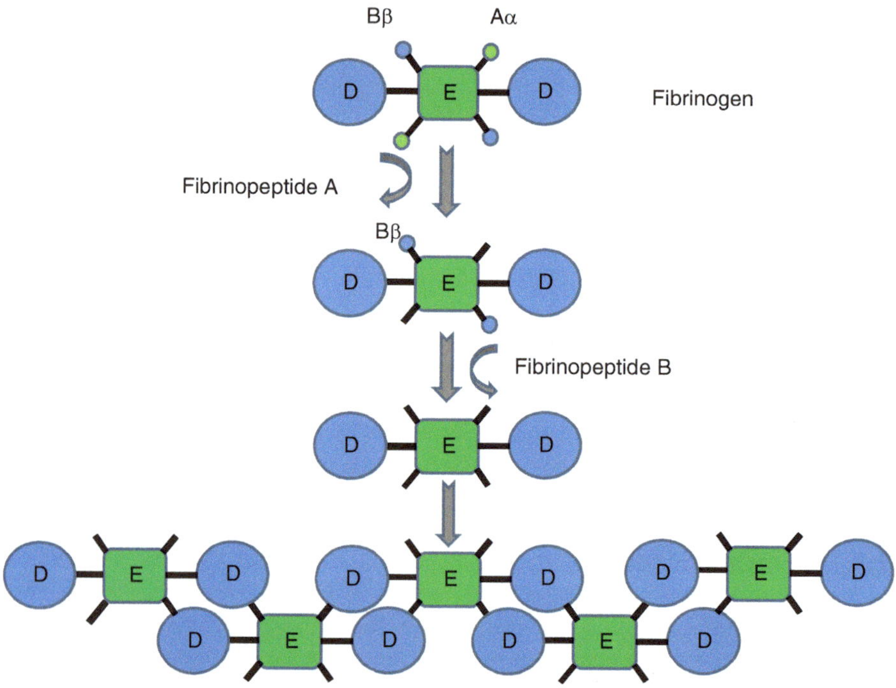

Fig. 7.3 Thrombin binds to the central E nodule of fibrinogen and cleaves this protein at four specific Arg-Gly bonds at the N-terminal of Aα and Bβ chains. This reaction leads to release of fibrinopeptide A (FPA) and B (FPB), respectively. Following the cleavage of FPA, a fibrin monomer which is also termed as fibrin I is formed. Fibrin I polymerizes to protofibrils. The deposition of fibrin leads to extensive meshwork formation (please refer to Chap. 6)

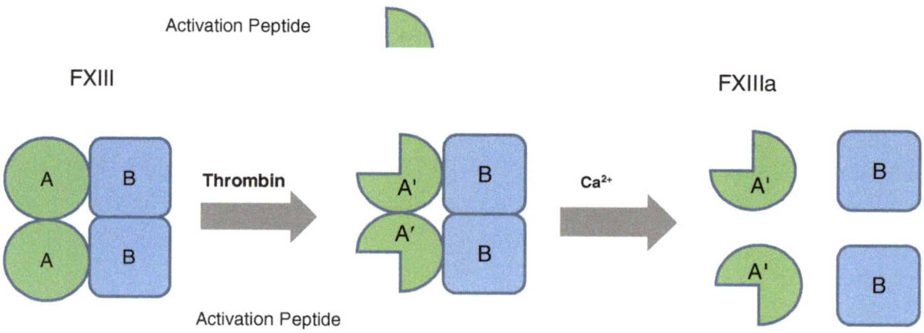

Fig. 7.4 FXIII activation. Thrombin cleaves FXIII-A subunit (Arg37). Following the cleavage, the activation peptide is released and the active site is exposed. FXIII-A and FXIII-B subunits are separated from each other in the presence of Ca^{++}, and therefore FXIII became activated

cleavage sites in FV are Arg709, Arg1018, and Arg1545. Following the cleavages, the A1-A2 domain ionically binds to A3-C1-C2 (Fig. 7.5a). FVIII is cleaved in Arg740, Arg1649, and Arg1689 residues (Fig. 7.5b). Then the A1-A2 fragments associated noncovalently with A3-C1-C2. The residues Lys70, Arg73, and Trp76 are important for binding of thrombin to FV and

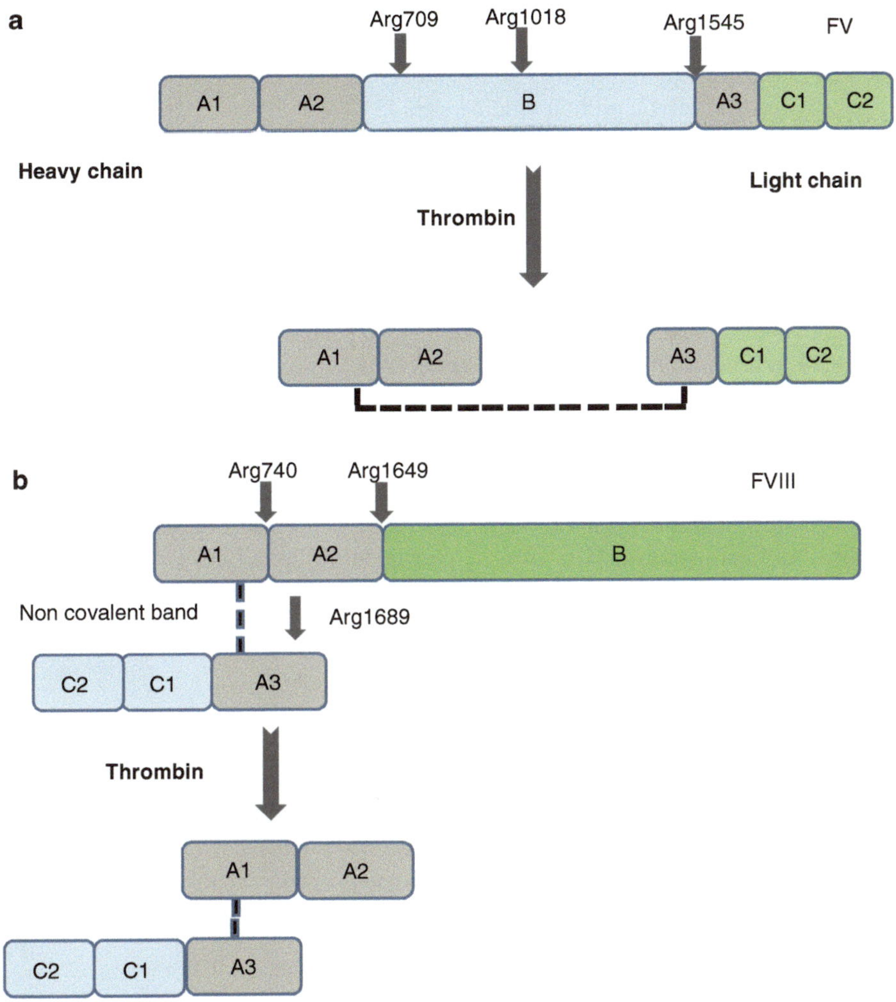

Fig. 7.5 FV and FVIII activation. (**a**) FVIII consists of the heavy and light chains (A1, A2, and B domains) and light chains (C1, C2, and A3) that noncovalently linked to each other. Thrombin activates FVIII through cleavage between A1-A2, A2-B, and at the A3 domains (shown by arrows). Following the cleavages, the B domain is released and FVIII became activated. (**b**) Thrombin cleaves FV in three sites including Arg709, Arg1018, and Arg1545 that leads to FV activation. Activated FV (FVa) consists of two chains including heavy (A1 and A2 domains) and light (A3, C1, and C2 domains) chains

FVIII, whereas Arg101 is important only for binding to FV (please refer to Chaps. 4 and 8) [29, 30].

7.5.4 Thrombin-Activated Fibrinolysis Inhibitors

Thrombin-thrombomodulin (TM) complex inhibits fibrinolysis through activation of thrombin-activatable fibrinolysis inhibitor (TAFI). The activation of TAFI by thrombin occurs via single cleavage at Arg92 and subsequently release of a glycosylated activation peptide. This process requires high concentration of thrombin and is stimulated about 1250-folds by the TM. Activated TAFI (TAFIa) suppresses fibrinolysis by removing C-terminal lysine residues of fibrin that results in disruption of fibrinolytic protein binding sites [31].

7.5.5 Platelet Activation

Thrombin plays an essential role in platelet activation. It causes shape change and release of platelet activators including adenine di-phosphate (ADP), serotonin, thromboxane 2, cytokines, and growth factors [32]. Thrombin-mediated effects are preceded by activation of G protein-coupled PAR. Among the PAR, PAR1, PAR3, and PAR4 are activated by thrombin; however, PAR1 and PAR4 are the major human platelet thrombin receptors [33].

PAR1 is activated when thrombin cleaves its amino-terminal exodomain to unmask a new receptor amino terminus. Then the new N-terminus serves as a tethered peptide ligand, binds intramolecularly to the receptor, and causes receptor activation. PAR1 activation leads to rapid increase in intracellular calcium concentration, while PAR4 induces a more slowly increased and prolonged response in low and high thrombin concentrations, respectively [32].

7.5.6 Protein C Activation

Thrombin binds to the transmembrane protein TM on the surface of endothelial cells and represents its anticoagulant role in coagulation system. In fact, formation of the thrombin-TM complex results in change of substrate specificity of thrombin from procoagulant to anticoagulant reactions by activation of protein C. Procoagulant activity of thrombin stopped by occupancy of exosite I, while cleavage of protein C (PC) at

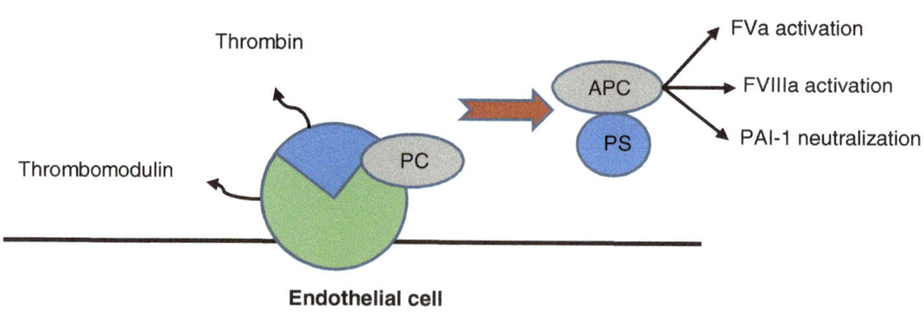

Fig. 7.6 Role of TM complex. Thrombin binds to the TM on the endothelial cells and shows its anticoagulant roles. In fact, thrombin-TM complex formation results in activation of PC. Activated PC (APC) with its cofactor, protein S (PS), inactivates the factor (F) V and FVIII and therefore inhibits the further thrombin formation. In addition, APC inhibits the function of plasminogen-activated inhibitor-1(PAI-1). *PC* protein C, *PS* protein S, *APC* activated protein C, *FVa* activated factor V, *FVIIIa* activated factor VIII, *PAI-1* plasminogen activator inhibitor-1

Arg169 leads to activation of this protein. Activated PC (APC) in association with its cofactor, protein S (PS), inactivates the FV and FVIII and therefore inhibits the further thrombin formation. APC also neutralizes the plasminogen-activated inhibitor-1(PAI-1) and therefore inhibits fibrinolysis (Fig. 7.6) (please refer to Chap. 1) [14, 34].

7.6 Congenital Factor II (Prothrombin) Deficiency

Congenital FII (Prothrombin) deficiency is a very rare autosomal recessive coagulation disorder with estimated incidence of 1 per 2 million in the general population. The incidence of FII deficiency is higher in regions with high rates of parental consanguinity. Prothrombin deficiency was described by Quick et al. in 1947, while the first case of this disorder was reported by Shapiro in 1969 [5]. Prothrombin deficiency is classified in two main phenotypes including hypoprothrombinemia which is also known as a type I deficiency with low levels of both FII activity and antigen (homozygotes and compound heterozygotes) and dysprothrombinemia (type II) characterized by normal or slightly decreased level of FII antigen, but low level of FII activity (homozygotes or heterozygotes), hypo–dys or dys–dys forms (compound heterozygotes), and combined deficiency of prothrombin and other γ-carboxylated coagulation factors [6, 7]. The ratio of type I which is also known as a true deficiency to type II is 1/2 to 1/3. The complete prothrombin deficiency is incompatible with life. This issue is confirmed in knockout mouse models with experimental prothrombin gene inactivation which results in embryonic lethality. Moreover, based on FII activity, this disorder is classified in three forms. The severe form of diseases is characterized by undetectable FII activity, while the mile and moderate forms of disease are characterized by FII activity >10% and <10%, respectively. Congenital FII disorders represent approximately 3% of all rare bleeding disorders (RBD) [35, 36].

7.7 Acquired FII Deficiency

Acquired FII deficiency is a rare disorder which presents with various clinical manifestations. In acquired FII deficiency, antibodies act direct against FII and cause degradation or activity's blocking of this protein. FII inhibitors occur in different conditions including lupus anticoagulant, hypoprothrombinemia syndrome, liver disease, use of anticoagulant drugs, vitamin K deficiency, hematological malignancies, nephritic syndromes, and infections. To evaluate the causes of FII inhibitor, an extensive workup is recommended [37].

7.8 Clinical Manifestations

The clinical manifestations among patients with FII deficiency are highly variable. Patients affected by severe FII deficiency presented with more severe bleeding episodes. The most common bleeding features in patients affected by FII deficiency are

Table 7.1 Clinical manifestations of patients affected by congenital prothrombin deficiency

Bleeding features	Girolami et al. (*n*: 26) (%)	Acharya et al. (*n*: 16) (%)		Stefano Lancellotti et al. [39] (%)
Umbilical cord bleeding	15.4	Homozygous subject (*n*: 10)	Heterozygous subject (*n*: 6)	–
Epistaxis	53.8			–
Hematoma and ecchymosis	68	40[a]	83[a]	60
Gingival bleeding	12			–
Post tooth extraction bleeding	36	–	–	36
Gastrointestinal bleeding	11	13	–	12
Hemarthrosis	44	26	–	42
Hematuria	8	–	–	–
Menorrhagia	100[b]	–	–	20
Postpartum hemorrhage	100[b]	–	–	–
Intracranial hemorrhage	12	20	–	12

[a]This study does not report the frequency of mucocutaneous bleeding (ecchymosis, epistaxis, and gingival bleeding) individually

[b]These bleeding features were observed in all three women who were included in the study

mucosal bleeding, post-trauma bleeding, and hematoma. Life-threatening episodes including gastrointestinal bleeding and central nervous system (CNS) bleeding were reported in few patients (Table 7.1) [3, 8]. Heterozygote patients (with plasma thrombin level of 40–60%) are usually asymptomatic and in some occasions present with postsurgical bleeding. Patients with dysprothrombinemia usually show milder bleeding episodes in comparing with true FII deficiency (type I deficiency) [3]. There is no exact correlation between coagulation test results and clinical manifestations in patients with dysprothrombinemia. However severity of bleeding episodes depends on FII activity, type of FII defect, and FII mutation [3].

Based on different studies, homozygous cases with Arg382His mutation show prothrombin activity lower than 20% with minimal bleeding tendency [38]. Moreover, prothrombin Salakta or Himi is not associated with bleeding tendency [39]. Patients with dysprothrombins Yukuhashi and Scranton have mutation in Na^+ binding loop and do not show hemorrhagic phenotypes [40, 41]. Some cases of FII with mutations of C20209T in 3′ UTR present with thrombosis [42].

7.9 Molecular Basis

Congenital prothrombin deficiency results from different mutations in *F2* gene. These causing mutations are missense mutations (80%), insertion/deletion (10%), nonsense (6%), and splice site mutations (4%) [9].

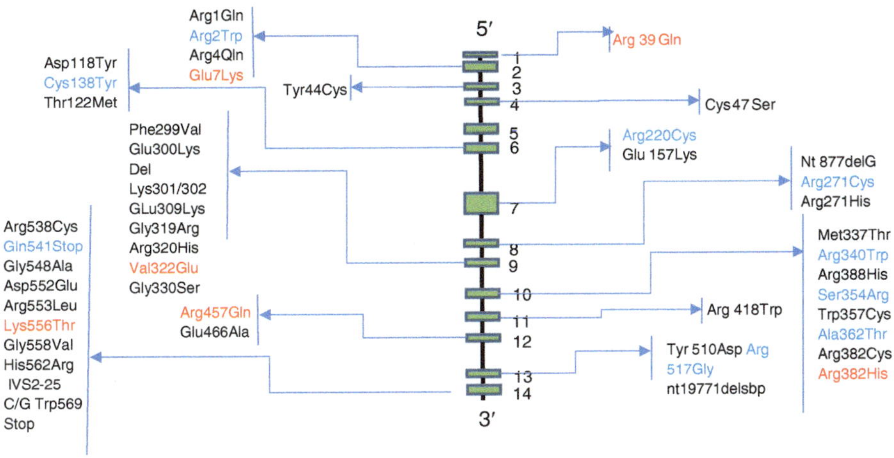

Fig. 7.7 The mutational spectrum of factor II deficiency. Almost all 60 variants (46 missenses, 3 splicing, 4 regulatory, and 7 frameshift) are represented. Exons and introns are shown by boxes and lines, respectively

Approximately 60 variants (46 missense, 3 splicing, 4 regulatory, and 7 frameshift) are accompanied with prothrombin deficiency that listed in the Human Gene Mutation Database (HGMD) http://www.hgmd.cf.ac.uk/ac/all.Php [9]. These mutations are shown in (Fig. 7.7). Although mutations involved different exons, the prevalence of them is higher in exon 8 to exon 14 [3]. Dysfunctional defects are classified in two groups including activation mechanism defects such as FII Barcelona (Arg271Cys) and Padua (Arg271His) or thrombin's protease activity defects [43–45].

Defects in protease activity of thrombin result from:

(1) Amidolytic activity defects for both low and macromolecular substrates which result from impaired catalytic activity of thrombin. FII Molise (Arg418Trp and Stop codon 174) and FII Vellore (Ala362(56)Thr) cause this type of defect.
(2) Defective interaction of thrombin with macromolecular substrates including fibrinogen, TM, and PAR1 which occurs due to mutations in molecular recognition domain of enzyme or insertion loop. FII Quick (Arg382(67)Cys and stop codon Gln541(209)), FII Salakta (Glu466(146)Ala), FII Himi II (Arg388(73) His), and Arg382(67)His lead to this type of defect [3].

Heterozygous prothrombin mutations are found in approximately 2% of US white population, while it is rare in other populations (African-Americans, Asian, and Native American) [46]. Some polymorphisms in *F2* gene lead to increases of FII level. The most common polymorphism of this type is G20210A in the 3′ UTR of gene. This substitution (G to A) is associated with higher prothrombin levels. The prevalence of FII G20210A heterozygotes is higher in Caucasian population. This substitution alters processing, stability, and translocation of prothrombin mRNA. Another polymorphism is A19911G polymorphism located within the last intron of prothrombin [47–49]. 19911G allele is associated with mildly elevated plasma prothrombin level (4 UdL^{-1} higher than A allele) and increases the venous thrombosis risk [50].

7.10 Laboratory Diagnosis

In general, family history, clinical manifestations, and screening laboratory tests are pivotal for diagnosis of FII deficiency. The presence of family history for bleeding disorders can be helpful, but their absence does not exclude the existence of these disorders. FII deficiency is suspected in the presence of prolonged PT and aPTT. For confirmation of FII deficiency, FII activity and antigen level should be performed [51, 52].

7.10.1 Measurement of Factor II Activity

Following the prolonged PT and aPTT, specific assays should be performed. Several assays including PT-based one-stage assay, tiger snake venom assay, taipan viper venom assay, Textarin time, *Echis carinatus* venom assay, and staphylocoagulase assay are available which today the PT-based one-stage assay is the most widely used method. Each assay has an especial activating substance which converts prothrombin to thrombin in different ways. In classical one-stage assay, the presence of FV, phospholipids, and calcium is necessary, and tissue thromboplastin acts as an activating agent. Tiger snake venom acts as an activating agent in the presence of FV, calcium, and phospholipids while *Echis carinatus* venom activates prothrombin without need of other factors. Taipan viper venom activates the prothrombin to thrombin in the presence of calcium and phospholipids [53, 54].

7.10.2 PT-Based One-Stage Assay

PT-based one-stage assay is a specific test which determines the FII activity. This assay is based on PT test and compared the ability of patient's plasma with standard plasma to correct the PT of substrate (prothrombin-depleted plasma). In this assay equal volume of dilution of patient's plasma and standard's plasma (1 in 5, 1 in 10, 1 in 20, and 1 in 40) is mixed with substrate plasma and is warmed in 37 °C. Then by adding the equal volume of diluted thromboplastin (recombinant and re-lipidated tissue factor), the clotting time is recorded. For calculation of the FII activity, the clotting time of each dilution of test plasma and standard plasma is plotted against concentration of FII [3, 10].

7.10.3 Chromogenic Assay

The chromogenic/fluorogenic assays can also be used for measurement of thrombin level. In this assay the amidolytic activity of thrombin in presence of chromogenic substances such as anilides or fluorogenic peptide including 7-amino-4-methylcoumarin amides is measured. These chromogenic/fluorogenic substances interact with thrombin's active side pocket. This method is able to detect any difference between the level of FII in this assay and the level of it in the coagulation assay. Therefore, the result of chromogenic activity is not always the same as coagulation activity. Any difference between this assay and PT-based one-stage assay suggests the presence of dysprothrombin which results from mutation of recognition domain of thrombin especially fibrinogen recognition domain [37].

7.11 Determination of Factor II Antigen Level

Enzyme-linked immunosorbent assay (ELISA) is used conventionally for measurement of FII antigen level. In this assay, a specific antibody is coated on the plate. Following the addition of standard and patient's plasma, antihuman prothrombin primary antibody binds to captured protein. Then unbounded antibodies are washed away, and the secondary antibody which is conjugated with horseradish peroxidase (HRP) is added. By adding the substrate, the color change is spectrophotometrically assessed at 450 nm. The concentration of FII in sample is determined by comparing the optical density (OD) of sample via standard curve [10, 55].

7.12 Factor II Inhibitor Assay

For detection of inhibitor against FII, the patient's plasma is mixed with normal pooled plasma (50:50). When the results of PT and aPTT do not normalize, the presence of an inhibitor is suspected. Then inhibitor should be titrated by Bethesda method.

For this method, two tubes are prepared for normal plasma and patient's plasma, respectively, and two tubes are prepared for equal mixture of patient and normal plasma (time-dependent and immediate inhibitors, respectively). APTT and PT should be performed duplicate for all tubes (please refer to Chap. 8) (Table 7.2) [56].

7.12.1 Bethesda Assay

For inhibitor titration, the Bethesda method is used. The Bethesda unit is defined as amount of inhibitor which neutralized 50% of 1 unit of FII in normal plasma. In this method two dilution series are prepared as follows and incubated at 37 °C for 0 hour (h), 1 h, or 2 h:

(1) Dilutions of patient's plasma with an equal volume of normal plasma (normally contain 100% FII)
(2) Dilutions of control plasma which contain no inhibitors (equal volume of normal plasma and buffer)

The residual FII is determined based on one-stage PT assay for each mixture. The dilution with residual FII activity about 50% is considered for determination of

Table 7.2 Interpretation of the inhibitor screen for factor II deficiency based on PT and aPTT

		The results of clotting time		
Tube	Content	FII deficiency	Immediate inhibitors	Time-dependent inhibitors
1	Normal plasma	Normal	Normal	Normal
2	Patient's plasma	Prolonged	Prolonged	Prolonged
3	Equal volume of normal and patient's plasma (2 h incubation)	Normal	Prolonged	Prolonged
4	Equal volume of normal and patient's plasma (without incubation)	Normal	Normal	Prolonged

APTT activated partial thromboplastin time
PT prothrombin time

inhibitor strength. For calculation of FII inhibitor, the standard graph of residual FII activity versus inhibitor units is used [10, 55].

7.13 Treatment

Replacement therapy is required in the homozygous cases with bleeding or prior to surgical procedures. The minimum level of FII needed for hemostasis is >10% [57].

As no prothrombin-specific concentrate is available for replacement therapy of FII, PCC or FFP is currently used for on-demand therapy and long-term prophylaxis in patients with FII deficiency. Moreover in cases with mild bleeding, antifibrinolytic agents (tranexamic acid and epsilon-aminocaproic acid) are also recommended (Table 7.3) [10].

Although PCC is a mainstay of therapy in prothrombin, high or repeated doses of PCC have been associated with arterial and venous thrombosis; therefore patients require close monitoring [10]. PCC contains three factors including FII, FIX, and FX. This product is known as three-factor PCC. If the amount of FVII is more than 10%, this product is labeled as a four-factor PCC (please refer to Chap. 10) [58].

As the incidence of severe bleeding is not high during the neonatal periods, prophylactic replacement therapy is not routinely recommended for this group. On the other hand, prophylactic replacement therapy should be used according to the frequency and type of bleeding [59]. Although it is difficult to make firm recommendations on pregnancy management, it had been suggested that a FII level up to 25 IU/dL minimizes the bleeding complications during labor and delivery [60].

Table 7.3 Doses and target therapeutic levels in patients with factor II deficiency

Kind of treatment	Recommend level	Dosage of therapeutic level
On-demand therapy	>10%	15–25 mL/kg: FFP
		20–40 U/kg: PCC
Long-term prophylaxis	>10%	20–40 U/kg once a week
Major surgery	>20% (maintaining level)	20–40 IU/kg (before surgery)
		10–20 IU/kg every48 h

References

1. Pozzi N, Chen Z, Gohara DW, Niu W, Heyduk T, Di Cera E. Crystal structure of prothrombin reveals conformational flexibility and mechanism of activation. J Biol Chem. 2013;288(31):22734–44.
2. Kamath P, Krishnaswamy S. Fate of membrane-bound reactants and products during the activation of human prothrombin by prothrombinase. J Biol Chem. 2008;283(44):30164–73.
3. Lancellotti S, Basso M, De Cristofaro R. Congenital prothrombin deficiency: an update. Semin Thromb Hemost. 2013;39(6):596–606.
4. Hassanian SM, Dinarvand P, Rezaie AR. Adenosine regulates the proinflammatory signaling function of thrombin in endothelial cells. J Cell Physiol. 2014;229(9):1292–300.
5. Mannucci PM, Duga S, Peyvandi F. Recessively inherited coagulation disorders. Blood. 2004;104(5):1243–52.
6. Peyvandi F, Duga S, Akhavan S, Mannucci P. Rare coagulation deficiencies. Haemophilia. 2002;8(3):308–21.
7. Akhavan S, Luciani M, Lavoretano S, Mannucci PM. Phenotypic and genetic analysis of a compound heterozygote for dys-and hypoprothrombinaemia. Br J Haematol. 2003;120(1):142–4.
8. Rodriguez V, Warad D. Pediatric coagulation disorders. Pediatr Rev. 2016;37(7):279.
9. Su K, Jin Y, Miao Z, Cheng X, Yang L, Wang M. Phenotypic and genetic analysis of dysprothrombinemia due to a novel homozygous mutation. Hematology. 2017;22(6):380–5.
10. Mumford AD, Ackroyd S, Alikhan R, Bowles L, Chowdary P, Grainger J, et al. Guideline for the diagnosis and management of the rare coagulation disorders. Br J Haematol. 2014;167(3):304–26.
11. Huntington JA. How Na^+ activates thrombin–a review of the functional and structural data. Biol Chem. 2008;389(8):1025–35.
12. Bode W. The structure of thrombin: a janus-headed proteinase. Semin Thromb Hemost. 2006;32(Suppl 1):16–31.
13. Bode W, Turk D, Karshikov A. The refined 1.9-A X-ray crystal structure of D-Phe-Pro-Arg chloromethylketone-inhibited human alpha-thrombin: structure analysis, overall structure, electrostatic properties, detailed active-site geometry, and structure-function relationships. Protein Sci. 1992;1(4):426–71.
14. Adams TE, Huntington JA. Thrombin-cofactor interactions: structural insights into regulatory mechanisms. Arterioscler Thromb Vasc Biol. 2006;26(8):1738–45.
15. Crawley J, Zanardelli S, Chion C, Lane D. The central role of thrombin in hemostasis. J Thromb Haemost. 2007;5(s1):95–101.
16. Carter IS, Vanden Hoek AL, Pryzdial EL, MacGillivray RT. Thrombin a-chain: activation remnant or allosteric effector? Thrombosis. 2010;2010:416167.
17. Hansson K, Stenflo J. Post-translational modifications in proteins involved in blood coagulation. J Thromb Haemost. 2005;3(12):2633–48.
18. Davie EW, Kulman JD. An overview of the structure and function of thrombin. Semin Thromb Hemost. 2006;32(Suppl 1):3–15.
19. Mizuochi T, Fujii J, Kisiel W, Kobata A. Studies on the structures of the carbohydrate moiety of human prothrombin. J Biochem. 1981;90(4):1023–31.
20. Krishnaswamy S. Prothrombinase complex assembly. Contributions of protein-protein and protein-membrane interactions toward complex formation. J Biol Chem. 1990;265(7):3708–18.
21. Krishnaswamy S. The transition of prothrombin to thrombin. J Thromb Haemost. 2013;11(s1):265–76.
22. Haynes LM, Bouchard BA, Tracy PB, Mann KG. Prothrombin activation by platelet-associated prothrombinase proceeds through the prethrombin-2 pathway via a concerted mechanism. J Biol Chem. 2012;287(46):38647–55.
23. Di Cera E, Dang Q, Ayala Y. Molecular mechanisms of thrombin function. CMLS. 1997;53(9):701–30.
24. Boissel J, Le Bonniec B, Rabiet M, Labie D, Elion J. Covalent structures of beta and gamma autolytic derivatives of human alpha-thrombin. J Biol Chem. 1984;259(9):5691–7.

25. Mullin JL, Gorkun OV, Binnie CG, Lord ST. Recombinant fibrinogen studies reveal that thrombin specificity dictates order of fibrinopeptide release. J Biol Chem. 2000;275(33):25239–46.
26. Wolberg AS. Thrombin generation and fibrin clot structure. Blood Rev. 2007;21(3):131–42.
27. Standeven KF, Ariëns RA, Whitaker P, Ashcroft AE, Weisel JW, Grant PJ. The effect of dimethylbiguanide on thrombin activity, FXIII activation, fibrin polymerization, and fibrin clot formation. Diabetes. 2002;51(1):189–97.
28. Narayanan S. Multifunctional roles of thrombin. Ann Clin Lab Sci. 1999;29(4):275–80.
29. Camire R, Bos M. The molecular basis of factor V and VIII procofactor activation. J Thromb Haemost. 2009;7(12):1951–61.
30. Myles T, Yun TH, Leung LL. Structural requirements for the activation of human factor VIII by thrombin. Blood. 2002;100(8):2820–6.
31. Bouma BN, Mosnier LO. Thrombin activatable fibrinolysis inhibitor (TAFI)—how does thrombin regulate fibrinolysis? Ann Med. 2006;38(6):378–88.
32. Coughlin SR. Thrombin signalling and protease-activated receptors. Nature. 2000;407(6801):258–65.
33. Andersen H, Greenberg DL, Fujikawa K, Xu W, Chung DW, Davie EW. Protease-activated receptor 1 is the primary mediator of thrombin-stimulated platelet procoagulant activity. Proc Natl Acad Sci. 1999;96(20):11189–93.
34. Yang L, Manithody C, Rezaie AR. Activation of protein C by the thrombin–thrombomodulin complex: cooperative roles of Arg-35 of thrombin and Arg-67 of protein C. Proc Natl Acad Sci U S A. 2006;103(4):879–84.
35. Girolami A, Santarossa L, Scarparo P, Candeo N, Girolami B. True congenital prothrombin deficiency due to a 'new' mutation in the pre-propeptide (ARG-39 GLN). Acta Haematol. 2008;120(2):82–6.
36. Acharya SS. Rare bleeding disorders in children: identification and primary care management. Pediatrics. 2013;132(5):882–92.
37. Bajaj S, Rapaport S, Barclay S, Herbst K. Acquired hypoprothrombinemia due to non-neutralizing antibodies to prothrombin: mechanism and management. Blood. 1985;65(6):1538–43.
38. O'Marcaigh AS, Nichols WL, Hassinger NL, Mullins JD, Mallouh AA, Gilchrist GS, et al. Genetic analysis and functional characterization of prothrombins Corpus Christi (Arg382-Cys), Dhahran (Arg271-His), and hypoprothrombinemia. Blood. 1996;88(7):2611–8.
39. Lancellotti S, De Cristofaro R. Congenital prothrombin deficiency. Semin Thromb Hemost. 2009;35(4):367–81.
40. Miyawaki Y, Suzuki A, Fujita J, Maki A, Okuyama E, Murata M, et al. Thrombosis from a prothrombin mutation conveying antithrombin resistance. N Engl J Med. 2012;366(25):2390–6.
41. Sun WY, Smirnow D, Jenkins ML, Degen SJ. Prothrombin scranton: substitution of an amino acid residue involved in the binding of Na+ (LYS-556 to THR) leads to dysprothrombinemia. Thromb Haemost. 2001;85(4):651–4.
42. Flaujac C, Conard J, Horellou M, Le Flem L, Samama M. Atypical mutations of the prothrombin gene at positions 20 209 and 20 218, and a novel mutation at position 20 219. Report on 10 patients. J Thromb Haemost. 2007;5(5):1064–8.
43. Rabiet MJ, Furie BC, Furie B. Molecular defect of prothrombin Barcelona. Substitution of cysteine for arginine at residue 273. J Biol Chem. 1986;261(32):15045–8.
44. Lefkowitz JB, Haver T, Clarke S, Jacobson L, Weller A, Nuss R, et al. The prothrombin Denver patient has two different prothrombin point mutations resulting in Glu-300→ Lys and Glu-309→ Lys substitutions. Br J Haematol. 2000;108(1):182–7.
45. Bezeaud A, Vidaud D, Guillin M-C. Les déficits constitutionnels en prothrombine et les informations qu'ils peuvent nous apporter sur la structure et les fonctions de la prothrombine. Hématologie. 2005;11(6):397–407.
46. Varga EA, Moll S. Prothrombin 20210 mutation (factor II mutation). Circulation. 2004;110(3):e15-e8.
47. Zivelin A, Rosenberg N, Faier S, Kornbrot N, Peretz H, Mannhalter C, et al. A single genetic origin for the common prothrombotic G20210A polymorphism in the prothrombin gene. Blood. 1998;92(4):1119–24.

48. Pihusch R, Hiller E, Buchholz T, Rogenhofer N, Hasbargen U, Thaler CJ, et al. Thrombophilic gene mutations and recurrent spontaneous abortion: prothrombin mutation increases the risk in the first trimester. Am J Reprod Immunol. 2001;46(2):124–31.
49. Carter AM, Sachchithananthan M, Stasinopoulos S, Maurer F, Medcalf RL. Prothrombin G20210A is a bifunctional gene polymorphism. Thromb Haemost. 2002;87(5):846–53.
50. Warshawsky I, Makkar V, Rimmerman C, Kottke-Marchant K. Prothrombin 20209C> T: 16 new cases, association with the 19911A> G polymorphism, and literature review. J Thromb Haemost. 2009;7(9):1585–7.
51. Peyvandi F, Menegatti M, Palla R. Rare bleeding disorders: worldwide efforts for classification, diagnosis, and management. Semin Thromb Hemost. 2013;39(6):579–84.
52. Meeks S, Abshire T. Abnormalities of prothrombin: a review of the pathophysiology, diagnosis, and treatment. Haemophilia. 2008;14(6):1159–63.
53. Denson K, Borrett R, Biggs R. The specific assay of prothrombin using the Taipan snake venom. Br J Haematol. 1971;21(2):219–26.
54. Girolami A, Scarano L, Saggiorato G, Girolami B, Bertomoro A, Marchiori A. Congenital deficiencies and abnormalities of prothrombin. Blood Coagul Fibrinolysis. 1998;9(7):557–70.
55. Acharya S, Coughlin A, Dimichele DM. Rare Bleeding Disorder Registry: deficiencies of factors II, V, VII, X, XIII, fibrinogen and dysfibrinogenemias. J Thromb Haemost. 2004;2(2):248–56.
56. Kershaw G, Favaloro EJ. Laboratory identification of factor inhibitors: an update. Pathology. 2012;44(4):293–302.
57. Peyvandi F, Di Michele D, Bolton-Maggs P, Lee C, Tripodi A, Srivastava A. Classification of rare bleeding disorders (RBDs) based on the association between coagulant factor activity and clinical bleeding severity. J Thromb Haemost. 2012;10(9):1938–43.
58. Deangelo J, Jarrell D, Cosgrove R, Camamo J, Edwards C, Patanwala AE. Comparison of 3-factor versus 4-factor prothrombin complex concentrate with regard to warfarin reversal, blood product use, and costs. Am J Ther. 2017. https://doi.org/10.1097/MJT.0000000000000643.
59. Bolton-Maggs P, Perry D, Chalmers E, Parapia L, Wilde J, Williams M, et al. The rare coagulation disorders–review with guidelines for management from the United Kingdom Haemophilia Centre Doctors' Organisation. Haemophilia. 2004;10(5):593–628.
60. Kadir R, Chi C, Bolton-Maggs P. Pregnancy and rare bleeding disorders. Haemophilia. 2009;15(5):990–1005.

Congenital Factor V Deficiency

8

Shadi Tabibian, Akbar Dorgalaleh, and Rodney M. Camire

8.1 Introduction

Coagulation factor V (FV), also known as labile factor or proaccelarin, circulates in the blood as an inactive pro-cofactor protein [1]. FV was discovered in 1943 by Paul Owren [2] through study of a woman affected by a syndrome resembling hemophilia. Following coagulation activation, FV converts to its active form, FVa, via limited proteolysis at discrete sites by thrombin or factor Xa (FXa). FVa is a cofactor that binds to the serine protease FXa on activated cells to form the prothrombinase complex, which rapidly converts prothrombin to thrombin [1]. FV is synthetized by hepatocytes and circulates as a precursor molecule in plasma. However, approximately 20% to 25% of the total FV is stored in platelet α-granules, which originate from the endocytosis of plasma FV by megakaryocytes [3]. In addition to procoagulant activity, FV is thought to have anticoagulant activity via participation in the downregulation of FVIII [4].

FV deficiency is a rare bleeding disorder (RBD) with an estimated prevalence of one per million in the general population. This disorder mostly presents in regions where parental consanguinity is common [5]. FV deficiency is classified into two types: type I deficiency (parallel reduction in antigen and activity level) and type II deficiency (normal or mildly reduced antigen level with reduced activity) [6]. FV deficiency most often presents at birth or during early childhood, but some cases remain undiagnosed until later in life because of mild clinical presentations. The most common clinical manifestations affecting patients are mucosal bleeds

S. Tabibian · A. Dorgalaleh
Department of Hematology and Blood Transfusion, School of Allied Medicine, Iran University of Medical Sciences, Tehran, Iran

R. M. Camire (✉)
Division of Hematology, Department of Pediatrics, Children's Hospital of Philadelphia, University of Pennsylvania, Perelman School of Medicine, Philadelphia, PA, USA
e-mail: rcamire@pennmedicine.upenn.edu

A. Dorgalaleh (ed.), *Congenital Bleeding Disorders*,
https://doi.org/10.1007/978-3-319-76723-9_8

(epistaxis, gum bleeding, and menorrhagia in women) and postsurgical bleeding. Hematoma and hemarthrosis are present in about one fourth of patients. Life-threatening episodes including central nervous system (CNS) bleeding and gastrointestinal (GI) bleeding present rarely in these patients and most often present in patients with an undetectable FV level [5, 7]. FV deficiency is suspected in the presence of a positive family history, bleeding episodes, and prolonged prothrombin time (PT) and activated partial thromboplastin time (aPTT). To confirm diagnosis, the measurement of activity, via mixing studies, and level of FV antigen is necessary. In cases with low factor activity and low antigen level, the measurement of FVIII antigen and activity is necessary to exclude FV deficiency from combined FV and FVIII deficiency [7]. It has been found that patients with severe FV deficiency have markedly reduced levels of tissue factor pathway inhibitor (TFPI) [8]. It is suggested that this may explain the amelioration of the bleeding phenotype in many severely FV-deficient patients. For FV deficiency, the sharp decrease in TFPI levels seems to be related to the finding that FV and TFPI interact with each other and, to a certain degree, are bound together in plasma [8].

Acquired FV deficiency is a rare condition that mostly results from previous exposure to bovine thrombin or antibiotic administration, surgery, and malignancies. Acquired FV deficiency is associated with prolonged PT and aPTT without correction in a mixing study. In this condition, the presence of an inhibitor is confirmed by the Bethesda method [9]. Because FV concentrate is not available, fresh frozen plasma (FFP) is the only available treatment option for patients affected by FV deficiency. The dose of FFP depends on the kind of treatment (on-demand or prophylaxis) and on the severity of bleeding episodes. Platelet transfusion in some situations is another option for treatment of patients with FV deficiency, but the risk of allo-immunization should be considered [10].

8.2 Factor V Structure and Function

The FV gene (*F5*) is composed of 25 exons and 24 introns covering a region of approximately 80 kb mapped on the long arm of chromosome 1 (1q24.2), not far from the antithrombin gene [11]. Cloning of the human coagulation FV cDNA leads to the identification of a 6672-bp transcript encoding a protein with 2224 amino acids. Following removal of a signal sequence, FV circulates in the plasma as a single-chain precursor protein that consists of 2196 amino acids with a molecular weight of approximately 330 kDa. FV contains a 28-residue leader peptide and six different domains oriented in A1, A2, B, A3, C1, or C2 conformations [1]. FV and FVIII have about 40% homology in domains A and C [12]. The three A domains are homologous to the copper-binding protein ceruloplasmin and the C domains belong to the lipid-binding discoidin-like protein family [13, 14]. The B domain has no similarity to other known proteins and contains a 2-tandem repeat with 17 amino acids and a 31-tandem repeat with 9 amino acids, which are not conserved among species [15–17]. FV has 19 cysteines, of which 14 are involved in disulfide bridges. The FV precursor undergoes posttranslational modifications and circulates in the blood as an inactive 330-kDa single-chain pro-cofactor protein [6]. Structural information derived from inactivated bovine FVa and snake FV indicate that the three A domains are arranged in a triangular fashion, sitting atop the two C domains [18].

8.3 Factor V Activation and Inactivation

FV circulates in blood in an inactive form and is converted to an active cofactor (FVa) by thrombin or activated FX (FXa) following proteolysis at arginine $(Arg)^{709}$, Arg^{1018}, and Arg^{1545}. Subsequently, the large central B domain is entirely removed, leaving the active cofactor that is composed of a 105-kDa heavy chain (A1, A2) and a 74- to 71-kDa light chain (A3, C1, C2). These two fragments are stabilized by noncovalent association by Ca^{2+} ion and also by hydrophobic interactions (Fig. 8.1a, b) [19, 20]. A key aspect of this pro-cofactor to cofactor transition is the removal of important B-domain sequences, consisting of a basic and acidic sequence that are essential for keeping FV inactive [20].

Downregulation of FV/FVa is mediated by activated protein C (APC). APC is a vitamin K-dependent serine protease that inhibits FVa and FVIIIa through

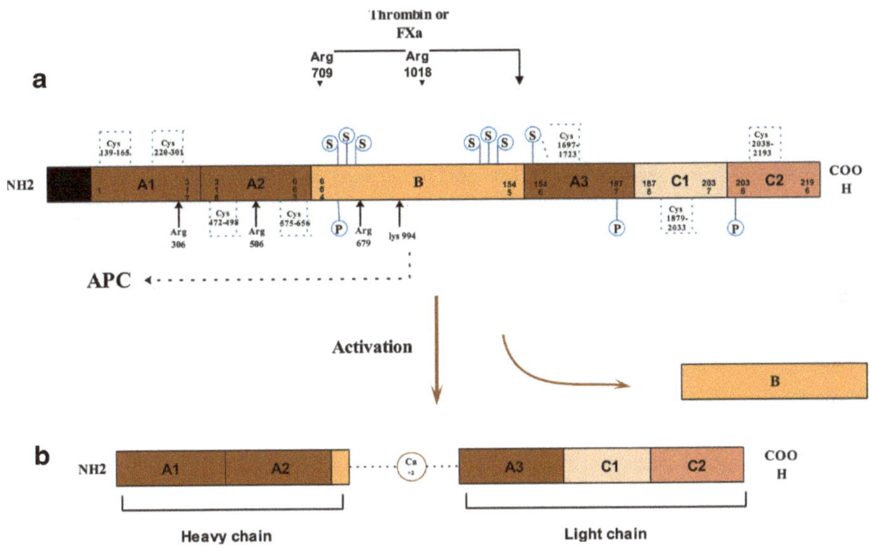

Fig. 8.1 Structure and activation of factor V. (**a**) Schematic presentation of factor V protein. Factor V precursor protein consists of 2224 amino acids and six different domains including A1, A2, B, A3, C1, and C2. The *dark box* located at the N-terminus is the 28-residue signal peptide. The A1, A2, and A3 domains are homologous to copper-binding protein ceruloplasmin whereas the B2 domain belongs to the lipid-binding discoidin-like protein family. Positions of proteolytic cleavage sites responsible for the activation and inactivation of factor V. The *arrows on the top* represent activation of factor V by thrombin or activated FX (FXa) and *arrows on the bottom* represent inactivation sites by APC. (**b**) Activated form of factor V. Factor V activation occurs by cleavage by thrombin or activated factor X in Arg^{709}, Arg^{1018}, and Arg^{1545}. After the cleavages the B domain is removed; FVa consists of two fragments including the 105-kDa heavy chain and the 74- or 71-kDa light chain, which are stabilized by Ca^{2+} ions and also by hydrophobic interaction

limited proteolysis. APC with its cofactor (protein S) cleaves FV/FVa at three residues including Arg^{506}, Arg^{306}, and Arg^{679} or Lys^{994} (Fig. 8.1a). The first cleavage occurring at Arg^{506} leads to decreased FV cofactor activity and also to the affinity of this protein to FXa, which results in partial FVa inactivation. The next cleavage takes place in Arg^{306} and leads to complete FVa inactivation. The functional implications of cleavage of FV/FVa at Arg^{679}/Lys^{994} are not very well understood [21]. Following cleavage of FV/FVa by APC, the A2 domain, divided into two fragments, dissociates from the rest of the molecule. The remaining FV molecule (FVai) consists of the A1 domain, which is noncovalently associated with the light chain (A3, C1, C2) [22]. The significance of FV/FVa inactivation by APC is illustrated by prothrombotic clinical manifestations in FV Leiden (Arg^{506} to Gln), which is resistant to APC cleavage at the 506 site [23].

FVa also can be inactivated by other proteases such as thrombin or the fibrinolytic protease plasmin. Thrombin cleavage of FVa at Arg^{643} reduces the affinity between the two chains [24]. Plasmin is another inactivator of FVa, and the amino acid region of 307–348 of FV is critical for this inactivation [25]. However, the physiological significance of these reactions is not clear.

8.4 Role of Factor V in the Coagulation Cascade

Approximately 80% of FV is synthetized by hepatocytes and circulates in plasma at a concentration of 7–10 μg/ml; the remaining 20% originates from the plasma pool via endocytosis by megakaryocytes and is stored in platelet α-granules (4600–14,000 molecules/platelet) in association with soluble protein multimerin 1 (MMRN). Platelet FV appears to be processed by certain enzymes (e.g., FXa and APC) differently compared to its plasma counterpart, which may contribute to some differently functional properties of the platelet FV following its release from α-granules upon platelet activation [26–28].

FVa has *procoagulant activity*, acting as a cofactor for the serine protease FXa in a prothrombinase complex (FVa-FXa). This complex rapidly converts prothrombin to thrombin at the platelet membrane surface or on other activated cells that expose negatively charged phospholipids. FVa accelerates the rate of conversion of prothrombin to thrombin by several orders of magnitude. Because FXa alone is not a potent activator and because there is no alternative pathway to generate thrombin, FVa is essential for rapid thrombin generation (Fig. 8.2) [3]. In addition, following platelet activation, platelet FV is disassociated from the MMRN and then exposed on the platelet membrane surface. Exposing FV enhances theassembly and activity of the prothrombinase complex [29].

In addition to its procoagulant function, FV protein is thought to have an *anticoagulant role*. The anticoagulant capacity of FV is related to APC-mediated inactivation of FVIII. FV appears to act as an APC cofactor to stimulate the inactivation of FVIIIa by APC/protein S complex (Fig. 8.2) [4].

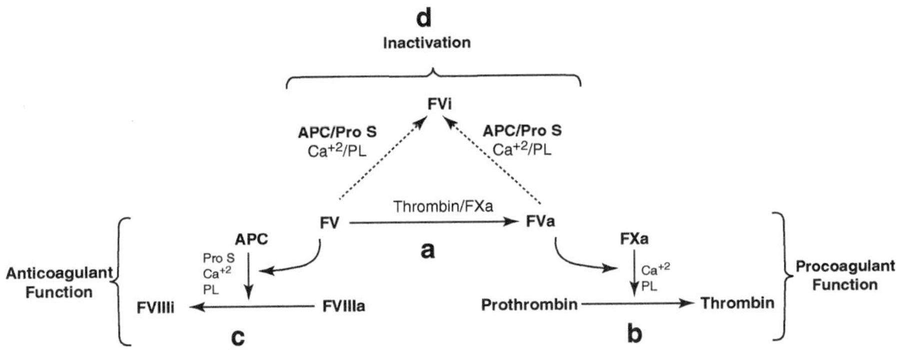

Fig. 8.2 Different functions of factor V. (**a**) Factor V (FV) is activated via proteolysis mediated by activated factor X (FXa) or thrombin. (**b**) After activation of FV, this factor acts as a cofactor for the conversion of prothrombin to thrombin by FXa in the presence of calcium ion (Ca^{2+}) and phospholipid (PL) in the prothrombinase complex. (**c**) FV (before activation) acts as a cofactor for activated protein C (APC) in the presence of protein S (ProS), calcium ion, and phospholipid to inactive FVIII (anticoagulant function). (**d**) Activated FV (FVa) and FV inactivated by APC and in the presence of ProS, calcium, and phospholipid

8.5 Congenital Factor V Deficiency

Congenital FV deficiency is a RBD with a frequency of about 1 per million in the general population [30]. This disorder, also named Owren parahemophilia, was first described in 1947 by Paul Owern in a Norwegian woman who suffered from lifelong epistaxis and menorrhagia [2]. FV deficiency, similar to other RBDs, is most common in regions with a high frequency of parental consanguinity. FV deficiency is inherited in an autosomal recessive pattern and results from the near complete absence of FV in plasma or platelets [30, 31].

FV deficiency can be classified as either a type I deficiency or cross-reacting material negative (CRM−), which presents with a low or undetectable antigen level (quantitative defect), or a type II deficiency or cross-reacting material positive (CRM+) with normal or mildly reduced antigen level but reduced coagulant activity (qualitative defect) [6]. Based on the residual factor level, the severity of FV deficiency is classified as mild (FV level ≥10%), moderate (FV level <10%), or severe (FV level is undetectable) [32]. Individuals with homozygous or compound heterozygous deficiency typically have FV levels less than 10%, whereas patients affected by the heterozygote state have mild or moderate FV deficiency with a FV level around 50% [33].

8.6 Clinical Manifestations

Several studies have evaluated the clinical aspects of patients affected by FV deficiency. Based on these studies, mucocutaneous (epistaxis and menorrhagia in women), soft-tissue, and posttraumatic are the most common bleeding features

Table 8.1 Clinical manifestations of patients affected by factor V deficiency

Bleeding episodes	Iran (%)[a] *n* = 35	Iran (%)[a] *n* = 16	USA and Canada (%) Severe *n* = 18	Mild *n* = 19
Epistaxis	57	68.7	42	62
Oral cavity bleeding		31.25		
Menorrhagia	50	83.3		
Gastrointestinal bleeding	6	6.25	6	–
Genitourinary bleeding	6	12.5	19	19
Hemarthrosis	26	18.75	23	19
Hematoma	29	–	–	–
Central nervous system bleeding	6	–	8	–
Umbilical cord bleeding	3	–	–	–
Post-operative bleeding/post-partum bleeding	43	6.25		

[a]The severity of factor V deficiency is not mentioned in these studies

(Table 8.1). Hematoma and hemarthrosis, which are mostly related to trauma rather than spontaneous development, are present in one fourth of patients. There have been occasional reports of spontaneous life-threatening bleeding episodes including CNS bleeding, umbilical cord bleeding (UCB), and GI bleeding [34–36]. In fact, spontaneous minor bleeding including epistaxis, bruising, oral cavity bleeding, minor bruising, ecchymosis, and menorrhagia are the most common bleeding diathesis and account for 34% of all clinical manifestations. About 32% of FV-deficient patients are asymptomatic. Spontaneous major bleedings including CNS bleeding, UCB, GI bleeding, hematoma, and hemarthrosis, and provoked bleedings including post-trauma bleeding, postsurgical bleeding, and antiplatelet or anticoagulant therapy account for 14% and 20%, respectively, of all bleeding features [37].

Patients with FV deficiency develop a bleeding diathesis early in life. Although most patients with a mild deficiency present no clinical features, these can manifest later in life and may be accidentally diagnosed in routine coagulation laboratory tests [6]. Homozygous or compound heterozygous patients have moderate to severe bleeding features based on residual factor level whereas most heterozygote cases present with a mild degree of clinical manifestations [33]. Based on a European network of rare bleeding disorders (EN-RBD), there is a weak association between residual FV and clinical bleeding severity [38]. It can be concluded that undetectable FV level does not necessarily result in life-threatening bleeding episodes and also that a higher level of FV does not guarantee patients will present with life-threatening episodes. Whether these observations are related to the potential protective effect of having low TFPI levels in some of these patients is currently not known; however, from a biochemical perspective, a low TFPI should provide a compensatory mechanism to limit severe bleeding. Despite an overall benign phenotype of FV deficiency, different cases affected by neonatal and prenatal and neonatal intracranial hemorrhage (ICH) have been reported. In addition, an Iranian study conducted on six patients with moderate FV deficiency reported 20 episodes of miscarriage. The significant point here is that recurrent miscarriage is not reported as a clinical manifestation of FV deficiency in available clinical studies [39]. Therefore, different types of bleeding diathesis at different FV levels could be observed.

8.7 Platelet Factor V Deficiency

The Quebec platelet disorder (QPD) is an inherited disorder that is transmitted in an autosomal dominant pattern. QPD results from increased expression (more than 100 fold) of urokinase-type plasminogen activator (u-PA), which leads to plasmin generation and the degradation of alpha granule proteins [40]. Affected patients experience a wide range of bleeding features ranging from easy bruising to joint bleeding. However, the most common bleeding episode in these patients is delayed-onset bleeding following surgery or trauma. The laboratory features of these patients are mild thrombocytopenia, defective response to platelet aggregation test, and reduced FV levels but normal plasma FV level [40, 41]. However, QPD is categorized as a platelet disorder. The only platelet FV deficiency characterized is $FV_{NewYork}$, which results from the defective activity of platelet prothrombinase without proteolysis in platelet granule proteins [42].

8.8 Acquired Factor V Deficiency

Acquired FV deficiency is a rare disorder that presents with different bleeding tendencies, ranging from complete absence of bleeding symptoms to life-threatening bleeding episodes [43]. In acquired FV deficiency, antibodies are directed against FV and lead to enhanced clearance or neutralization of procoagulant activity. Inhibitors directed against FV can occur at any age but generally are very rare; however, they represent a clinical challenge. There are two forms of inhibitors: (1) inhibitors that develop in patients with congenital FV deficiency who are exposed to exogenous FV (FFP) and (2) inhibitors which form in individuals from autoimmune or alloimmune events [9]. By comparison, the first type is rarely present in patients with FV deficiency. The second type of inhibitors mostly presents in elderly patients and has high titers. Risk factors that lead to development of inhibitors against FV include surgical procedures, exposure to bovine thrombin, antibiotics administration, blood transfusion, and malignancy [44–47]. Among all these risk factors, exposure to bovine thrombin represents the most prevalent risk. Bovine thrombin, which contains a trace amount of bovine FV, is used as a hemostatic agent in different surgical procedures. Bovine FV is a potent stimulus that leads to development of autoantibodies directed against it (anti-bovine FV). These antibodies cross react with human FV, resulting in acquired FV deficiency [48, 49]. The clinical manifestations and outcome of this disorder vary depending upon antibody titers, epitopes of the antibodies, and the access of antibody to platelet FV [50, 51]. Inhibitors against the C2 domain, which is responsible for binding of this factor to phospholipids, are associated with bleeding manifestations [52]. In cases in which inhibitors lead to inactivation of the anticoagulant function of FV, thrombotic manifestations are more common compared to hemorrhagic manifestations [53]. Although FV inhibitors generally spontaneously resolve in months, administration of FFP and platelet concentrate is recommended in the presence of acute bleeding episodes [54]. In addition, follow-up treatment including intravenous immunoglobulin injection, immunosuppression, and plasmapheresis to decrease the inhibitor titer is also recommended [6].

8.9 Molecular Basis of Congenital Factor V Deficiency

Although the first patient affected by FV deficiency was described in 1947, it was another half-century before the first causative mutation in the *F5* gene was found [2]. Currently, more than 150 different mutations have been reported in the *F5* gene (Human Genome Mutation Database; www.hgmd.cf.ac.uk) [55]. These mutations include missense, nonsense, splicing mutations, and small insertions/deletions (frameshift) covering the whole *F5* gene except the promoter region, which has not been sufficiently investigated. Table 8.2 shows the diversity of mutations in FV deficiency [37]. The only mutation that results in partial deficiency of FV is FV New Brunswick, which was reported in 1995 [56]. The first true null mutation was reported in 1997 in a patient who was pseudo-homozygous for activated protein C resistance in *F5* [57]. In addition to FV deficiency-casing mutations, different single-nucleotide polymorphisms (SNP) in *F5* are reported, which have been assembled in http://www.ncbi.nlm.nih.gov/SNP. These alterations of sequence may be (missense mutation) associated with changes in activity and antigen levels of FV [58]. Figure 8.3 shows most of the missense FV deficiencies causing mutations.

The distinction between innocuous polymorphisms and true protein-altering mutations represents a significant challenge. The difference between these two is rarely obvious, and a careful family history investigation is needed as well as biochemical work. The availability of different databases assembling all known polymorphisms (innocuous polymorphism and true mutations) is clearly helpful to make distinctions. Most FV-causing mutations have been reported as private mutations (the mutations are reported in unique families or one patient), and few of them are represented as recurrent [19]. P.Tyr1702Cys was reported as a mutation that was detected in several European and Asiatic patients [59]. The heterogeneity of mutations required the full genomic screening for molecular diagnosis. Almost one third

Table 8.2 Diversity of mutations in congenital factor V deficiency

		Premature termination			Splice	Small in	Other	
Mutation	Missense mutations (%)	Small deletion (%)	Small insertion (%)	Nonsense mutation (%)	site mutation (%)	frame deletion (%)	Major rearrangement (%)	Gross deletion (%)
	46.6	18.4	6.8	11.7	10.7	3.9	1	1
Total	46.8	36.9			10.7	3.9	2	

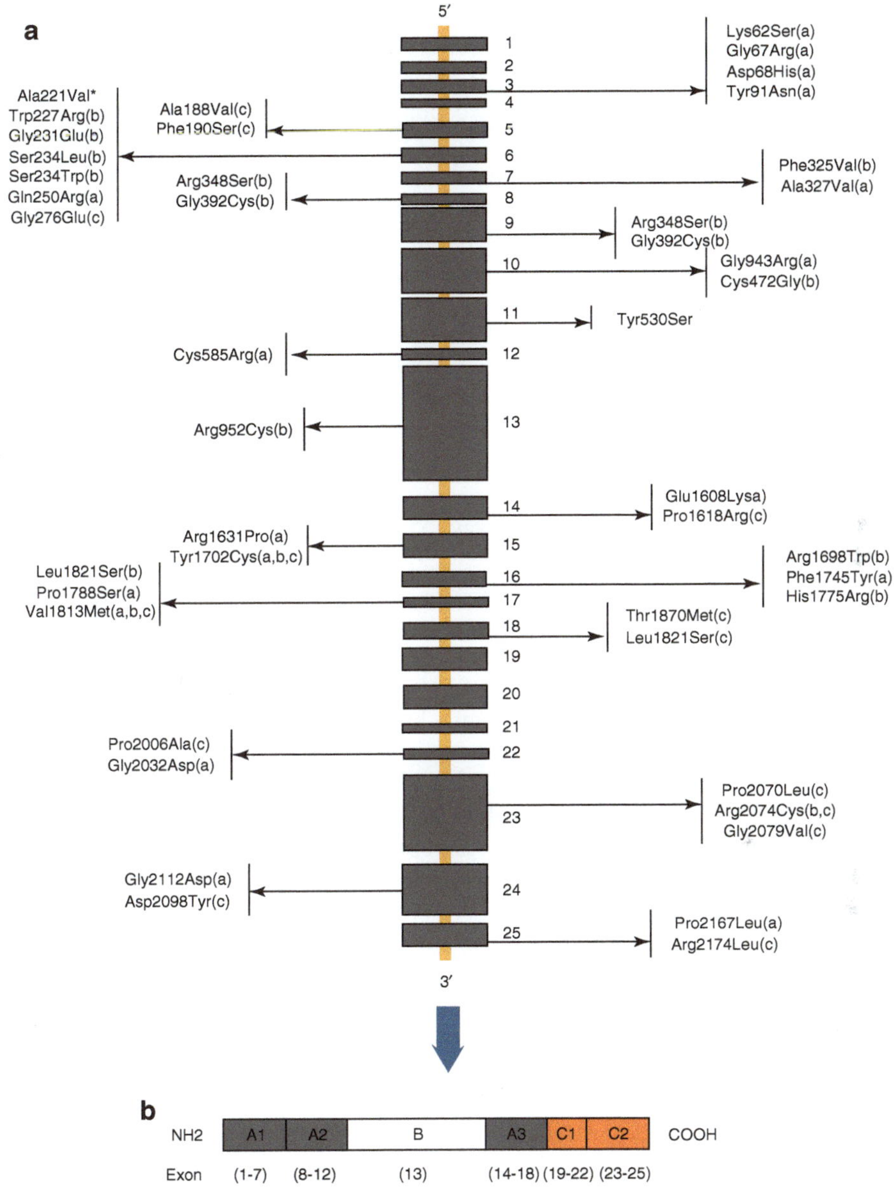

Fig. 8.3 (**a**) The mutational spectrum of factor V deficiency. Almost all causative missense mutations for type I and type II deficiency are represented. Exons and introns are shown by *boxes* and *lines*, respectively. Mutations are named at protein level, and the protein domains are also indicated. The mutation indicated by "asterisk" is the only mutation of type II deficiency. Mutations indicated by *a*, *b*, and *c* were detected in heterozygous, compound heterozygous, and homozygous patients, respectively. (**b**) Factor V domains and number of exons

of all mutations cause premature termination codons (PTCs). Investigation at the mRNA level showed degradation of corresponding transcripts by the nonsense-mediated mRNA decay pathway (NMD). It appears that mutations predicting a premature stop codon are overrepresented compared to other genes. Most of the nonsense mutations were detected in exon 13 (domain B) whereas the majority of missense mutations are clustered in the A and C domains; domain B is free of this type of mutation [37]. Expression of missense mutations in mammalian cells showed that these mutations lead to secretion defects or early intracellular degradation. Splicing mutations consist of approximately 10% of total mutations, but different studies showed that this frequency was probably underestimated because splicing mutations outside the canonical splice sites are not easily recognized. Splicing mutations disrupt splice sites and therefore result in mRNA degradation and exon skipping in the final protein [60, 61]. There are a few studies showing the relationship between the type of mutations and the severity of bleeding episodes. However, a study conducted in 2016 presented the association between *F5* splicing mutations and severe hemorrhagic diathesis, which is related to mRNA degradation by the nonsense-mediated decay pathway [55].

8.10 Diagnosis

Similar to other RBDs, the diagnosis of FV deficiency should include several key factors including bleeding episodes, family history, and routine and specific coagulation laboratory tests [34]. FV deficiency is suspected when routine coagulation laboratory tests including PT and aPTT have prolonged results. Because different coagulation disorders result in the prolongation of one or both of these tests, specific tests including mixing studies and measurement of FV antigen and activity level may be necessary. In situations with prolonged PT and aPTT, addition of normal plasma to the patient's plasma should correct these prolonged tests [6, 8]. In severe FV deficiency, bleeding time (BT) is also prolonged, which can be related to platelet FV [8]. In the presence of low FV, measurement of FVIII is necessary to exclude combined FV and FVIII deficiency. In addition, the low activity of FV should distinguished from liver disease and consumptive coagulopathy [8].

8.10.1 Factor V Antigen Assay

To quantitate FV levels in plasma, a FV antigen assay can be performed. The principle of the test is a sandwich enzyme immunoassay (ELISA). In this method, biotin-conjugated monoclonal antibody against FV is coated to a microplate. The FV and FVa in the sample or standard react with captured antibody. Then, after washing steps, avidin conjugated to horseradish peroxidase (HRP) is added to each plate. By adding the substrate, the color change is spectrophotometrically assessed at 450 nm. The concentration of FV in the sample is determined by comparing the optical density (OD) of the sample via the standard curve [62].

8.10.2 Factor V Activity Assay

Several manual and automated methods including PT-based assay, the Lewis and Ware method, EDTA method, and microplate activity assay were described to measure the activity of FV. These methods have different advantages and disadvantages.

8.10.3 One-Stage PT-Based Assay

The principle of this assay is based on the ability of patient plasma to correct the PT of factor-deficient plasma (substrate). Diluted patient plasma is mixed with an equal volume of FV-deficient plasma for correction of PT. Then, the factor activity in the patient's plasma is determined on a standard curve by using standard plasma.

In this assay, serial dilution of standard plasma (1 in 5, 10, 20, or 40) and test plasma in buffered saline is prepared. The equal amount of each dilution and deficient (substrate) plasma is mixed in another tube and warmed to 37 °C. By adding the equal amount of diluted thromboplastin, the clotting time is recorded. For calculation of the activity of FV, the clotting time of each dilution of test plasma and standard plasma is plotted against the concentration of FV.

8.10.4 Microplate Factor V Assay

In 1953, Lewis and Ware presented a technique for a FV assay in which a potassium oxalate sample is added at room temperature to diminish FV activity. The disadvantage of this method is the long incubation (4 weeks) time. In addition, this technique does not always produce usable substrate, and occasionally the prothrombin level is decreased to 60% of normal level [63]. In 1979, the EDTA method was introduced in which the incubation time is reduced to 5–10 h and yields satisfactory substrate. In addition, in contrast to the Lewis and Ware method, the EDTA method does not require a sterile environment and CO_2 atmosphere [63]. However, these manual techniques are time consuming because they can assess only one sample at a time. Subsequently, automated methods were introduced. The automated methods require expensive reagents and only show clotting time, not the rate and extend of clot formation.

In 2012, the rapid and convenient microplate assay for measurement of FV activity was introduced. In this method, a kinetic microplate reader is used to measure the increase in plasma turbidity. In fact, this assay monitors the absorbance change at 405 nm during fibrin formation at 0.35–0.45 unit. Then, between starting and maximal absorbance before and after addition of thromboplastin and calcium chloride, the activity of FV is measured [64, 65]. This method, unlike previously reported techniques, requires only a small amount of plasma and also measures the initial time, rate, and extent of fibrin formation in both nonactivated (FV1 stage assay) human plasma samples or plasma that has been activated with thrombin (FV2 stage assay) [64, 65]. These parameters provide more accurate information about the status of FV during clot formation. Compared to manual and automated methods, this assay has a higher sensitivity and detection limit (20–80 pM) and also has comparable clot time ranges (25–75 s) and corresponding FV levels in the sample (0.5–0.005 Units/ml). In addition, this technique is a quantitative method and accurately measures the time, rate, and extent of clotting, whereas manual techniques are based on visual assessment of clot formation. The microplate assay compared to an automated assay is inexpensive, and the required reagents can be provided commercially or be made in house. Another significant advantage of these methods is the simultaneous assessment of about 12 samples [64, 65].

This method utilizes a multichannel pipet to add FV-deficient plasma and diluted test or normal plasma in immunomodule strip wells simultaneously. After adding thromboplastin and a 1-min incubation at 25 °C, calcium chloride is added to initiate clotting. The clotting time is determined as the time between the minimum and maximum absorbance at 405 nm after addition of chloride calcium. The initial clotting rate is measured by using a curve in which absorbance is plotted versus time and defined as a rate of increase in absorbance at 405 nm (first five time points of clot formation) in the linear portion. In addition, the extent of clot formation is calculated by measuring the difference between maximal and minimal absorbance at 405 nm during clot formation [64, 65].

The FV activity of diluted test plasma in the one-stage assay is determined by use of the standard curve of initial rate of clot formation or clot times versus the activity of serial dilution of normal reference plasma. One unit of FV is defined as the activity of FV in 1 ml normal human plasma before activation by thrombin [64, 65].

The two-stage FV assay initially requires a pre-incubation of the plasma sample with thrombin to convert FV to FVa. After incubation, the plasma is further diluted and reassayed as already described. The two-stage FV activity is calculated from the one-stage standard curve. The total FV activity is calculated as two-stage FV activity minus one-stage FV activity [64, 65].

8.10.5 Factor V Inhibitor Assay

In the initial investigation, the prolonged PT and aPTT were further investigated by mixing patient plasma with normal pooled plasma (50:50). The inhibitor is suspected when PT and PTT are not corrected by mixing studies. Inhibitors were confirmed and titrated by the Bethesda method.

8.10.6 Mixing Study

For this method, normal plasma, patient plasma, and aPTT reagents are required. The normal plasma used for this purpose can be a commercial lyophilized plasma or a plasma pool of at least 20 donors.

In the first step, four tubes are prepared as follow:

1. Normal plasma
2. Patient's plasma
3. Equal mixture of patient and normal plasma (50:50) (time-dependent inhibitor: incubate 2 h at 37 C)
4. Equal mixture of patient and normal plasma (50:50) (immediate inhibitor)

APTT and PT should be performed in duplicate for all tubes.

Interpretation:
1. If both immediate and incubated PT and aPTT tests show correction, FV deficiency or multiple factor deficiencies are suspected.
2. If neither immediate nor incubated PT/aPTT shows correction, the presence of inhibitor is suspected.
3. If the immediate PT/aPTT results show correction, but the incubated tube results show no correction, a slow-acting inhibitor, including anti-FVIII, is suspected (Table 8.3) [9, 62].

An important issue that must be considered is that the activity of coagulation factors including FV and FVIII in potassium EDTA samples is factitiously decreased. Therefore, the mixing studies in these samples do not correct and the results of Bethesda assays are spuriously positive. Finding the inhibitors direct against FV and FVIII is a clue of potassium EDTA samples [66, 67].

8.10.7 Bethesda Assay

For quantitative measurement of FV inhibitor titer, the Bethesda method is used. The Bethesda unit is the amount of inhibitor that neutralized 50% 1 unit FV in normal plasma [68]. Dilution of patient plasma with an equal volume of normal plasma (normally contains 100% FV) incubated at 37 °C for 0 hour (h), 1 h, or 2 h at 37 °C. FV inhibitors, in contrast to FVIII inhibitors that need 1–2 h incubation to fully inactivate FVIII, immediately neutralize FV [69]. However, incubation up to 2 h to accurately quantify the FV inhibitor level is recommended [69]. Dilutions of

Table 8.3 Interpretation of the inhibitor screen for factor V deficiency

		Results of PT and aPTT		
Tube	Content	FVD	Immediate inhibitors	Time-dependent inhibitors
1	Normal plasma	Normal	Normal	Normal
2	Patient plasma	Prolonged	Prolonged	Prolonged
3	Mixed plasma: incubated 2 h	Normal	Prolonged	Prolonged
4	Mixed plasma: no incubation	Normal	Normal	Prolonged

FVD Factor V deficiency, *APTT* activated partial thromboplastin time, *PT* prothrombin time

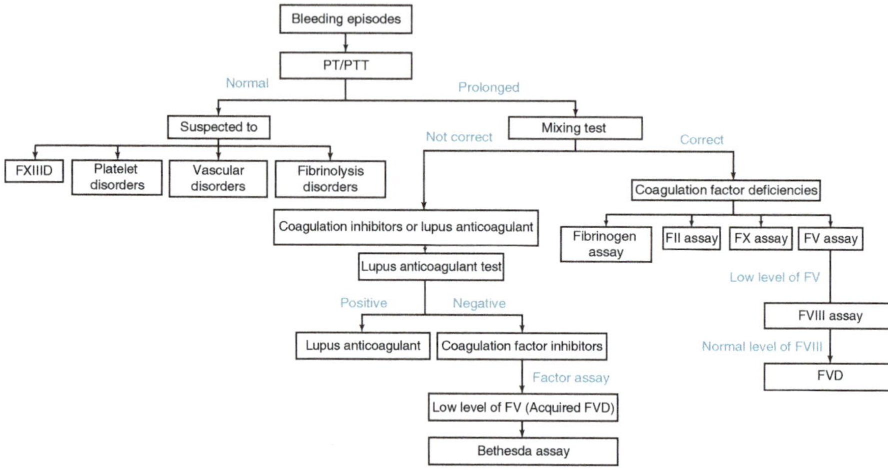

Fig. 8.4 An algorithmic approach for diagnosis of congenital and acquired factor (F) V deficiency. This algorithm has been developed by the authors based on different studies. The algorithm begins by presentation of bleeding diathesis and routine coagulation laboratory tests including PT and PTT. In the presence of normal PT and PTT with bleeding episodes, FXIII deficiency can be suspected, and further specific testes are required (for more information, refer to Chap. 13). If these two tests are prolonged, a mixing test is indicated with a mixture of equal volumes of patient plasma and normal plasma. *If correction is achieved*, there is a factor deficiency or multiple factor deficiencies. Therefore, performance of factor assays for coagulation factors in the common pathway is mandatory. In the presence of a low level of FV, the FVIII assay to distinguish FVD from combined FV and FVIII deficiency is necessary. A normal level of FVIII indicates FV deficiency. *If the mixing study does not correct*, inhibiters direct against coagulation factors of common pathway or lupus anticoagulant are suspected. A negative lupus anticoagulant test indicates the presence of coagulation factor inhibitors. A factor assay should be performed to find the coagulation factor against which the inhibitor is direct. A low level of FV indicates acquired FV deficiency. The Bethesda assay will quantify the inhibitor titer. *FXIIID* factor XIII deficiency, *FVD* factor V deficiency

control plasma that contain no inhibitors are treated as the same way (a control consists of an equal volume of normal plasma with buffer). After incubation, the residual FV for each mixture assay using the one-stage PT-based assay is measured. The dilution with residual FV activity about 50% is considered for determination of inhibitor strength. The strength of the FV inhibitor is calculated by using a standard graph of residual FV activity versus inhibitor units. The inhibitor titers from the graph are multiplied by dilution to give the final titer (Fig. 8.4) [9, 62].

8.11 Treatment

The mainstay of treatment in patients with congenital FV deficiency is on-demand therapy to alleviate the hemorrhage as soon as possible. As there is no commercially available FV concentrate, the only source of FV for patients affected by FV deficiency is virus-inactivated FFP. In addition, because platelets contain FV, platelet

Table 8.4 Doses and target therapeutic levels in patients with factor V deficiency

Kind of treatment	Recommended level	Dosage of therapeutic level
On-demand therapy	10%	15–25 ml/kg (FFP) Platelet transfusion
Long-term prophylaxis	10%	20 ml/kg 2 times/week
Major surgery	>15%–20% (maintaining level)	15–25 ml/kg)before surgery) 10 ml/kg every 12 h Platelet transfusion (if required)
Minor surgery	–	15–20 mg/kg or 1 g four times daily: tranexamic acid

transfusion can be helpful in some situations [70]. The required dosage in coagulation factor deficiencies depends on the kind of treatment (on demand and prophylaxis), the minimal hemostatic level, plasma half-life, and, most importantly, the type of bleeding episode [10]. The plasma half-life of FV is 36 h and, based on the EN-RBD study, 10% of FV is the minimum level need for patients to be asymptomatic [38]. Table 8.4 shows the doses and therapeutic target level in different treatments and major surgery [71].

A new FV concentrate has been developed for clinical trials, and related preclinical studies are being conducted for the orphan drug designation application [72].

References

1. Mann KG, Kalafatis M. Factor V. A combination of Dr Jekyll and Mr Hyde. Blood. 2003;101(1):20–30.
2. Owren P. Parahaemophilia: haemorrhagic diathesis due to absence of a previously unknown clotting factor. Lancet. 1947;249(6449):446–8.
3. Rosing J, Tans G, Govers-Riemslag J, Zwaal R, Hemker HC. The role of phospholipids and factor Va in the prothrombinase complex. J Biol Chem. 1980;255(1):274–83.
4. Shen L, Dahlbäck B, Factor V. protein S as synergistic cofactors to activated protein C in degradation of factor VIIIa. J Biol Chem. 1994;269(29):18735–8.
5. Bolton-Maggs P, Perry D, Chalmers E, Parapia L, Wilde J, Williams M, et al. The rare coagulation disorders–review with guidelines for management from the United Kingdom Haemophilia Centre Doctors' Organisation. Haemophilia. 2004;10(5):593–628.
6. Duckers C, Simioni P, Rosing J, Castoldi E. Advances in understanding the bleeding diathesis in factor V deficiency. Br J Haematol. 2009;146(1):17–26.
7. Tabibian S, Kazemi A, Dorgalaleh A. Laboratory diagnosis of congenital factor V deficiency, routine, specific coagulation tests with molecular methods. J Cell Mol Anesth. 2016;1(2):87–90.
8. Duckers C, Simioni P, Spiezia L, Radu C, Gavasso S, Rosing J, et al. Low plasma levels of tissue factor pathway inhibitor in patients with congenital factor V deficiency. Blood. 2008;112(9):3615–23.
9. Favaloro EJ, Posen J, Ramakrishna R, Soltani S, McRae S, Just S, et al. Factor V inhibitors: rare or not so uncommon? A multi-laboratory investigation. Blood Coagul Fibrinolysis. 2004;15(8):637–47.
10. Peyvandi F, Garagiola I, Biguzzi E. Advances in treatment of bleeding disorders. J Thromb Haemost. 2016;14(11):2095–106.

11. Cripe LD, Moore KD, Kane WH. Structure of the gene for human coagulation factor V. Biochemistry. 1992;31(15):3777–85.
12. William H, Earl W. Blood coagulation factor V and VIII: structural and functional similarities and their relationship to hemorrhagic and thrombotic disorders. Blood. 1988;71(71):539–55.
13. Ortel TL, Takahashi N, Putnam FW. Structural model of human ceruloplasmin based on internal triplication, hydrophilic/hydrophobic character, and secondary structure of domains. Proc Natl Acad Sci USA. 1984;81(15):4761–5.
14. Baumgartner S, Hofmann K, Bucher P, Chiquet-Ehrismann R. The discoidin domain family revisited: new members from prokaryotes and a homology-based fold prediction. Protein Sci. 1998;7(7):1626–31.
15. Nicolaes GA, Dahlbäck B. Factor V and thrombotic disease. Arterioscler Thromb Vasc Biol. 2002;22(4):530–8.
16. Macedo-Ribeiro S, Bode W, Huber R, Quinn-Allen MA. Crystal structures of the membrane-binding C2 domain of human coagulation factor V. Nature (Lond). 1999;402(6760):434.
17. Villoutreix BO, Dahlbäck B. Structural investigation of the A domains of human blood coagulation factor V by molecular modeling. Protein Sci. 1998;7(6):1317–25.
18. Lechtenberg BC, Murray-Rust TA, Johnson DJ, Adams TE, Krishnaswamy S, Camire RM, et al. Crystal structure of the prothrombinase complex from the venom of *Pseudonaja textilis*. Blood. 2013;122(16):2777–83.
19. Asselta R, Tenchini M, Duga S. Inherited defects of coagulation factor V: the hemorrhagic side. J Thromb Haemost. 2006;4(1):26–34.
20. Camire R, Bos M. The molecular basis of factor V and VIII procofactor activation. J Thromb Haemost. 2009;7(12):1951–61.
21. Kalafatis M, Rand MD, Mann KG. The mechanism of inactivation of human factor V and human factor Va by activated protein C. J Biol Chem. 1994;269(50):31869–80.
22. Mann KG, Hockin MF, Begin KJ, Kalafatis M. Activated protein C cleavage of factor Va leads to dissociation of the A2 domain. J Biol Chem. 1997;272(33):20678–83.
23. Thorelli E, Kaufman RJ, Dahlbäck B. Cleavage of factor V at Arg 506 by activated protein C and the expression of anticoagulant activity of factor V. Blood. 1999;93(8):2552–8.
24. Hockin M, Kalafatis M, Cawthern K, Simoni P, Mann K, editors. A novel cellular mechanism for factor Va inactivation. 40th Annual Meeting of the American Society of Hematology Blood; 1998.
25. Kalafatis M, Mann KG. The role of the membrane in the inactivation of factor va by plasmin. Amino acid region 307–348 of factor V plays a critical role in factor Va cofactor function. J Biol Chem. 2001;276(21):18614–23.
26. Christella M, Thomassen L, Castoldi E, Tans G, Magdeleyns E, Delaunoit C, et al. Endogenous factor V synthesis in megakaryocytes contributes negligibly to the platelet factor V pool. Haematologica. 2003;88(10):1150–6.
27. Gould WR, Silveira JR, Tracy PB. Unique in vivo modifications of coagulation factor V produce a physically and functionally distinct platelet-derived cofactor: characterization of purified platelet-derived factor V/Va. J Biol Chem. 2004;279(4):2383–93.
28. Camire RM, Kalafatis M, Cushman M, Tracy RP, Mann KG, Tracy PB. The mechanism of inactivation of human platelet factor Va from normal and activated protein C-resistant individuals. J Biol Chem. 1995;270(35):20794–800.
29. Lippi G, Favaloro EJ, Montagnana M, Manzato F, Guidi GC, Franchini M. Inherited and acquired factor V deficiency. Blood Coagul Fibrinolysis. 2011;22(3):160–6.
30. Naderi M, Tabibian S, Alizadeh S, Hosseini S, Zaker F, Bamedi T, et al. Congenital factor V deficiency: comparison of the severity of clinical presentations among patients with rare bleeding disorders. Acta Haematol. 2015;133(2):148–54.
31. Mannucci PM, Duga S, Peyvandi F. Recessively inherited coagulation disorders. Blood. 2004;104(5):1243–52.
32. Lippi G, Pasalic L, Favaloro EJ. Detection of mild inherited disorders of blood coagulation: current options and personal recommendations. Expert Rev Hematol. 2015;8(4):527–42.
33. Asselta R, Peyvandi F. Factor V deficiency. Semin Thromb Hemost. 2009;35(4):382–9.

34. Acharya S, Coughlin A, Dimichele DM. Rare bleeding disorder registry: deficiencies of factors II, V, VII, X, XIII, fibrinogen and dysfibrinogenemias. J Thromb Haemost. 2004;2(2):248–56.
35. Mansouritorghabeh H, Manavifar L, Mobalegh A, Shirdel A. Haemorrhagic manifestations and prevalence of factor V deficiency in North-Eastern Iran. Haemophilia. 2010;16(2):376–80.
36. Lak M, Sharifian R, Peyvandi F, Mannucci F. Symptoms of inherited factor V deficiency in 35 Iranian patients. Br J Haematol. 1998;103:1067–9.
37. Thalji N, Camire RM. Parahemophilia: new insights into factor V deficiency. Semin Thromb Hemost. 2013;39(6):607–12.
38. Peyvandi F, Palla R, Menegatti M, Siboni S, Halimeh S, Faeser B, et al. Coagulation factor activity and clinical bleeding severity in rare bleeding disorders: results from the European Network of Rare Bleeding Disorders. J Thromb Haemost. 2012;10(4):615–21.
39. Naderi M, Tabibian S, Shamsizadeh M, Dorgalaleh A. Miscarriage and recurrent miscarriage in patients with congenital factor V deficiency: a report of six cases in Iran. Int J Hematol. 2016;103(6):673–5.
40. Diamandis M, Adam F, Kahr W, Wang P, Chorneyko K, Arsenault A, et al. Insights into abnormal hemostasis in the Quebec platelet disorder from analyses of clot lysis. J Thromb Haemost. 2006;4(5):1086–94.
41. Blavignac J, Bunimov N, Rivard GE, Hayward CP. Quebec platelet disorder: update on pathogenesis, diagnosis, and treatment. Semin Thromb Hemost. 2011;37(6):713–20.
42. Weiss HJ, Lages B, Zheng S, Hayward CP. Platelet factor V New York: a defect in factor V distinct from that in factor V Quebec resulting in impaired prothrombinase generation. Am J Hematol. 2001;66(2):130–9.
43. Franchini M, Lippi G. Acquired factor V inhibitors: a systematic review. J Thromb Thrombolysis. 2011;31(4):449–57.
44. Miesbach W, Voigt J, Peetz D, Scharrer I. Massive bleeding symptoms in two patients with factor V inhibitor and antiphospholipid antibodies after treatment with ciprofloxacin. Med Klin. 2003;98(6):339–43.
45. Lucia J, Aguilar C. A case of an asymptomatic idiopathic inhibitor to coagulation factor V. Haemophilia. 2005;11(2):178–80.
46. Takahashi H, Fuse I, Abe T, Yoshino N, Aizawa Y. Acquired factor V inhibitor complicated by Hashimoto's thyroditis, primary biliary cirrhosis and membranous nephropathy. Blood Coagul Fibrinolysis. 2003;14(1):87–93.
47. Koyama T, Saito T, Kusano T, Hirosawa S. Factor V inhibitor associated with Sjögren's syndrome. Br J Haematol. 1995;89(4):893–6.
48. Streiff MB, Ness PM. Acquired FV inhibitors: a needless iatrogenic complication of bovine thrombin exposure. Transfusion. 2002;42(1):18–26.
49. Ortel TL, Mercer MC, Thames EH, Moore KD, Lawson JH. Immunologic impact and clinical outcomes after surgical exposure to bovine thrombin. Ann Surg. 2001;233(1):88–96.
50. Nesheim ME, Nichols WL, Cole TL, Houston JG, Schenk RB, Mann KG, et al. Isolation and study of an acquired inhibitor of human coagulation factor V. J Clin Invest. 1986;77(2):405.
51. Ajzner E, Balogh I, Haramura G, Boda Z, Kalmar K, Pfliegler G, et al. Anti-factor V autoantibody in the plasma and platelets of a patient with repeated gastrointestinal bleeding. J Thromb Haemost. 2003;1(5):943–9.
52. Ortel TL, Moore KD, Quinn-Allen MA, Okamura T, Sinclair AJ, Lazarchick J, et al. Inhibitory anti-factor V antibodies bind to the factor V C2 domain and are associated with hemorrhagic manifestations. Blood. 1998;91(11):4188–96.
53. Kalafatis M, Simioni P, Tormene D, Beck DO, Luni S, Girolami A. Isolation and characterization of an antifactor V antibody causing activated protein C resistance from a patient with severe thrombotic manifestations. Blood. 2002;99(11):3985–92.
54. de Raucourt E, Barbier C, Sinda P, Dib M, Peltier JY, Ternisien C. High-dose intravenous immunoglobulin treatment in two patients with acquired factor V inhibitors. Am J Hematol. 2003;74(3):187–90.
55. Nuzzo F, Beshlawi I, Wali Y, Castoldi E. High incidence of intracranial bleeding in factor V-deficient patients with homozygous F5 splicing mutations. Br J Haematol. 2017;179(1):163–6.

56. Murray JM, Rand MD, Egan J, Murphy S, Kim H, Mann K. Factor V New Brunswick: Ala221-to-Val substitution results in reduced cofactor activity. Blood. 1995;86(5):1820–7.
57. Guasch J, Lensen R, Bertina R. Molecular characterization of a type I quantitative factor V deficiency in a thrombosis patient that is "pseudo homozygous" for activated protein C resistance. Thromb Haemost. 1997;77(2):252–7.
58. Vos H. An online database of mutations and polymorphisms in and around the coagulation factor V gene. J Thromb Haemost. 2007;5(1):185–8.
59. Castoldi E, Lunghi B, Mingozzi F, Muleo G, Redaelli R, Mariani G, et al. A missense mutation (Y1702C) in the coagulation factor V gene is a frequent cause of factor V deficiency in the Italian population. Haematologica. 2001;86(6):629–33.
60. Nuzzo F, Bulato C, Nielsen B, Lee K, Wielders S, Simioni P, et al. Characterization of an apparently synonymous F5 mutation causing aberrant splicing and factor V deficiency. Haemophilia. 2015;21(2):241–8.
61. Castoldi E, Bulato C, Nuzzo F, Nielsen B, Lee K, Key N, et al. Characterisation of an apparently synonymous F5 mutation causing aberrant splicing and factor V deficiency. J Thromb Haemost. 2013;11:195.
62. Bain BJ, Bates I, Laffan MA. Dacie and Lewis practical haematology. Amsterdam: Elsevier; 2016.
63. Bloom JW, Nesheim ME, Mann KG. A rapid technique for the preparation of factor V deficient plasma. Thromb Res. 1979;15(5-6):595–9.
64. Tilley D, Levit I, Samis JA. Measurement of factor V activity in human plasma using a microplate coagulation assay. JoVE. 2012;67:3822.
65. Tilley D, Levit I, Samis JA. Development of a microplate coagulation assay for factor V in human plasma. Thromb J. 2011;9(1):11.
66. Favaloro EJ, Bonar R, Duncan E, Earl G, Low J, Aboud M, et al. Mis-identification of factor inhibitors by diagnostic haemostasis laboratories: recognition of pitfalls and elucidation of strategies. A follow up to a large multicentre evaluation. Pathology. 2007;39(5):504–11.
67. Favaloro EJ, Bonar R, Duncan E, Earl G, Low J, Aboud M, et al. Identification of factor inhibitors by diagnostic haemostasis laboratories. A large multi-centre evaluation. Thromb Haemost. 2006;96(1):73–8.
68. Knöbl P, Lechner K. Acquired factor V inhibitors. Baillieres Clin Haematol. 1998;11(2):305–18.
69. Ang AL, Kuperan P, Ng CH, Ng HJ. Acquired factor V inhibitor-A problem-based systematic review. Thromb Haemost. 2009;101(5):852–9.
70. Salooja N, Martin P, Khair K, Liesner R, Hann I. Severe factor V deficiency and neonatal intracranial haemorrhage: a case report. Haemophilia. 2000;6(1):44–6.
71. Peyvandi F, Menegatti M. Treatment of rare factor deficiencies in 2016. Hematology Am Soc Hematol Educ Program. 2016;2016(1):663–9.
72. Lawrie AS, Berbenni C, Menegatti M, Nardini I, Mackie I, Machin S, et al. In vitro characterizations of the first therapeutic factor V concentrate. Haemophilia. 2014;20:25–6.

Multiple Coagulation Factor Deficiency 9

Maryam Sadat Hosseini, Mahmood Shams,
Akbar Dorgalaleh, and Hassan Mansouritorghabeh

9.1 Combined Factor V and Factor VIII Deficiency

9.1.1 Introduction

Combined factor (F) V and FVIII deficiency (F5F8D) is a rare bleeding disorder (RBD) that comprises about 3% of all RBD and is the most common form of familial multiple coagulation factor deficiency (MCFD) (Table 9.1). The disorder has an incidence of about 1per 1,000,000 in general population and is far more prevalent (1 per 100,000) among Middle Eastern Jews and non-Jewish Iranians [1, 2]. This higher frequency may be explained by the high rate of consanguineous marriages in these regions [3]. The underlying cause of F5F8D is separated from isolated congenital deficiency of FV and FVIII, which are due to gene defect in *F5* and *F8* genes, respectively. It is an autosomal recessive disorder caused by mutations in either lectin

M. S. Hosseini
Department of Hematology and Blood transfusion, School of Allied Medicine,
Shahid Beheshti University of Medical Sciences, Tehran, Iran
e-mail: ms.hosseini@sbmu.ac.ir

M. Shams
Department of Laboratory Sciences, Paramedical Faculty,
Babol University of Medical Sciences, Babol, Iran

Department of Hematology and Blood transfusion, School of Allied Medicine,
Iran University of Medical Sciences, Tehran, Iran
e-mail: shams@mubabol.ac.ir

A. Dorgalaleh (✉)
Department of Hematology and Blood transfusion, School of Allied Medicine,
Iran University of Medical Sciences, Tehran, Iran

H. Mansouritorghabeh
Allergy Research Center, School of Medicine,
Mashhad University of Medical Sciences, Mashhad, Iran

A. Dorgalaleh (ed.), *Congenital Bleeding Disorders*,
https://doi.org/10.1007/978-3-319-76723-9_9

Table 9.1 Main characteristics of multiple coagulation factor deficiency (MCFD)

	Deficient factors	Underlying cause	OMIM designation
Acquired			
Liver disease	Variable global defect	Impaired synthesis	–
DIC	Variable global defect	Excessive consumption	–
Massive transfusion	Variable global defect	Dilutional effect	–
Cardiopulmonary bypass	Variable global defect	Dilutional effect	–
Familial (MCFD)			
Single genetic defect			
Defect of a gene implicated in production or activation of multiple factors			
F5F8D	FV + FVIII	Mutations in LMAN1 or MCFD2 genes	227300
Combined vitamin K-dependent factors deficiency	FII + FVII + FIX + FX	Mutations in GGCX or VKORC1 genes	2777450 607473
FMCFD as part of a syndrome			
Congenital disorders of glycosylation	Variable	Mutations in PMM2	212065 (CDG1a)
Noonan syndrome	Variable	Mutations in PTPN11, SOS1, RAF1, KRAS	163950
Inborn errors of liver metabolism	Variable	Mutations in GALT	230400 (Galactosaemia)
13q34 deletions syndromes	FVII + FX	Gene deletion 13q34	227500 227600
Independent segregation of two or more defects			

OMIM Online Mendelian Inheritance in Man. (http://www.ncbi.nlm.nih.gov/omim/), DIC disseminated intravascular coagulation, *FMCFD* Familial Multiple coagulation factor deficiencies, *F5F8D* combined FV and FVIII deficiency, *LMAN1* mannose binding lectin1, *MCFD2* multiple coagulation factor deficiency 2, *GGCX* γ-glutamyl carboxylase, *VKORC1* vitamin K epoxide reductase complex subunit 1, *PMM2* phosphomannomutase 2, *CDG1a* congenital disorder of glycosylation type 1a, *PTPN11* protein tyrosine phosphatase non-receptor type 11, *SOS1* Son of sevenless homolog 1, *GALT* galactose-1-phosphate uridylyltransferase

mannose-binding 1 (*LMAN1*) or multiple coagulation factor deficiency 2 (*MCFD2*) genes [4]. F5F8D is usually accompanied by mild bleeding tendency, mainly mucocutaneous hemorrhages. Therefore on-demand therapy is usually sufficient for management of the disorder, and generally prophylaxis is not required for patients with this disorder [5]. Diagnosis mainly is based on prolonged prothrombin time (PT) and activated partial thromboplastin time (aPTT) and parallel reduction in both FV and FVIII activity, but it is required to be distinguished from concomitant presence of FV deficiency with either hemophilia A or von Willebrand disease (VWD).

9.1.2 Structure and Function of LMAN1 and MCFD2

LMAN1 was previously known as a marker of the endoplasmic reticulum Golgi intermediate compartment 53 kDa (ERGIC-53). It acts as a cargo receptor for glycoproteins. It has been demonstrated that LMAN1 is a crucial component in the secretory pathway of FV and FVIII, as mediates transportation of both factors from endoplasmic reticulum (ER) to Golgi (Fig. 9.1) [4, 6, 7].

LMAN1 is a 53 kDa homo-hexameric transmembrane protein. LMAN1 contains three domains including (I) a luminal domain which is divided into a carbohydrate recognition domain (CRD) and α-helix coiled coil regions, (II) a transmembrane, and (III) a cytoplasmic domain (Fig. 9.2b). It has been established that there is a direct interaction between LMAN1 and MCFD2, as each LMAN1 hexamer is associated with six MCFD2 proteins (Fig. 9.1) [8]. MCFD2 is a 16 kDa monomeric protein. It has two Ca^{+2}-binding motifs called EF-hand domains which are separated by a linker region (Fig. 9.3b) [4, 7].

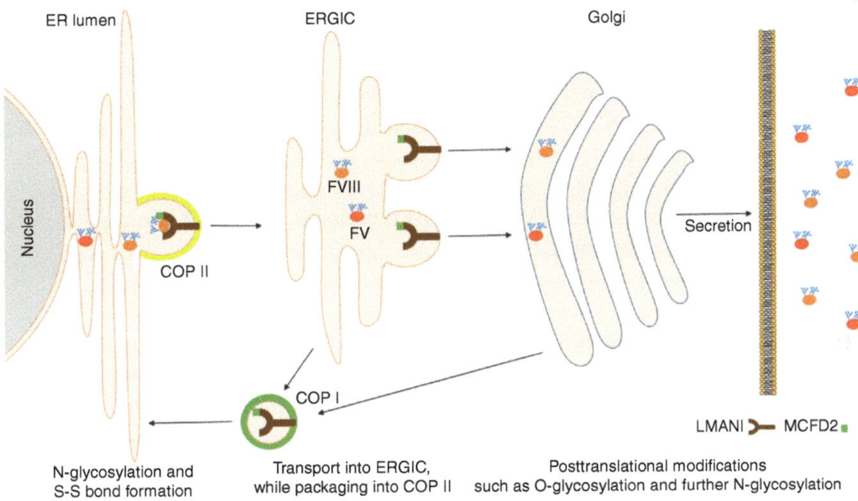

Fig. 9.1 FV and FVIII transportation by LMAN1 and MCFD2 complex. *N*-glycosylation and S-S bond formation of FV and FVIII occur in ER. The FV and FVIII bind to LMAN1-MCFD2 complex on distinct binding sites and transport into ERGIC, while packaging into COP II. Specific location of binding sites is not clear. However it seems that CRD has probably an important role in recognition of FV and FVIII. FV and FVIII are released to Golgi apparatus, where other post-translational modifications such as *O*-glycosylation and further processing of *N*-glycosylation occur. The LMAN1-MCFD2 complex is packaged into COP I and then recycled back to ER (known as retrograde transport). Finally, FV and FVIII are secreted outside of the cell. *FV* factor V, *FVIII* factor VIII, *LMAN1* lectin mannose-binding 1, *MCFD2* multiple coagulation factor deficiency 2, *ER* endoplasmic reticulum, *ERGIC* endoplasmic reticulum Golgi intermediate compartment, *COP II* coat protein II, *CRD* carbohydrate recognition domain, *COP I* coat protein I

9.1.3 Combined Factor V and Factor VIII Deficiency

F5F8D (OMIM #227300 and #61362522) was first described by *Oeri et al.* in 1954 [9]. The underlying cause of F5F8D is different from isolated deficiency of FV and FVIII, which is caused by *F5* and *F8* gene defects, respectively. Although the first case of F5F8D was reported in 1954, the underlying molecular basis remained unknown for more than 40 years [10]. In 1998 *Nichols et al.* introduced null mutations in the *ERGIC53* (currently known as *LMAN1*) gene, as the responsible genetic defect causing F5F8D [5, 11, 12]. Five years later, assessment of about 15% of affected families with no mutations in *ERGIC-53* was suggestive of another causative genetic defect [4].

9.1.4 Clinical Manifestations

Patients with F5F8D are not usually manifested by severe bleeding events. They commonly experience easy bruising, epistaxis, gingival bleeding, and excessive bleeding after trauma or invasive procedures such as tooth extraction. Affected females usually present menorrhagia and post-partum hemorrhages. Hemarthrosis and gastrointestinal bleeding (GI) may also occur in these patients but with much less frequency. Hematuria, muscle hematoma, and central nervous system (CNS) hemorrhages have been only described in few cases [1, 3, 13–15].

Generally, patients with F5F8D present various clinical presentations ranging from mild bleeding episodes such as epistaxis to severe bleeds including CNS bleeding (Table 9.2).

In comparison with isolated FV and FVIII deficiencies, F5F8D is not associated with a higher bleeding tendency [5].

9.1.5 Molecular Basis

It seems that mutations in *LMAN1* and *MCFD2* genes are responsible for almost all cases with F5F8D. The gene encoding for LMAN1 with about 29 kb length and 13 exons (Fig. 9.2a) is located on the long arm of chromosome 18 (18q21.32). MCFD2 is encoded by a 19 kb gene on the short arm of chromosome 2 (2p21), containing 4 exons (Fig. 9.3a).

Fig. 9.2 (**a**) *LMAN1* gene and F5F8D-causing mutations. *LMAN 1* gene comprises of 13 exons. Exons are shown in gray rectangles and are drawn to scale; and introns are indicated by yellow lines and are not to scale. White rectangles indicate 3′ UTR and 5′ UTR of gene. (**b**) Domains of LMAN1 protein. Signal peptide of LMAN1 contributes in translocation of LMAN1 into ER. The protein consists of three domains, a luminal, a transmembrane (TM), and a short cytoplasmic (**c**) domain. The luminal domain is divided into two sub-domains, an N-terminal CRD and a membrane-proximal α-helical coiled domain, known as stalk domain. *LMAN1* lectin mannose-binding 1, *UTR* untranslated region, *ER* endoplasmic reticulum, *CRD* carbohydrate recognition domain

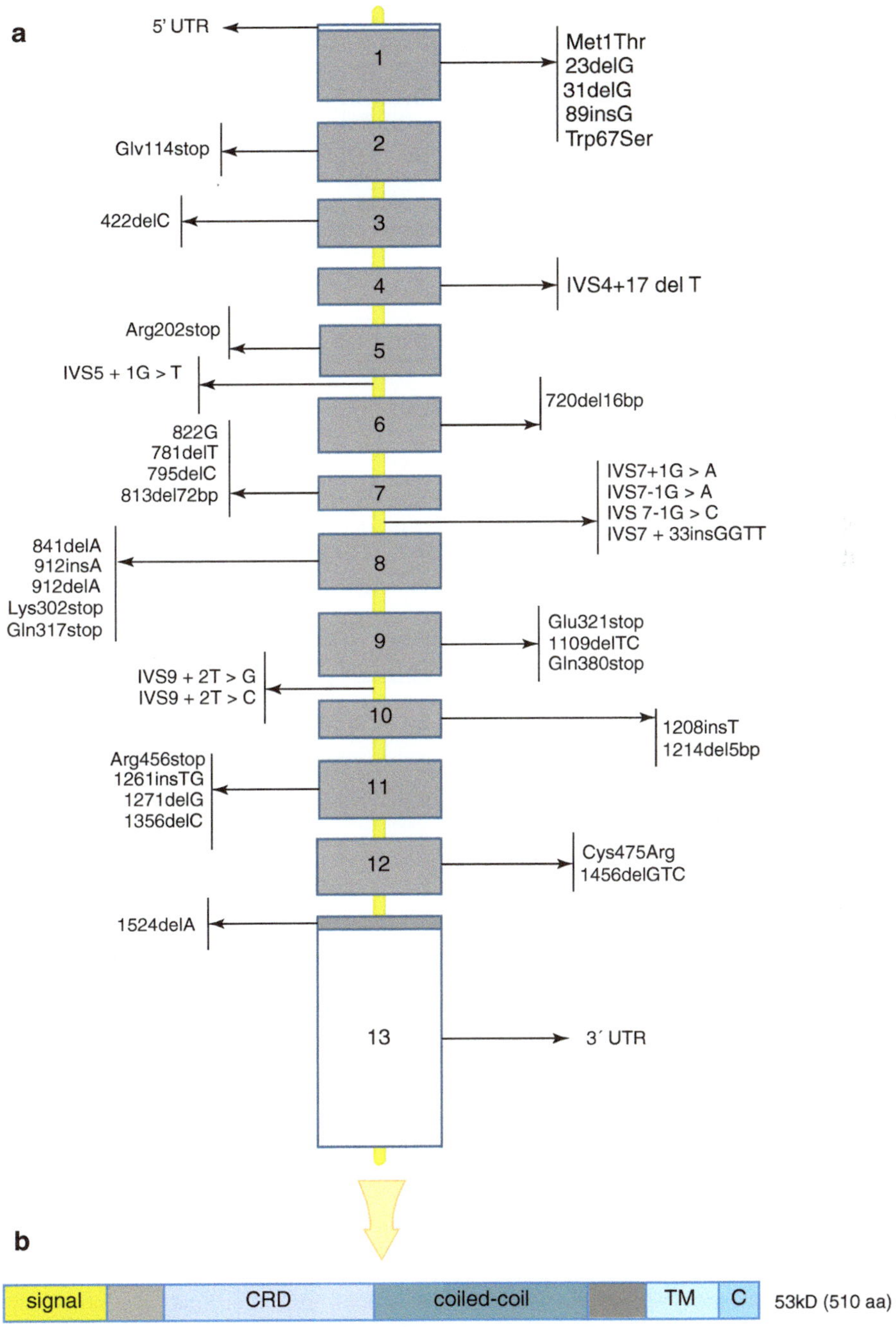
a
5' UTR
1
Met1Thr
23delG
31delG
89insG
Trp67Ser
Glv114stop
2
422delC
3
4
IVS4+17 del T
Arg202stop
5
IVS5 + 1G > T
6
720del16bp
822G
781delT
795delC
813del72bp
7
IVS7+1G > A
IVS7-1G > A
IVS 7-1G > C
IVS7 + 33insGGTT
841delA
912insA
912delA
Lys302stop
Gln317stop
8
9
Glu321stop
1109delTC
Gln380stop
IVS9 + 2T > G
IVS9 + 2T > C
10
1208insT
1214del5bp
Arg456stop
1261insTG
1271delG
1356delC
11
12
Cys475Arg
1456delGTC
1524delA
13
3´ UTR
b
signal
CRD
coiled-coil
TM
C
53kD (510 aa)

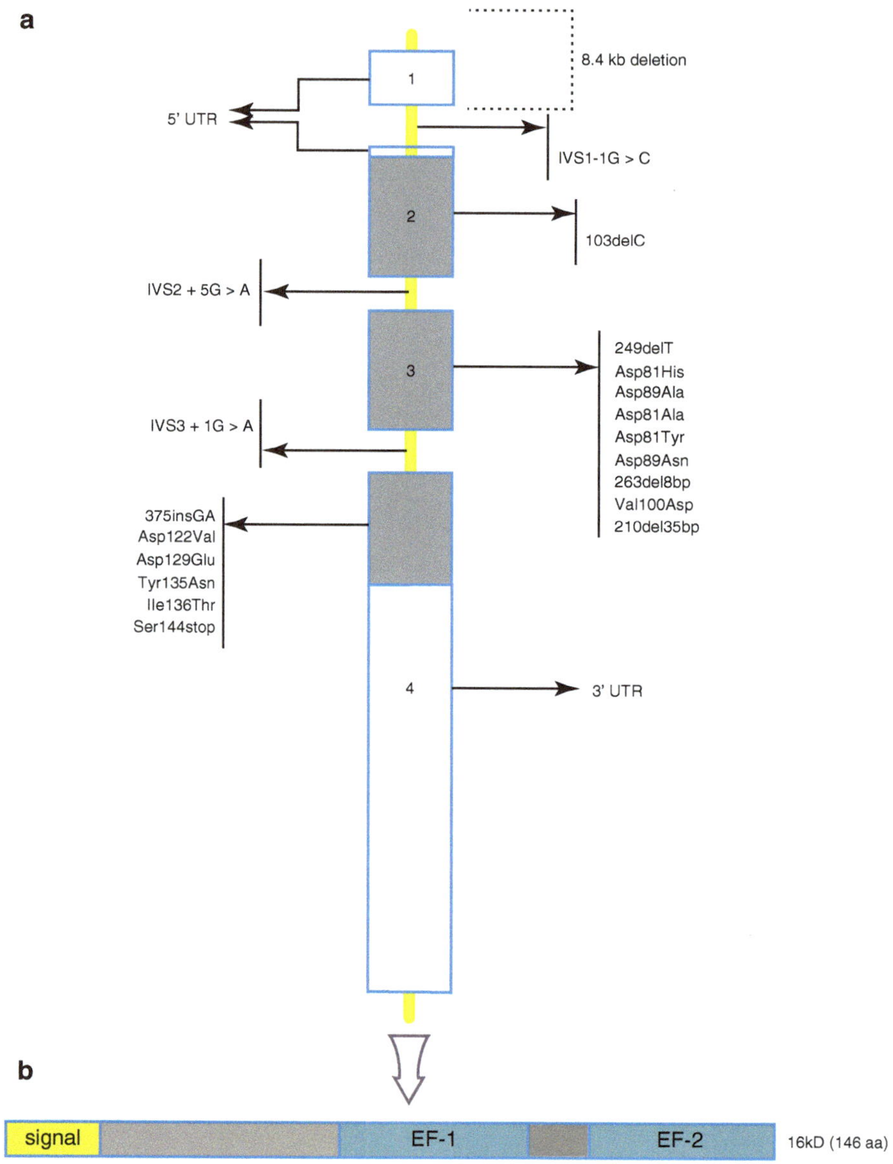

Fig. 9.3 (**a**) *MCDF2* gene and F5F8D causing mutations. Exons are indicated by gray rectangles and are drawn to scale. Introns are indicated by yellow lines and are not to scale. White rectangles indicate 3′ UTR and 5′ UTR of gene. (**b**) Domains of MCFD2 protein. MCFD2 is a small protein with 166 amino acids and 3 domains including a signal sequence for direction of MCFD2 into ER and two EF-hand motifs which probably can bind to Ca^{+2} ions. *MCFD2* multiple coagulation factor deficiency 2, *UTR* untranslated region, *ER* endoplasmic reticulum *EF-hand motif* calcium-binding motif composed of two helixes (E and F) joined by a loop (helix-loop-helix)

Table 9.2 Reported clinical manifestations of patients with combined factor V and factor VIII deficiency (F5F8D)

Clinical manifestations	Published references (number)				
	Seligsohn et al. (*n* = 14) (%)	*Peyvandi et al.* (*n* = 27) (%)	*Shetty et al.* (*n* = 9) (%)	*Mansouritorghabeh et al.* (*n* = 19) (%)	*Viswabandya et al.* (*n* = 37) (%)
Epistaxis	57	77.8	–	69.2	18.9
Gingival bleeding	64.3	–	44.4	–	48.6
Ecchymosis/easy bruising	28.6	–	44.4	–	29.7
Menorrhagia	100	58.3	50	33.3	66.7
Post-circumcision bleeding[a]	–[b]	66.7	–	46.1	–
Excessive post-dental extraction bleeding[a]	92.3	82.3	33.3	92.3	56.7
Excessive post-surgical bleeding[a]	75	75	–	83.3	62.2[c]
Excessive post-partum hemorrhage[a]	100	75	–	50	–
Post-lacerations bleeding[a]	42.8	–	–	–	–
Post-abortion bleeding[a]	80	–	–	–	–
Post-cutting bleeding[a]	–	–	77.8	57.9	–
Hemarthrosis	–	26	–	36.8	13.5
Gastrointestinal bleeding	21.4	7.4	–	10.5	2.7
Hematuria	14.3	–	–	–	–
Muscle hematoma	–	7.4	–	–	–
Intracranial hemorrhage	–	3.7	–	–	–

[a]These symptoms were evaluated among patients who underwent the related procedure.
[b]One infant died of post-circumcision bleeding (not examined in the mentioned study).
[c]This number also includes patients who experienced bleeding after trauma.

At least, 38 mutations in *LMAN1* and 20 mutations in *MCFD2* genes have been described so far (Tables 9.3 and 9.4) (Figs. 9.2a and 9.3a) [16–22]. The most common mutations in *LMAN1* gene are insertion/deletion, nonsense, and splice site mutations which lead to complete destruction of protein function (Table 9.3). The majority of mutations involving *MCFD2* gene is insertion/deletion, missense, and splice site (Table 9.4).

Some mutations such as 89insG (Frameshift), IVS9+2 T>C (Splicing), and M1T (c.2T > C) (abolish initiation codon), which are exclusively seen in Middle Eastern

Table 9.3 *LMAN1* gene mutations in patients with combined factor V and factor VIII deficiency (F5F8D)

Type of mutations	Nomenclature	Gene location
Initiation codon	Met1Thr	Exon 1
Frameshift	23delG	Exon 1
Frameshift	31delG	Exon 1
Frameshift	89insG	Exon 1
Missense	Trp67Ser	Exon 1
Nonsense	Gly114stop	Exon 2
Frameshift	422delC	Exon 3
Frameshift	IVS4+17 del T	Exon 4
Non-sense	Arg202stop	Exon 5
Splicing	IVS5+1G>T	Intron 5
Frameshift	720del16bp	Exon 6
Frameshift	781delT	Exon 7
Frameshift	795delC	Exon 7
Frameshift	813del72bp	Exon 7
Splicing	822G>A	Exon 7
Splicing	IVS7+1G>A	Intron 7
Splicing	IVS7-1G>A	Intron 7
Splicing	IVS7–1G>C	Intron 7
Splicing	IVS7 + 33insGGTT	Intron 7
Nonsense	Lys302stop	Exon 8
Nonsense	Gln317stop	Exon 8
Frameshift	841delA	Exon 8
Frameshift	912insA	Exon 8
Frameshift	912delA	Exon 8
Nonsense	Glu321stop	Exon 9
Frameshift	1109delTC	Exon 9
Nonsense	Gln380stop	Exon 9
Splicing	IVS9+2T>G	Intron 9
Splicing	IVS9+2T>C	Intron 9
Frameshift	1208insT	Exon 10
Frameshift	1214del5bp	Exon 10
Frameshift	1261insTG	Exon 11
Nonsense	Arg456stop	Exon 11
Splicing	1271delG	Exon 11
Frameshift	1356delC	Exon 11
Missense	Cys475Arg	Exon 12
Deletion	1456delGTG	Exon 12
Frameshift	1524delA	Exon 13

LMAN1 lectin mannose-binding 1

Jewish, Tunisian Jewish and Italian origin, respectively, are suggestive of funder effect [16, 20].

According to a study by *Zhang et al.*, it was suggested that mutations involving *MCFD2* are associated with lower levels of FV and FVIII, compared with *LMAN1* mutations. This finding supports a genotype-phenotype relationship in patients with

Table 9.4 *MCFD2* gene mutations in patients with combined factor V and factor VIII deficiency (F5F8D)

Type of mutations	Nomenclature	Location
Large deletion	8.4 kb deletion	Promoter and exon 1
Splicing	IVS1–1G>C	Intron 1
Frameshift	103delC	Exon 2
Splicing	IVS2+5G>A	Intron 2
Frameshift	249delT	Exon 3
Frameshift	263del8bp	Exon 3
Frameshift	210del35bp	Exon 3
Missense	Asp81Tyr	Exon 3
Missense	Asp81His	Exon 3
Missense	Asp81Ala	Exon 3
Missense	Asp89Asn	Exon 3
Missense	Asp89Ala	Exon 3
Missense	Val100Asp	Exon 3
Splicing	IVS3+1G>A	Intron 3
Frameshift	375insGA	Exon 4
Missense	Asp122Val	Exon 4
Missense	Asp129Glu	Exon 4
Missense	Tyr135Asn	Exon 4
Missense	Ile136Thr	Exon 4
Nonsense	Ser144stop	Exon 4

MCFD2 multiple coagulation factor deficiency 2

F5F8D [23]. In F5F8D there is a poor relationship between FV and FVIII activity and severity of clinical phenotype. Heterozygous of F5F8D is usually asymptomatic [5].

9.1.6 Diagnosis

Bleeding phenotype of F5F8D is relatively similar to the clinical pictures of isolated FV and FVIII deficiencies; therefore some cases may be misdiagnosed as mild hemophilia A or FV deficiency and one of the factor defects may be overlooked [4]. Such errors revealed that there may be a bias in the exact number of patients with F5F8D in some countries specially where there are poor laboratory and genetic assays.

The concomitant presence of FV deficiency with either hemophilia A or VWD is the main differential diagnosis of F5F8D. Rely on VWD-specific tests, F5F8D, and coinheritance of FV deficiency and VWD can be distinguished. Differentiation of F5F8D from coinheritance of FV deficiency and hemophilia A is mainly based on family history. In F5F8D there may be no evidence of a positive family history; however if present, the inheritance pattern is autosomal recessive [24].

F5F8D is ordinarily suspected after simultaneous decrease of FV and FVIII plasma levels, usually between 5 and 20%. In general, prolongation of PT and aPTT, with normal thrombin time (TT), is suggestive of deficiency of coagulation factors of common pathway. Mixing study (50:50) can rule out presence of inhibitors, and reduced activity of 0.05–0.2 IU/mL and rarely <0.05 IU/mL of both FV and FVIII confirms the disorder [2, 5]. Finally, molecular analysis of *MCFD2* and *LMAN1* genes can be used for confirmation of F5F8D, although it is not routinely performed [16].

Due to the mild bleeding phenotype of F5F8D, prenatal diagnosis is not usually recommended. However if wish to be performed, both parents should be carriers of the disorder, and it may be known by already having an affected child. Chorionic villus sampling (CVS) has to be performed at 10–12 gestational weeks. Then fetal DNA is evaluated for the specific mutations which were found in parents and affected child [25].

9.1.7 Management

The bleeding tendency in combined deficiency is not more severe than single FV or FVIII defect. Clinical presentations are usually mild; thus on-demand therapy is usually preferred for management of bleeding in surgical procedures or in time of delivery and in cases of traumatic bleeding events. In F5F8D, there is no need for prophylaxis except for specific cases with severe recurrent bleeding events [25].

Both FV and FVIII are labile factors and have a short half-life of about 16–36 h and 10–14 h, respectively; therefore fresh frozen plasma (FFP) infusion is usually sufficient to restore FV activity to hemostatic level, but may not be enough for FVIII activity. On-demand therapy consists of virally inactivated FFP for compensation of FV in combination with 1-desamino-8D-arginine vasopressin (DDAVP) in cases of mild FVIII deficiency or with plasma-derived/recombinant FVIII concentrates in cases of moderate/severe FVIII deficiency (Table 9.5) [27].

Circulating target level of FV and FVIII for surgery must be more than 20% and 50%, respectively [27]. For severe bleeding events or major surgeries, it is recommended to compensate FV and FVIII levels by 15–25 mL/kg solvent-detergent FFP (SD-FFP) and further replacement of FVIII by 20–40 IU/kg recombinant FVIII (rFVIII) concentrates or 0.3 μg/kg desmopressin. To maintain FV and FVIII activities at target levels for major surgeries, continuous treatment with 12 h intervals is necessary [5]. For mild bleeding events and minor surgeries, 15–20 mL/kg tranexamic acid or 1 g four times daily alone is recommended [5].

During pregnancy, FVIII level progressively increases although FV remains unchanged; thus in pregnant women with F5F8D, FVIII activity is usually enough for hemostasis, but hemostatic level of FV is not usually sufficient at delivery [28]. Women with F5F8D are at risk of post-partum hemorrhage; therefore they must be managed during and after pregnancy. In women with FV activity <20% in the third trimester, administration of one dose of SD-FFP (15–25 mL/kg) at the time of delivery or before caesarean section is recommended. Further treatment with SD-FFP with a dose of 10 mL/kg at 12 h intervals should be considered to maintain FV activity more than 20% for at least 72 h. In cases with FVIII activity below 50% in the third trimester, additional rFVIII is also recommended [5].

Table 9.5 Different therapeutic choices for management of patients with combined factor V and factor VIII deficiency (F5F8D) in different conditions

Condition	Recommended dosages
Mild bleeding events/ minor surgeries	Tranexamic acid (15–20 mL/kg or 1 g four times daily)
Severe bleeding events/ major surgeries	SD-FFP (15–25 mL/kg) + (DDAVP) desmopressin (0.3 μg/kg) [26] for mild FVIII deficiency or rFVIII concentrates (20–40 IU/kg) for moderate/severe FVIII deficiency
Pregnancy (FV activity <20% in the third trimester)	SD-FFP (15–25 mL/kg), one dose at the time of delivery or before cesarean section + SD-FFP (10 mL/kg) at 12 h intervals for at least 3 days If FVIII activity <50% in the third trimester: + additional rFVIII

SD-FFP solvent-detergent fresh frozen plasma, *rFVIII* recombinant factor VIII, *FV* factor V, *FVIII* factor VIII, DDAVP 1-desamino-8-d-vasopressin.

9.2 Vitamin K-Dependent Coagulation Factor Deficiency

9.2.1 Introduction

Vitamin K-dependent coagulation factor deficiency (VKCFD) is a rare bleeding disorder with less than 50 reported families so far [29]. Literature is only restricted to few case reports and small case series. It is an autosomal recessive disorder which arises from defects in either γ-glutamyl carboxylase (*GGCX*) or subunit 1 of vitamin K epoxide reductase complex (*VKORC1*) genes. If there is a mutation in the former enzyme, it will be considered as type I disorder, and if the responsible mutation involves the latter, it will be considered as type II [30]. These genes are encoding proteins which are involved in the γ-carboxylation of the glutamate (Glu) residues of vitamin K-dependent coagulation factors, including FII, FVII, FIX, and FX. VKCFD is usually represented in infancy with life-threatening bleeding events [31]. VKCFD can be diagnosed by prolongation of PT, aPTT with normal TT, and parallel reduction of vitamin K-dependent coagulation factors, usually around 1–30%. Management of the disorder is mainly through administration of vitamin K1 or four-factor prothrombin complex concentrate (PCC) (Table 10.6 of Chap. 10) [5].

9.2.2 Structure and Function of GGCX and VKOR

GGCX is an integral transmembrane protein which is located on the ER membrane. It consists of 758 amino acids, and there is a disulfide bond between cysteines 99 and 450 [31]. There is limited information on the structure of GGCX. However, it seems that GGCX contains five transmembrane domains. The amino terminal of this enzyme is located in cytoplasm, and the carboxyl terminal is exposed to ER lumen [32]. Based on the studies on the structure and mechanism of action, different binding and catalytic sites are considered for GGCX. Accordingly, GGCX contains a propeptide binding site, a glutamate binding site, a vitamin K binding site, a carboxylation active site, an epoxidation active site, and, probably, a CO_2 binding site. But the information on the exact location of these functional regions is limited [32].

The VKOR protein is also an integral protein in the ER membrane with 163 amino acids [31]. There are two topology models which consider three or four transmembrane domains for the protein. According to the different studies, three transmembrane models are more reasonable. In this model, the amino terminal of VKOR is located in the ER lumen and the carboxy-terminal located in the cytoplasm [32]. For a long period, it was assumed that the VKOR was a multi-enzyme complex, a theory which is now questioned [32].

9.2.2.1 Vitamin K Cycle

Vitamin K-dependent carboxylation is a post-translational modification which is critical for proper function of vitamin K-dependent proteins. The most important vitamin K-dependent proteins are coagulation FII, FVII, FIX, and FX; natural anticoagulants protein C, protein S, and protein Z; and bone proteins including osteocalcin, matrix Gla protein, and growth arrest-specific protein 6 (Gas6) [33].

In vitamin K-dependent carboxylation, specific glutamate (Glu) residues are modified to gamma-carboxyglutamate (Gla). Each vitamin K-dependent factor contains 10–12 Gla residues in the amino terminus which is called Gla domain. The responsible enzyme for this conversion is GGCX which requires reduced vitamin K (KH2), CO_2, and O_2 as cofactors. When each Glu is modified, one KH_2 molecule is oxidized to vitamin K 2, 3 epoxide (KO). For restoration of KH2, this KO molecule needs to be converted back to the reduced form (Fig. 9.4). This conversion occurs in a two-step reaction, first KO is reduced to vitamin K using VKOR and then vitamin K reduced to KH_2 using vitamin K reductase [32, 34].

Gamma-carboxylation of the Glu residues is necessary for binding of calcium ions which then allows binding of vitamin K-dependent factors to phospholipid membranes such as surface of activated platelets or damaged endothelium. This phenomenon leads to concentration of clotting factors at the site of vascular injury [32].

9.2.3 Vitamin K-Dependent Coagulation Factor Deficiency

VKCFD (OMIM #277450 and #607473) was first described in 1966 by *McMillan* and *Robert* in a 4-month-old girl [36]. She presented with several bruises and bleeding events, a prolonged PT and aPTT, and undetectable levels of FII, FVII, FIX, and FX by clotting assays. However, neither liver disease nor malabsorption had been detected. Low level of coagulation factors showed a partial recovery following administration of high doses of vitamin K [36]. The patient was further investigated at age of 15 years, and the clotting factors were re-evaluated by immunologic assays [37]. However the molecular mechanism remained unclear.

Now, VKCFD is known as an autosomal recessive bleeding disorder which arises from defects in either *GGCX* or *VKORC1* genes. Plasma level of vitamin K-dependent coagulation factors in VKCFD may be around 1–30% [2]. VKCFD has been reported in less than 50 families so far [2, 29].

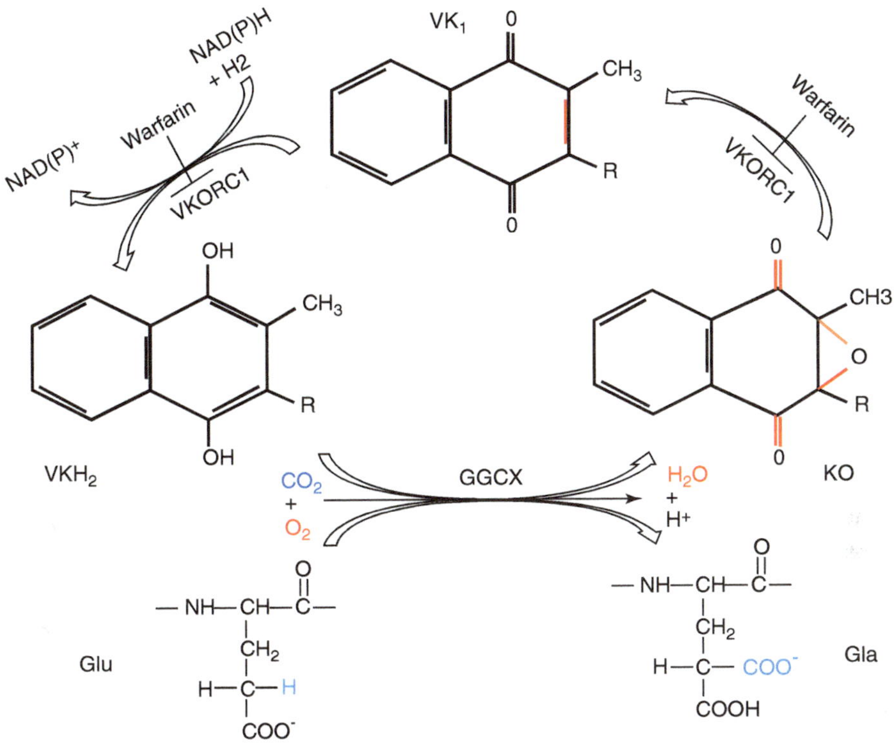

Fig. 9.4 Carboxylation of glutamate (Glu) to carboxyglutamate (Gla) residues by GGCX is necessary for the activation of vitamin K-dependent coagulation factors. VKH_2 is the cofactor of this conversion. In this process, VKH_2 is oxidized into KO and then reduced to vitamin K quinone and VKH_2, respectively, by VKORC1. Warfarin can block the VKORC1. Another reductase, NQO1, can also convert VK to VKH_2. Warfarin can inhibit VKORC1 but not NQO1 [35]. *GGCX* γ-glutamyl carboxylase, *VKH2* vitamin K hydroquinone, *KO* vitamin K epoxide, *VKORC1* vitamin K epoxide reductase complex subunit 1, *NQO1* NADPH quinone oxidoreductase, *VK* vitamin K

9.2.4 Clinical Manifestations

VKCFD usually manifests in infancy, although it may also remain latent for a short time. Severity of clinical manifestations depends on the level of reduced coagulation factors [6]. However the clinical picture is not closely correlated to the activity of vitamin K-dependent coagulation factors [5]. Severe bleeding such as ICH or umbilical cord bleeding has been described in affected neonates [38–40]. Mucocutaneous and soft tissue bleeding and post-traumatic hemorrhages are also reported in these patients (Table 9.6) [39, 41]. Less commonly, VKCFD may present with hemorrhagic events in adulthood or even may be found incidentally [5].

Some affected individuals may also suffer from mental retardation and skeletal abnormalities which is attributed to the impaired γ-carboxylation of other vitamin K-dependent proteins [38, 42]. Skeletal abnormalities including nasal hypoplasia, distal digital hypoplasia, and epiphyseal stippling are similar to those seen in

Table 9.6 Clinical manifestations of vitamin K-dependent coagulation factor deficiency

Clinical manifestations	Frequency (%)
Intracranial hemorrhage	34
Ecchymoses/easy bruising	21
Skeletal abnormalities/growth or developmental retardation	21
Umbilical cord bleeding	17
Post-trauma/post-operative bleeding	17
Epistaxis	17
Gingival/oral cavity bleeding	12
Hemarthrosis	4

warfarin embryopathy [43]. Pseudoxanthoma elasticum-like disorders have also been reported in patients affected by VKCFD with GGCX mutations [44].

Some natural anticoagulants including protein C, protein S, and protein Z also require Glu residues to be modified into γ-carboxyglutamate (Gla) residues, and therefore there are also low levels of protein C and protein S in the deficiencies of GGCX or VKOR. This fact that no cases with thrombosis have been reported in the literature so far may suggest the dominant effect of these two enzymes in procoagulant activities [29, 45].

9.2.5 Molecular Basis

The gene encoding for GGCX with 13 kb length is located on chromosome 2p11.2 and comprises of 15 exons. The responsible gene for VKORC1 protein that is called *VKORC1* is located on chromosome 16p11.2. It is a small gene with 5126 bp length and includes 3 exons [6]. Defect in GGCX is known as type I VKCFD. Another enzyme playing an important role in this cycle is VKORC1. VKORC1 catalyzes reconversion of vitamin K epoxide (KO), which is produced during the last reaction, to KH2 (Fig. 9.4). Defect in VKORC1 is known as type II VKCFD [5, 33].

To date, at least 18 mutations have been reported in the *GGCX* gene which are associated with VKCFD, and the majority of them are point mutations (Table 9.7) [6, 29, 46]. It seems that a missense mutation that leads to the substitution of tryptophan to arginine at amino acid number 98 is the only reported mutation involving *VKORC1* (Table 9.7).

More recently, *Jin et al.* showed that 1657delA and IVS13-6G>A are the underlying mutations of the first case of VKCFD which was reported by *McMillan* and *Robert* [10].

9.2.6 Diagnosis

There is a weak relationship between severity of clinical manifestations and laboratory results of VKCFD [5]. VKCFD can be diagnosed by prolongation of PT, aPTT with normal TT, and parallel reduction of FII, FVII, FIX, and FX activity

Table 9.7 Vitamin K-dependent coagulation factors deficiency causing mutations in the *GGCX* and *VKORC1* genes

	Type	Nomenclature	Gene region
Mutations in *GGCX* gene (type I disorder)	Undefined[a]	IVS1del14bp	Intron 1
	Splicing	IVS1 − 1G > A	Intron 1
	Missense	Asp31Asn	Exon 2
	Splicing	IVS2 + 1G > T	Intron 2
	Splicing	IVS2 − 1G > T	Intron 2
	Missense	Pro80Leu	Exon 3
	Missense	Asp153Gly	Exon 4
	Missense	Trp157Arg	Exon 4
	Missense	Met174Arg	Exon 4
	Missense	Leu394Arg	Exon 9
	Missense	His404Pro	Exon 9
	Missense	Arg485Pro	Exon 11
	Missense	Trp501Ser	Exon 11
	Missense	Ile532Thr	Exon 11
	Splicing	IVS11 + 3A > G	Intron 11
	Frameshift	1657delA	Exon 12
	Missense	Thr591Lys	Exon 13
	Splicing	IVS13 − 6G > A	Intron 13
Mutations in *VKORC1* gene (type II disorder)	Missense	Arg98Trp	Exon 3

[a]It seems that the deleted region in intron 1 is probably associated with cis-acting elements and thereby is involved in gene regulation [45]
GGCX γ-glutamyl carboxylase, *VKORC1* vitamin K epoxide reductase complex subunit 1

[2, 5]. Although both PT and aPTT are prolonged in VKCFD, PT test is slightly more affected. Factor activities are usually around 0.2–0.6 IU/ml and less commonly are <0.1 IU/mL at baseline [5]. Presence of inhibitors can be excluded by mixing study.

Differentiation of VKCFD and acquired vitamin K deficiency must be intentioned with normal fasting serum KH_2 (reduced vitamin K) concentration in VKCFD. Acquired vitamin K deficiency may arise from intestinal malabsorption of vitamin K in the inflammatory bowel disease or celiac disease, liver cirrhosis, and exposure to coumarin anticoagulants [5]. The differential diagnosis of the disorder in neonates mainly includes vitamin K deficiency. In healthy newborns the levels of vitamin K-dependent coagulation factors gradually increase up to the age of 6 months. Therefore, the diagnosis in neonates has to be confirmed by repeating the test in 6 months old [5].

In the subject of type I and II of the disorder, it should be considered that oxidized vitamin K (KO) is typically undetectable in VKCFD type I, even after vitamin K supplementation, but in VKCFD type II, an elevation of KO level can be observed following vitamin K supplementation [5, 30]. In addition, VKCFD must be distinguished from congenital factor deficiency including FII deficiency, isolated FVII and FIX deficiencies and FX deficiency, as well as combined FVII and FX deficiency. In this setting, study about presence of inhibitor against FIX (acquired hemophilia) and FVII is mandatory [30]. For definite diagnosis, molecular analysis for mutations of *VKORC* or *GGCX* is necessary.

9.2.7 Management

Management of the disorder is mainly through administration of vitamin K1 (phytomenadione), but in severely affected patients and in major surgeries, four-factor prothrombin complex concentrate (PCC) (containing prothrombin, FVII, FIX, and FX) is also required (Table 9.8) [27]. Most of the cases (not all) may show a partial restoration in the level of deficient factors with high doses of vitamin K [6].

As VKCFD may lead to life-threatening hemorrhagic events, prophylaxis at diagnosis is highly recommended. Dose of treatment for long-term prophylaxis is 5–20 mg/day of oral vitamin K1, and when response is poor, 5–20 mg/week of parenteral vitamin K1 is recommended [5, 27]. In the subject of mild bleeding or minor surgery, 15–20 mL/kg tranexamic acid or 1 g four times daily alone is recommended [5]. In connection with severe bleeding or major surgery, 20–30 IU/kg of four-factor PCC combined with 5–20 mg of vitamin K1 is recommended. In the lack of four-factor PCC, 15–25 mL/kg of virus-inactivated FFP can be substituted [5, 27].

In normal pregnancy, the level of FVII and FX usually increases, while FII and FIX levels do not alter. The level of FVII in some pregnant women may elevate even up to tenfold [47]. However, in some pregnant women affected by VKCFD, the physiologic increase in the deficient factors may be inadequate for an uneventful delivery. Pregnant women in whom each of the vitamin K-dependent factors has an activity below 20 IU/mL in the third trimester must be managed carefully in time of delivery. In this condition, one dose of four-factor PCC 20–30 IU/kg before

Table 9.8 Different therapeutic choices for management of patients with vitamin K-dependent coagulation factor deficiency (VKCFD) in different conditions

Conditions	Recommended drugs and dosages
Long-term prophylaxis	Oral vitamin K1 (5–20 mg/day) *If response is poor* parenteral vitamin K1 (5–20 mg/week)
Mild bleeding events/minor surgeries	Tranexamic acid (15–20 mL/kg or 1 g four times daily)
Severe bleeding events/major surgeries	Four-factor PCC (20–30 IU/kg) + Vitamin K1 (5–20 mg) *Four-factor PCC can be substituted by virus inactivated FFP* (15–25 mL/kg)
Pregnancy (each of the vitamin K-dependent factor activity <20 IU/mL in the third trimester)	Four-factor PCC (20–30 IU/kg), one dose at the time of delivery or before caesarean section and continued for at least 3 days

PCC prothrombin complex concentrate

delivery or before cesarean section is recommended which should be continued for at least 72 h [5].

It seems that prenatal diagnosis of VKCFD is not preferred. Considering the potential bleeding risk of the procedure and because major hemorrhagic events in the affected newborn can be prevented by administration of vitamin K in the third trimester of pregnancy in mothers which are prone to have a child with VKCFD, prenatal diagnosis is not generally essential [30].

9.3 Multiple Coagulation Factor Deficiency as a Part of a Syndrome

9.3.1 Noonan Syndrome

Noonan syndrome (NS) is an autosomal dominant disorder with an estimated prevalence of about 1 in 1000–2500 lived born children worldwide. It is a heterogeneous disorder, and mutations in *PTPN11*, *SOS1*, *KRAS*, and *RAF1* genes are usually responsible for the disorder. NS is associated with multiple abnormalities in the physical appearance and also internal organs. Heart defects, facial malformation, growth retardation, and hematologic abnormalities are few features of the wide range characteristics which have been described in NS [48, 49]. On the subject of hematologic abnormalities, the problem is generally related to clotting disorders. FXI deficiency is the most common coagulation factor deficiency, which has been reported in about 37% of patients with NS. FXI deficiency may represent alone or in combination with other clotting factors mainly including FVIII, FIX, FXII, and VWF [50]. These deficiencies as well as low platelet count, platelet dysfunction, and an unbalance activity of plasminogen activator inhibitor-1 (PAI-1) and tissue plasminogen activator (t-PA) lead to a bleeding tendency in patients with NS [48, 49].

9.3.2 13q34 Deletion Syndrome

FVII and FX have many similarities in structural and functional properties. Both factors belong to the family of vitamin K-dependent coagulation factors and related encoding genes located on the same chromosome (13q34) with short distance from each other. Deletion of the long arm of chromosome 13 leads to a syndrome (-13q syndrome) with multiple abnormalities such as mental retardation and heart failure. Bleeding diathesis is another manifestation which arises from haplo-insufficiency of *F7* and *F10* genes [51, 52].

Reduction in coagulant activity of FVII and FX is not proportional in some cases with 13q34 deletion, as FVII deficiency is much more severe. It may be due to an independent mutation in the intact haplotype of *F7* gene which results in a lower level of FVII and deterioration of the bleeding tendency [53].

9.4 Multiple Coagulation Factor Deficiency Due to Independent Segregation of Two or More Defects

In differential diagnosis of patients with concomitant reduction in the level of two or more clotting factors, a simple chance in co-inheritance of mutant alleles must also be considered, although it is an ultra rare phenomenon, particularly in regions with a high rate of consanguinity. For example, combined deficiency of FVII and FX may result from heritable or acquired deficiency of vitamin K-dependent clotting factors, may be caused by chance inheritance of independent abnormalities in the *F7* and *F10* genes, or may be observed in 13q34 deletion syndrome. It seems that a comprehensive family study is a good way for differential diagnosis, as in the family study of many cases who suffer from independent segregation of two or more defects, there are some members affected by one of the deficiencies and some by the others.

References

1. Seligsohn U, Zivelin A, Zwang E. Combined factor V and factor VIII deficiency among non-Ashkenazi Jews. N Engl J Med. 1982;307(19):1191.
2. Castaman G, Linari S. Diagnosis and treatment of von Willebrand disease and rare bleeding disorders. J Clin Med. 2017;6(4):45.
3. Peyvandi F, Tuddenham E, Akhtari A, Lak M, Mannucci P. Bleeding symptoms in 27 Iranian patients with the combined deficiency of factor V and factor VIII. Br J Haematol. 1998;100(4):733–4.
4. Zhang B. Recent developments in the understanding of the combined deficiency of FV and FVIII. Br J Haematol. 2009;145(1):15–23.
5. Mumford AD, Ackroyd S, Alikhan R, Bowles L, Chowdary P, Grainger J, et al. Guideline for the diagnosis and management of the rare coagulation disorders. Br J Haematol. 2014;167(3):304–26.
6. Zhang B, Ginsburg D. Familial multiple coagulation factor deficiencies: new biologic insight from rare genetic bleeding disorders. J Thromb Haemost. 2004;2(9):1564–72.
7. Zheng C, Liu H-H, Yuan S, Zhou J, Zhang B. Molecular basis of LMAN1 in coordinating LMAN1-MCFD2 cargo receptor formation and ER-to-Golgi transport of FV/FVIII. Blood. 2010;116(25):5698–706.
8. Zheng C, Liu H-H, Zhou J, Zhang B. EF-hand domains of MCFD2 mediate interactions with both LMAN1 and coagulation factor V or VIII. Blood. 2010;115(5):1081–7.
9. Oeri J, Matter M, Isenschmid H, Hauser F, Koller F. Congenital factor V deficiency (parahemophilia) with true hemophilia in two brothers. Bibl Paediatr. 1954;58:575.
10. Jin D-Y, Ingram BO, Stafford DW, Tie J-K. Molecular basis of the first reported clinical case of congenital combined deficiency of coagulation factors. Blood. 2017;130(7):948–51.
11. Nichols WC, Seligsohn U, Zivelin A, Terry VH, Arnold ND, Siemieniak DR, et al. Linkage of combined factors V and VIII deficiency to chromosome 18q by homozygosity mapping. J Clin Investig. 1997;99(4):596.
12. Nichols WC, Seligsohn U, Zivelin A, Terry VH, Hertel CE, Wheatley MA, et al. Mutations in the ER–Golgi intermediate compartment protein ERGIC-53 cause combined deficiency of coagulation factors V and VIII. Cell. 1998;93(1):61–70.
13. Shetty S, Madkaikar M, Nair S, Pawar A, Baindur S, Pathare A, et al. Combined factor V and VIII deficiency in Indian population. Haemophilia. 2000;6:504–7.

14. Mansouritorgabeh H, Rezaieyazdi Z, Pourfathollah A, Rezai J, Esamaili H. Haemorrhagic symptoms in patients with combined factors V and VIII deficiency in North-Eastern Iran. Haemophilia. 2004;10(3):271–5.
15. Viswabandya A, Baidya S, Nair SC, Lakshmi KM, Mathews V, George B, et al. Clinical manifestations of combined factor V and VIII deficiency: a series of 37 cases from a single center in India. Am J Hematol. 2010;85(7):538–9.
16. Zheng C, Zhang B. Combined deficiency of coagulation factors V and VIII: an update. Semin Thromb Hemost. 2013;39(6):613–20.
17. Karimi M, Cairo A, Safarpour MM, Haghpanah S, Ekramzadeh M, Afrasiabi A, et al. Genotype and phenotype report on patients with combined deficiency of factor V and factor VIII in Iran. Blood Coagul Fibrinolysis. 2014;25(4):360–3.
18. Hejer E, Adnen L, Asma J, Ibtihel M, Benammar-Elgaaied A, Gouider E. Identification of a novel mutation in the MCFD2 gene in a Tunisian family with combined factor V and VIII deficiency. Tunis Med. 2012;90(4):343–4.
19. Wang A, Liu X, Wu J, Cai X, Zhu W, Sun Z. Combined FV and FVIII deficiency (F5F8D) in a Chinese family with a novel missense mutation in MCFD2 gene. Haemophilia. 2014;20(6):e436–8.
20. Genotypes of patients with combined factor V and VIII deficiency [internet]. 2011. https://c.ymcdn.com/sites/www.isth.org/resource/resmgr/publications/fv_and_viii_mutations-2011.pdf.
21. Wang A, Duan Q, Ding K, Liu X, Wu J, Sun Z. Successful abdominal operation without replacement therapy in a patient with combined factor V (FV) and FVIII deficiency due to novel homozygous mutation in LMAN1. Haemophilia. 2015;21(6):e492–4.
22. Elmahmoudi H, Wigren E, Laatiri A, Jlizi A, Elgaaied A, Gouider E, et al. Analysis of newly detected mutations in the MCFD2 gene giving rise to combined deficiency of coagulation factors V and VIII. Haemophilia. 2011;17(5):e923–7.
23. Zhang B, Spreafico M, Zheng C, Yang A, Platzer P, Callaghan MU, et al. Genotype-phenotype correlation in combined deficiency of factor V and factor VIII. Blood. 2008;111(12):5592–600.
24. Khoriaty R, Vasievich MP, Ginsburg D. The COPII pathway and hematologic disease. Blood. 2012;120(1):31–8.
25. Latif A, Aledort L. Inherited combined factor deficiency states. In: Hemostasis and thrombosis. Oxford: Wiley; 2014. p. 127–36.
26. Mansouritorghabeh H, Shirdel A. Desmopressin acetate as a haemostatic elevator in individuals with combined deficiency of factors V and VIII: a clinical trial. J Thromb Haemost. 2016;14(2):336–9.
27. Peyvandi F, Menegatti M. Treatment of rare factor deficiencies in 2016. Hematology Am Soc Hematol Educ Program. 2016;2016(1):663–9.
28. Oukkache B, El Graoui O, Zafad S. Combined factor V and VIII deficiency and pregnancy. Int J Hematol. 2012;96(6):786–8.
29. Brenner B, Kuperman AA, Watzka M, Oldenburg J. Vitamin K-dependent coagulation factors deficiency. Semin Thromb Hemost. 2009;35(4):439–46.
30. Napolitano M, Mariani G, Lapecorella M. Hereditary combined deficiency of the vitamin K-dependent clotting factors. Orphanet J Rare Dis. 2010;5(1):21.
31. Stafford D. The vitamin K cycle. J Thromb Haemost. 2005;3(8):1873–8.
32. Tie JK, Stafford DW. Structural and functional insights into enzymes of the vitamin K cycle. J Thromb Haemost. 2016;14(2):236–47.
33. Oldenburg J, Marinova M, Müller-Reible C, Watzka M. The vitamin K cycle. Vitam Horm. 2008;78:35–62.
34. Oldenburg J, Bevans CG, Müller CR, Watzka M. Vitamin K epoxide reductase complex subunit 1 (VKORC1): the key protein of the vitamin K cycle. Antioxid Redox Signal. 2006;8(3-4):347–53.
35. Gallieni M, Fusaro M. Vitamin K and cardiovascular calcification in CKD: is patient supplementation on the horizon? Kidney Int. 2014;86(2):232.
36. McMillan CW, Roberts HR. Congenital combined deficiency of coagulation factors II, VII, IX and X: report of a case. N Engl J Med. 1966;274(23):1313–5.

37. Chung K-S, Bezeaud A, Goldsmith JC, McMillan CW, Menache D, Roberts HR. Congenital deficiency of blood clotting factors II, VII, IX, and X. Blood. 1979;53(4):776–87.
38. Oldenburg J, Von Brederlow B, Fregin A, Rost S, Wolz W, Eberl W, et al. Congenital deficiency of vitamin K-dependent coagulation factors in two families presents as a genetic defect of the vitamin K-epoxide-reductase-complex. Thromb Haemost. 2000;84(6):937–41.
39. Brenner B, Sánchez-Vega B, Wu S-M, Lanir N, Stafford DW, Solera J. A missense mutation in γ-glutamyl carboxylase gene causes combined deficiency of all vitamin K-dependent blood coagulation factors. Blood. 1998;92(12):4554–9.
40. Spronk HM, Farah RA, Buchanan GR, Vermeer C, Soute BA. Novel mutation in the γ-glutamyl carboxylase gene resulting in congenital combined deficiency of all vitamin K–dependent blood coagulation factors. Blood. 2000;96(10):3650–2.
41. Lunghi B, Redaelli R, Caimi T, Corno A, Bernardi F, Marchetti G. Novel phenotype and γ-glutamyl carboxylase mutations in combined deficiency of vitamin K-dependent coagulation factors. Haemophilia. 2011;17(5):822–4.
42. Hauschka PV, Lian JB, Cole D, Gundberg CM. Osteocalcin and matrix Gla protein: vitamin K-dependent proteins in bone. Physiol Rev. 1989;69(3):990–1047.
43. Pauli R, Lian J, Mosher D, Suttie J. Association of congenital deficiency of multiple vitamin K-dependent coagulation factors and the phenotype of the warfarin embryopathy: clues to the mechanism of teratogenicity of coumarin derivatives. Am J Hum Genet. 1987;41(4):566.
44. Vanakker OM, Martin L, Gheduzzi D, Leroy BP, Loeys BL, Guerci VI, et al. Pseudoxanthoma elasticum-like phenotype with cutis laxa and multiple coagulation factor deficiency represents a separate genetic entity. J Investig Dermatol. 2007;127(3):581–7.
45. Palla R, Peyvandi F, Shapiro AD. Rare bleeding disorders: diagnosis and treatment. Blood. 2015;125(13):2052–61.
46. Thomas A, Stirling D. Four factor deficiency. Blood Coagul Fibrinolysis. 2003;14:S55–S7.
47. Prisco D, Ciuti G, Falciani M. Hemostatic changes in normal pregnancy. Haematol Rep. 2009;1:1–5.
48. Tartaglia M, Gelb BD, Zenker M. Noonan syndrome and clinically related disorders. Best Pract Res Clin Endocrinol Metab. 2011;25(1):161–79.
49. Roberts AE, Allanson JE, Tartaglia M, Gelb BD. Noonan syndrome. Lancet. 2013;381(9863):333–42.
50. Briggs BJ, Dickerman JD. Bleeding disorders in Noonan syndrome. Pediatr Blood Cancer. 2012;58(2):167–72.
51. Kurosawa H, Suzumura H, Okuya M, Fukushima K, Sugita K, Fujiwara T, et al. Haemostatic management of surgery for imperforate anus in a patient with 13q deletion syndrome with combined deficiency of factors VII and X. Haemophilia. 2009;15(1):398–400.
52. Pfeiffer R, Ott R, Gilgenkrantz S, Alexandre P. Deficiency of coagulation factors VII and X associated with deletion of a chromosome 13 (q34). Evidence from two cases with 46, XY, t (13; Y)(q11; q34). Hum Genet. 1982;62(4):358–60.
53. Chilcott J, Russell G, Mumford A. Combined deficiency of factors VII and X: clinical description of two cases and management of spinal surgery. Haemophilia. 2006;12(5):555–8.

Congenital Factor VII Deficiency

10

Mahmood Shams and Akbar Dorgalaleh

10.1 Introduction

Congenital factor FVII (FVII) deficiency is a rare autosomal recessive bleeding disorder with the estimated prevalence of 1 per 500,000 in the general population, without ethnic or gender predilection [1, 2], but the prevalence is higher in regions with the high rate of consanguinity marriage [1, 3]. Clinical pictures in these patients range from asymptomatic condition to severe life-threatening hemorrhages [4, 5]. There is a relatively poor correlation between FVII coagulant activity (FVII:C) and bleeding tendency and mutation profile in congenital FVII deficiency [3, 6]. Severe clinical symptoms usually present in patients with less than 1% FVII:C, but some patients with severe deficiency don't experience severe bleeding episodes. The complete absence of functional FVII in knockout mice is incompatible with life, suggesting FVII deficiency is not associated with complete absence of functional FVII, but patients with residual FVII level can survive and are able to prevent lethal bleeding [7, 8]. The disorder is accompanied with a wide spectrum of bleeding problems including mild symptoms such as mucous membranes and skin hemorrhages and life-threatening hemorrhages such as central nervous system (CNS) bleeding. Iron deficiency due to menorrhagia is common in women with FVII deficiency [3]. This disorder can be managed by different therapeutic options including fresh frozen

M. Shams
Department of Laboratory Sciences, Paramedical Faculty,
Babol University of Medical Sciences, Babol, Iran

Department of Hematology and Blood transfusion, School of Allied Medicine,
Iran University of Medical Sciences, Tehran, Iran
e-mail: shams@mubabol.ac.ir

A. Dorgalaleh (✉)
Department of Hematology and Blood transfusion, School of Allied Medicine,
Iran University of Medical Sciences, Tehran, Iran

A. Dorgalaleh (ed.), *Congenital Bleeding Disorders*,
https://doi.org/10.1007/978-3-319-76723-9_10

plasma (FFP), prothrombin complex concentrate (PCC), plasma-derived FVII (pd-FVII) products, and recombinant activated FVII (rFVIIa).

10.2 Factor VII Structure and Function

FVII is a low molecular weight protein (50 kDa) composed of 406 amino acids that is synthesized as single-chain molecule in the endoplasmic reticulum of hepatocytes. FVII has homology with FIX, FX, and protein C on the catalytic site and amino-terminal region [9]. In hepatocytes, FVII has a signal peptide that is required for secretion and a propeptide (removed intracellularly) that is necessary for γ-carboxylation of all glutamate residues within ~45 amino acids in N-terminus of FVII protein [10]. Coagulation FVII consists of four domains including one gamma-carboxyglutamic acid (*Gla*) domain on the N-terminal with ten glutamic acid residues (at residues 6, 7, 14, 16, 19, 20, 25, 26, 29, and 35). These ten glutamic acid residues undergo post-translational modification; convert to γ-carboxyglutamic acid with calcium-binding capacity. Binding of calcium to Gla domain leads to conformational changes and exposure of new epitopes that facilitate its subsequent binding to TF and phospholipid. Other FVII domains are two epidermal growth factor-like domains (*EGF1, EGF2*) and a catalytic serine protease (*SP*) domain in C-terminal (Fig. 10.1) [1, 10].

FVII in zymogen has the plasma half-life of 5 h that is the shortest half-life among the clotting factors, but the half-life of free FVIIa is 2 h, whereas the plasma half-life of most other activated coagulation factors is very short [1, 10]. FVII reversibly in a Ca^{2+}-dependent manner can bind to membranes with negatively charged phospholipids such as phosphatidylserine or phosphatidic via Gla domain [11, 12]. The majority of plasma FVII circulates as the single-chain inert zymogen (10 nmol/L (0.5 μg/mL)), and the minority circulates in the plasma as two-chain active protein (~10 to 110 pmol/L) [1, 3, 10, 13]. The key event in the activation of FVII is proteolysis of a single peptide bond between Arg-c15 (amino acid 152) and Ile-c16 (amino acid 153) in the connecting region of EGF2 and SP domains. This results in formation of two polypeptide chains: heavy chain with 254 amino acids (30 kDa) (residues 153–406), comprised of serine protease domain with Trypsin homology at C terminus, and light chain with 152 amino acids (20 kDa) (residues 1–152), composed of Gla and 2 EGF-like domains [1, 10, 14–16].

FVII chiefly interacts with TF via the Gla and EGF1 domains; however, two other domains can also interact with TF [15, 17]. FVII/TF complex is necessary for the restructuring of active site and full enzymatic activity of FVIIa, because free FVIIa has very weak catalytic activity [14, 15]. In addition to FVII/TF complex, several other coagulation factors including FXa, FIIa, and FIXa contribute to FVII activation; however, it seems that membrane-bound FXa is the most effective [18]. Once formed, the TF/FVIIa complex results in proteolytic activation of FIX and FX to FIXa and FXa, respectively, and generating few amount of thrombin that is able to produce a strong feedback amplification of coagulation cascade [10, 19]. Tissue factor pathway inhibitor (TFPI) and antithrombin (AT) are inhibitors of FVIIa, but only in complex form (FVIIa/TF) can it inhibit FVII [20, 21]. The TFPI is a Kunitz-type proteinase inhibitor and

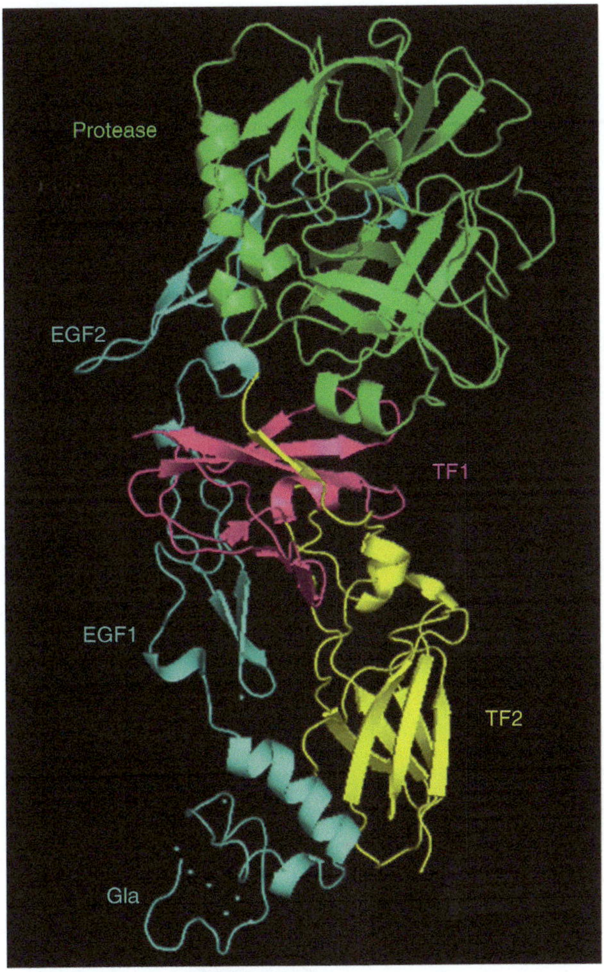

Fig. 10.1 The cartoon representation of activated factor VII (FVIIa)/soluble tissue factor (sTF) complex. FVII has four domains including gamma-carboxyglutamic acid (Gla), two epidermal growth like factor (EGF1, EGF2) domains, and serine protease domain. sTF contains two fibronectin type III domains (TF1 and TF2 represent of N- and C-terminal of sTF)

attaches to membrane surface via glycophosphatidylinositol (GPI)-linked. TFPI mainly is expressed by endothelial cells and partly by platelets [22]. The TFPI/FXa complex can inhibit FVIIa/TF complex and prevents further FX activation via inactivation of tetra-molecular (TF-FVIIa-TFPI-FXa) complex formation that rapidly inhibits the extrinsic coagulation pathway [20, 22]. Inhibitory function of TFPI/FXa, at least in part, is by inducing of TF-expressing cells to internalize the TF/FVIIa complexes, which leads to degradation of the majority of FVIIa [22, 23]. TFPI is synthesized by microvascular endothelial cells, megakaryocytes, and the liver [3, 24]. Heparin and various platelet agonists can increase the release of TFPI from the surface of endothelial cells. AT reaction is heparin dependent, and its reactivity with FVIIa is increased after FVIIa/TF complex formation. After binding of AT to FVIIa/TF complex, the affinity of FVIIa to TF is decreased and then FVIIa/AT complex releases into the bloodstream (Fig. 10.2) [3, 20]. FVIIa/AT complex is increased in many prothrombotic situations and seems to be the early marker of coagulation cascade activation [20].

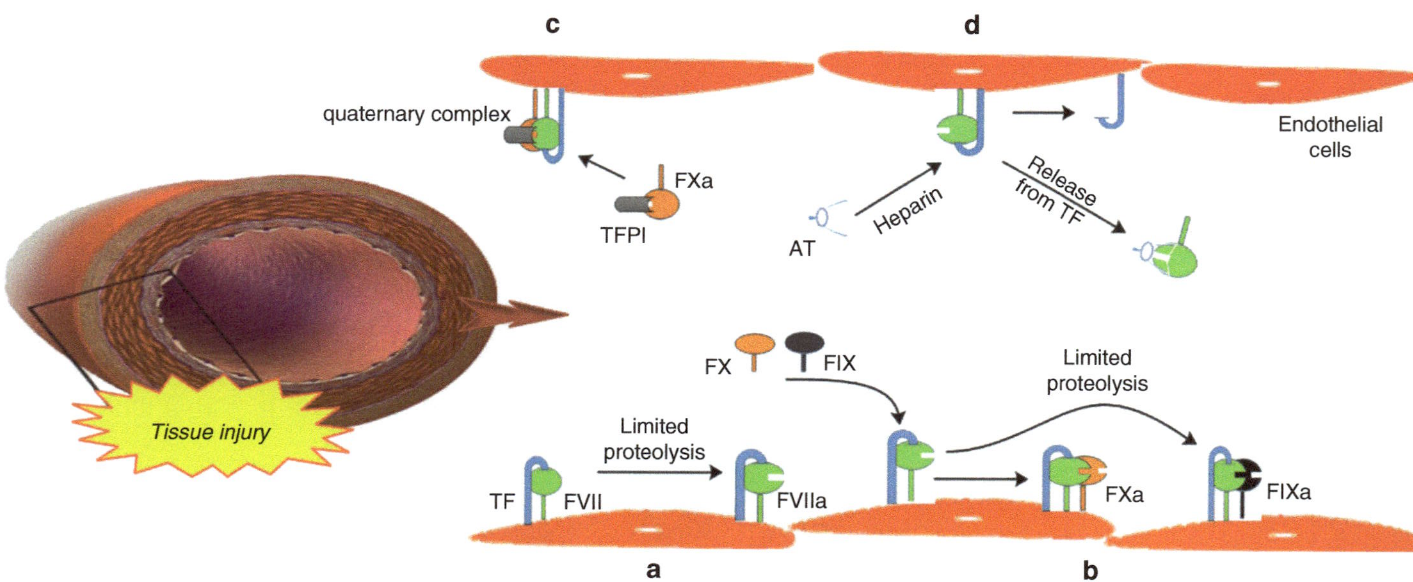

Fig. 10.2 In vivo activation and inhibition of factor VII (FVII). (**a**, **b**) FVII binds to tissue factor (TF) and is converted to its active form, FVIIa, by minor proteolysis and then activates factor X (FX) and factor IX (FIX). (**c**, **d**) Tissue factor pathway inhibitor (TFPI) and antithrombin (AT) are inhibitors of FVII/TF complex. TFPI/FXa complex can form an inactive tetra-molecular (TF-FVIIa-TFPI-FXa) complex that results in extrinsic coagulation pathway inhibition. In addition to direct deactivation of FXa, TFPI can prevent further FX activation after TFPI/TF/FVIIa complex formation. TFPI/FXa can induce internalization of TF/FVIIa complex that results in degradation of the majority of FVIIa (not shown). TFPI can also inhibit the early forms of prothrombinase (not shown). AT directly attaches to TF/FVIIa complex and causes segregation of FVIIa from TF by losing affinity of FVIIa for TF resulting in a release of FVIIa/AT into the bloodstream and therefore causing extrinsic coagulation pathway inhibition. AT activity can be strengthened by heparin

FVII with the initiation of coagulation pathway following complex formation with TF at injury site has a critical role in the coagulation cascade. This complex is an important activator of both extrinsic and intrinsic coagulation pathways by activating FVII, FIX, and FX [4]. It was shown that complete deletion of *F7* gene leads to mouse perinatal death, while mice and human with very low FVII level could survive [7, 25, 26]. Although the normal perinatal course was observed in FVII knockout mouse, major abdominal and intracranial hemorrhages (ICH) lead to death in such cases at birth or shortly after birth [8]. Generally, it is accepted that absence of FVII is incompatible with life [3, 19, 27].

TF also known as thromboplastin, coagulation FIII, or CD142 is a glycosylated, transmembrane protein that doesn't require proteolysis for activation [10]. It is well known that normal hemostasis process in some tissues with high TF-expression such as the brain, bowel, uterus, placenta, lungs, and heart mainly depends on the extrinsic pathway; therefore, decrease or absence of FVII can result in bleeding in some of these tissues [4, 7]. In addition to well-known role of TF in coagulation process, in complex with FVIIa, other functions including embryonic angiogenesis, oncogenic angiogenesis, tumor progression, leukocyte diapedesis, and regulation of inflammation and sepsis are described. This complex can also change cellular physiology in the TF-expression cells [28, 29].

10.3 Congenital Factor VII Deficiency

Congenital FVII deficiency (OMIM 227500) is an autosomal recessive bleeding disorder, for the first time described by Alexander in 1951 in a 4-year-old white girl who experienced prolonged umbilical cord bleeding at birth [30]. This bleeding disorder with a prevalence of 1 per 500,000 individuals is the most common rare bleeding disorders (RBD) [1, 5, 30]. Although the disorder has distributed over the world, it is more frequent in some areas such as the United Kingdom, United States, Brazil, Turkey, Italy, Slovak Republic, and Iran, according to the annual global survey of World Federation of Hemophilia (WFH). Although consanguinity is the main cause for high rate of disorder, in some countries like the United Kingdom, this was attributed to noticeable grow up of hygienic surveillance and the improved quality of life. The number of patients with congenital FVII deficiency might be underestimated probably due to undiagnosed asymptomatic patients and those with the mild bleeding tendency. FVII deficiency is categorized in two groups, including type I (quantitative deficiencies), which is characterized by simultaneous decreases in FVII activity and antigen levels, and type II (qualitative defects) with only decreases in factor activity with normal or near-normal FVII antigen level (Table 10.1) [5]. Clinical manifestations of the disorder are highly variable both in severity and type of bleeding, with poor correlation between residual plasma factor activity and severity of bleeding [4, 31]. The FVII reference range is between 70% and 140%, and usually, less than 2% FVII activity (FVII:C) is related to increased risk of severe bleeds during the newborn and young childhood periods [1, 6]. The disorder is due to mutations in *F7* gene, and a wide spectrum of mutations has been identified

Table 10.1 Classification of congenital factor VII deficiency and results of coagulation tests

	aPTT	PT	FVII:C	FVII:Ag
Normal people	Normal	Normal	Normal	Normal
FVII deficiency (type I)	Normal	Prolonged	Decreased	Decreased
FVII deficiency (type II)	Normal	Prolonged	Decreased	Normal or nearly normal

aPTT activated partial thromboplastin time, *PT* prothrombin time, *FVII:C* factor VII coagulant activity, *FVII:Ag* factor VII antigen

within this gene. Most of the identified mutations are new and restricted to the special area or specific family and could be used for carrier detection, precise diagnosis, and prenatal diagnosis in affected families.

The presence of abnormal bleeding, accompanied by isolated prolonged PT, is the first clue for suspicion to FVII deficiency, but in general, clinical presentations, physical examination, family history, and laboratory assessments can be used for precise diagnosis of the disorder. Several therapeutic options such as fresh frozen plasma (FFP), plasma-derived FVII (pd-FVII), prothrombin complex concentrate (PCC), activated PCC (aPCC), and more recently recombinant FVIIa (rFVIIa) are available for patients with FVII deficiency.

10.4 Acquired Factor VII Deficiency

Acquired FVII deficiency can be present as the isolated or combined deficiency as a part of vitamin K-dependent coagulation factors deficiency [1, 32, 33]. Acquired isolated FVII deficiency is an extremely rare disorder, but the frequency was underestimated, because clinical symptoms of the disorder may be mild to moderate with slightly prolonged PT [32–34]. Different conditions such as malignancies, severe systemic sepsis, infectious agents, drugs (penicillin), and aplastic anemia as well as stem cell transplantation and presence of an inhibitory antibody may be accompanied with acquired isolated FVII deficiency [1, 33, 35, 36]. In some cases, no underlying condition of FVII deficiency (idiopathic) was identified [33]. The pathogenesis and the possible mechanism of FVII deficiency are not clear in these situations [33]. Simultaneous deficiency of FVII with other coagulation factors may arise in different conditions including [1]:

- Problem in synthesis, particular in liver failure that leads to decrease of all coagulation factors.
- A defective synthesis, especially during hypovitaminosis K syndrome caused by insufficient intake, malabsorption, or anticoagulant therapy with vitamin K antagonists such as warfarin, acenocoumarol (Sinthromin), and phenprocoumon (Marcoumar). These conditions only lead to vitamin K-dependent coagulation factor deficiency (FII, FVII, FIX, and FX) and the decrease of protein C and protein S levels. Warfarin inhibits the vitamin K-dependent reductase and the vitamin K-dependent quinone reductase and leads to disturbing in the recycling of vitamin K to its enzymatically active form and its carboxylation activity (Fig. 9.4).

- Consumption syndromes, especially disseminated intravascular coagulation (DIC) or hyperfibrinolysis that leads to consuming of all coagulation factors.

As mentioned, FVII has the shortest plasma half-life among clotting factors; thus, decrease in plasma level of FVII occurs faster than other coagulation factors. Therefore, diagnosis of isolated FVII deficiency should be made with caution [1].

10.5 Clinical Manifestations

Patients with congenital FVII deficiency have variable bleeding diathesis with poor correlation between FVII activity and bleeding tendency [1, 33]. The clinical phenotype is very heterogeneous and ranges from asymptomatic condition to life-threatening diathesis. The clinical phenotype of these patients could be categorized into two main categories [1, 3, 37]:

- Asymptomatic that composed about one-third of patients
- Symptomatic with two subgroups:
  - Nonsevere: Mild to moderate with mucocutaneous bleeding (mimic platelet disorders) including approximately two-third of affected patients. These patients usually don't require medical intervention.
  - Severe with life- or limb-threatening hemorrhages (CNS bleeding, gastrointestinal (GI) bleeding, or hemarthrosis) that composed about 10–15% of patients [1, 3, 37].

Asymptomatic patients might be randomly diagnosed or identified during family studies, especially in cases with other affected family member (s). According to a large study, 71% of homozygous and 50% of compound heterozygous patients are symptomatic, while only 19% of heterozygous subjects are symptomatic [2]. Based on another large study, most common bleeding features among patients with FVII deficiency are epistaxis, easy bruising, gum bleeding, hematoma, hemarthrosis, post-operative bleeding, and menorrhagia, and less common bleeding features are hematuria, GI bleeding, and CNS bleeding (Table 10.2) [2, 6, 27, 37–40]. Severe clinical presentations generally occur at young ages (soon after birth or when they are toddler) in severely affected patients [9, 37]. Severe chronic iron deficiency due to menorrhagia is common in women with FVII deficiency [3]. Patients with plasma FVII level <2% may present severe bleeding, while those with >20% are generally asymptomatic. Interestingly, bleeding can be observed among patients with plasma levels between 20% and 50%, while asymptomatic subjects with plasma level <1% were also reported [9]. Prediction of hemorrhagic risk may not be possible, even in the presence of laboratory assays such as thrombin generation test, FVIIa and FVII antigen level (FVII:Ag) assays, and TFPI measurement [41]. CNS bleeding is less common condition and is an important problem, mainly in children under 6 months with severe FVII deficiency and associated with high rate of morbidity and mortality [3, 9]. Bleeding episodes in FVII deficiency may mimic hemophilia (hemophilia

Table 10.2 Clinical manifestations of patients with congenital factor VII deficiency

	Mariani et al. (*n*: 174[a]) (%)	Mariani et al. (*n*: 139[b]) (%)	Mariani et al. (*n*: 228) (%)	Herrmann et al. (*n*: 217) (%)	Peyvandi et al. (*n*: 28) (%)	Mariani et al. (*n*: 24) (%)
CNS bleeding	4.6	6.5	7	1	17	–
GI bleeding	13.8	14.4	14	9	–	17
Hemarthrosis	16.1	21.6	22	12	21	67
Epistaxis	56.3	66.2	83	58	64	62
Easy bruising	47.7	43.2	62	37	32	29
Gum bleeding	33.9	25.9	42	25	–	33
Menorrhagia	62.9	–	–	57 (of 106 female)	60 (of 10 female)	90 (of 10 female)
Hematomas	16.1	20.9	21	20	12	46
Hematuria	5.2	12.2	12	7	10	29
Post-operative bleeding	29.8	30.4	34	–	55	–
Thrombosis	3	–	–	–	–	–

CNS central nervous system, *GI* gastrointestinal

[a]The incidence of menorrhagia has been reported in female aged >10 and <50 years and all of patients are female

[b]Only males

type) with the present of hemarthrosis and hematoma or may mimic primary hemostasis defects with menorrhagia, epistaxis, or ecchymosis [9]. In addition to bleeding episodes, thrombotic events with the unknown mechanism (particularly deep vein thrombosis) also may occur in ~3% of patients with severe FVII deficiency, especially those patients undergoing surgical interventions or those under replacement therapy; however, spontaneous thrombosis also may occur [42, 43]. Although severe clinical events were observed in homozygous or compound heterozygotes, heterozygous are usually asymptomatic [2, 27].

10.6 Diagnosis

The first case with congenital FVII deficiency was described by prolonged PT in 1951 [30]. The diagnosis was made based on clinical presentations, physical examination, family history, and laboratory assessments [38]. Occasionally, the disorder could be identified during routine work up. In general, the mean age of diagnosis in inherited FVII deficiency is 8 years [1]. FVII deficiency is usually suspected by the presence of isolated prolonged PT that is corrected by 50:50 mixing of patient's plasma with normal pooled plasma. In this setting, the activated partial thromboplastin time (aPTT), thrombin time (TT), fibrinogen concentration, and platelet count are usually normal. Evaluation of FVII coagulant activity (FVII:C) (with twice repeating) leads to confirmation of disorder [3, 38]. In general, the mainstay in the diagnosis of FVII deficiency is FVII:C assay. Exclusion of vitamin K deficiency or other acquired causes of clotting factor deficiencies is useful, but not necessary, because concomitant prolongation of aPTT is observed in these conditions [3].

In patients with acquired isolated FVII deficiency, isolated prolongation of PT was occurred, while aPTT is normal. However, prolonged aPTT might have occurred in some patients with the presence of lupus anticoagulant (LA). In this situation, FVII:C should be determined and isolated FVII deficiency should be confirmed. Evaluation of other vitamin K-dependent clotting factors might be helpful to rule out other disorders. For further investigation, mixing study should be performed. After mixing study, if PT was prolonged, the presence of specific FVII inhibitor is suspected, and the Bethesda assay could confirm the presence of specific FVII inhibitor [33]. In this way, the absence of bleeding history, the presence of malignancy (or other underlying conditions), as well as absence of family history of congenital FVII deficiency could be useful during the process of diagnosis.

10.6.1 Factor VII Coagulant Activity

FVII:C should be performed for diagnosis of FVII deficiency. FVII:C usually determines by one-stage prothrombin time-based assay [44]. The source of thromboplastin, calibration materials, and quality of the reagents can affect the results of FVII:C [45]. Three types of thromboplastin reagents with different sensitivities including rabbit brain, ox[1] brain, or human recombinant thromboplastin are available [44, 46].

According to the type of thromboplastin, different results might be obtained; however, variability that is caused by qualitative FVII defects such as FVII Padua, FVII Nagoya, and FVII Tondabayashi is more profound. For example, in Padua variant (Arg304Gln in exon 8) which usually associates with no bleeding history and the normal range of FVII:Ag, disparate results toward different thromboplastins could be obtained, so that normal results using ox brain thromboplastin and abnormal results by use of rabbit brain thromboplastin might be obtained [1, 47]. It should be noted that variable reactivity of different thromboplastins only occurs in type II deficiency such as Padua, not type I deficiency [1, 47]. In this setting, based on structural similarity of recombinant thromboplastins and human TF, use of this product is more reliable than other thromboplastins for FVII assay.

In spite of the presence of certified reference materials for the accuracy of calibrators, the different calibration materials may have variable interlaboratory precision, especially in cases with FVII level below 20% [1].

The quality of the FVII-deficient reagents impresses accuracy of FVII:C assay, especially when FVII-deficient plasma has residual FVII:C. This issue can lead to overestimation of FVII:C in patients with low plasma level of FVII [45]. According to 2016 Clinical and Laboratory Standards Institute (CLSI) document H48-Ed2, the mean activity of FVII-deficient plasma in the one-stage clotting assay should be less than 1% [48]. Indeed, contamination of thromboplastin with small amounts of FVIIa can decrease sensitivity to patient's plasma FVII:C, while it increases sensitivity to patient's plasma level of FV, FX, and prothrombin [1, 49]. Finally, it should be noted that plasma FVII level is raised in some circumstances, such as female gender, increasing age, and hyperlipidemia, especially hypertriglyceridemia [50].

[1] Ox is derived from oxen and commonly referred as castrated adult male cattle.

10.6.2 Factor VIIa Assay

In addition to the pivotal role of TF-FVIIa pathway in the initiation of the coagulation cascade, it has the important effect on the inflammatory pathway, regulation of inflammation and sepsis [28].

When recombinant activated FVII (rFVIIa) was introduced for treatment of patients with hemophilia having inhibitor, FVII deficiency, and other bleeding events such as retropubic prostatectomy, the interest for concentrates FVIIa assay was increased [1, 51, 52]. Although PT and FVII:C assay could also be used for monitoring of rFVIIa treatment, but as mentioned above, the FVII:C and PT results vary greatly among laboratories (mostly due to type of thromboplastin), even if different assays used thromboplastins with similar sensitivity. Therefore, FVIIa assay may be more effective than PT and FVII:C for monitoring of these patients [1, 51]. FVIIa assay is not recommended for diagnosis of FVII deficiency [1, 51]. The assessment of FVIIa could be performed by different methods: the first method relies on clotting-based assay using recombinant soluble mutant TF molecule (sTF1–219), a TF without transmembrane and cytoplasmic domains. STF cannot activate FVII, but its FVIIa cofactor activity is conserved [53, 54]. Normal plasma FVIIa level using this technique is 0.5–8.4 ng/mL (mean 3.6 ng/mL), encompassing 1–3% of the total inactive zymogen form [3, 54], based on the specificity of the FVIIa assay [55]. The second method is based on enzyme linked immunosorbent assay (ELISA), using the high specific antibody against two-chain FVIIa that cannot reactive with FVII. An obvious discrepancy might be observed between results of these two methods [54, 55]. The ELISA can detect approximately 0.0125 ng/mL (±0.01 ng/mL) of FVIIa, but the correlation between both methods is excellent [3].

The FVII:Ag could be determined by different methods including ELISA or immunoturbidimetric assays (IRMAs) with epitope-specific monoclonal antibodies against free-circulating FVII. Distinguish between type I and II defects is feasible, by using the FVII:Ag assay. The FVII:Ag level is not a good predictor of severity of bleeding tendency, but it can help understanding of mutational mechanisms of FVII deficiency [1, 38].

10.7 Molecular Basis

The *F7* gene spans 12.8 kb on chromosome 13q34 and contains nine exons and five short tandem repeats. These minisatellite DNA sequences cover more than a quarter of the intron sequence and more than one-third of 3′ untranslated region (UTR) of mRNA. The *F7* gene is located approximately 2.8 kb upstream of the *F10* gene and located near another vitamin K-dependent protein *Z* gene [4, 16, 27, 56]. *F7* gene and protein are structurally homologous with other vitamin K-dependent coagulation factors, particularly FIX, FX, and protein C. The overall base compositions of the *F7* gene in exons and introns are similar (60% G-C and 40% A-T), which is similar to the protein C and the *F10* genes [16]. *F7* gene consists of nine exons. Exons 1a and 1b (the latter is an alternatively spliced target in 90% of factor VII mRNA transcripts) and a part of exon 2 encode 5′ UTR and mainly a part of the pre-pro leader. Exon 2 encodes Gla domain. Exon 3 encodes the hydrophobic aromatic stack, exons 4 and 5 encode two epidermal-like growth factor (EGF) domains, exons 6 and 7 are responsible for encoding of activation region, and, finally, exon 8 encodes the catalytic domain and 3′ UTR including poly (A) tail (Fig. 10.3) [3].

A wide spectrum of mutations was identified within *F7* gene, and whole gene sequencing including exons, introns, boundaries, and the promoter regions is recommended for mutation detection in patients with congenital FVII deficiency. This is mostly due to a large number of identified mutations within *F7* gene, the short length of the gene, and merely possibility in detection of a recurrence mutation [1]. In general, 90–92% of mutated alleles could be identified with the current routine direct sequencing methods, and ~10% of gene mutation could not be found. Although new techniques, such as next-generation sequencing (NGS), certainly can improve this situation, some of the cases with congenital FVII deficiency may occur due to mutations in different another genes that can make FVII deficiency still an open question [1, 19]. A wide spectrum of normal gene variations and disease-causing mutations, including missense, nonsense, splice site mutations, and insertions/deletions, were observed in *F7* gene. Several functional and nonfunctional polymorphisms have also been observed (Table 10.3) [3, 19, 57–64]. For example, functional promoter polymorphism at position −402 (G > A) of the ATG codon leads to increased FVII:C, while promoter polymorphism at position −401 (G > T) associated with decreased plasma FVII level [58]. Arg413Gln substitution in exon 7 (classically known as R353Q variant) arises from G to A substitution at nucleotide 10,976 and generally associated with another polymorphism, a decanucleotide (10-bp sequence) insertion at position −323 in the 5′-flanking region of the *F7* gene, resulting in 20 to 30% reduction in FVII level [3, 58]. In vitro functional analysis of two adenine (g.11293_11294insAA) insertion polymorphisms located in the 3' UTR of *F7* gene revealed the steady-state decreases of FVII mRNA level [57].

According to available data, most of the mutations in *F7* gene, similar to other congenital bleeding disorders, are point mutation. Missense mutations (79%) are the most frequent while nonsense mutations are the rarest mutations (4%) (Fig. 10.4). Exon 8 as the largest exon (1.6 kb) [16] in *F7* gene that is responsible for encoding of the catalytic domain has a considerable number of mutations.

Prenatal diagnosis (PND) can be used in patients with congenital FVII deficiency, but it is more suitable for those families with severe factor deficiency and history of life-threatening bleeding such ICH [1, 65].

10.8 Management

Due to highly variable clinical presentations and low correlation between severity of clinical presentations and FVII:C level, bleeding risk prediction and management of these patients remained debated. The mainstay of treatment in patients with

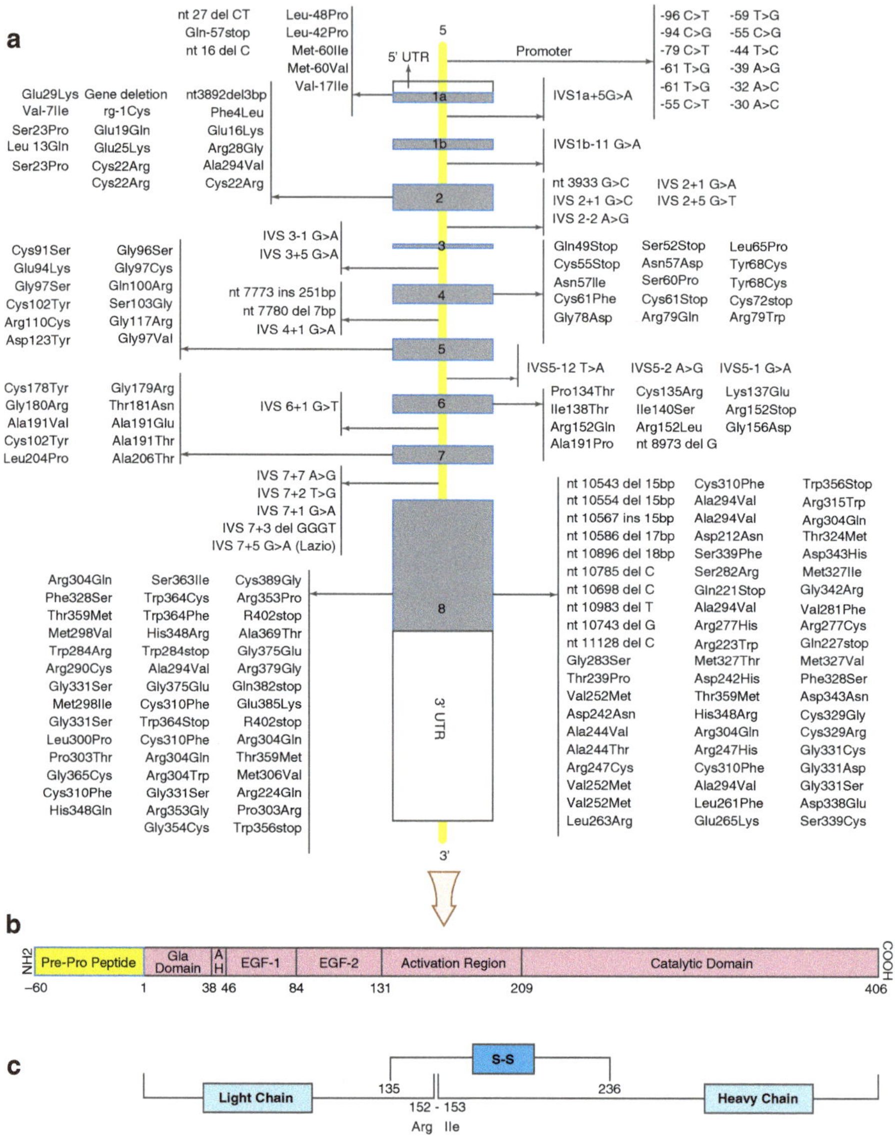

Fig. 10.3 *F7* gene and FVII protein structures and spectrum of gene mutations in *F7* gene. (**a**) *F7* gene contains nine exons that encode FVII protein. Exon 1b, usually alternatively spliced in 90% of FVII mRNA transcript. (**b**) The FVII protein contains pre-pro sequence, Gla, EGF1, EGF2, and catalytic serine protease domains. (**c**) Cleavage at Arg152-Ile153 location, leads to generation of two-chain active molecule which join together by a disulfide bond between Cys135 and Cys236. Light chain contains residues +1 to 152 and heavy chain contains residues 153 to 406. *FVII* factor VII, *Gla* gamma-carboxyglutamic acid, *EGF* epidermal growth factor

Table 10.3 *F7* gene polymorphisms

Polymorphism type	Location	Frequency	Effect on FVII:C
Decanucleotide [CCTATATCCT] insert	5′ region (−323)	0.77 0.23	Decrease[a]
G/T dimorphism	5′ region (−401)	0.91 0.09	Decrease
G/A dimorphism	5′ region (−402)	0.71 0.29	Increase
Intron 1a (G73A)	Intron 1a	0.79 0.21	Decrease[a]
Dimorphism (his 115)	Exon 5	0.80 0.20	–
VNTR repeat (37 bp monomer repeat, 9716ins)	Intron 7	0.30 0.70	Increase[b]
G/A dimorphism	Intron 7	0.82 0.18	NM
Arg353Gln polymorphism	Exon 8	0.80 0.20	Decrease[a]
G/A dimorphism (Ser 333)	Exon 8	0.99 0.01	–
2 adenine (g.11293_11294 insAA) insert	3′ UTR	0.85 0.15	Decrease[c]

NM not mentioned

[a]The 10 bp insertion, and the Arg353Gln polymorphism indicate a strong linkage disequilibrium and therfore it is not clear whether the G73A allele or 10 bp insertion contributed per se to lowering FVII:C

[b]The high mRNA expression in quantitative mRNA analysis has shown that this polymorphism probably is associated with incresed plasma FVII level, although there are contradictory results in this regard

[c]The effect of other polymorphisms was not excluded

congenital FVII deficiency is on-demand replacement therapy that means the stop of bleeding as soon as possible after the occurrence of bleeding. In patients with the history of life-threatening bleeding such as ICH, secondary prophylaxis is recommended. Primary prophylaxis could be used for those patients with severe factor deficiency and risk of life-threatening bleeding. Different therapeutic choices including FFP, pd-FVII, PCC, aPCC, and rFVIIa are available for patients with FVII deficiency (Table 10.4) [1, 27].

The recommended dose and therapeutic target levels of FVII for on-demand, prophylaxis, and in surgeries are summarized in Table 10.5 [66].

rFVIIa (eptacog alfa) is the structurally similar product to plasma-derived coagulation factor VIIa but is manufactured using DNA biotechnology [67, 68]. The first report of successful treatment with rFVIIa was in 1988 with NovoSeven® (rFVIIa; NovoSeven, Novo Nordisk, Copenhagen, Denmark) in patient with severe

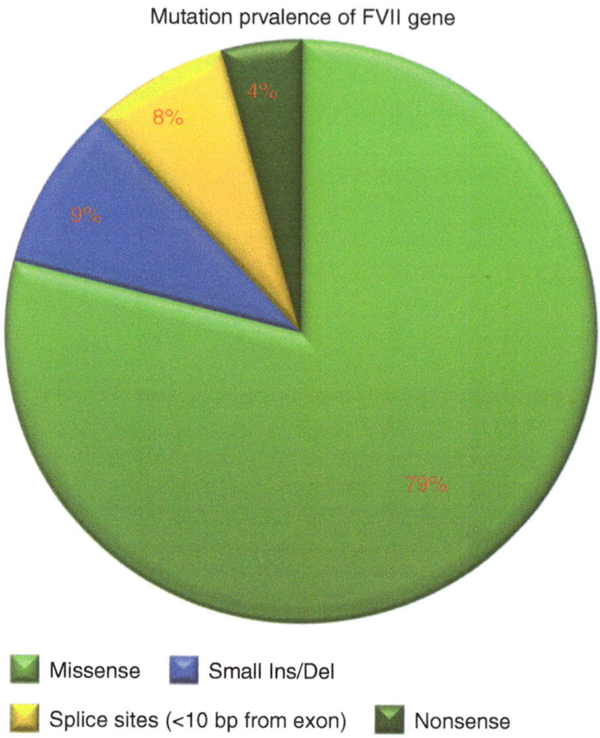

Fig. 10.4 Mutation prevalence of *F7* gene. Most common mutations of *F7* gene are missense mutations (79%), while small Ins/Del (9%), splice sites (8%), and nonsense (4%) mutations form other mutations in *F7* gene

Table 10.4 Available therapeutic options for patients with factor VII deficiency

Factor	Advantage	Disadvantage
FFP	Easily available, cheap	Limited effectiveness, need to high volumes for treatment, fluid overload, risk of viral transmission
Pd-FVII	Effective; suitable for surgery	Unavailable in some countries, other vitamin K-dependent factor concentrations are higher than factor VII, risk of viral transmission, risk of TE
rFVIIa	Very effective Low dosage requirement for treatment No risk of viral transmission Not immunogenic in patients with hemophilia Not produces an anamnestic response in hemophilia patients with inhibitors Very low thrombogenicity	Risk of TE, expensive
PCC	Suitable for surgery	Risk of TE, concentration of other vitamin K-dependent factors is higher than factor VII and presence of activated factors Variable amount of factor VII

Pd-FVII plasma-derived FVII, *FFP* fresh frozen plasma, *rFVIIa* recombinant FVIIa, *TE* thrombotic events, *PCC* prothrombin complex concentrates

Table 10.5 Recommended dose and therapeutic target levels for factor VII on on-demand and prophylaxis treatment in patients with factor VII deficiency

Recommended and maintaining level	Plasma half-life	On-demand dosages	Major surgery	Minor surgery	Long-term prophylaxis dosages
>20%	2–4 h	Pd-FVII concentrate (30–40 U/kg)	rFVIIa: Before surgery: 15–30 μg/kg After surgery: continue the same dose for first day with 4–6 h interval, and then change interval to 8–12 h or Pd-FVII concentrate: 8–40 IU/kg with similar intervals	Tranexamic acid 15–20 mg/kg or 1 g 4 times daily or antifibrinolytics[a]	FFP: 10–15 mL/kg 2 times/week Pd-FVII: 30–40 U/kg 3 times/week

Pd-FVII plasma-derived FVII, *FFP* fresh frozen plasma, *rFVIIa* recombinant FVIIa
[a]This recommendation needs further research because the quality of evidence is moderate

hemophilia A during synovectomy [69]. AryoSeven™ as a new generic rFVIIa claimed that it has biosimilarity with NovoSeven® and is similar in clinical safety and efficacy with NovoSeven® [70–72]. rFVIIa has been approved for treatment of patients with congenital FVII deficiency, congenital hemophilia B with high-responding inhibitors, acquired hemophilia, and Glanzmann thrombasthenia with refractoriness to platelet transfusions, with or without antibodies to platelets and recommended as the first-line therapeutic option for hemophilia A patients with high-responder inhibitors [67, 68]. rFVIIa also was used in surgical bleeding related to dilutional or consumptive coagulopathies or in patients with impaired liver function [73]. In addition, the rFVIIa could be used in various conditions, such as spontaneous bleeding, hemarthrosis, and major surgical procedures. Inhibitor development is one of the most important problems in the administration of rFVIIa [74]. According to FDA report, the risk of the thrombotic events associated with rFVIIa is 2% of treated patients in rFVIIa clinical trials. The very low frequency of thrombotic events, no virus transmission, and scarce production of inhibitory antibodies are advantages of rFVIIa, and expensiveness and short half-life of rFVIIa even than FVII and FVIIa are disadvantages of rFVIIa [1].

PCC is another therapeutic choice for patients with FVII deficiency. PCC usually contains FII (prothrombin), FIX, FX, and the variable amount of FVII. In general, two commercially types of PCC are available, including 3-factor PCC (with absent or low levels of FVII) and 4-factor PCC (with high level of FVII) (Table 10.6), [75–81] and another form is activated PCC (FEIBA) which contains 4-factors in

Table 10.6 Characteristics of some available four-factor prothrombin complex concentrates (PCC)

PCC	Manufacturer/country	Hemophilia B (factor IX)	Acquired deficiency (e.g., VKA)	Congenital deficiency (specific factor not available)	Other factor deficiency, such as factor II, VII, X
Beriplex P/N	CSL Behring GmbH/Germany		√	√	
Kcentra[a]	CSL Behring GmbH/Germany		√		
Cofact	Sanquin/the Netherlands		√	√	
Kaskadil	LFB/France		√		√ (FII & FX)
Octaplex	Octapharma/Vienna, Austria		√		√ (FII & FX)
Prothromplex Total 600 IU	Baxalta Innovations GmbH/Vienna, Austria		√	√	
Proplex T[b]	Baxter/Glendale, USA	√			√ (FVII)

PCC prothrombin complex concentrates, *VKA* vitamin K antagonists, *FIX* factor IX, *FII* factor II, *FVII* factor VII, *FX* factor X

[a]Kcentra is indicated for the urgent reversal of acquired coagulation factor deficiency induced by vitamin K antagonist therapy in adult patients during acute major bleeding (it does not have indication in patients without acute major bleeding)

[b]Proplex T is indicated for the treatment of bleeding episodes in patients with factor VIII deficiency with inhibitors

inactive (FII, FIX, and FX) and activated (FVII) forms [82–84]. The amount of FVII is variable in different manufactured PCC that is usually indicated by the manufacturer; thus, after requirement calculation could be administered [3]. Some PCC may contain the additional components such as anticoagulants, protein C, protein S, protein Z, and antithrombin III as well as heparin, to mitigate thrombotic risk [83, 85, 86]. Overall clotting factors of these concentrates are approximately 25 times higher than normal plasma [87]. Some advantages of PCC over the FFP include relatively constant high level of vitamin K-dependent coagulation factors (FII, FVII, FIX and FX), a more rapid decrease in INR value, and no need for matching the blood groups, or thawing the product [84, 88]. Several reports indicated both venous and arterial thrombosis associated with PCC; therefore, utilization of these concentrates in patients with liver disease and major trauma and neonates (because of relatively immature livers) is not recommended. The incidence of thrombotic events in patients treated with 4-factor and 3-factor PCC is 1.8% and 0.7%, respectively [84]. Another disadvantage of PCC is high concentration of other vitamin K-dependent factors than FVII [1, 27, 89–91].

The pd-FVII is the useful product for prophylaxis in children with severe FVII deficiency and for long-term prophylaxis in the range of 30–40 U/Kg, 3 times/week. Pd-FVII was successfully used for surgery with doses ranging from 8 to 40 U/Kg every 4–6 h. For major surgeries, FVII level must be kept above 20 U/dl. Similar to PCC, FVII concentration of pd-FVII is less than other vitamin K-dependent coagulation factors [3, 27, 92]. Acquired FVII deficiency is usually treated as same as inherited FVII deficiency by FFP, PCC, aPCC, and pd-FVII or rFVIIa. However, in these cases, underlying disease should be treated.

References

1. Sevenet P-O, Kaczor DA, Depasse F. Factor VII deficiency: from basics to clinical laboratory diagnosis and patient management. Clin Appl Thromb Hemost. 2016. https://doi.org/10.1177/1076029616670257.
2. Herrmann F, Wulff K, Auerswald G, Schulman S, Astermark J, Batorova A, et al. Factor VII deficiency: clinical manifestation of 717 subjects from Europe and Latin America with mutations in the factor 7 gene. Haemophilia. 2009;15(1):267–80.
3. Perry DJ. Factor VII deficiency. Br J Haematol. 2002;118(3):689–700.
4. Lapecorella M, Mariani G. Factor VII deficiency: defining the clinical picture and optimizing therapeutic options. Haemophilia. 2008;14(6):1170–5.
5. Peyvandi F, James P, Salomon O, Mikovic D. Rare bleeding disorders. Haemophilia. 2014;20(4):71.
6. Mariani G, Herrmann FH, Dolce A, Batorova A, Etro D, Peyvandi F, et al. Clinical phenotypes and factor VII genotype in congenital factor VII deficiency. Thromb Haemost. 2005;93(3):481.
7. Mackman N. The role of tissue factor and factor VIIa in hemostasis. Anesth Analg. 2009;108(5):1447.
8. Rosen ED, Chan JC, Idusogie E, Clotman F. Mice lacking factor VII develop normally but suffer fatal perinatal bleeding. Nature. 1997;390(6657):290.
9. Moerloose P, Schved JF, Nugent D. Rare coagulation disorders: fibrinogen, factor VII and factor XIII. Haemophilia. 2016;22(S5):61–5.
10. Smith SA, Travers RJ, Morrissey JH. How it all starts: initiation of the clotting cascade. Crit Rev Biochem Mol Biol. 2015;50(4):326–36.

11. Neuenschwander PF, Morrissey JH. Roles of the membrane-interactive regions of factor VIIa and tissue factor. The factor VIIa Gla domain is dispensable for binding to tissue factor but important for activation of factor X. J Biol Chem. 1994;269(11):8007–13.
12. Tavoosi N, Smith SA, Davis-Harrison RL, Morrissey JH. Factor VII and protein C are phosphatidic acid-binding proteins. Biochemistry. 2013;52(33):5545–52.
13. Fair DS. Quantitation of factor VII in the plasma of normal and warfarin-treated individuals by radioimmunoassay. Blood. 1983;62(4):784–91.
14. Vadivel K, Bajaj SP. Structural biology of factor VIIa/tissue factor initiated coagulation. Front Biosci. 2012;17:2476.
15. Eigenbrot C, Kirchhofer D, Dennis MS, Santell L, Lazarus RA, Stamos J, et al. The factor VII zymogen structure reveals reregistration of β strands during activation. Structure. 2001;9(7):627–36.
16. O'Hara PJ, Grant FJ, Haldeman BA, Gray CL, Insley MY, Hagen FS, et al. Nucleotide sequence of the gene coding for human factor VII, a vitamin K-dependent protein participating in blood coagulation. Proc Natl Acad Sci. 1987;84(15):5158–62.
17. Banner DW, D'arcy A, Chene C, Winkler FK, Guha A, Konigsberg WH, et al. The crystal structure of the complex of blood coagulation factor VIIa with soluble tissue factor. Nature. 1996;380(6569):41–6.
18. Butenas S, Mann KG. Kinetics of human factor VII activation. Biochemistry. 1996;35(6):1904–10.
19. McVey JH, Boswell E, Mumford AD, Kemball-Cook G, Tuddenham EG. Factor VII deficiency and the FVII mutation database. Hum Mutat. 2001;17(1):3–17.
20. Spiezia L, Campello E, Dalla Valle F, Woodhams B, Simioni P. Factor VIIa-antithrombin complex: a possible new biomarker for activated coagulation. Clin Chem Lab Med. 2017;55(4):484–8.
21. Rao L, Nordfang O, Hoang A, Pendurthi U. Mechanism of antithrombin III inhibition of factor VIIa/tissue factor activity on cell surfaces. Comparison with tissue factor pathway inhibitor/factor Xa-induced inhibition of factor VIIa/tissue factor activity. Blood. 1995;85(1):121–9.
22. Monroe DM, Key N. The tissue factor–factor VIIa complex: procoagulant activity, regulation, and multitasking. J Thromb Haemost. 2007;5(6):1097–105.
23. Iakhiaev A, Pendurthi UR, Voigt J, Ezban M, Rao LVM. Catabolism of factor VIIa bound to tissue factor in fibroblasts in the presence and absence of tissue factor pathway inhibitor. J Biol Chem. 1999;274(52):36995–7003.
24. Lwaleed BA, Bass PS. Tissue factor pathway inhibitor: structure, biology and involvement in disease. J Pathol. 2006;208(3):327–39.
25. Rosen ED, Xu H, Liang Z, Martin JA, Suckow M, Castellino FJ. Generation of genetically-altered mice producing very low levels of coagulation factor VII. Thromb Haemost. 2005;94(3):493–7.
26. Tuddenham EGD, Pemberton S, Cooper DN. Inherited factor VII deficiency: genetics and molecular pathology article in thrombosis and haemostasis. Thromb Haemost. 1995;74(1):313–21.
27. Mariani G, Bernardi F. Factor VII deficiency. Semin Thromb Hemost. 2009;35:400.
28. Versteeg HH, Peppelenbosch MP, Spek CA. Tissue factor signal transduction in angiogenesis. Carcinogenesis. 2003;24(6):1009–13.
29. Krikun G, Schatz F, Taylor H, Lockwood CJ. Endometriosis and tissue factor. Ann N Y Acad Sci. 2008;1127(1):101–5.
30. Alexander B, Goldstein R, Landwehr G, Cook C, Addelson E, Wilson C. Congenital SPCA deficiency: a hitherto unrecognized coagulation defect with hemorrhage rectified by serum and serum fractions. J Clin Invest. 1951;30(6):596.
31. Triplett DA, Brandt JT, Batard M, Dixon J, Fair DS. Hereditary factor VII deficiency: heterogeneity defined by combined functional and immunochemical analysis. Blood. 1985;66(6):1284–7.
32. Girolami A, Santarossa C, Cosi E, Ferrari S, Lombardi AM. Acquired isolated FVII deficiency: an underestimated and potentially important laboratory finding. Clin Appl Thromb Hemost. 2016;22(8):705–11.

33. Mulliez SM, Devreese KM. Isolated acquired factor VII deficiency: review of the literature. Acta Clin Belg. 2016;71(2):63–70.
34. Toor A, Slungaard A, Hedner U, Weisdorf D, Key N. Acquired factor VII deficiency in hematopoietic stem cell transplant recipients. Bone Marrow Transplant. 2002;29(5):403.
35. Biron C, Bengler C, Gris J, Schved J. Acquired isolated factor VII deficiency during sepsis. Pathophysiol Haemost Thromb. 1997;27(2):51–6.
36. Delmer A, Horellou M, Andreu G, Lecompte T, Rossi F, Kazatchkine M, et al. Life-threatening intracranial bleeding associated with the presence of an antifactor VII autoantibody. Blood. 1989;74(1):229–32.
37. Napolitano M, Giansily-Blaizot M, Dolce A, Schved JF, Auerswald G, Ingerslev J, et al. Prophylaxis in congenital factor VII deficiency: indications, efficacy and safety. Results from the Seven Treatment Evaluation Registry (STER). Haematologica. 2013;98(4):538–44.
38. Napolitano M, Siragusa S, Mariani G. Factor VII deficiency: clinical phenotype, genotype and therapy. J Clin Med. 2017;6(4):38.
39. Mariani G, Mazzucconi M. Factor VII congenital deficiency. Pathophysiol Haemost Thromb. 1983;13(3):169–77.
40. Peyvandi F, Mannucci P, Asti D, Abdoullahi M, Di Rocco N, Sharifian R. Clinical manifestations in 28 Italian and Iranian patients with severe factor VII deficiency. Haemophilia. 1997;3(4):242–6.
41. Giansily-Blaizot M, Verdier R, Biron-Adreani C, Schved J-F, Bertrand M, Borg J, et al. Analysis of biological phenotypes from 42 patients with inherited factor VII deficiency: can biological tests predict the bleeding risk? Haematologica. 2004;89(6):704–9.
42. Mariani G, Herrmann F, Schulman S, Batorova A, Wulff K, Etro D, et al. Thrombosis in inherited factor VII deficiency. J Thromb Haemost. 2003;1(10):2153–8.
43. Marty S, Barro C, Chatelain B, Fimbel B, Tribout B, Reynaud J, et al. The paradoxical association between inherited factor VII deficiency and venous thrombosis. Haemophilia. 2008;14(3):564–70.
44. Poggio M, Tripodi A, Mariani G, Mannucci PM. Factor VII clotting assay: influence of different thromboplastins and factor VII-deficient plasmas. CISMEL Study Group. Thromb Haemost. 1991;65(2):160–4.
45. Takamiya O, Ishikawa S, Ohnuma O, Suehisa H, Iijima K, Kayamori Y, et al. Japanese collaborative study to assess inter-laboratory variation in factor VII activity assays. J Thromb Haemost. 2007;5(8):1686–92.
46. Bleavins MR, Carini C, Jurima-Romet M, Rahbari R. Biomarkers in drug development: a handbook of practice, application, and strategy. Hoboken: Wiley; 2011.
47. Girolami A, Fabris F, Dal Bo ZR, Ghiotto G, Burul A. Factor VII Padua: a congenital coagulation disorder due to an abnormal factor VII with a peculiar activation pattern. J Lab Clin Med. 1978;91(3):387–95.
48. Clinical and Laboratory Standard Institute. Determination of coagulation factor activities using the one-stage clotting assay. Wayne: Clinical and Laboratory Institute; 2016.
49. Smith S, Comp P, Morrissey J. Traces of factor VIIa modulate thromboplastin sensitivity to factors V, VII, X, and prothrombin. J Thromb Haemost. 2006;4(7):1553–8.
50. Simpson H, Meade T, Stirling Y, Mann J, Chakrabarti R, Woolf L. Hypertriglyceridaemia and hypercoagulability. Lancet. 1983;321(8328):786–90.
51. Cid A, Lorenzo J, Haya S, Montoro J, Casana P, Aznar J. A comparison of FVII: C and FVIIa assays for the monitoring of recombinant factor VIIa treatment. Haemophilia. 2001;7(1):39–41.
52. Friederich PW, Henny CP, Messelink EJ, Geerdink MG, Keller T, Kurth K-H, et al. Effect of recombinant activated factor VII on perioperative blood loss in patients undergoing retropubic prostatectomy: a double-blind placebo-controlled randomised trial. Lancet. 2003;361(9353):201–5.
53. Neuenschwander PF, Morrissey JH. Deletion of the membrane anchoring region of tissue factor abolishes autoactivation of factor VII but not cofactor function. Analysis of a mutant with a selective deficiency in activity. J Biol Chem. 1992;267(20):14477–82.

54. Morrissey JH, Macik BG, Neuenschwander PF. Quantitation of activated factor VII levels in plasma using a tissue factor mutant selectively deficient in promoting factor VII activation. Blood. 1993;81(3):734–44.
55. Philippou H, Adami A, Amersey RA, Stubbs PJ, Lane DA. A novel specific immunoassay for plasma two-chain factor VIIa: investigation of FVIIa levels in normal individuals and in patients with acute coronary syndromes. Blood. 1997;89(3):767–75.
56. Colman RW. Hemostasis and thrombosis: basic principles and clinical practice. Philadelphia: Lippincott Williams & Wilkins; 2006.
57. Peyvandi F, Garagiola I, Palla R, Marziliano N, Mannucci P. Role of the 2 adenine (g. 11293_11294insAA) insertion polymorphism in the 3' untranslated region of the factor VII (FVII) gene: molecular characterization of a patient with severe FVII deficiency. Hum Mutat. 2005;26(5):455–61.
58. van't Hooft FM, Silveira A, Tornvall P, Iliadou A, Ehrenborg E, Eriksson P, et al. Two common functional polymorphisms in the promoter region of the coagulation factor VII gene determining plasma factor VII activity and mass concentration. Blood. 1999;93(10):3432–41.
59. Marchetti G, Patracchini P, Papacchini M, Ferrati M, Bernardi F. A polymorphism in the 5' region of coagulation factor VII gene (F7) caused by an inserted decanucleotide. Hum Genet. 1993;90(5):575–6.
60. Peyvandi F, Mannucci P, Bucciarelli P, Zeinali S, Akhavan S, Sacchi E, et al. A novel polymorphism in intron 1a of the human factor VII gene (G73A): study of a healthy Italian population and of 190 young survivors of myocardial infarction. Br J Haematol. 2000;108(2):247–53.
61. Marchetti G, Ferrati M, Patracchini P, Redaelli R, Bernardi F. A missense mutation (178Cys-> Tyr) and two neutral dimorphisms (115His and 333Ser) in the human coagulation factor VII gene. Hum Mol Genet. 1993;2(7):1055–6.
62. Marchetti G, Patracchini P, Gemmati D, DeRosa V, Pinotti M, Rodorigo G, et al. Detection of two missense mutations and characterization of a repeat polymorphism in the factor VII gene (F7). Hum Genet. 1992;89(5):497–502.
63. Tamary H, Fromovich Y, Shalmon L, Reich Z, Dym O, Lanir N, et al. Ala244Val is a common, probably ancient mutation causing factor VII deficiency in Moroccan and Iranian Jews. Thromb Haemost. 1996;76:283.
64. Green F, Kelleher C, Wilkes H, Temple A, Meade T, Humphries S. A common genetic polymorphism associated with lower coagulation factor VII levels in healthy individuals. Arterioscler Thromb Vasc Biol. 1991;11(3):540–6.
65. Tabibian S, Shams M, Naderi M, Dorgalaleh A. Prenatal diagnosis in rare bleeding disorders-An unresolved issue? Int J Lab Hematol. 2018. https://doi.org/10.1111/ijlh.12789.
66. Peyvandi F, Menegatti M. Treatment of rare factor deficiencies in 2016. Hematology Am Soc Hematol Educ Program. 2016;2016(1):663–9.
67. Asif M, Siddiqui A, Scott LJ. Recombinant factor VIIa (Eptacog Alfa): a review of its use in congenital or acquired haemophilia and other congenital bleeding disorders. Drugs. 2005;65(8):1161–78.
68. Croom KF, McCormack PL. Recombinant factor VIIa (eptacog alfa): a review of its use in congenital hemophilia with inhibitors, acquired hemophilia, and other congenital bleeding disorders. BioDrugs. 2008;22(2):121–36.
69. Hedner U, Glazer S, Pingel K, Alberts KA, Blonback M, Schulman S, et al. Successful use of recombinant factor VIIa in patient with severe haemophilia A during synovectomy. Lancet. 1988;332:1193.
70. Sadeghi N, Kahn D, Syed D, Iqbal O, Abro S, Eshraghi R, et al. Comparative biochemical and functional studies on a branded human recombinant factor VIIa and a biosimilar equivalent product. Clin Appl Thromb Hemost. 2014;20(6):565–72.
71. Faranoush M, Abolghasemi H, Toogeh G, Karimi M, Eshghi P, Managhchi M, et al. A comparison between recombinant activated factor VII (Aryoseven) and Novoseven in patients with congenital factor VII deficiency. Clin Appl Thromb Hemost. 2015;21(8):724–8.
72. Faranoush M, Abolghasemi H, Mahboudi F, Toogeh G, Karimi M, Eshghi P, et al. A comparison of efficacy between recombinant activated factor VII (Aryoseven) and Novoseven

in patients with hereditary FVIII deficiency with inhibitor. Clin Appl Thromb Hemost. 2016;22(2):184–90.
73. Miller RD, Eriksson LI, Fleisher LA, Wiener-Kronish JP, Cohen NH, Young WL. Miller's anesthesia. London: Elsevier Health Sciences; 2014.
74. Bauer KA. Treatment of factor VII deficiency with recombinant factor VIIa. Pathophysiol Haemost Thromb. 1996;26(Suppl. 1):155–8.
75. CSL Behring. Beriplex® P/N 250, 500 and 1000 IU [package leaflet]. CSL Behring GmbH, Marburg. 2014.
76. CSL Behring. KCENTRA (Prothrombin complex concentrate (human), [package insert]. CSL Behring GmbH, Marburg. 2013.
77. Sanquin. Cofact 250, 500 IU [information for use]. Sanquin Plasma Products B.V., Amsterdam. 2016.
78. LFB-BIOMEDICAMENTS. KASKADIL (human coagulation factor II) [patient information leaflet]. Courtaboeuf Cedex. 2010.
79. Octapharma. Octaplex 500, 1000. [package leaflet]. Octapharma Pharmazeutika Produktionsges.m.b.H., Vienna. 2015.
80. Baxalta. Prothromplex TOTAL 600 IU [package leaflet]. Baxalta Innovations GmbH, Vienna. 2015.
81. Baxter. Proplex-T (factor IX complex). Baxter Healthcare Corporation, Glendale. 2000.
82. Awad NI, Cocchio C. Activated prothrombin complex concentrates for the reversal of anticoagulant-associated coagulopathy. Pharm Ther. 2013;38(11):696.
83. Sørensen B, Spahn DR, Innerhofer P, Spannagl M, Rossaint R. Clinical review: prothrombin complex concentrates-evaluation of safety and thrombogenicity. Crit Care. 2011;15(1):201.
84. Dentali F, Marchesi C, Pierfranceschi MG, Crowther M, Garcia D, Hylek E, et al. Safety of prothrombin complex concentrates for rapid anticoagulation reversal of vitamin K antagonists. Thromb Haemost. 2011;106(3):429–38.
85. Grottke O, Rossaint R, Henskens Y, van Oerle R, ten Cate H, Spronk HM. Thrombin generation capacity of prothrombin complex concentrate in an in vitro dilutional model. PLoS One. 2013;8(5):e64100.
86. Pabinger I, Brenner B, Kalina U, Knaub S, Nagy A, Ostermann H. Prothrombin complex concentrate (Beriplex® P/N) for emergency anticoagulation reversal: a prospective multinational clinical trial. J Thromb Haemost. 2008;6(4):622–31.
87. Schulman S, Bijsterveld NR. Anticoagulants and their reversal. Transfus Med Rev. 2007;21(1):37–48.
88. Strengers P, Drenth J. PPSB as first choice treatment in the reversal of oral anticoagulant therapy. Acta Anaesthesiol Belg. 2001;53(3):183–6.
89. Lusher J. Thrombogenicity associated with factor IX complex concentrates. Semin Hematol. 1991;28:3.
90. Schulman S, Johnsson H, Lindmarker P. Thrombotic complications after substitution with a FVII concentrate. Thromb Haemost. 1991;66(5):619.
91. Escoffre M, Zini J, Schuamser L, Mazoyer E, Soria C, Tobelem G, et al. Severe arterial thrombosis in a congenitally factor VII deficient patient. Br J Haematol. 1995;91(3):739–41.
92. Ferster A, Capouet V, Deville A, Fondu P, Corazza F. Cardiac surgery with extracorporeal circulation in severe factor VII deficiency. Pathophysiol Haemost Thromb. 1993;23(1):65–8.

Congenital Factor X Deficiency

11

Fateme Roshanzamir and Akbar Dorgalaleh

11.1 Introduction

Coagulation factor X (FX) is a vitamin K-dependent glycoprotein which plays a pivotal role in the coagulation cascade. After its activation, activated FX (FXa) is the first enzyme in the common coagulation pathway. Congenital FX deficiency is a rare bleeding disorder that is inherited in autosomal recessive manner; therefore it equally affects both genders. It is estimated to occur in 1:1,000,000 individuals, although the prevalence is much greater in areas with high rate of consanguineous marriage [1, 2]. Although, bleeding manifestations usually occur in homozygous and compound heterozygous cases, heterozygous cases generally are symptomatic. Regardless to severity of FX deficiency, the most common bleeding symptoms are mucocutaneous bleedings including epistaxis, gum bleeding, and easy bruising. The patients with severe FX deficiency have a high incidence of spontaneous major bleeding. The bleeding may occur at any age; however, the cases with severe FX deficiency with FX coagulatn activity (FX:C) <1% may be diagnosed early in life with abnormal bleeding tendency. The affected women at reproductive age may present with menorrhagia [1–4].

F. Roshanzamir
Blood Transfusion Research Center, High Institute for Research and Education in Transfusion Medicine, Tehran, Iran
e-mail: F-Roshanzamir@alumnus.tums.ac.ir

A. Dorgalaleh (✉)
Department of Hematology and Blood transfusion, School of Allied Medicine, Iran University of Medical Sciences, Tehran, Iran

A. Dorgalaleh (ed.), *Congenital Bleeding Disorders*,
https://doi.org/10.1007/978-3-319-76723-9_11

11.2 Factor X Structure and Function

FX that is also known as autoprothrombin III and Stuart-Prower factor is a serine protease which mainly is synthesized in the liver. Its zymogen form secretes to plasma and circulates as a two-chain molecule with a concentration of 8–10 μg/ml (Table 11.1) [5].

FX contains a 40-residue pre-propeptide and hydrophobic signal sequence (−37 to −22) in homology with the other vitamin K-dependent coagulation factors. The signal sequence is cleaved in a two-step process. The first cleavage occurs after Leu-29 and then the propeptide (−1 to −18) is removed from the N-terminus of light chain by second peptidase (between −1Arg and +1Ala). It seems that the propeptide is important for intracellular post-translational modifications in FX that is essential for its function. The light chain of FX contains 11 glutamic acid residues which are modified to γ-carboxyglutamic acid (Gla) domains. Ten residues are encoded by exon II and the last one encoded by exon III. The Gla domains are necessary for the binding of Ca^{2+} ions and negatively charged phospholipid membranes.

Mature FX consists of two light (17 kDa) and heavy chains (45 kDa) that are covalently linked to each other by a disulfide bond between residues Cys89 and Cys124 and a tripeptide (Arg-Lys-Arg). The light chain consists of 139 amino acids which form Gla domain, a high proportion of aromatic amino acids segment (aromatic stack) and two epidermal growth factor (EGF)-like domains. There are three conserved Gly and six Cys residues forming three unique disulfide bonds in each EGF-like domain. These domains are important for maintaining the correct conformation of FXa. The heavy chain consists of 346 residues that form catalytic serine protease domain and activation peptide. The catalytic domain contains the catalytic site—His236, Asp282, and Ser379 which is homologous with other vitamin K-dependent factors and trypsin-like enzymes. The activation peptide is cleaved when FX is activated (Fig. 11.1) [1, 6, 7].

11.3 Factor X Activation

The zymogen form of coagulation FX is cleaved in Arg194-Ile195 peptide bond of the heavy chain. This cleavage releases a 52-residues activation peptide and produces the active form of FX (FXa). Then second cleavage occurs at the C-terminus to produce FXaβ [7].

Table 11.1 General characterizations of coagulation factor X

Name	OMIM no	Prevalence of homozygous form	Gene (kb)	Chromosoe location	Number of exon	Hemostatic level	Plasma half-life (h)
FX	227,600	1 in 1,000,000	*F10* (26.7)	13q34	8	15–20%	40–60

FX factor X, *OMIM no* *O*nline *M*endelian *I*nheritance in *M*an is the largest registry of human genetics disease (http://www.ncbi.nlm.nih.gov/entrez/query.fcgi?db=OMIM)

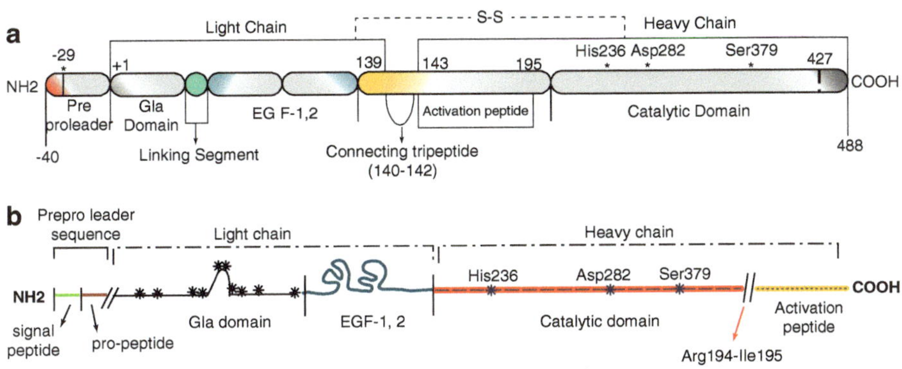

Fig. 11.1 (**a**) Factor (F) X polypeptide structure and its functional domains. The signal peptidase probably cleavages FX protein at residue −29 and the mature protein initiates from residue +1. The light chain consists of 139 amino acids (residues +1 to 139) containing Gla domain and EGF-1, 2 domains, while the heavy chain consists of 364 residues (143–448) containing activation peptide and catalytic domain in which activation peptide is located at residues 143–195. The position of connecting tripeptide (Arg-Lys-Arg) is between residues 140 and 142. Clotting FX is activated by cleavage at Arg194-Ile195. The second cleavage at residue 427 generates FXaβ. The catalytic site within the catalytic domain is formed by His236, Asp282, and Ser379. (**b**) Schematic of FX structure. Separated part indicates the cleavage of pre-pro-leader sequence. The Gla domain is shown with Gla residues and the active sites His, Asp, and Ser are shown in the catalytic domain. Two light and heavy chains are linked by a disulfide bond. The cleavage site of activation peptide (yellow part) is indicated by the red arrow. *EGF* epidermal growth factor

FX may be activated either in vivo or in vitro. A complex of tissue factor (TF), FVIIa, Ca^{2+} ion, and appropriate phospholipid membrane is required for in vivo activation of FX and FIX (extrinsic pathway of coagulation cascade) (please refer to Chap. 1). Physiologically activation of FIX by TF/FVIIa complex is more important than direct activation of FX. Generation of FVIIa is amplified via a positive feedback loop by produced of FXa. Phospholipid membrane may be provided by a variety of cell types such as fibroblast, monocyte-macrophage, and endothelial cells as well as tumor cells. Conversion of FX to FXa also occurs through coagulation intrinsic pathway by interaction of FIXa, FVIIIa, Ca^{2+} ion, and phospholipid membrane (platelet and/or endothelial cells) (Fig. 11.2). In vitro activation of FX may occur by Russell viper venom of the snake *Vipera russelli.* It contains a metalloproteinase which can directly activate FX without Ca^{2+} ion or phospholipid membrane [1, 7, 8].

FXa could be generated independent of either TF/FVIIa or FIXa/FVIIIa, Ca^{2+} ion, and phospholipid membrane. For instance, some malignant cells cysteine proteinase may be involved in FX activation [1, 7].

FXa is the major activator of prothrombin. A complex of FXa, FVa, and Ca^{2+} ion at a suitable phospholipid membrane (prothrombinase complex) can 280,000-fold accelerate prothrombin conversion. This complex may assemble on the surface of platelets, lymphocytes, monocytes, neutrophils, and endothelial cells. The suggested model for prothrombinase complex shows that, initially, FVa binds to the negatively charged phospholipid membrane through its light chain and provides a

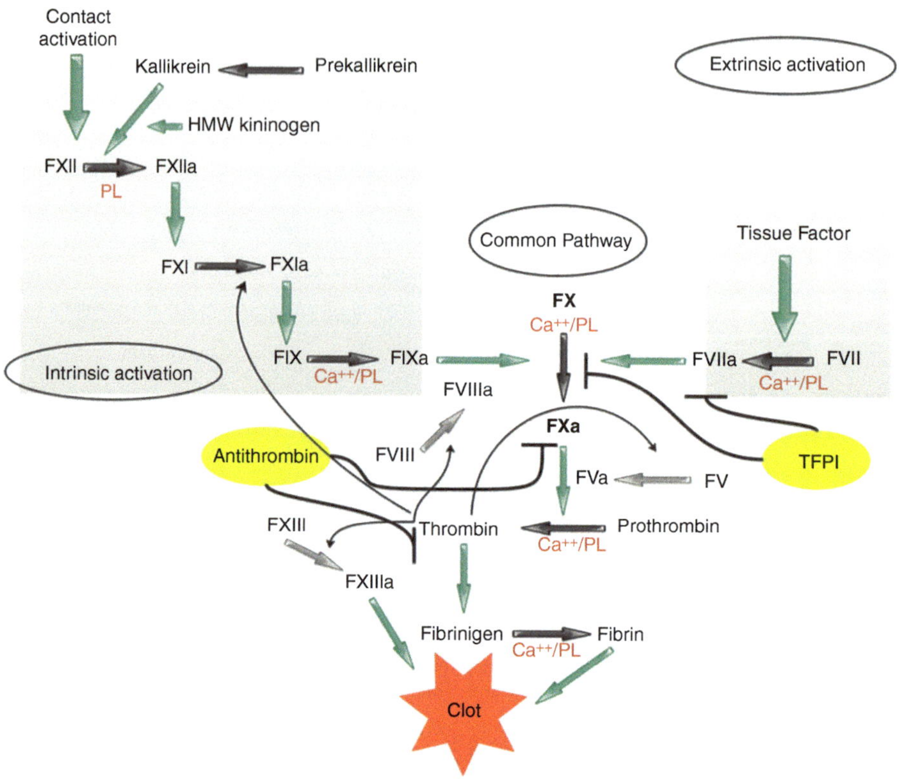

Fig. 11.2 Coagulation cascade. This illustration represents role and activation of clotting factor (F) X in the coagulation cascade. FX is the first enzyme of common pathway activating by a complex of TF/FVIIa/Ca^{2+}/PL through extrinsic pathway and FIXa/FVIIIa/Ca^{2+}/PL via intrinsic route. Then a complex of FXa/FVa/Ca^{2+}/PL (prothrombinase complex) cleavages prothrombin to the thrombin that subsequently leads to cleavage of fibrinogen to fibrin. Finally FXIIIa stabilizes the generated clot. FV, FVIII, FIX, and FXIII also are activated by thrombin. Activation of FX may be inhibited by tissue factor pathway inhibitor (TFPI) and antithrombin. TFPI is a pivotal inhibitor of extrinsic pathway that in complex with FXa/TF/FVIIa inhibits their catalytic activity. Antithrombin also affects FXa and generates a stable inactive complex (please refer to Chap. 1). TF, tissue Factor; FVII, factor VII; FVIIa, activated factor VII; FX, factor X; FXa, activated factor X; FXII, factor XII; FXIIa, activated factor XII; FXI, factor IX; FIXa, activated factor IX; FXa, activated factor IX; FVIII, factor VIII; FVIIIa, activated factor VIII; FV, factor V; FVa, activated factor V; FXIII, factor XIII; FXIIIa, activated factor XIII; TFPI, tissue factor pathway inhibitor; PL, phospholipid

suitable receptor for FXa. Then FXa binds to the membrane surface via Gla domains of its light chain and interacts with FVa by its heavy chain. FVa also interacts with prothrombin through its heavy chain without Ca^{2+} ion. Then prothrombin binds to the membrane surface by formation of Ca^{2+} bridges (Gla residues). Finally, prothrombin is cleaved by prothrombinase complex and is converted to the thrombin. Actually, FVa is cofactor of FXa which enhances the catalytic efficacy of FXa, and the negatively charged phospholipid membrane is an appropriate surface that increases the local concentration of FXa, FVa, and prothrombin to accelerate conversion of prothrombin to the active serine protease, thrombin. FV, FVII, and FVIII are other substrates of FXa. FXa may cleave both FV and FVIII to generate their active form. Activation of FVII and FX is a reciprocal pathway. FXa is generated by TF/FVIIa complex and then FVIIa is increased by FXa in a positive feedback loop [1].

11.4 Regulation of Factor X Activity

Antithrombin (III) Antithrombin affects FXa and forms a stable inactive complex. Therefore FXa is inhibited by antithrombin. Generated inactive complexes of FX are removed from the circulation by the liver. Low molecular weight heparin (LMWH) enhances the anti-Xa activity of antithrombin. Various sulfated glycosaminoglycans may accelerate the antithrombin activity.

Tissue Factor Pathway Inhibitor (TFPI) TFPI is the pivotal inhibitor of coagulation extrinsic pathway. It binds to FXa in a 1:1 ratio and then forms a quaternary complex with TF-FVIIa. The complex of TFPI/FXa/TF/FVIIa lacks TF/FVIIa catalytic activity, so the coagulation cascade is turned off (please refer to Chap. 10).

Factor VIII and Activated Factor X FXa is involved in inactivation of FVIIIa. Therefore FXa is inhibited via a negative feedback loop [7].

11.5 Congenital Factor X Deficiency

Congenital FX deficiency is one of the rarest coagulation bleeding disorders that was identified by two independent groups in the 1950s [7]. First, Telfer et al. described a significant bleeding tendency in a 22-year-old patient (Prower) in 1956; then 1 year later, Hougie et al. reported a 36-year-old man (Stuart) with abnormal clotting assays. At first they thought that bleeding tendency in these patients is due to FVII deficiency, but later they found that direct mixing of the patient plasma with FVII-deficient plasma led to correction of prolonged prothrombin time (PT). Hougie et al. found that aPTT, Russell viper venom (RVVT), and thromboplastin generation test are prolonged in the patient, while in patients with FVII deficiency, both aPTT and thromboplastin generation tests are normal. So it became clear that there is deficiency in a clotting factor other than FVII. It was named Stuart-Prower factor by Telfer and Hougie. Then in 1954, Duckert et al. described a type of factor deficiency that was distinct from FVII and FIX deficiency in a patient who received coumarin anticoagulants. Finally it was officially named FX in 1962 [1–3, 7, 9].

FX deficiency or Sturt-Prower disease is inherited in autosomal recessive manner, so it equally affects both genders.

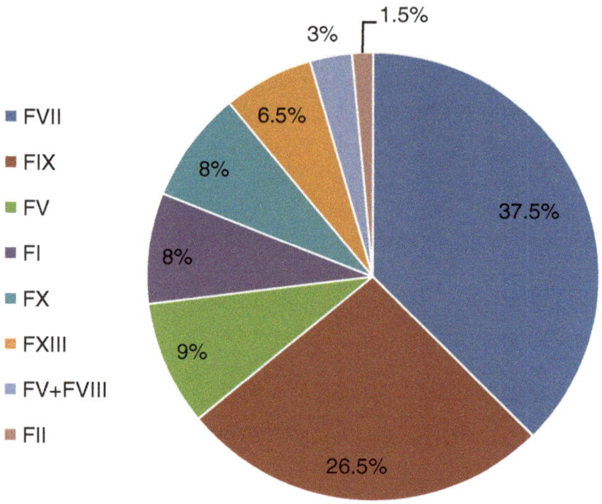

Fig. 11.3 Relative percent of rare bleeding disorders

Estimated incidence of FX deficiency in homozygous form is 1:1,000,000, while the prevalence of heterozygotes is ~1:500. It encompassed 8% of all rare bleeding disorders (Fig. 11.3). Similar to other autosomal recessive diseases, it is more frequent in areas with high rate of consanguineous marriages [2, 10, 11]. FX is activated through extrinsic and intrinsic coagulation pathways and has a pivotal role in common pathway. It is a key part of prothrombinase complex, so FX deficiency causes defects in formation of prothrombinase complex and leads to bleeding. Congenital FX deficiency presents with variable bleeding tendency. Heterozygotes usually are asymptomatic, but bleeding symptoms may occur due to insufficient enzymatic activity or interference of mutant gene product with normal reaction of coagulation pathway [7, 9].

11.6 Classification

FX deficiency could be simply classified in two types: type 1 is described by concomitant reduction in antigenic and functional levels of FX, whereas type 2 is demonstrated with decrease in FX:C and normal or nearly normal antigenic level of FX (FX:Ag) [1]. The first classification of FX deficiency was established in 1969–1970 including type I or cross-reacting maternal negative (CRM^-) (Stuart family), type II or CRM^+ (Prower family), and CRM Friuli form. CRM^- type is described by simultaneous reduction of both FX:Ag and FX:C levels as a result of abnormal synthesis or secretion of the protein, while CRM^+ form is characterized by normal or nearly normal FX:Ag and reduction of FX:C. During years a wide range of *F10* gene defects have been identified that affect only extrinsic or intrinsic coagulation pathway. So it became clear that type II or CRM^+ is heterogeneous type with various presentations in different families. Therefore this classification was insufficient to describe all types of FX deficiency. Establishing molecular biology techniques studying *F10* gene in the last two decades leads to identification of several mutations in association with different types of FX deficiency. According to molecular studies, FX deficiency could be classified based on the type of mutations, e.g., nonsense, missense, insertion, deletion, etc. There is also a classification on the basis of the site that mutations occur including promoter, Gla domain, EGF domain, activation peptide, and catalytic domain. Despite of these investigations, no obvious correlation has been found between genotype and phenotype in FX deficiency. Mutations in the same area may accompany with different phenotypes, whereas the same phenotypes may be due to different mutations. The only exception is variants in Gla domain of the light chain that accompany with similar phenotypes in different cases.

In conclusion because of the great heterogeneity in genotype and phenotype of FX deficiency, it seems that more suitable classification could be achieved by using immunological, functional, and clotting assays as well as molecular biology studies. According to these considerations, the following classification has been proposed by Denson, Fair, Edgington, and then by Girolamt et al. that is more acceptable and practical:

Type I: CRM negative or Stuart like (classic form of congenital FX deficiency)
Type II: CRM positive or Prower like, inert protein
Type III: CRM positive with disreactive protein that is categorized in four levels:
- CRM positive Friuli like: defects in all clotting assays except for RVVT
- CRM positive Padua like: defects only or mainly in extrinsic pathway
- CRM positive Melbourne like: defects only or mainly in intrinsic pathway
- Defects with contradiction in chromogenic assay

Type IV: concurrent deficiency in FX and other coagulation factors mostly FVII as a result of abnormality in chromosome 13 (Table 11.2) [9, 12]

It is worth noting that the pattern of clotting assays is variable among different patients based on involved area of *F10* gene and protein. For instance, Girolamis et al. in 2008 described some cases of mutations in catalytic domain and light chain

Table 11.2 Classification of factor X deficiency

Type		Clotting assay			Chromogenic assay	Antigenic assay (FX:Ag)
		PT	aPTT	RVVT		
I	CRM negative	↓	↓	↓	↓	↓
II	CRM positive	↓	↓	↓	↓	N or nearly N
III	Friuli like	↓	↓	N	↓	N or nearly N
	Padua like	↓	N	N	↓	N or nearly N
	Melbourne like	N	↓	N	↓	N or nearly N
	–	↑	↑	↑	H	N or nearly N
IV[a]	–	↓	↓	↓	↓	↓

[a]FX deficiency concomitant deficiency of other clotting factors especially factor VII, *CRM* cross-reacting material, *PT* prothrombin time, *aPTT* activated partial thromboplastin time, *RVVT* Russell viper venom time, *FX* factor X, *FX:Ag* factor X Antigen, *N* normal, *H* high

C-terminal of FX protein which affect mainly intrinsic pathway. They also reported some variants in Gla domain of light chain, EGF domain, and catalytic domain that predominantly affect extrinsic pathway [1, 7, 12].

11.7 Clinical Manifestations

Clinical features of the patients with FX deficiency are in association with the plasma level of FX protein, but the correlation between the plasma level of FX and bleeding tendency is not as strong as hemophilia A and B [3, 4]. The severity of disease could be classified into three grades according to the FX:C [2, 3, 13]:

1. Severe: FX:C <1 U/dL
2. Moderate: FX:C 1–5 U/dL
3. Mild: FX:C 6–10 U/dL

Although the bleeding may occur at any ages, the most severely affected patients with FX:C less than 1% can present with life-threatening manifestations such as umbilical cord bleeding or intracranial hemorrhage (ICH) in the neonatal period [2–4, 13]. Patients with different FX:C levels demonstrate variable bleeding tendency. Moderately affected individuals with 1–5% FX:C level may bleed due to hemostatic challenges such as operation or trauma, while mildly affected cases (FX:C: 6–10%) generally are asymptomatic and identified based on family studies or occasionally on routine laboratory evaluations, but easy bruising and menorrhagia may occur in some patients (Table 11.3) [1, 3, 13]. Symptomatic patients of clotting factor deficiencies are usually homozygous or compound heterozygous; however, there are some reports of post-dental extraction and post-delivery bleeding in heterozygote of FX deficiency [4].

Generally, regardless of severity of the disease, mucosal bleeding, particularly epistaxis, and easy bruising are the most common symptoms in congenital FX deficiency. Menorrhagia is an unusual symptom of affected women at reproductive ages, while recurrent miscarriages and placental abrupt rarely occurred. Other clinical manifestations including central nervous system (CNS) bleeding, umbilical cord bleedings (usually during neonatal period), and gastrointestinal (GI) bleeding as

Table 11.3 Classification and clinical presentations of patients with congenital factor X deficiency

Severity	Factor X level	Clinical features (predominantly)
Mild	6–10 U/dL	Usually asymptomatic or occasionally present easy bruising, epistaxis, and menorrhagia
Moderate	1–5 U/dL	Mucosal bleeding and traumatic or surgical bleedings
Severe	<1 U/dL	Mucosal bleeding, ICH and umbilical cord bleeding especially during neonatal period, hemarthrosis, hematoma, hematuria, and GI bleeding

ICH intracranial hemorrhage, *GI* gastrointestinal

well as recurrent hemarthrosis, hematoma, and hematuria usually present in the most severely deficient patients [2, 3, 13]. Some life-threatening and limb-endangering clinical manifestations such as umbilical cord bleeding, hemarthrosis, and soft tissue hematoma occur more frequently in the cases with FII, FX, and FXIII deficiencies (please refer to Chap. 2) [5].

Herrmann et al. analyzed clinical manifestations of 102 patients with FX deficiency from Europe and Latin America with *F10* gene mutations in 2006. The most severe bleeding symptoms among 42 symptomatic patients (homozygous, heterozygous, and compound heterozygous) were ICH, GI bleeding, and hemarthrosis that were observed in cases with FX:C <2%. However there were differences among the bleeding patterns of the patients due to corresponding genotypes and the type of mutation. Among clinically symptomatic subjects, 13% were heterozygous, mainly with mucocutaneous hemorrhage. It could occur either due to insufficient enzymatic activity of FX wild type or inhibition of one reaction in the clotting cascade by FX mutant protein [14].

The most common bleeding symptom among 32 Iranian patients, regardless of the disorder severity, was epistaxis (72%). Other clinical manifestations including GI bleeding and hematuria were mainly observed in the cases with undetectable level of FX. In this study, umbilical stump bleeding was found unexpectedly in 9 patients occurring at the time of stump detachment (7–10 day after birth). A direct correlation between FX level and bleeding diathesis was observed in this study (Table 11.4) [2, 14–16].

Table 11.4 Prevalence of bleeding symptoms in patients with congenital factor X deficiency

Symptom	Herrmann et al. (*n* = 42) (%)	Peyvandi et al. (*n* = 32) (%)	Acharya et al. Homo (*n* = 19) (%)	Acharya et al. S Hetero (*n* = 15) (%)	Anwar et al. (*n* = 20) (%)
Epistaxis	36	72	45[a]	75[a]	35
Gum bleeding	31	–	–	–	35
Easy bruising	55	–	–	–	45
Hematoma	43	66	27	–	–
Hematuria	7	25	–	–	5
Hemarthrosis	33	69	–	–	5
GI bleeding	12	38	4–9	12	10
CNS bleeding	21	9	15	–	–
Umbilical cord bleeding	–	28	–	–	15
Post-circumcision bleeding	–	–	–	–	30
Menorrhagia[b]	71	505	–	–	10
Post-operative hemorrhage	–	–	4	13	–

Homo homozygous, *S Hetero* symptomatic heterozygous, *GI* gastrointestinal, *CNS* central nerves system

[a]Skin and mucus membrane bleeding

[b]Women in reproductive age

11.8 Acquired Factor X Deficiency

In addition to inherited form of disease, FX deficiency may occur secondary to other disorders such as AL amyloidosis, myeloma, tumors, infections, and drug consumption as well as liver disease [1]. Acquired deficiency of FX may present either as isolated deficiency or along with other factors deficiencies, e.g., FV [3, 10].

1. Liver disease or vitamin K deficiency

   Deficiency of vitamin K due to malabsorption or oral anticoagulants may result in FX deficiency. On the other hand, affected patients with dysfunction liver or hepatocellular damages such as hepatocellular carcinoma (HCC) are also at risk of acquired FX deficiency. However, in such disorders, there is concomitant decrease of other hepatic-derived or vitamin K-dependent coagulation factors [3, 4].
2. AL amyloidosis

   For the first time, Korsan-Bengsten et al. reported a case of amyloidosis with concomitant FX deficiency. They described an association between amyloidosis and FX deficiency. Since then more similar cases were reported in several studies, and the correlation between systemic amyloidosis and FX deficiency became more clear [1].

   Amyloidosis is a general name to define some clinical disorders in which insoluble abnormal fibril proteins are aggregated extra- or intracellularly on the affected tissues that leads to functional defects of involved organs. Primary or systemic light chain amyloidosis that is also called AL amyloidosis is a myeloma-associated disorder. It is characterized by deposition of immunoglobulin abnormal light chain that involves variable organs and may lead to thrombotic and hemorrhagic complications [17]. Isolated FX deficiency is the most clinically significant coagulopathy in association with primary amyloidosis that occurs in 6.3–14% of cases [18]. It seems that irreversible binding of FX to the abnormal amyloid fibrils that usually occurs in the liver, spleen, and vasculature leads to rapid clearance of both endogenous and exogenous FX from plasma. Therefore in this situation, either antigenic or functional levels of FX are reduced, although reduction in the level of FX:C is more profound than FX:Ag [3, 10]. The most common clinical manifestations in acquired isolated FX deficiency similar to congenital form of disease are epistaxis, easy bruising, and menorrhagia. Amyloidosis is usually accompanied by other hemostatic disorders such as other clotting factor deficiencies due to liver damages, vascular fragility because of amyloid infiltration, and defects in platelet aggregation as well as fibrin polymerization. Therefore, it is not practically possible to determine an obvious correlation between severity of disorder and the FX:C level. Acquired FX deficiency in relation with secondary or AA amyloidosis is very rare [1, 3, 18].
3. Miscellaneous

   In addition to acquired FX deficiency due to AL amyloidosis, there are few reports of non-amyloid deficiency of FX [10]. Some malignancies such as myeloma without amyloidosis, acute myeloid leukemia, thymoma, as well as renal, adrenal, and gastric carcinoma may lead to reduction of FX level. However, the exact mechanism is not clear. In addition to malignancies, a transient FX deficiency has been reported in relation to viral or bacterial upper respiratory tract infections, especially due to mycoplasma pneumonia. It is probably due to similar antigenic determinants of FX and the infectious agents. Therefore, circulatory FX is cleared by patient's immune system [1, 3, 10, 18]. Some medicines may also be in association with isolated reduction of FX, e.g., exposure to sodium valproate or treatment with fungicides and amsacrine [18]. Warfarin and other oral anticoagulants could be in charge of acquired FX deficiency along with reduction of other coagulation factors [3].

11.9 Factor X Inhibitors

Inhibitor formation in patients with congenital FX deficiency is a very rare phenomenon, but is more frequent in acquired deficiency. Observation of abnormally prolonged PT, aPTT, without correction in mixing study in a symptomatic case without prior history of bleeding or immune disease is doubtful to existence of an inhibitor. The inhibitor of FX may be either specific or nonspecific due to presence of lupus anticoagulant or may occur as a result of burns, leprosy, and respiratory tract infections [1, 13, 18].

11.10 Factor X Deficiency in Pregnancy

Normally the level of FX enhances in childbearing women, but severely affected women with FX deficiency in fertility ages are at high risk of abortion or preterm delivery [1]. To optimize the outcomes of pregnancy, careful prophylaxis and replacement therapy may be useful. There are some concerns about FX-deficient women who are at childbearing ages. First, it should be considered that their opportunity for fertilization is lower than normal population because of either higher frequency of bleeding in some organs such as ovary or prolonged menstruation especially in women with FX level less than 1%. Second, affected pregnant women are at high risk of severe hemorrhagic complications following some necessary invasive procedures, e.g., chorionic villus sampling (CVS), amniocentesis, or axillary reproductive techniques. Sampling of CVS and amniocentesis are required for prenatal diagnosis (PND). Another concern is about heritability of FX deficiency. Since deficiency of FX is inherited in traditional Mendelian behavior, in regions with high rate of consanguinity, either affected or mandatory carrier offspring would be expected more than other areas [19].

Therefore, for FX-deficient pregnant women or who want to try pregnancy, a team of experts and adequately equipped center are required for appropriate management of patients during pregnancy and within labor. In such conditions, more affected women are able to experience low-risk pregnancy and delivery healthy infant [1, 19].

11.11 Molecular Basis

The human FX gene (*F10*) is 22 kb, mapping on long arm of chromosome 13 at 13q34, 2.8 kb downstream of *F7*gene (Fig. 11.4) [3].

As there is significant homology in *F10* gene and the other vitamin K-dependent clotting factors, both in structure and organization, an evaluation from a common ancestral gene is suggested. The *F10* gene spread approximately 27 kb of genomic sequence. It has eight exons which each exon encodes a specific part of FX protein (Fig. 11.5) [20]. Exon I encodes the signal peptide; exon II codes the propeptide and γ-carboxyglutamic acid-rich (Gla) domain. Exon III codes a short linking segment of aromatic amino acid (aromatic stack), exons IV and V encode two regions homologous to EGF, and exon VI codes activation peptide at the amino-terminus of the heavy chain. Exons VII and VIII encode two active serine protease domains containing the residues for the catalytic triad (His236, Asp282, and Ser379) (Table 11.5) [7].

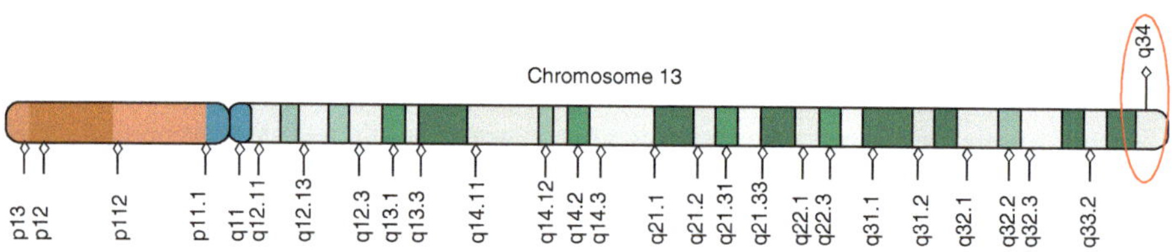

Fig. 11.4 Chromosomal location of *F10* gene. The *F10* gene is located in long arm of chromosome 13 at 13q34

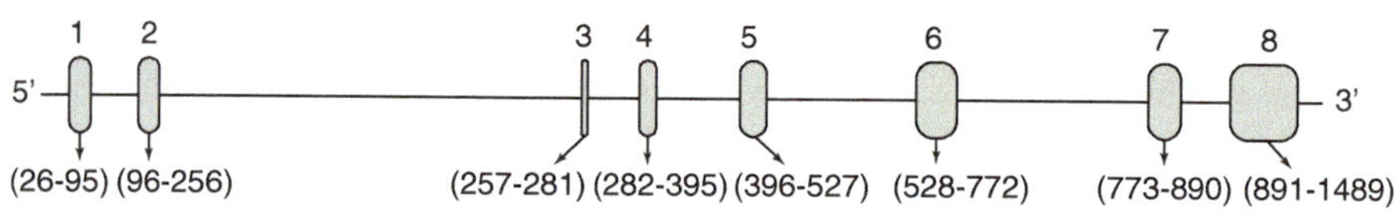

Fig. 11.5 *F10* gene organization. The *F10* gene consists of eight exons. The illustration shows the location of first and last nucleotides of each exon

Table 11.5 Characteristics of *F10* gene

Exon	Size (bp)	Domain
1	70	Pre-pro-leader sequence (aa-40 to −17)
2	161	Propeptide region containing Gla domain (aa-17 to +37)
3	25	Linking region (aa38 to 46)
4	114	EGF-1 (aa46 to 84)
5	132	EGF-2 (aa84 to 128)
6	245	Connecting region and activation peptide (aa128 to 209)
7	118	Catalytic domain (aa210 to 249)
8	599	Catalytic domain (aa249 to 448)

bp base pair, *aa* amino acid, *Gla* γ-carboxyglutamic acid rich, *EGF* epidermal growth factor

The *F10* cDNA consists of 120 bp encoding 40 amino acids pre-pro-leader sequence and 1344 bp coding 488 amino acids of the mature protein. There is a short 3′ untranslated region of 10 bp preceding the poly (A) tail. An obvious TATA box has not been identified at 5′ end of *F10* gene, but almost six different transcription initiation sites have been detected at 5′ region like other TATA-less promoter genes. Analysis of *F10* gene promoter shows that a 200-bp region upstream of the coding region is vital for its function. *F10* gene has been cloned by different groups. Isolated *F10* colons with a lack of 9-bp sequence encoding a tripeptide (Lys-Val-Arg) have been detected by different groups. At first, it was considered as an artifact but later Tuddenham and Copper suggested that it is as a result of formation of a "semi-cryptic" splice site that led to alternative processing. Several polymorphisms also have been detected within *F10* gene [1, 7].

Since FX has a leading role in coagulation cascade common pathway, absolute lack of FX seems to be incompatible with life. Some surveys on *F10* gene knockout mice have proven that complete absence of FX is lethal for mice, but it is different in human. Patients with undetectable activity of FX as a result of null mutations can survive, although they are dependent on constant replacement therapy [1, 7]. There is no hot spot region in *F10* gene, and the number of mutations occurring in each exon relatively is proportional to its length; however, most mutations happen in exon 8 (Fig. 11.6) [1, 13, 20]. Almost all types of mutations such as deletion, nonsense, missense, splice site, and frame shift have been reported in *F10* gene so far. However, missense single point mutations, mostly localized in Gla and catalytic domains (exons 2, 7, 8), are the most reported *F10* gene lesions (Fig. 11.7) [21]. Generally missense mutations are the most frequent gene effects in most of congenital bleeding disorders.

There are also some reports of FX deficiency as a part of vitamin K-dependent clotting factors deficiency due to some defects in either γ-glutamyl carboxylase (*GGCX*) or subunit 1 of vitamin K epoxide reductase complex (*VKORC1*) (please refer to Chap. 9). Among different reported *F10* gene mutations, some mutations are in association with severe and life-endangering manifestations. Gly380Arg, IVS7-1G > A, and Tyr163delAT are such mutations that are associated with high incidence of ICH, and Gly-20Arg is in association with severe hemarthrosis. A number of mutations such as Leu-32pro, Glu102Lys, and Gly114Arg are more common in patients with mild deficiency [1–4, 7, 13, 14, 22].

1. Chromosomal abnormalities/gene deletions

   The first molecular abnormality effecting *F10* gene was 13q34 monosomy reported by Scambler and Williamson. They described a patient who suffered from concomitant deficiency of FX and FVII, while her brother was trisomic for 13q34 and had increased levels of FX and FVII. *FX San Antonio* arises from an 838-T single nucleotide deletion that leads to a frame shift and production of a stop codon at residue 232. *San Giovanni Rotondo FX* is also due to a single nucleotide deletion (556-C) that leads to the creation of a stop codon in residue 226.

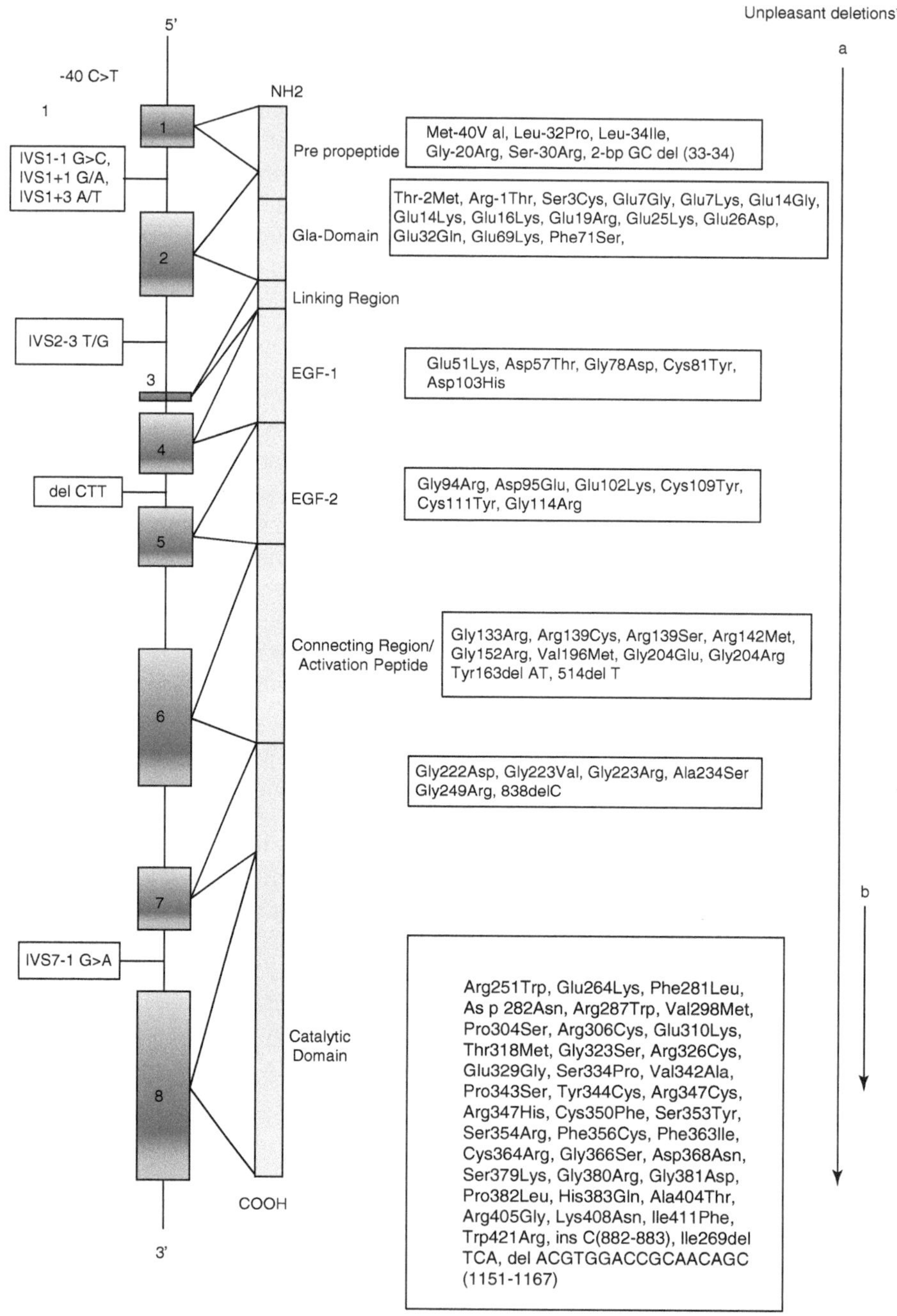

Fig. 11.6 *F10* gene mutations. The first filled boxes show exons of *F10* gene and the second one shows the protein domains. The number of mutations in exon 8 is more than others. Frequency of mutations in each exon is relatively proportional to its length, suggesting that there is no hot spot in *F10* gene. *Unpleasant deletions: (**a**) complete deletion of gene and partial deletion of exons 7 and 8, (**b**) deletion of exon 7 and part of exon 8

Fig. 11.7 Frequency of different type of mutations in *F10* gene (141 mutations)

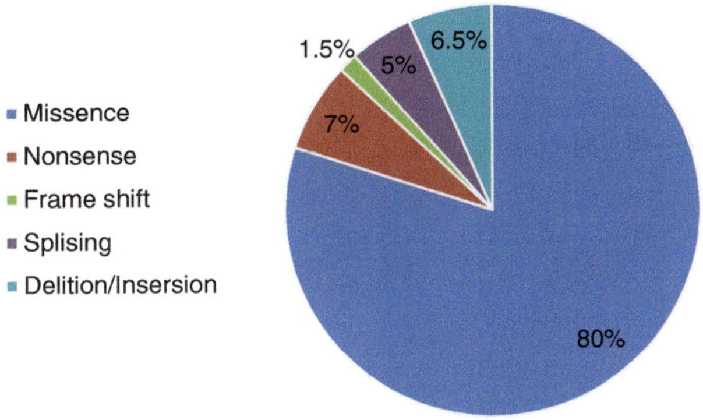

2. Missense mutations

FX Nice I: It arises from Met-40Val substitution. FX Nice I usually occurs in concomitant with *FX Nice II* (Pro304Ser). The FX:C and FX:Ag levels are 4% (based on PT assay) and 7%, respectively. The replacement of methionine by valine results in the complete loss of translation of FX, while the Pro304Ser mutation leads to defective FX secretion [1, 7].

FX Santo Domingo: It is a variant that results from a G-A substitution leading to replacement of glycine at position −20 to arginine (Gly20Arg). The FX activity is <1% and the antigenic level is <5% in the homozygous state. This mutation affects signal peptide of FX protein, so the FX protein is not processed by signal peptidase into the endoplasmic reticulum [1].

A compound heterozygous of Thr2Met and Cys111Tyr has been reported by Miller et al. that former affects propeptide sequence. These variants were observed in an asymptomatic patient with the FX:C and the FX:Ag levels of 12% and 26%, respectively.

FX St. Louis II: In this variant, replacement of the Gla residue by a glycine at residue 7 results in the loss of one Gla residue of the Gla domain, which affects Ca^{2+} binding of the molecule. This mutation is characterized with the normal level of FX:Ag; however, the activity level is <1%.

Factor X Voralberg and Factor X Frankfurt I: Two variants Glu14Lys and Glu102Lys that reduce the FX affinity to calcium ion were identified in *FX Voralberg* cases. In homozygous cases of *FX Voralberg*, the FX activity is <10% (PT based) and the antigen level is about 20%. *FX Frankfurt* results from Glu25Lys replacement. It was reported in a patient with a FX:C and FX:Ag of 56% and 55%, respectively.

FX Friuli: FX Friuli was the first dysfunctional mutant FX and the most well-characterized mutation in FX. Pro343Ser replacement causes new hydrogen bridge formation between Ser343 and Thr318 in the catalytic domain. So the tertiary structure of the domain and its catalytic potential is affected. FX Friuli is characterized by FX normal antigen level and near-normal Stypven time, but prolonged PT and aPTT-based clotting assays. It occurs in both heterozygous and homozygous states (Table 11.6) [1, 7, 23].

Table 11.6 Characterizations of some FX gene mutations

Name	Mutation	Involved exon and domain	Clotting assay			FX:C	FX:Ag	Comment
			PT	aPTT	RVVT			
Nice I Nice II	ATG > GTG Met-40Val CCC > TCC Pro304Ser	Exon 1, preproregion Exon 8, catalytic domain	↓	ND	ND	ND	↓	Start codon is destroyed by loss of Met Hydrophobic core is destabilized, problem in secretion
Stuart	GTG > ATG Val246Met	Exon 7, catalytic domain	↓	↓	↓	↓	↓	–
Santo Domingo	GGG > AGG Gly-20Arg	Exon 1, pre-propeptide	↓	↓	↓	↓	↓	Prevents from secretion
St Louis II	GAG > GGG Glu7Gly	Exon 2, Gla domain	↓	↓	ND	ND	N	Affects Ca^{2+} binding
Ketchikan	GAA > GGA Glu14Gly	Exon 2, Gla domain	↓	↓	↓	ND	↓	Affects Ca^{2+} binding
Vienna	GGG > GAG Gly204Glu	Exon 6, activation domain	↓	↓	ND	↓	↓	–
Voralberg	GAA > AAA Glu14Lys GAG>AAG Glu102Lys	Exon 2, Gla domain	↓	↓	↓	↓	↓	–
Malmo 4	GAG > GAC Glu26Asp	Exon 2, Gla domain	↓	↓	ND	↓	ND	–
Tokyo	GAG >CAG Glu32Gln	Exon 2, Gla domain	↓	NN	↓	ND	N	Affects Ca^{2+} binding
Wenatchee II Wenatchee I	AAC > AC Asn57Thr CGC > TGC Arg139Cys	Exon 4, EGF Exon 6, activation domain	↓	↓	↓ND	↓	↓	Compound heterozygote
Kurayoshi	CGC > AGC Arg139Ser	Exon 6, activation domain	↓	↓	↓	N	N	Interaction with FVa and FVIIIa is changed
Nagoya I	CGT > TGT Arg306Cys	Exon 8, catalytic domain	↓	↓	ND	ND	↓	Alpha-helix is destroyed
Nottingham	GCC > ACC Ala404Thr	Exon 8, catalytic domain	↓	↓	↓	ND	N	Unfolding of protein

Table 11.6 (continued)

Name	Mutation	Involved exon and domain	Clotting assay PT	aPTT	RVVT	FX:C	FX:Ag	Comment
Taunton	CGT > GGT Arg405Gly	Exon 8, catalytic domain	BL	BL	BL	ND	N	–
Marseille	TCC > CCC Ser334Pro	Exon 8, catalytic domain	↓	↓	↓	↓	N	–
Stockton	GAC > AAC Asp282Asn	Exon 8, catalytic domain	↓	↓	ND	↓	N	–
Friuli	CCC > TCC Pro343Ser	Exon 8, catalytic domain	↓	↓	NN	↓	N	–
Roma	ACG > ATG Thr318Met	Exon 8, catalytic domain	↓	↓	N	↓	N	–
Frankfurt1	GAA > AAA Gla25Lys	Exon 2, Gla domain	↓	N	↓	ND	↓	–
Unnamed	CTC > ATC Leu-34Ile GGC > GGT Gly323ser GAC > AAC Asp368Asn GGC > GAC Gly381Asp	Exon 1, preproregion Exon 8, catalytic domain	↓	↓	ND	ND	↓	Substitution of serine at residue 323 causes protein misfolding, Ag levels not affected by others
Unnamed	AGG > ACG Arg-1Thr	Exon 2, preproregion	↓	↓	↓	N	N	–
Unnamed	TGT > TAT Cys81Tyr	Exon 4, EGF	↓	↓	↓	↓	↓	Disulfide bond is disrupted
Unnamed	GGG > AGG Gly94Asp GAC > GAA Asp95Glu	Exon 5, EGF	↓	↓	↓	↓	↓	Problem in folding of protein
Unnamed	TGC > TAC Cys109Tyr	Exon 5, EGF	↓	ND	ND	ND	↓	Disulfide bond is disrupted
Unnamed	ACG > ATG Thr-2Met TGC > TAC Cys111Tyr	Exon 2 Exon 5, EGF	↓	ND	ND	ND	↓	Disulfide bond is disrupted
Unnamed	GGG > AGG Gly204Arg	Exon 6, activation domain	↓	↓	ND	ND	↓	–

(continued)

Table 11.6 (continued)

Unnamed	GAG > AAG Glu264Lys	Exon 8, catalytic domain	NN	ND	ND	ND	NN	Affects FVa binding
Unnamed	CGG > TGG Arg287Trp	Exon 8, catalytic domain	↓	ND	ND	ND	ND	Doubly homozygous with Asp282Asn, affects FVa binding
Unnamed	GAG > AAG Glu310Lys	Exon 8, catalytic domain	↓	ND	ND	ND	↓	–
Unnamed	GGC > AGC Gly323Ser	Exon 8, catalytic domain	↓	ND	ND	ND	N	Doubly heterozygous with Thr318Met
Unnamed	TGT > CGT Cys364Arg	Exon 8, catalytic domain	↓	ND	ND	ND	↓	Disulfide bond is disrupted
Unnamed	CAC > CAG His383Gln TGG > CGG Trp421Arg	Exon 8, catalytic domain	ND	ND	ND	↓	ND	Substitution of His is near to catalytic domain
Unnamed	Gly380Arg	Exon 8, catalytic domain						Immediately after the active site, causes formation of a new hydrogen bond with Ala234, causes ICH
Unnamed	Tyr163delAT	Exon 6, activation domain	↓	↓	↓	↓	↓	Interruption with reading frame leading to a stop codon 163 in exon 6, causes ICH
Deletion	Complete deletion of gene and partial deletion including exon 7–8	–	↓	↓	↓	ND	↓	Probable germline mosaicism in the father

Table 11.6 (continued)

Name	Mutation	Involved exon and domain	Clotting assay PT	aPTT	RVVT	FX:C	FX:Ag	Comment
San Antonio	838-T leading to stop codon at position 232	Exon 8, catalytic domain	↓	N	ND	↓	↓	Additional mutation at CGC > TGC Arg326Cys
San Giovanni Rotondo	556-C leading to stop codon at residue 226	Exon 8, catalytic domain	↓	↓	↓	↓	N	Additional mutation at AAG > AAC Lys408Asn
Deletion	17 bp deletion in exon 8	Exon 8, catalytic domain	↓	ND	ND	ND	↓	Additional mutation at GTG > ATG Val298Met

PT prothrombin Time, *aPTT* activated partial thromboplastin time, *RVVT* Russell viper venom rime, *FVa* activated factor V, *FVIIIa* activated factor VIII, *FX:Ag* factor X antigenic assay, *FX:C* factor X activity by chromogenic assay, *FX* factor X, *N* normal, *ND* no data, *BL* borderline, *ICH* intracranial hemorrhage, *NN* near normal

11.12 Diagnosis

Similar to other rare bleeding disorders for the diagnosis of FX deficiency, a general approach consists of three main steps could be followed: (1) precise assessment of patient's clinical manifestations and family history, (2) first-line screening tests, and (3) specific coagulation tests:

1. A full clinical examination including determination of site, type, and duration of bleeding as well as other clinical diathesis has a great value in the diagnosis of the disorder. Personal and family history of bleeding and other criteria should be taken for every suspected patient to FX deficiency [24].
2. Following clinical assessment, laboratory screening should be performed. Complete blood count (CBC) and peripheral blood smear examination is necessary to determine any abnormality in number and morphology of platelets. PT, aPTT, mixing study, and thrombin time (TT) as well as RVVT should be established for a case suspected to FX deficiency. Since coagulation FX has a pivotal role in the both coagulation pathways, prolonged PT and aPTT as well as RVVT are observed, while TT is normal in case of FX deficiency. However, a number of patients with FX deficiency harbor mutants that affect just extrinsic coagulation pathway that exhibits as prolonged PT and normal aPTT, while other patients who harbor mutations in which only intrinsic pathway is affected will display a prolonged aPTT and normal PT. There have been also some mutants in FX that have a normal RVV test. In patients suspected to presence of inhibitor, mixing study should be performed. Corrected mixing study in 50:50 mixture of normal plasma with patient's plasma represents reduction in the coagulation factor level, while prolonged mixing test may be an evidence of inhibitor presence [1, 2, 24, 25].

   RVVT is an available clotting assay to assess deficiency of FX. RVV is a metalloproteinase unlike FX activator of other snakes' venom such as king cobra which is a serine proteinase. It cleaves a specific peptide in N-terminal domain of FX heavy chain and then directly activates FX similar to proteolytic enzymes. Therefore, RVV starts up the common pathway of coagulation cascade. Prolonged RVVT may be associated with deficiency in FX, FV, prothrombin, and fibrinogen [2, 26], although, by using of FX-deficient plasma as substrate in RVVT, this assay would be specific for FX deficiency [3].

3. If a patient is suspected to FX deficiency based on first-line screening tests, more specific analyses should be considered in the next step. There are various methods for measurement of both antigenic and functional levels of FX. Plasma levels of FX:Ag may be determined by several immunological assays such as electroimmunoassay, immunodiffusion, radioimmunoassay, antibody neutralization, and laser nephelometry as well as enzyme-linked immunosorbent assay (ELISA) (Fig. 11.8).

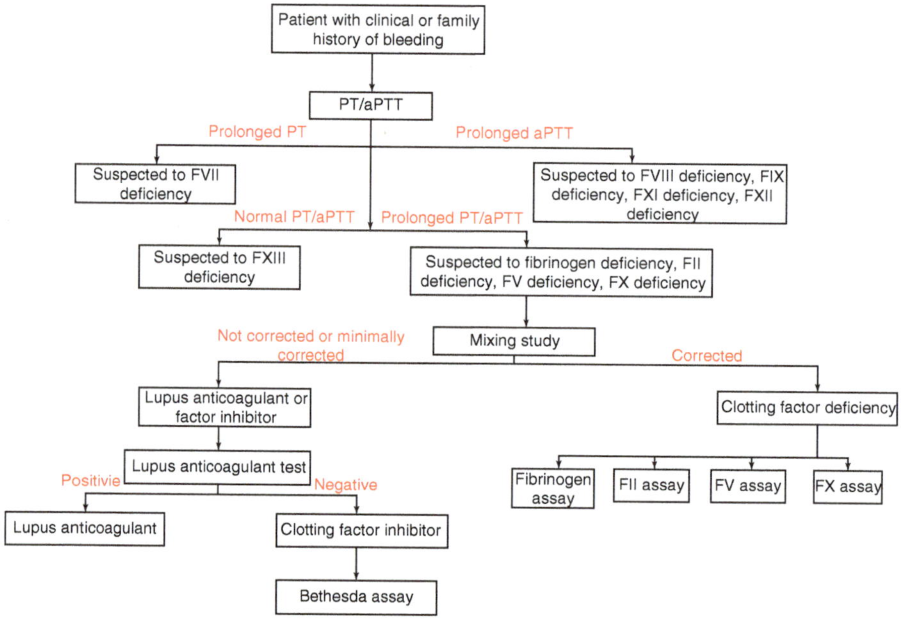

Fig. 11.8 An algorithm approach to diagnose congenital factor (F) X deficiency. To evaluate a patient presenting clinical or family history of bleeding, screening tests such as PT and aPTT are the first step. Prolonged PT with normal aPTT is suspected to FVII deficiency (extrinsic pathway), while normal PT with prolonged aPTT may be due to FVIII deficiency, FIX deficiency, FXI deficiency, or FXII deficiency (intrinsic pathway). Normal PT and aPTT along with bleeding symptom may be suspected to FXIII deficiency or other bleeding disorders that further specific assays are required. In presence of prolonged PT and aPTT, deficiency in fibrinogen, FII, FV, or FX is suspected (common pathway). Then the mixing study by using equal volume of normal and patient plasma could be performed to determine presence of an inhibitor or deficiency in the coagulation factors. Uncorrected or minimally corrected mixing test should be checked for the presence of lupus anticoagulant or coagulation factor inhibitors, while corrected mixing study is an evidence for one or more than one factor deficiency. In the next step, specific assays for the coagulation factors in common pathway are required. *PT* prothrombin time, *aPTT* activated partial thromboplastin time, *FII* factor II, *FV* factor V, *FVII* factor VII, *FVIII* factor VIII, *FIX* factor IX, *FX* factor X, *FXI* factor XI, *FXII* factor XII, *FXIII* factor XIII

One-stage FX assay is one of the most common methods to determine FX:C level. It is based on using FX-deficient plasma as substrate in mixing with normal or patient plasma. Then PT and aPTT are retested on the substrate and correlated ratio of the clotting times is calculated [2, 3].

Chromogenic assay is another trustable method to assess plasma FX:C level, in which FX is activated in plasma and then generated FXa affects FXa-sensitive chromogenic substrate to produce color. Finally, produced color is detected by spectrophotometer. More activity levels of FX result in more FXa, so the color will be more intense [1]. It is important to know that because of nonspecific nature in using of chromogenic substrate, the FX level may be estimated higher in some cases [3].

Besides routine coagulation assessments, using other processes including thrombin generation and fibrin polymerization as well as thromboelastography to evaluate total blood coagulation pathway dynamically is useful in the diagnosis of FX deficiency.

It is noteworthy that the reliability of results of FX assays depends on both pre-analytical and analytical variables, e.g., amount and type of anticoagulant, sampling, centrifuging of sample, preservation of reagents and instruments, as well as using suitable quality controls in analytical phase [13].

Anti-FXa assay is a chromogenic method monitoring the level of low molecular weight heparin (LMWH). LMWH binds to antithrombin specifically and more effectively inactivates FXa than thrombin. Remaining FXa in patient's plasma cleaves a chromogenic substrate and produces color. Intensity of produced color is measured by spectrophotometer. The intensity of color is inversely associated to the amount of LMWH. It should be noticed that in the case with renal failure or due to contamination of sample with heparin, the level of anti-Xa may be overestimated. This method is also appropriate to monitor direct oral FXa inhibitors, if a suitable standard curve be available [27].

11.13 Considerations

1. As immunological assays measure only antigenic level of FX, the cases with dysfunctional FX protein without any reduction of antigenic level may be missed. During warfarin therapy, both antigenic and activity levels of FX are decreased to about 50%, although the functional levels may be lower [3].
2. It is noticeable that the FX level in newborn and infants under 6 month is lower than adults. Therefore, FX assay results should be calculated according to age- and gestational age-matched reference intervals. The FX level in healthy term newborns has a wide range of 0.12–0.68 IU/ml and increases gradually during 6 months.
3. Since the FX level is affected either by liver disease or vitamin K deficiency, it is necessary to rule out such disorders or other acquired cause of FX deficiency. On the other hand, vitamin K deficiency in preterm or young neonates may complicate diagnosis of FX deficiency, especially in cases with mild deficiency. Therefore, reassessment should be done after replacement therapy for vitamin K and also at 6 months of age [2, 3].

11.14 Molecular Basis

During last two decades, several *F10* gene mutations have been identified that majority of them were unique and restricted to special family. DNA amplification and direct sequencing mostly are used to find underlying mutations. Therefore establishing a genetic diagnosis method is challenging and costly, identification of recurrent variants of each population is more practical and also is helpful to reduce using of direct sequencing, but it's not applicable because in most families the mutations are unique.

11.15 Prenatal Diagnosis (PND)

Prenatal diagnosis (PND) can be used for families with risk of having a severely affected infant, e.g., when both parents are carriers or having at least one affected child. To diagnose an affected fetus, CVS is performed at weeks of 10–12 of gestation and then extracted DNA is analyzed to find parents underlying mutations. In especial geographic areas with recurrent mutations, establishing a mutation-screening method may be helpful to reduce the rate of affected offspring [13].

11.16 Treatment

The proportion of the patients with FX deficiency that require treatment is higher than most of other rare bleeding disorders according to UK Hemophilia Centre Doctors' Organisation (UKHCDO) registry data. Main therapeutic choice in patients with congenital FX deficiency is on-demand therapy (stopping of hemorrhage as soon as possible), while regular prophylaxis can be used for those with risk of severe hemorrhagic manifestations. Replacement therapy in congenital FX deficiency is guided by the particular hemorrhagic episode. Current policies for the management of patients are on the basis of two general options: (1) antifibrinolytic agents including tranexamic acid and aminocaproic acid and (2) blood-derived products such as FFP, prothrombin complex concentrate (PCC), FIX products, and plasma-derived FX concentrate (pdFX) [2, 3, 11, 28, 29].

11.16.1 Antifibrinolytic Agents

Generally, these medicines are used to manage minor mucosal bleeding such as epistaxis, mouth bleeding, and menorrhagia.

Aminocaproic acid is usually administrated either as mouthwash (15 mL every 6 h) or orally taken (50–100 mg/kg every 6 h) to control nose and mouth bleeds.

Tranexamic acid is effective to manage idiopathic menorrhagia. It is prescribed orally in dosage of 15 mg/kg every 6–8 h.

Nosebleeds Quick Release™ powder (Biolife; LLC, Sarasota, FL, USA) is a hydrophilic polymer that is administrated for the management of epistaxis [2, 13].

11.16.2 Blood-Derived Products

11.16.2.1 Nonspecific FX Replacement Therapy

Fresh Frozen Plasma (FFP) Virus-inactivated FFP is used widely to control both traumatic and spontaneous bleeding. A level of 10–20% of FX:C is sufficient for normal hemostasis, so given that the half-life of FX is 20–40 h in plasma, doses of 3–6 ml/kg twice a day increase FX:C level to 10–20%. In cases of active bleeding, a dosage of 15–20 ml/kg of FFP is required [1, 2, 10, 13]. Since a low concentration of each clotting factor exists in FFP, a large volume is required to achieve hemostatic level of FX. Therefore a related issue is fluid overload, especially in children and elderly patients suffering from cardiovascular disease. Allergic reaction and transfusion-associated lung injury (TRALI) are also the other main complications of FFP [2, 3, 13].

Prothrombin Complex Concentrates (PCC) Virally inactivated PCC are plasma-derived concentrates in which there are three (FII, FIX, and FX) or four (FII, FIX, FVII, and FX) clotting factors and also protein C and protein S (please refer to Chap. 10).

PCC contains a 1:1 ratio of FX:FIX that is administrated to manage bleeding diathesis in patients with FX deficiency. By a dose of 1 IU/kg, PCC increases the level of FX:C to 1.5%, and due to FX long half-life, daily infusion is not necessary. In the case of severe deficiency, a daily dosage of 20–30 IU/kg PCC is required; however, the optimal dose should be determined with regard to the type of bleeding and remaining level of FX:C [1, 2, 13]. It is worth to know that PCC also contains other activated clotting factors (FVIIa, FIIa, and FIXa), so it may be in association with high risk of thrombotic complications. Therefore, during long-term treatment or in case of orderly prophylaxis, regular monitoring of FIX and FX as well as D-dimer is required. PCC also should be administrated with caution in cases of liver disease, major trauma, large hematoma, and antithrombin deficiency as well as neonates [30]. It is noticeable that concomitant using of fibrinolytic inhibitors such as tranexamic acid and PCC is contraindicated due to high risk of thromboembolism [2, 3, 13].

Factor IX Products The concentrates of FIX containing approximately 1200 IU of FIX and 800 IU of FX (therapeutic amounts) have been administrated in patients with FX deficiency prophylactically. There is the risk of thrombosis by using FIX products [29].

- A freeze-dried concentrate of human clotting FIX and FX (factor X P Behring; CSL Behring, Marburg, Germany) was developed that is an alternative source of PCC. It is especially helpful in the cases where using of PCC should be avoided [13].

Fibrin Glue Fibrin glue is generally used to facilitate a local hemostasis, particularly in sites of surgery [2, 10].

11.16.2.2 Specific Factor X Products

High-Purity Human Plasma-Derived Factor X Concentrate (pdFX) pdFX or Coagadex (the commercial name) was approved by the Food and Drug Administration (FDA) in 2015. It is the first single-factor FX concentrate used in the FX-deficient patients to achieve sufficient hemostasis. Coagadex is manufactured from plasma of healthy and virally negative (hepatitis A, B, and C and HIV-1 and HIV-2 viruses) donors. Virus-inactivated pdFX is produced as lyophilized powder that is injected after reconstitution with sterile water. It contains 100 IU/ml FX, less than 1 IU/ml of FII and FIX, and no added proteins. pdFX activity level is more than 100 IU/mg protein by using the chromogenic FX activity assay.

The safety and clinical efficacy of pdFX were assessed in two open-label, multicenter, and nonrandomized phase III trials, Ten01 and Ten03 (Table 11.7) [29].

Table 11.7 Completed clinical studies of Coagadex

Name of study	Ten01	Ten03
Design	Multicenter, nonrandomized, open-label, and prospective phase III trial	Multicenter, nonrandomized, open-label, and prospective phase III trial
Patients	16 patients aged ≥12 years with plasma FX:C < 5 IU/dL	2 patients aged ≥12 years with plasma FX:C < 20 IU/dL
Aim of study	Overall efficacy assessment and safety in the management of bleeding diathesis up to 2 years PK after a single dose of 25 IU/kg Peri-operative management for the surgical patients	Peri-operative management for the surgical patients
Findings	Mean dose per injection: 25.3 IU/kg Mean half-life: 29.4 h Mean IR: 2.00 IU/dL per IU/kg Excellent or good efficacy of on-demand management of episodes: 98% of cases Common complication: mild headache Possibly complications: one subject with pain in the injection site and one subject with erythema in the injection site, fatigue and back pain	Excellent efficacy for the management of blood loss before surgery: 100% No bleeding after surgery No needing for blood transfusion Expected or less than expected blood loss No possibly complications

FX factor X, *FX:C* factor X functional activity, *PK* pharmacokinetic, *IR* incremental recovery

The first study (Ten01) was conducted on a population of 16 patients (208 bleeding episodes) aged >12 years with moderate to severe FX deficiency (<5 IU/dL) that experienced ≥1 bleeds in the last year. pdFX was administrated in a dose of 25 IU/kg for the baseline pharmacokinetics (PK1) measurement including recovery rate and half-life. Then the patients are treated on-demand for spontaneous, traumatic, and heavy menorrhagia bleeding diathesis for more than 6 months and till >1 bleeding episodes had been treated. After which, the secondary endpoints including PK2, the number of required infusions, were evaluated. The mean recovery rate was 2.0 IU/dL per IU/kg, and the terminal half-life ($t_{½}$) of pdFX was approximately 30 h suggesting that a prophylactic regime once or twice infused weekly is adequate (depending on the required activity level of FX). Clearance (CL) of pdFX through hepatic route is slow so it remains in plasma for long time.

It is noteworthy that the PK of pdFX depends on plasma volume as well as body weight of patients. Therefore, it varies from younger children to older children and adults.

The second study investigated pre-operatively treatment of Coagadex in two surgical patients aged >12 years with mild to severe FX deficiency (FX:C <20 IU/dL).

The most common adverse event was mild headache in the first study, while erythema and pain in the site of fusion, back pain, and fatigue were observed in the both studies.

Indication of Coagadex Coagadex is indicated in the patients aged >12 years for the management of bleeding diathesis and on-demand treatment. It is also could be administrated as pre-operative management in the patients with mild FX deficiency. Efficacy of Coagadex for major surgery in the patients with moderate and severe deficiency has not been investigated. It should be avoided in patients with allergy to any components of the product.

- As Coagadex is manufactured from human plasma, there may be contamination with infectious agents such as viruses or the agent of Creutzfeldt-Jakob disease (theoretically). Also formation of FX inhibitors is possible by using Coagadex so monitoring of the patients taking Coagadex via suitable laboratory assays is necessary [28, 29, 31, 32].

11.17 Management of Factor X Deficiency in Surgery

Target level of FX in surgery is variable in different patients according to the residual FX level in the plasma and based on type and duration of surgery. A satisfactory surgery could be achieved in severely affected patients with FX deficiency (FX <1%) by carefully using of FFP, PCC, or other products. A level of 20 IU/dL FX in plasma seems to be adequate for stable hemostasis and controlling of bleeding, so a loading dose of 15–20 IU/kg PCC followed by 10–15 IU/kg daily or every other day for minor surgery is recommended (Table 11.8) [3, 13, 30].

Table 11.8 Recommended dose of different products for the management of patients with factor X deficiency

	Products	Recommended dose
Mucosal bleeding	TA	10 mL of a 5% solution as mouthwash every 8 h
	FFP	A loading dose of 10–20 mL/kg followed by 3–6 mL/kg twice a day to keep FX:C level above 10–20 IU/dL[a]
	PCC	1 IU/kg, PCC raises FX:C level by 1.5%[b]
Acute bleeding in severe factor X deficiency	FFP	A loading dose of 10–20 mL/kg followed by 3–6 mL/kg twice a day to keep FX:C level above 10–20 IU/dL
	PCC	20–30 IU/kg once a day
	pdFX	25 IU/kg (patients aged ≥12 years)
Surgery in severe factor X deficiency[c]	FFP	15–25 mL/kg, an alternative if PCC is unavailable
	PCC	A loading dose of 15–20 IU/kg followed by 10–15 IU/kg after surgery[d]
Prophylaxis	PCC (FIX)	15–40 IU/mL two or three times per week 20–70 IU/mL weekly
	FX	15–20 IU/kg weekly

[a]Level of 10–20 IU/dL FX seems to be sufficient for hemostasis; however, some reports suggest that 5 IU/dL FX may also be adequate

[b]As biologic half-life of FX is 20–40 h daily infusion is not usually required

[c]Replacement therapy is not required in patients with factor IX level >10% without significant bleeding history

[d]Generally a daily dose is sufficient; however, in minor surgery, a dose every other day may be adequate

TA tranexamic acid, *FFP* fresh frozen plasma, *PCC* prothrombin complex concentrate, *pdFX* plasma-derived factor X, *FX* factor X

11.18 Obstetric and Pediatric Care

As mentioned, menorrhagia and long-term menses occur frequently in women with FX deficiency, while recurrent abortion and placental abruption appear only in cases with severe deficiency. Affected women are also at risk of gynecologic problems including hemoperitoneum and corpus luteum bleeding in relation with ovulation. Factor replacement therapy and fibrinolytic inhibitors are usually administrated to manage menorrhagia. During pregnancy sufficient replacement therapy is required to prevent adverse outcomes such as miscarriage, preterm birth, and placental abruption. In severely affected patients (FX:C <2 IU/dL), who are at third trimester of pregnancy and require cesarean section, loading dose of 20–40 IU/kg, PCC is required to achieve FX:C >4 IU/dL and then followed by 10–20 IU/kg once a day to keep FX:C >3 IU/dL for at least 3 days [33].

According to some reports, bleeding-related childbirth may occur in heterozygous individuals; therefore, prophylactic therapy should be considered in such cases. On the other hand, the risk of thromboembolism must be assessed attentively by using PCC [13].

FX evaluation is required either before delivery or at birth (cord blood sample) to reduce the risk of hemorrhage in neonates. Further, severely affected neonates should carefully be evaluated by cranial ultrasound due to high risk of ICH. Prophylactic care also must be considered in necessity during neonatal [3, 34].

Replacement therapy is not usually required to manage moderately factor X deficiency (FX:C >2 IU/dL) without significant bleeding history (despite hemostatic challenges). Although any prior hemostatic challenges related bleeding history and the kind of surgery must be considered.

11.19 Prophylaxis

As FX deficiency is one of the most severe rare bleeding disorders, prophylaxis is recommended for those patients at risk of severe bleeding, to prevent intense bleeding diathesis including CNS, GI bleeding, hematoma, and hemarthrosis particularly in patients with FX <0.05 IU/ml. According to Greifswald registry, 5% of FX is mightily sufficient to generate at least 50% thrombin in patients; therefore, a dose of 15–20 IU/kg FX once a week leads to a significant reduction of hemorrhage especially in children [3, 13]. If PCC is used, doses of 15–40 IU/ml twice or three times a week are shown as more effective than 20–70 IU/ml weekly [33].

11.20 Prognosis

By early identification and diagnosis of patients, bleeding complications of FX deficiency would be effectively managed. Special consideration is also required for affected women and children. On the other hand, in heterozygous cases, genetic counseling may be greatly helpful to prevent birth of affected offspring [2].

11.21 Management of Acquired Factor X Deficiency

Treatment of underlying cause of acquired FX deficiency is first step in the management of acquired FX deficiency. Then based on the severity of deficiency, suitable therapeutic choice should be selected. However, due to shortened half-life of infused FX, as it is adsorbed by amyloid fibrils, administration of FFP, PCC, or other products increases FX level transiently and so improves the bleeding tendency just for short time; therefore, they are not actually useful. On the other hand, possible risk of thrombosis and hepatitis may increase by overuse of these products. Antifibrinolytic agents may also be useful to improve hemostatic system in some cases [18, 35]. Recombinant FVII (rFVII) is another useful product for primary amyloid-associated FX deficiency [3]. Splenectomy is also a highly beneficial therapeutic choice for AL amyloid-related FX deficiency. Since large amount of amyloid deposition fibrils aggregate in the spleen, removal of involved spleen leads to reduction of ruptured FX and so increases the level of factor in plasma. Melphalan and corticosteroids are also used in AL amyloidosis [18, 35].

There are some reports of successful management of acquired FX deficiency associated with inhibitors by using plasmapheresis and steroid therapy as well as intravenous immunoglobulins [1, 18, 36].

References

1. Uprichard J, Perry DJ. Factor X deficiency. Blood Rev. 2002;16(2):97–110.
2. Brown D, Kouides P. Diagnosis and treatment of inherited factor X deficiency. Haemophilia. 2008;14(6):1176–82.
3. Lee CA, Berntorp EE, Keith Hoots W. Textbook of hemophilia. Oxford: Blackwell; 2010. [cited 2017 2017].
4. Peyvandi F, Menegatti M. Inherited deficiencies of coagulation factors II, V, V+VIII, VII, X, XI, and XIII. In: Williams hematology. 9th ed. New York: McGraw-Hill; 2016. p. 40.
5. Mannucci PM, Duga S, Peyvandi F. Recessively inherited coagulation disorders. Blood. 2004;104(5):1243–52.
6. Karimi M, Menegatti M, Afrasiabi A, Sarikhani S, Peyvandi F. Phenotype and genotype report on homozygous and heterozygous patients with congenital factor X deficiency. Haematologica. 2008;93(6):934–8.
7. Perry D. Factor X and its deficiency states. Haemophilia. 1997;3(3):159–72.
8. Versteeg HH, Spek CA, Peppelenbosch MP, Richel DJ. Tissue factor and cancer metastasis: the role of intracellular and extracellular signaling pathways. Mol Med. 2004;10(1-6):6.
9. Girolami A, Vettore S, Scarparo P, Lombardi A. Persistent validity of a classification of congenital factor X defects based on clotting, chromogenic and immunological assays even in the molecular biology era. Haemophilia. 2011;17(1):17–20.
10. Lee G, DUAN-PORTER W, Metjian A. Acquired, non-amyloid related factor X deficiency: review of the literature. Haemophilia. 2012;18(5):655–63.
11. Palla R, Peyvandi F, Shapiro AD. Rare bleeding disorders: diagnosis and treatment. Blood. 2015. https://doi.org/10.1182/blood-2014-08-532820.
12. Girolami A, Scarparo P, Scandellari R, Allemand E. Congenital factor X deficiencies with a defect only or predominantly in the extrinsic or in the intrinsic system: a critical evaluation. Am J Hematol. 2008;83(8):668–71.
13. Menegatti M, Peyvandi F. Factor X deficiency. Semin Thromb Hemost. 2009;35:407.
14. Herrmann F, Auerswald G, RUIZ-SAEZ A, Navarrete M, Pollmann H, Lopaciuk S, et al. Factor X deficiency: clinical manifestation of 102 subjects from Europe and Latin America with mutations in the factor 10 gene. Haemophilia. 2006;12(5):479–89.
15. Peyvandi F, Mannucci P, Lak M, Abdoullahi M, Zeinali S, Sharifian R, et al. Congenital factor X deficiency: spectrum of bleeding symptoms in 32 Iranian patients. Br J Haematol. 1998;102(2):626–8.
16. Acharya S, Coughlin A, Dimichele DM. Rare bleeding disorder registry: deficiencies of factors II, V, VII, X, XIII, fibrinogen and dysfibrinogenemias. J Thromb Haemost. 2004;2(2):248–56.
17. Thompson CA, Kyle R, Gertz M, Heit J, Pruthi R, Pardanani A. Systemic AL amyloidosis with acquired factor X deficiency: a study of perioperative bleeding risk and treatment outcomes in 60 patients. Am J Hematol. 2010;85(3):171–3.
18. Vaidya K, Arnott C, Biscoe A, Eggleton S, Brighton T. Differential diagnosis and therapeutic limitations in a rare case of acquired factor X deficiency. Case Rep Intern Med. 2015;2(4):55.
19. Nance D, Josephson N, Paulyson-Nunez K, James A. Factor X deficiency and pregnancy: preconception counselling and therapeutic options. Haemophilia. 2012;18(3):e277.
20. Mariani G, Herrmann F, Schulman S, Batorova A, Wulff K, Etro D, et al. Thrombosis in inherited factor VII deficiency. J Thromb Haemost. 2003;1(10):2153–8.
21. Genotype of patients with factor X deficiency. 2011. http://c.ymcdn.com/sites/www.isth.org/resource/resmgr/publications/fx_mutations-2011.pdf?hhSearchTerms=%22coagulation+and+factor+and+X%22
22. Mota L, Shetty S, Idicula-Thomas S, Ghosh K. Molecular basis of factor X deficiency cases from India. Haemophilia. 2010;16(4):693–7.
23. Herrmann FH, Navarette M, Salazar-Sanchez L, Carillo JM, Auerswald G, Wulff K. Homozygous factor X gene mutations Gly380Arg and Tyr163delAT are associated with perinatal intracranial hemorrhage. J Pediatr. 2005;146(1):128–30.

24. Borhany M, Shamsi T, Moiz B, Hasan K, Hashmi KZ, Ayyub M, et al. Guidelines on the laboratory diagnosis of congenital bleeding disorders in Pakistan. JPMA J Pak Med Assoc. 2012;62(5):477.
25. Kaushansky K, Williams WJ, Joseph W. Williams hematology. New York: McGraw-Hill Medical; 2010.
26. Markland FS. Snake venoms and the hemostatic system. Toxicon. 1998;36(12):1749–800.
27. Fareed J, Hoppensteadt DA, Fareed D, Demir M, Wahi R, Clarke M, et al. Survival of heparins, oral anticoagulants, and aspirin after the year 2010. Semin Thromb Hemost. 2008;34:58.
28. Austin S, Brindley C, Kavakli K, Norton M, Shapiro A. Pharmacokinetics of a high-purity plasma-derived factor X concentrate in subjects with moderate or severe hereditary factor X deficiency. Haemophilia. 2016;22(3):426–32.
29. Shapiro A. Plasma-derived human factor X concentrate for on-demand and perioperative treatment in factor X-deficient patients: pharmacology, pharmacokinetics, efficacy, and safety. Expert Opin Drug Metab Toxicol. 2017;13(1):97–104.
30. Bolton-Maggs P, Perry D, Chalmers E, Parapia L, Wilde J, Williams M, et al. The rare coagulation disorders–review with guidelines for management from the United Kingdom Haemophilia Centre Doctors' Organisation. Haemophilia. 2004;10(5):593–628.
31. io Products Laboratory Receives FDA approval for Coagadex® (Coagulation Factor X, Human). 2015. http://www.businesswire.com/news/home/20151021005989/en/Bio-Products-Laboratory-Receives-FDA-approval-Coagadex%C2%AE
32. FDA Approves Coagadex®. First factor X concentrate. 2015. https://www.hemophilia.org/Newsroom/Medical-News/FDA-Approves-Coagadex-First-Factor-X-Concentrate
33. Mumford AD, Ackroyd S, Alikhan R, Bowles L, Chowdary P, Grainger J, et al. Guideline for the diagnosis and management of the rare coagulation disorders. Br J Haematol. 2014;167(3):304–26.
34. Tabibian S, Motlagh H, Naderi M, Dorgalaleh A. Intracranial hemorrhage in congenital bleeding disorders. Blood Coagul Fibrinolysis. 2018;29:1.
35. Greipp PR, Kyle RA, Bowie E. Factor-X deficiency in amyloidosis: a critical review. Am J Hematol. 1981;11(4):443–50.
36. Di Paola J, Nugent D, Young G. Current therapy for rare factor deficiencies. Haemophilia. 2001;7(s1):16–22.

12 Congenital Factor XI Deficiency

Tahere Tabatabaei and Akbar Dorgalaleh

12.1 Introduction

Factor XI (FXI) deficiency is a rare autosomal recessive injury-related hemorrhagic disorder, but some autosomal dominant cases were also reported. Worldwide prevalence of disorder is 1:1,000,000, but this rate is higher in some ethnicities such as Ashkenazi Jews with a prevalence of 1:450 [1–3]. The clinical symptoms are highly heterogeneous, and there is no direct relationship between bleeding tendency and residual plasma FXI level. Bleeding usually is observed in homozygotes and combined heterozygotes, while heterozygotes are usually asymptomatic. Sometimes, patients never experience any bleeding diathesis in their life. Bleedings are usually post-traumatic, post-surgical, and post-partum and occur in areas with high fibrinolytic activity such as the mucosal surface of oral cavity [3–5]. FXI deficiency is classified in two phenotypes: in type I or CRM−, both FXI coagulant activity (FXI:C) and FXI antigen (FXI:Ag) are low, and in type II or CRM+, FXI:Ag is normal, while FXI:C is lower than the normal range. A wide spectrum of mutations has been identified within *F11* gene. FXI deficiency in Ashkenazi Jews is mostly due to four common causative mutations that were categorized as types I to IV. The disorder based on FX:C level is classified in three types including mild, moderate, and severe [6–8]. FXI level is less than 20 U/dL in severe deficiency, while in mild and moderate deficiency, FXI level is usually between 20 and 70 U/dL. Due to mild phenotype of the disorder, in most cases, the disorder is diagnosed based on family history or randomly in routine work-up [3, 9, 10]. The main therapeutic strategy in these patients is on-demand therapy, and the main therapeutic products that can be used in these patients are fresh frozen plasma (FFP), FXI concentrate, and desmopressin [1, 2, 10].

T. Tabatabaei · A. Dorgalaleh (✉)
Department of Hematology and Blood transfusion, School of Allied Medicine, Iran University of Medical Sciences, Tehran, Iran

A. Dorgalaleh (ed.), *Congenital Bleeding Disorders*,
https://doi.org/10.1007/978-3-319-76723-9_12

12.2 Factor XI Structure

F11 gene is located at the distal end of the long arm of chromosome 4 (4q35) and consists of 15 exons and 14 introns that span a 23-kb region. FXI protein has an 18-amino acid leader peptide. Exon 1, exon 2, exons 3–10, and exons 11–15 encode the promoter region, signal peptide, four N-terminal apple domains, and C-terminal catalytic domain, respectively [9, 11–14]. FXI has a distinguished structure from other coagulation proteases. It is a 160-kDa homodimer with a similar 607-amino acid sequence in both subunits. These two subunits are joined together by covalent and non-covalent bounds. Each subunit has four 90- to 91-amino acid sequences at the N-terminal that named apple domain (Ap1–Ap4) and a catalytic domain with 238 amino acids at the C-terminal with serine protease (SP) role that is homologous to the serine protease domains of other coagulation factors (Fig. 12.1) [9–11, 13, 14].

Apple domains form a disk structure in each subunit that provide a surface for binding of platelet, high molecular weight kininogen (HMWK), and FIX. Prekallikrein has a homolog structure with FXI in their apple domains. In monomeric structure of FXI, each apple domain contains seven β-strands that form an antiparallel sheet, and an α-helix is attached to the concave side of the sheet by two disulfide bonds. Another bound connects N-terminal to C-terminal. These four apple domains are adhesion sites for other molecules [14–16]. These include Ap1 and Ap2 that are adhesion sites for thrombin and HMWK, respectively, and Ap3 is a binding site for glycoprotein (Gp) Ib, FIX, and heparin [1]. Ap4 is adhesion site for activated FXII (FXIIa) [1, 3, 11]. Ap4 is also necessary for dimerization of FXI. Catalytic domain that is in C-terminal site on the apple domains in a "cup and saucer" arrangement comprised of His413, Asp462, and Ser557 in a trypsin catalytic domain [9, 11, 15, 17, 18].

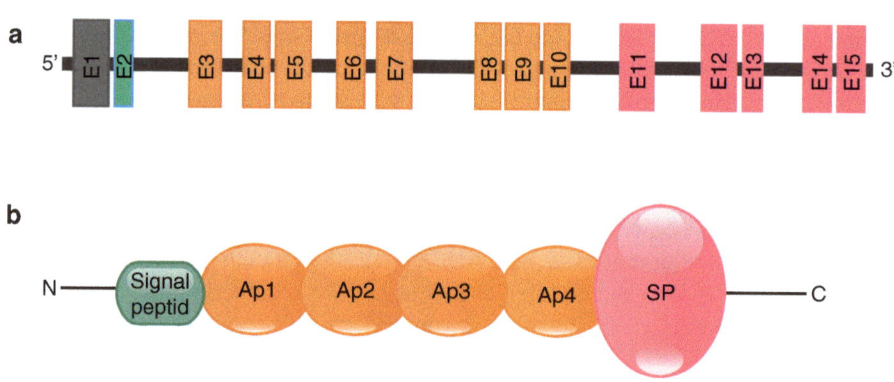

Fig. 12.1 (**a**) *F11* gene structure: *F11* gene consists of 15 exons and 14 introns. Exon 1 and exon 2 encode promoter and signal peptide, respectively. Exons 3–10 encode four apple domains and exons 11–15 encode serine protease domain. (**b**) Schematic structure of factor XI protein: factor XI protein is composed of a signal peptide, four apple domains (Ap1–4) at the N-terminal, and a catalytic domain with serine protease activity at C-terminal. *N* N-terminal, *C* C-terminal, *Ap* apple domain, *SP* serine protease domain, *E* exon

In bloodstream, FXI is the only serine protease in dimeric form that is active in this form. Ap4 is a major domain for FXI dimerization. Two Ap4 domains develop an interface disulfide bond between two FXI monomer subunits. This bond is formed through Cys321 at fingerlike loop in Ap4 domain. Moreover, hydrophobic interaction between Tyr329, Ile 290, and Leu284 of the Ap4 domain interface and a salt bridge between Lys331 in one subunit and Glu287 on another subunit is necessary for dimerization [4, 14]. FXI has five N-linked glycosylation sites including Asn residues at positions 72, 108, and 335 in heavy chain and Asn residues at 432 and 473 of light chain. Almost all circulating FXI is in complex with HMWK. HMWK is a multifunctional plasma protein with six domains (D1 to D6), that D6 domain is a binding site of FXI Ap2 domain. Also for activation of FIX, Ap3 in one monomers of FXI connect to platelet via Gp1b and HMWK in presence of zink ionse and another Ap3 connect to FIX. [11, 19, 20].

12.3 Factor XI Activation and Function

Plasma activators of FXI are FXIIa, thrombin, meizothrombin, and FXIa (auto activation). Platelet polyphosphate (polyP) affects FXI activation via α-thrombin, β-thrombin, and FXIa that all of them cleave FXI monomers at Arg369-Ile370 site between Ap4 and catalytic domain. The dimeric form of FXI is necessary for effective activation and function of FXI. FXI activators bind to one monomer and activate another subunit [7, 16]. HMWK is required for optimal FXI binding to GPIb on activated platelet. Indeed, FXI binds to platelet, as a negative charge surface, through one monomer and binds to substrate (FIX, FV, FVIII) through another subunit that is an explanation for its dimeric structure [21]. FXIa composed of two N-terminal heavy chains contain four apple domains, and two C-terminal light chains contain catalytic domain. Dimeric structure of FXIa is maintained by three disulfide bonds: heavy chains bind to light chains by two bounds in each monomers, and two monomers connect together by one disulfide bound [22].

Along with activation of FXI by thrombin and FXII, an intermediate product is generated that has one activation subunit. This intermediate named 1/2FXIa. Inhibition of FXI by antithrombin in the presence of 1/2 molar heparin shows that each of FXI subunits has independent catalytic function, so 1/2FXIa can be the main form of activated FXIa (Fig. 12.2) [23].

In the initiation phase of coagulation cascade, tissue factor (TF)/FVII complex activates FX and produces small amount of thrombin. Then tissue factor pathway inhibitor (TFPI) inhibits TF and blocks the extrinsic coagulation pathway. At this time, amplification phase is begun with conversion of FXII to FXIIa. Then FXII with its cofactor, HMWK, or other activators convert FXI to FXIa in intrinsic pathway. Since there is no bleeding tendency in patients with FXII deficiency, this fact is demonstrated that an alternative mechanism is the presence of FXI activation [24]. Thrombin-mediated FXI activation reinforces common pathway of coagulation with feedback mechanism [25]. Since, in the initiation phase of coagulation cascade, TF/FVII complex is inhibited by circulating TFPI, only

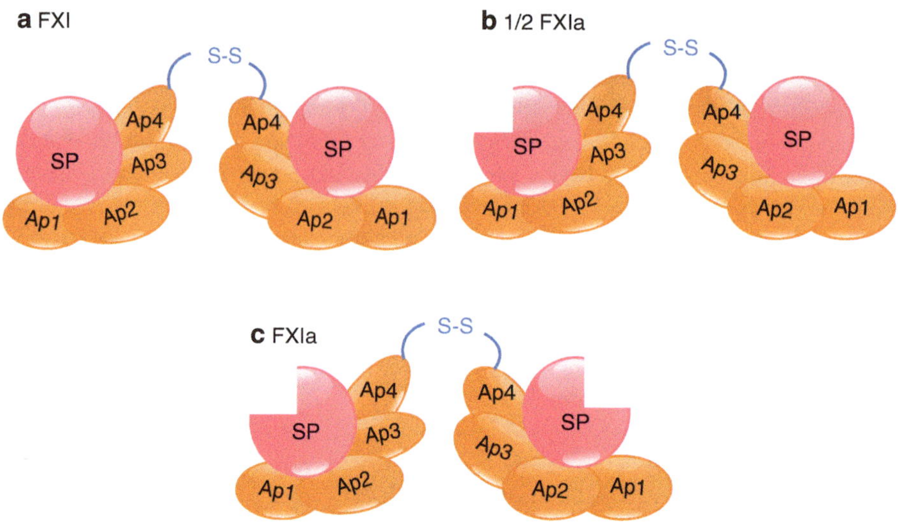

Fig. 12.2 (**a**) Each monomer of factor (F) XI consists of four apple domains (Ap1–Ap4) and a serine protease (SP) domain. The FXI dimer is linked by Cys321 interchain disulfide bond between AP4 of two subunits. (**b**) All FXI activators cleave FXI between Arg369 and Ile370 site and develop an intermediate form named 1/2FXIa. (**c**) With cleavage in another subunit, 1/2FXIa is changed to activated FXI. *FXI* factor XI, *FXIa* activated factor XI, *Ap* apple domain, *SP* serine protease domain

a small amount of thrombin can be produced, and the extrinsic pathway is stopped. At this time, generated thrombin can activate FV, FVIII, FXI and pelatelets. FXI dimeric structure is necessary, because FIX cannot bind to monomeric FXI on the platelet surface; therefore, one of apple3 domains is required to bind the surface of the platelet and the AP3 domain on another monomer available for binding of FIX [19, 26]. Therefore, after dimerization and conversion of FXI to FXIa, FXI binding site contains amino acids 183 to 191 at Ap3 is exposed, and FXIa can bind to FIX [2]. Then FXIa cleaves FIX at Arg145-Ala146 and Arg180-Val181 sites and releases active peptide (Ala146-Arg180); at this time, FIX converts to its active forms (FIXaα and FIXβ) [27]. Activated FIX activates FVIII that can activate common pathway and generates thrombin. Thrombin generation will continue even after clot formation. This additional thrombin activates thrombin-activable fibrinolysis inhibitor (TAFI) that protects clot form fibrinolysis system. Therefore, FXI has both procoagulation and antifibrinolysis atributies (please refer to Chap. 1) (Fig. 12.3) [11, 19, 20, 28].

Antithrombin, protease nexin-2 (PN-2), C1 inhibitor, aprotinin, leupeptin, *P*-aminobenzamidine, and protein Z-dependent protease inhibitor are FXI negative inhibitors [29–31]. Heparin also binds to serpin and A3 domain of FXI and inhibits FXI. Heparin also inhibits FXI via binding to catalytic domain through a charge neutralization mechanism [3]. PN-2 that is released from active platelets inhibits FXI through binding of its Kunitz-type domain to FXI catalytic domain [4, 32–35].

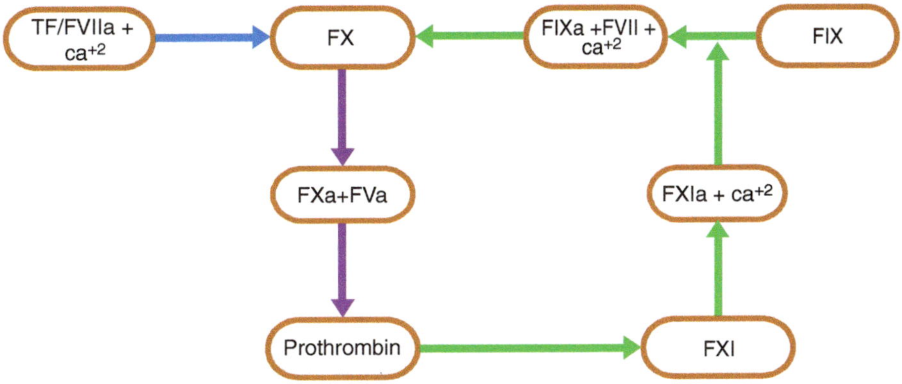

Fig. 12.3 Prothrombin feedback loop. In extrinsic coagulation pathway, a little amount of prothrombin is generated by TF/FVII + Ca^{+2} complex in the initiation phase. Then, TFPI inhibits TF/FVII complex. In the amplification phase, prothrombin activates intrinsic pathway through conversion of FXI to FXIa. FXIa cleaves FIX to FIXa, and then FIXa activates FX. At this time, a large amount of prothrombin is generated in common pathway. *TFPI* tissue factor pathway inhibitor, *FXI* factor XI, *FXIa* activated factor XI, *FXa* activated factor X, *FIX* factor IX, *FIXa* activated factor IX, *TF* tissue factor, *FVII* factor VII, *FV* factor V

12.4 Factor XI Deficiency

FXI deficiency, hemophilia C, plasma thromboplastin antecedent deficiency, or Rosenthal syndrome is a rare hemorrhagic disorders with variable clinical symptoms that for the first time was described by Rosenthal in 1953 [36, 37]. The incidence of disorder is equal in both genders and is ~1 per 1 million in the general population, but it is more common among Ashkenazi Jews with ~5% carriers and 1 per 450 homozygotes [15, 18]. The bleeding tendency is mild in this disorder. Patients with FXI deficiency may not experience abnormal bleeding in their life. Although severe bleeding is rare, menorrhagia and epistaxis are relatively common. Due to high fibrinolytic activity in oral and nasal cavities or the urinary tract, bleeding risk is higher in these areas. Some patients may experience bleeding after some surgeries such as tooth extraction and tonsillectomy. Postpartum hemorrhage may occur in this disorder [15, 38, 39].

The normal range of FXI coagulant activity (FXI:C) is 70–150 U/dL. Severe FXI-deficient patients have 1–20 U/dL of FXI:C level, while those with partially deficient FXI have 20–60 U/dL FXI:C levels, and patients with mild deficiency have 61–80 U/dL FXI plasma level. Individuals with severe FXI deficiency are homozygous or compound heterozygous for causative mutations, while those with partial deficiency are heterozygous, with one mutated allele [1, 2, 5]. Activated partial thromboplastin time (aPTT) is the screening test for FXII-mediated FXI activation and is prolonged in FXI deficiency. Thrombin-mediated FXI activation is assayed via FXIIa-inhibited diluted thromboplastin time (FXII ai DTT). FXI antigen level (FIX:Ag) is measured via enzyme-linked immunosorbent assay (ELISA). Generally, the mainstay of treatment in these patients is on-demand therapy. Replacement therapy is used in invasive operations, but it is not required for minor surgeries such as tooth extraction. Desmopressin elevates endogenous FXI level and can be used in severe FXI deficiency. Recombinant FVII (rFVII) can be used for patients with inhibitor (plasma FXI level <1%). Oral antifibrinolytic agents such as tranexamic acid can be used in pregnant women and in minor surgeries such as tooth extraction [2, 5, 6].

12.5 Molecular Basis

F11 gene is located at the distal end of the long arm of chromosome 4 (4q35) and consists of 15 exons and 14 introns that span a 23-kb region [40]. This gene is expressed in hepatocytes and regulated via transcription factor hepatocyte nuclear factor-4a (HNF4-α). Blood mononuclear cells, granulocytes, pancreas, and kidney also express a little *F11* gene. FXI deficiency mostly is an autosomal recessive injury-related hemorrhagic disorder, but autosomal dominant forms of disease also were reported. FXI deficiency is due to mutation in *F11* gene (Fig. 12.4). Most of mutations are accompanied with CRM− phenotype and fewer associated with CRM+ phenotype [21]. In type I, CRM−, FXI:C, and FXI:Ag levels are decreased [11, 41]. In this type, the mutant protein level is low or absent that can be due to reduced translation, secretion, or stability of the protein. There are three subgroups in type I (CRM−) (Fig. 12.4) [42]:

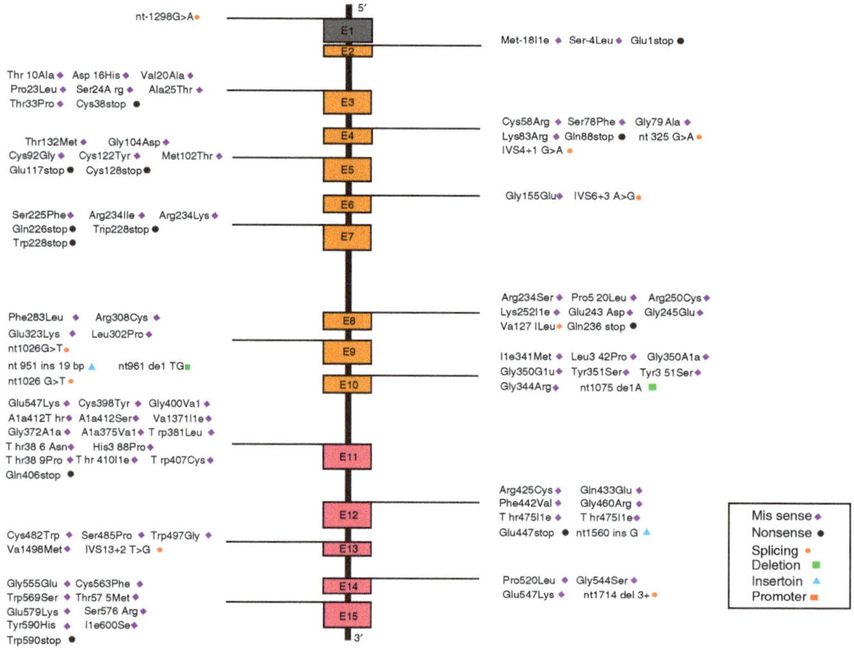

Fig. 12.4 A number of *F11* gene mutations. Missense mutations are the most common mutations within *F11* gene. Most of mutations occur in catalytic domain. *E* exon

(1) Mutations that affect protein synthesis; therefore the production of polypeptide is decreased or stopped. Glu117stop mutation is common in this group.
(2) Mutations that disrupt dimerization within two Ap4 domains; therefore polypeptide remains in monomeric form in the cell that results in decreased plasma level of FXI. Phe283Leu mutation is common in this group.
(3) Mutations that cause production of nonsecretable homodimers. Mutations that decrease homodimers secretion of wild-type FXI, also resulting in decreased plasma level of FXI. Ser225Phe and Trp596Ser mutations are common in this group.

In type II, CRM+, the FXI:C is low but FXI:Ag is normal. In other words, although the activity is decreased, the plasma protein level is normal or close to normal [38, 43]. A total of twelve CRM+ variants, eight in catalytic domain and four in apple domains, have been identified [6, 11].

Inhibitor formation against exogenous FXI is another problem in patients with FXI deficiency, mostly in severely affected patients. Patients with severe deficiency are at higher risk of inhibitor generation. FXI inhibitors are polyclonal IgG alloantibodies against various epitopes of the FXI molecule and inhibit FXI activation. The prevalence of antibody in patients with FXI deficiency is 3–5%. Most of patients with inhibitor are homozygotes, with <1% FXI plasma level and positive history of replacement therapy or injection of RH immunoglobulin. Glu117Stop is the most common mutation in patients with FXI deficiency and inhibitor [6, 11, 39, 44].

FXI deficiency in the Jewish population is due to four common causative mutations that are categorized as types I to IV. Type I, a point mutation, occurs at the donor splice site of the last intron (intron N) that is a G → A substitution. Type II, a nonsense mutation, Glu117stop in exon 5, results in early chain termination. Type III, a missense mutation, Phe283Leu substation in exon 9, results in the partial defect in dimerization and monomers of FXI hold over the cell [45]. Type IV is caused by a 14bp deletion in exon 14/intron N splice site. Types II and III account for >90% of causative mutations in Jews population [46]. Other frequent mutations were observed in other populations including type II in Iraqi, Arab, and other Middle Eastern Jews. Type III mutation more frequently is found in recent European origin, Cys88Stopp mutation in French Basques and the Cys128Stop mutation in the United Kingdom [46–48]. More than 220 mutations were observed in *F11* gene. *F11* mutations include missense (67%), nonsense (11.9%), splice site (10.6%), deletion/insertion (9.4%), and promoter mutations (0.8%) [45, 49, 50].

Most of mutations occur at the catalytic domain with about 31% frequency and then Ap1, Ap4, Ap3, intronic region, Ap2, signal peptide, and linker region, respectively (Fig. 12.5) [11, 12].

12.6 Clinical Manifestations

Patients with FXI deficiency present variable clinical phenotypes [51]. Patients with homozygote and compound heterozygote mutations usually have less than 15–20 U/dL FXI level, while heterozygotes usually have FXI level between 20 and 70 U/dL (mild to moderate deficiency) [52]. Generally there is no direct correlation between

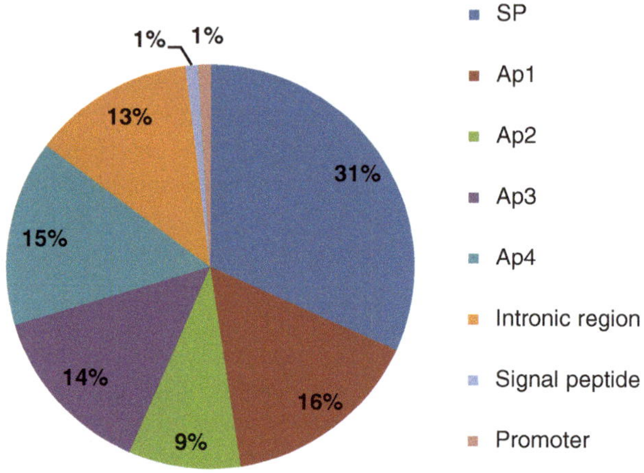

Fig. 12.5 Distribution of different mutations within *F11* gene, *Ap* apple domain, *SP* serine protease domain

bleeding tendency and FXI plasma level, bleeding tendency is more profound in homozygotes and compound heterozygotes than heterozygotes, and heterozygotes are usually asymptomatic. Some homozygotes may not experience abnormal bleeding in their life. FXI deficiency usually is detected in preoperative work-up, in hemostatic challenges, and in patients with positive family history of FXI deficiency. Although spontaneous bleeding is rare in this disorder, life-threatening bleeds after surgery or post-trauma may occur [50, 53]. Excessive bleeding often occurs in tonsillectomy, dental extraction, and sinus surgery. There is a mild to moderate bleeding tendency in hemostatic fluctuations at the sites with high fibrinolytic activity such as the oral cavity, nasal cavity, or genitourinary tract. Postpartum hemorrhage only occurs in ~20% of affected women [17, 54–57]. Abnormal bleeding due to obstetric and menstruation can occur in females (Table 12.1) [58]. Other contributing factors for bleeding tendency are type of mutations, plasmatic factors, platelet and endothelial disturbance, von Willebrand disease, hemophilia A or B, and other bleeding disorders [59]. These variable clinical symptoms make the diagnosis and management of FXI deficiences potentially difficult [60].

12.7 Diagnosis

Due to mild phenotype of the disorder, diagnosis of FXI deficiency is difficult, and in most cases, diagnosis is made based on family history or presurgery laboratory work-up. Routine and specific coagulation tests can be used for appropriate and timely diagnosis of the disorder. These tests include PT, aPTT, FXI:Ag, and FXI:C assays. FXII ai DTT can determine thrombin-mediated FXI activation [11].

- When PT is normal and aPTT is prolonged, there is probably FXI or other intrinsic coagulation pathway factor deficiencies. Differential diagnosis can be made by FXI:Ag and FXI:C assays.

Table 12.1 Clinical manifestations of patients with congenital factor XI deficiency

Bleeding symptom	Santorol et al. (*N*: 95)	Shao et al. (*N*: 57)	Peyvandi et al. (*N*: 18)
Ecchymosis	28		–
Epistaxis	24	5.3	27
Gastrointestinal bleeding	15	–	–
Hematuria	4	–	0
Hematoma	2	–	22
Menometrorrhagia	7 of women	7.5 of women	0.3 of women
Post-traumatic intracranial hemorrhage	1	–	–
Pulmonary hemorrhage	1	–	–
Gum bleeding	1	–	–
Bleeding from minor wounds	–	1.8	–
Postdental extraction bleeding	–	3.5	–
Postsurgical bleeding	–	2.5 of women	66
Hemarthrosis	–	–	27
Oral cavity bleeding	–	–	78
Easy bruising	–	8.8	–

- FXI plasma level (FXI:Ag) assay can be carried out by ELISA with a FXI polyclonal antibody in order to determine qualitative FXI deficiency [61, 62].
- FXI:C can be measured via a modified aPTT and FXII ai DTT.

aPTT reflects the FXII-imitated FXI activation and this test is prolonged in FXI deficiency. Patient's plasma is mixed with normal plasma. Correction percentage shows amount of FXI in patient's plasma [63, 64].

Factor XII-Inhibited Dilute Thromboplastin Time (FXII ai DTT)
Thromboplastin is diluted with normal saline to make different dilutions. Corn trypsin inhibitor (CTI) is a FXII inhibitor that is added immediately before assay. Diluted thromboplastin and plasma are mixed in identical proportion and are incubated for 2 min. Then, pre-warmed $CaCl_2$ is added in the mixture and clotting time is measured. FXII ai DTT is markedly prolonged in severe FXI deficiency at 1:1000 concentration of thromboplastin and has a good correlation with severity of bleeding [11, 63, 65, 66].

- *Thrombin generation assay (TGA) and thromboelastometry (TEM)* can be used to measure the effect of treatment with preferably solvent-detergent fresh frozen plasma (SD-FFP) or FXI concentrate in patient with FXI deficiency undergoing surgery and to limit monitoring the treatment with FVIIa and FXI concentrate in a small number of individuals [67, 68]. TGA is also a global test for hemostatic state of bleeder and non-bleeder. There is a miningful correlation between bleedin tendency and FXI level in patient with sever FXI deficiency [69, 70].

- *The mixing study* is used to find inhibitors in patients with severe FXI deficiency (<1%). The lack of aPTT correction after mixing of patient and control plasma probably is due to presence of inhibitors that required quantitative inhibitor assay. Patients with >5 Bethesda unit (BU) are classified as high-titration inhibitor [69, 70].
- *Molecular diagnosis*: Generally similar to other rare bleeding disorders, ther is no hot spot in *FII* gene, and therfore there is no recurrent mutation (s) that can be used a general marker for molecular diagnosis of FXI deficiency in all populations. Most of *FII* gene mutations are restricted to spesific family or population. Different molecular strategies were used in some areas. A four-color multiplex real time polymerase chain reaction (PCR) assay is used for detection of common mutations in specific population. Generally, for population without common mutation, coventional PCR and whole genom sequensing should be performed, but that is a costly and sophesticated process [47, 71–73].

12.8 Recommendations and Precautions in Laboratory Investigation

Although lipemic plasma may affect some coagulation tests in a number of automated analyzers, fasting is not necessary for routine coagulation tests. Patients should avoid stressful conditions, strenuous exercise, and some drugs that can affect the results. Anticoagulant drugs can also affect the results of coagulation tests [74].

Different aPTT reagents have been shown to give rise to variations in the aPTT sensitivity; therefore, reference ranges should be established locally [75, 76].

Some mutations such as large deletion or mutations in those regions that are not covered by conventional mutational screening may not be detected and should be analyzed with precauions. To predict effect of some of these mutations such as splice site mutations is difficult and required to be assessed either by reverse transcription (RT)-PCR or by using in vitro assessment by transfection of appropriate minigene construct [77].

Differential diagnoses should include presence of lupus anticoagulant, liver dysfunction, heparin contamination, VWD, and other coagulation factor deficiencies [11, 78].

12.9 Treatment

Most of patients with FXI deficiency have few problems during their life. Spontaneous bleeding except for menorrhagia is rare and usually reflow without treatment [79]. The mainstay of treatment in FXI deficiency similar to most other rare bleeding disorders is on-demand treatment that means stop the bleeding as soon as possible after onset of bleeding. Presence of FXI inhibitors should be also evaluated in patients with severe deficiency (<1%), particularly those that received plasma, FXI concentrates, or immunoglobulin. In addition to assessment the risk of thrombotic events in specific type of surgeries should carefully be evaluated. Age and underlying disease such as heart and renal failures can also affect the treatment [54, 77].

For patients with major surgeries, replacement therapy is used with FFP or FXI concentrate to achieve through levels of 45 U/dL for 5–7 days prior to surgery in areas with high fibrinolytic activity such as the nose, tonsils, oral cavity, and urinary tract [64, 80, 81]. The use of FFP may result in overload and related adverse consequences that are more important in patients with congestive heart failure and chronic renal failure. FXI concentrates have several advantages including (1) shorter infusion times and (2) level of other coagulation factors that are not increased and lower rate of transfusion-related reactions. Special precautions should be considered when these products are used in elderly and patients with cardiovascular disease, because of their potent thrombotic risk [81–83]. The dose should not exceed 30 U/kg and peak levels should not exceed 70 U/dL. Tranexamic acid should be avoided in patients receiving FXI concentrates, because it may pose thrombotic risk [59]. Replacement therapy is not necessary in minor surgeries. For minor surgeries such as tooth extraction and cataract extraction, antifibrinolytic agents such as *tranexamic acid* can be used. For this purpose, 1 g four times daily prescribed pre-operatively and then until 7 days post-operatively. 6-aminocaproic acid can be used 5–6 g four times daily at same time periods [84]. *Fibrin glue* can be used in resection of skin lesions and local hemostasis [64]. rFVII is used in patients with FXI deficiency and inhibitor [81]. *Desmopressin (DDAVP)*, a synthetic analogue of the natural antidiuretic hormone vasopressin, as a supplementary agent can elevate endogenous FXI level that can be used in patients with bleeding history (please refer to Chap. 3). Indeed, desmopressin can normalize coagulation parameters in heterozygous FXI deficiency by slightly increasing both FXI activity and antigen levels. Replacement therapy is not necessary in patients undergoing surgeries without history of bleeding tendency, but tranexamic acid and/or fibrin glue is used in high-risk surgeries such as prostatectomy [64, 84].

Patients with severe FXI deficiency may develop inhibitor after replacement therapy. *rFVIIa* or *prothrombin complex* is used in these patients [89, 90]. rFVIIa is effective at low dose of 15 μg/kg with *oral tranexamic acid* for major surgeries [91, 92]. It is also used in patients with history of allergic reaction to replacement therapy or those with IgA deficiency [77].

Menorrhagia

Oral antifibrinolytic agents such as *tranexamic acid* are used in women with prolong menorrhagia, but caution is required in elderly [64, 85].

Pregnant Women

In vaginal delivery women with partial FXI deficiency without previous bleeding history, wait and watch is recommended [55]. but In women with significant bleeding history, tranexamic acid for 3 days with the first dose being administered during vaginal delivery is used. FXI is prescribed for women with severe FXI deficiency during vaginal delivery. In caesarean section delivery, patients with severe FXI deficiency should receive FXI concentrate during labor. Oral antifibrinolytic agents can be used to prevent bleeding after surgery. FFP is advisable only when there is excessive bleeding during caesarean or vaginal delivery [55, 60, 86].

Circumcision

FXI deficiency may be observed first at this procedure. It is important to check newborn males in populations with high rate of FXI deficiency such as Ashkenazi Jews and Iraqi. For diagnosis of FXI deficiency in infants with FXI level of <10 U/dL, FXI level should be rechecked until 6 months. If the FXI level remained low, procedure should be performed by cover of either FFP or FXI concentrate. The boys with FXI levels >10 U/dL should receive tranexamic acid in a dose of 15 mg/kg every 8 h for 3 days under circumcision procedure [59, 87, 88].

Acknowledgment We appreciate the valuable work of Maryam Tabatabaei Shoja on this chapter that significantly improved the quality of this chapter.

References

1. Baglia FA, Gailani D, López JA, Walsh PN. Identification of a binding site for glycoprotein Ibα in the Apple 3 domain of factor XI. J Biol Chem. 2004;279(44):45470–6.
2. Sun M-F, Zhao M, Gailani D. Identification of amino acids in the factor XI apple 3 domain required for activation of factor IX. J Biol Chem. 1999;274(51):36373–8.
3. Zhao M, Abdel-Razek T, Sun M-F, Gailani D. Characterization of a heparin binding site on the heavy chain of factor XI. J Biol Chem. 1998;273(47):31153–9.
4. Emsley J, McEwan PA, Gailani D. Structure and function of factor XI. Blood. 2010;115(13):2569–77.
5. Jin L, Pandey P, Babine RE, Gorga JC, Seidl KJ, Gelfand E, et al. Crystal structures of the FXIa catalytic domain in complex with ecotin mutants reveal substrate-like interactions. J Biol Chem. 2005;280(6):4704–12.
6. Berber E. Molecular characterization of FXI deficiency. Clin Appl Thromb Hemost. 2011;17(1):27–32.
7. Papagrigoriou E, McEwan PA, Walsh PN, Emsley J. Crystal structure of the factor XI zymogen reveals a pathway for transactivation. Nat Struct Mol Biol. 2006;13(6):557–9.
8. Cheng Q, Sun MF, Kravtsov D, Aktimur L, Gailani D. Factor XI apple domains and protein dimerization. J Thromb Haemost. 2003;1(11):2340–7.

9. Gailani D, Smith S. Structural and functional features of factor XI. J Thromb Haemost. 2009;7(S1):75–8.
10. Bouma B, Griffin JH. Human blood coagulation factor XI. J Biol Chem. 1977;252(18):6432–7.
11. He R, Chen D, He S. Factor XI: hemostasis, thrombosis, and antithrombosis. Thromb Res. 2012;129(5):541–50.
12. McVey JH, Lal K, Imanaka Y, Kemball-Cook G, Bolton-Maggs P, Tuddenham EG. Characterisation of blood coagulation factor XI T475I. Thromb Haemost. 2005;93(6):1082–8.
13. Guella I, Soldà G, Spena S, Asselta R, Ghiotto R, Tenchini ML, et al. Molecular characterization of two novel mutations causing factor XI deficiency: a splicing defect and a missense mutation responsible for a CRM+ defect. Thromb Haemost. 2008;99(3):523–30.
14. O'connell NM. Factor XI deficiency-from molecular genetics to clinical management. Blood Coagul Fibrinolysis. 2003;14:S59–64.
15. Peretz H, Mulai A, Usher S, Zivelin A, Segal A, Weisman Z, et al. The two common mutations causing factor XI deficiency in Jews stem from distinct founders: one of ancient Middle Eastern origin and another of more recent European origin. Blood. 1997;90(7):2654–9.
16. Wu W, Sinha D, Shikov S, Yip CK, Walz T, Billings PC, et al. Factor XI homodimer structure is essential for normal proteolytic activation by factor XIIa, thrombin, and factor XIa. J Biol Chem. 2008;283:18655–64.
17. Peyvandi F, Duga S, Akhavan S, Mannucci P. Rare coagulation deficiencies. Haemophilia. 2002;8(3):308–21.
18. Asakai R, Chung DW, Davie EW, Seligsohn U. Factor XI deficiency in Ashkenazi Jews in Israel. N Engl J Med. 1991;325(3):153–8.
19. Zucker M, Zivelin A, Landau M, Rosenberg N, Seligsohn U. Three residues at the interface of factor XI (FXI) monomers augment covalent dimerization of FXI. J Thromb Haemost. 2009;7(6):970–5.
20. Sinha D, Marcinkiewicz M, Lear JD, Walsh PN. Factor XIa dimer in the activation of factor IX. Biochemistry. 2005;44(30):10416–22.
21. Gailani D, Broze GJ. Factor XI activation in a revised model of blood coagulation. Science. 1991;253(5022):909–12.
22. Fujikawa K, Chung DW, Hendrickson LE, Davie EW. Amino acid sequence of human factor XI, a blood coagulation factor with four tandem repeats that are highly homologous with plasma prekallikrein. Biochemistry. 1986;25(9):2417–24.
23. Smith SB, Verhamme IM, Sun M-F, Bock PE, Gailani D. Characterization of novel forms of coagulation factor XIa. J Biol Chem. 2008;283(11):6696–705.
24. Ratnoff OD, Saito H. Interactions among Hageman factor, plasma prekallikrein, high molecular weight kininogen, and plasma thromboplastin antecedent. Proc Natl Acad Sci. 1979;76(2):958–61.
25. Naito K, Fujikawa K. Activation of human blood coagulation factor XI independent of factor XII. Factor XI is activated by thrombin and factor XIa in the presence of negatively charged surfaces. J Biol Chem. 1991;266(12):7353–8.
26. Baglia FA, Jameson BA, Walsh PN. Identification and characterization of a binding site for platelets in the Apple 3 domain of coagulation factor XI. J Biol Chem. 1995;270(12):6734–40.
27. Bajaj SP, Rapaport SI, Russell WA. Redetermination of the rate-limiting step in the activation of factor IX by factor XIa and by factor VIIa/tissue factor: explanation for different electrophoretic radioactivity profiles obtained on activation of 3Hand 125I-labeled factor IX. Biochemistry. 1983;22(17):4047–53.
28. Von dem Borne PA, Meijers JC, Bouma BN. Feedback activation of factor XI by thrombin in plasma results in additional formation of thrombin that protects fibrin clots from fibrinolysis. Blood. 1995;86:3035–42.
29. Curling J, Goss N, Bertolini J, Chtourou S, Poulle M, Turecek P, et al. Production of plasma proteins for therapeutic use. Hoboken: John Wiley & Sons, Inc.; 2012.
30. Wuillemin WA, Minnema M, Meijers J, Roem D, Eerenberg A, Nuijens J, et al. Inactivation of factor XIa in human plasma assessed by measuring factor XIa-protease inhibitor complexes: major role for C1-inhibitor. Blood. 1995;85(6):1517–26.

31. Nielsen V. Effects of aprotinin on plasma coagulation kinetics determined by thrombelastography: role of Factor XI. Acta Anaesthesiol Scand. 2006;50(2):168–72.
32. Scandura JM, Zhang Y, Van Nostrand WE, Walsh PN. Progress curve analysis of the kinetics with which blood coagulation factor XIa is inhibited by protease nexin-2. Biochemistry. 1997;36:412–20.
33. Navaneetham D, Jin L, Pandey P, Strickler JE, Babine RE, Abdel-Meguid SS, et al. Structural and mutational analyses of the molecular interactions between the catalytic domain of factor XIa and the Kunitz protease inhibitor domain of protease nexin 2. J Biol Chem. 2005;280(43):36165–75.
34. Zhang J, Tu Y, Lu L, Lasky N, Broze GJ Jr. Protein Z-dependent protease inhibitor deficiency produces a more severe murine phenotype than protein Z deficiency. Blood. 2008;111:4973–8.
35. Yang L, Sun MF, Gailani D, Rezaie AR. Characterization of a heparin-binding site on the catalytic domain of factor XIa: mechanism of heparin acceleration of factor XIa inhibition by the serpins antithrombin and C1-inhibitor. Biochemistry. 2009;48:1517–24.
36. Guéguen P, Galinat H, Blouch MT, Bridey F, Duchemin J, Le Gal G, et al. Biological determinants of bleeding in patients with heterozygous factor XI deficiency. Br J Haematol. 2012;156(2):245–51.
37. Rosenthal RL, Dreskin OH, Rosenthal N. New hemophilia-like disease caused by deficiency of a third plasma thromboplastin factor. Proc Soc Exp Biol Med. 1953;82:171–4.
38. Saunders RE, O'Connell NM, Lee CA, Perry DJ, Perkins SJ. Factor XI deficiency database: an interactive web database of mutations, phenotypes, and structural analysis tools. Hum Mutat. 2005;26:192–8.
39. Zucker M, Zivelin A, Teitel J, Seligsohn U. Induction of an inhibitor antibody to factor XI in a patient with severe inherited factor XI deficiency by Rh immune globulin. Blood. 2008;111(3):1306–8.
40. Kato A, Asakai R, Davie E, Aoki N. Factor XI gene (F11) is located on the distal end of the long arm of human chromosome 4. Cytogenet Genome Res. 1989;52(1–2):77–8.
41. Saito H, Ratnoff OD, Bouma BN, Seligsohn U. Failure to detect variant (CRM+) plasma thromboplastin antecedent (factor XI) molecules in hereditary plasma thromboplastin antecedent deficiency: a study of 125 patients of several ethnic backgrounds. J Lab Clin Med. 1985;106(6):718–22.
42. Kravtsov DV, Monahan PE, Gailani D. A classification system for cross-reactive material-negative factor XI deficiency. Blood. 2005;105:4671–3.
43. Mannhalter C, Hellstern P, Deutsch E. Identification of a defective factor XI cross-reacting material in a factor XI deficient patient. Blood. 1987;70:31–7.
44. Salomon O, Zivelin A, Livnat T, Dardik R, Loewenthal R, Avishai O, et al. Prevalence, causes, and characterization of factor XI inhibitors in patients with inherited factor XI deficiency. Blood. 2003;101(12):4783–8.
45. Hancock JF, Wieland K, Pugh R, Martinowitz U, Schulman S, Kakkar V, et al. A molecular genetic study of factor XI deficiency. Blood. 1991;77(9):1942–8.
46. Shpilberg O, Peretz H, Zivelin A, Yatuv R, Chetrit A, Kulka T, et al. One of the two common mutations causing factor XI deficiency in Ashkenazi Jews (type II) is also prevalent in Iraqi Jews, who represent the ancient gene pool of Jews. Blood. 1995;85(2):429–32.
47. Zivelin A, Bauduer F, Ducout L, Peretz H, Rosenberg N, Yatuv R, et al. Factor XI deficiency in French Basques is caused predominantly by an ancestral Cys38Arg mutation in the factor XI gene. Blood. 2002;99(7):2448–54.
48. Bolton-Maggs P, Peretz H, Butler R, Mountford R, Keeney S, Zacharski L, et al. A common ancestral mutation (C128X) occurring in 11 non-Jewish families from the UK with factor XI deficiency. J Thromb Haemost. 2004;2(6):918–24.
49. Bouma BN, Meijers JC. Role of blood coagulation factor XI in downregulation of fibrinolysis. Curr Opin Hematol. 2000;7(5):266–72.
50. International Society on Thrombosis and Haemostasis. [internet] 2015 [cited 22 Sept 2017]. http://www.isth.org/?MutationsRareBleedin.

51. Peyvandi F, Lak M, Mannucci PM. Factor XI deficiency in Iranians: its clinical manifestations in comparison with those of classic hemophilia. Haematologica. 2002;87(5):512–4.
52. Chi C, Kulkarni A, Lee CA, Kadir RA. The obstetric experience of women with factor XI deficiency. Acta Obstet Gynecol Scand. 2009;88(10):1095–100.
53. Mannucci PM, Duga S, Peyvandi F. Recessively inherited coagulation disorders. Blood. 2004;104(5):1243–52.
54. Bolton-Maggs P, Patterson D, Wensley R, Tuddenham E. Definition of the bleeding tendency in factor XI-deficient kindredsDOUBLEHYPHENa clinical and laboratory study. Thromb Haemost. 1995;73(2):194–202.
55. Salomon O, Steinberg DM, Tamarin I, Zivelin A, Seligsohn U. Plasma replacement therapy during labor is not mandatory for women with severe factor XI deficiency. Blood Coagul Fibrinolysis. 2005;16(1):37–41.
56. Martincic D, Zimmerman SA, Ware RE, Sun M-F, Whitlock JA, Gailani D. Identification of mutations and polymorphisms in the factor XI genes of an African American family by dideoxyfingerprinting. Blood. 1998;92(9):3309–17.
57. Shao Y, Cao Y, Lu Y, Dai J, Ding Q, Wang X, et al. Clinical manifestations and mutation spectrum of 57 subjects with congenital factor XI deficiency in China. Blood Cells Mol Dis. 2016;58:29–34.
58. Santoro C, Di Mauro R, Baldacci E, De Angelis F, Abbruzzese R, Barone F, et al. Bleeding phenotype and correlation with factor XI (FXI) activity in congenital FXI deficiency: results of a retrospective study from a single centre. Haemophilia. 2015;21(4):496–501.
59. Bolton-Maggs P, Perry D, Chalmers E, Parapia L, Wilde J, Williams M, et al. The rare coagulation disorders–review with guidelines for management from the United Kingdom Haemophilia Centre Doctors' Organisation. Haemophilia. 2004;10(5):593–628.
60. Mumford AD, Ackroyd S, Alikhan R, Bowles L, Chowdary P, Grainger J, et al. Guideline for the diagnosis and management of the rare coagulation disorders. Br J Haematol. 2014;167(3):304–26.
61. Wilmot H, Hockley J, Rigsby P, Gray E. Establishment of the World Health Organization 2nd international standard for factor XI, plasma, human. Front Med. 2017;4:28.
62. Zadra G, Asselta R, Malcovati M, Santagostino E, Peyvandi F, Mannucci PM, et al. Molecular genetic analysis of severe coagulation factor XI deficiency in six Italian patients. Haematologica. 2004;89(11):1332–40.
63. Wheeler AP, Gailani D. Why factor XI deficiency is a clinical concern. Expert Rev Hematol. 2016;9(7):629–37.
64. Seligsohn U. Factor XI deficiency in humans. J Thromb Haemost. 2009;7(s1):84–7.
65. He S, Xiong S, He R, He X, Liu F, Han J, et al. Factor XIIa-inhibited diluted thromboplastin time can reflect coagulation process. Zhonghua Xue Ye Xue Za Zhi. 2000;21(3):118–21.
66. He R, Xiong S, He X, Liu F, Han J, Li J, et al. The role of factor XI in a dilute thromboplastin assay of extrinsic coagulation pathway. Thromb Haemost. 2001;85(6):1055–9.
67. Pike G, Cumming A, Thachil J, Hay C, Bolton-Maggs P, Burthem J. Evaluation of the use of rotational thromboelastometry in the assessment of FXI deficiency. Haemophilia. 2017;23(3):449–57.
68. Pike G, Cumming A, Thachil J, Hay C, Burthem J, Bolton-Maggs P. Evaluation of the use of global haemostasis assays to monitor treatment in factor XI deficiency. Haemophilia. 2017;23(2):273–83.
69. Livnat T, Martinowitz U, Mansharov R, Ariella Z. Thrombin generation test can predict bleeding tendency in patients with severe factor XI deficiency. Am Soc Hematology. 2013;122:3600.
70. James P, Salomon O, Mikovic D, Peyvandi F. Rare bleeding disorders–bleeding assessment tools, laboratory aspects and phenotype and therapy of FXI deficiency. Haemophilia. 2014;20(s4):71–5.
71. Mitchell M, Harrington P, Cutler J, Rangarajan S, Savidge G, Alhaq A. Eighteen unrelated patients with factor XI deficiency, four novel mutations and a 100% detection rate by denaturing highperformance liquid chromatography. Br J Haematol. 2003;121(3):500–2.

72. Zucker M, Rosenberg N, Peretz H, et al. Point mutations regarded asmissense mutations cause splicing defects in the factor XI gene. J Thromb Haemost. 2011;9(10):1977–84.
73. Weaver JM, Edwards PA. Targeted next-generation sequencing for routine clinical screening of mutations. Genome Med. 2011;3(9):58.
74. Lippi G, Salvagno GL, Montagnana M, Lima-Oliveira G, Guidi GC, Favaloro EJ. Quality standards for sample collection in coagulation testing. Semin Thromb Hemost. 2012;38(6):565–75.
75. Srivastava A, Brewer A, Mauser-Bunschoten E, Key N, Kitchen S, Llinas A, et al. Guidelines for the management of hemophilia. Haemophilia. 2013;19(1):e1–47.
76. Gomez K, Bolton-Maggs P. Factor XI deficiency. Haemophilia. 2008;14(6):1183–9.
77. Duga S, Salomon O. Factor XI deficiency. Semin Thromb Hemost. 2009;35(4):416–25.
78. Bortoli R, Monticielo OA, Chakr RM, Palominos PE, Rohsig LM, Kohem CL, et al., editors. Acquired factor XI inhibitor in systemic lupus erythematosus—case report and literature review, Seminars in arthritis and rheumatism. New York: Elsevier; 2009.
79. Kadir R, Economides D, Lee C. Factor XI deficiency in women. Am J Hematol. 1999;60(1):48–54.
80. Salomon O, Steinberg D, Seligshon U. Variable bleeding manifestations characterize different types of surgery in patients with severe factor XI deficiency enabling parsimonious use of replacement therapy. Haemophilia. 2006;12(5):490–3.
81. Bolton-Maggs PH. Factor XI deficiency and its management. Haemophilia. 2000;6:100–9.
82. Bolton-Maggs P, Colvin B, Satchi B, Lee C. Thrombogenic potential of factor XI concentrate. Lancet. 1994;344(8924):748.
83. Mannucci PM, Bauer KA, Santagostino E, et al. Activation of the coagulation cascade after infusion of a factor XI concentrate in congenitally deficient patients. Blood. 1994;84:1314–9.
84. Berliner S, Horowitz I, Martinowitz U, Brenner B, Seligsohn U. Dental surgery in patients with severe factor XI deficiency without plasma replacement. Blood Coagul Fibrinolysis. 1992;3(4):465–8.
85. Bonnar J, Sheppard BL. Treatment of menorrhagia during menstruation: randomised controlled trial of ethamsylate, mefenamic acid, and tranexamic acid. BMJ. 1996;313(7057):579–82.
86. Davies J, Kadir R, editors. The management of factor XI deficiency in pregnancy. Seminars in thrombosis and hemostasis. Stuttgart: Thieme Medical Publishers; 2016.
87. Kadir R, Kingman C, Chi C, O'connell N, Riddell A, Lee C, et al. Screening for factor XI deficiency amongst pregnant women of Ashkenazi Jewish origin. Haemophilia. 2006;12(6):625–8.
88. Ben-Nun L. Fatal condition related to male circumcision. Israel: B.N. Publications House; 2011.
89. Kenet G, Lubetsky A, Luboshitz J, Ravid B, Tamarin I, Varon D, et al. Lower doses of rFVIIa therapy are safe and effective for surgical interventions in patients with severe FXI deficiency and inhibitors. Haemophilia. 2009;15(5):1065–73.
90. Lawler P, White B, Pye S, Hermans C, Riddell A, Costello C, et al. Successful use of recombinant factor VIIa in a patient with inhibitor secondary to severe factor XI deficiency. Haemophilia. 2002;8(2):145–8.
91. Livnat T, Tamarin I, Mor Y, Winckler H, Horowitz Z, Korianski Y, et al. Recombinant activated factor VII and tranexamic acid are haemostatically effective during major surgery in factor XI-deficient patients with inhibitor antibodies. Thromb Haemost. 2009;102(3):487–92.
92. O'connell N, Riddell A, Pascoe G, Perry D, Lee C. Recombinant factor VIIa to prevent surgical bleeding in factor XI deficiency. Haemophilia. 2008;14(4):775–81.

Congenital Factor XIII Deficiency 13

Akbar Dorgalaleh, Majid Naderi, and Majid Safa

13.1 Introduction

Coagulation factor XIII (FXIII) is a transglutaminase (EC 2.3.2.13) composed of two carrier subunits (FXIII-B_2) and two catalytic subunits (FXIII-A_2) which circulates in the bloodstream as a heterotetramer (FXIII-A_2B_2) [1]. FXIII has a crucial role in hemostasis and in the final step of coagulation cascade, with the cross-linking of unstable primary fibrin, makes it firm and stable [1, 2]. In addition to the well-known role of FXIII in coagulation cascade, this factor has several crucial roles in other processes including angiogenesis, wound healing, and pregnancy maintenance as well as bone metabolism and cardiac protection [1, 3–6]. Congenital FXIII deficiency is an extremely rare hemorrhagic disorder with estimated incidence of 1 per 2 million in the general population. Patients with this disorder present severe clinical presentations including umbilical cord bleeding, recurrent pregnancy loss, and intracranial hemorrhage (ICH) [7]. Patients with severe FXIII deficiency (<1%) should receive regular primary prophylaxis from the time of diagnosis, even in the absence of severe clinical presentations. Different therapeutic choices are available for this disorder, including fresh frozen plasma (FFP), cryoprecipitate, FXIII concentrate (Corifact™/Fibrogammin®P), and recombinant FXIII (rFXIII) (NovoThirteen, Tretten) [7–9]. Today FXIII concentrate is the treatment of choice,

A. Dorgalaleh (✉) · M. Safa
Department of Hematology and Blood Transfusion, School of Allied Medicine, Iran University of Medical Sciences, Tehran, Iran

M. Naderi
Department of Pediatrics Hematology and Oncology, Ali Ebn-e Abitaleb Hospital Research Centre for Children and Adolescents Health [RCCAH], Zahedan University of Medical Sciences, Zahedan, Iran

A. Dorgalaleh (ed.), *Congenital Bleeding Disorders*,
https://doi.org/10.1007/978-3-319-76723-9_13

and FFP and cryoprecipitate are not recommended due to the risk of transfusion-transmitted diseases. In addition to primary prophylaxis, these patients may require on-demand therapy in different situations. Dose of replacement therapy in these conditions such as acute bleeding, ICH, and major and minor surgeries varies in case to case. FXIII deficiency is the most underdiagnosed bleeding disorder that accompanies with normal results in routine coagulation tests. FXIII functional assay is recommended as the first-line screening test, but clot solubility test remained as the only diagnostic test in a considerable number of countries [7, 8]. The available used assays for the measurement of FXIII activity are ammonia release assays that can potentially overestimate FXIII activity in the absence of plasma blank [2, 9]. Diagnosis of the disorder can be made based on clinical presentations, family history, and appropriate laboratory diagnosis. With timely diagnosis and appropriate management of the disorder, severe diathesis of the disorder and fetal consequences can be significantly decreased or even be alleviated [2, 8].

13.2 Factor XIII Structure and Function

FXIII or fibrin-stabilizing factor is a 37 kDa circulating protein in plasma as a tetramer (FXIII-A_2B_2) composed of two subunits including catalytic FXIII-A_2 and carrier FXIII-B_2. FXIII-A is mainly synthesized by bone marrow origin cells, while FXIII-B is mainly produced by hepatocytes [2, 10–13]. FXIII-A as a tetramer is present in plasma (FXIII-A_2B_2), while dimeric form of protein (FXIII-A_2) is present in platelets, monocytes, megakaryocytes, and macrophages [12, 13]. About 50% of FXIII-B presents in plasma in dimeric non-complex form [2].

FXIII-A is a 731-amino acid transglutaminase (732 amino acids with initiator methionine) and consists of an activation peptide in the N-terminal and four other domains: β-sandwich, catalytic core, β-barrel 1, and β-barrel 2 (Fig. 13.1) [2, 3].

Activation peptide, composed of first 37 amino acids in N-terminal of FXIII-A, buries cysteine 34 in catalytic core to prevent its access to substrate and keeps FXIII-A in inactivation form [2, 3]. Tyrosine 560 side chain in β-barrel 1 also has a similar function. Therefore, for the activation of FXIII-A, the activation peptide should be cleaved, and tyrosine 560 should be dislocated. This cleavage is done by

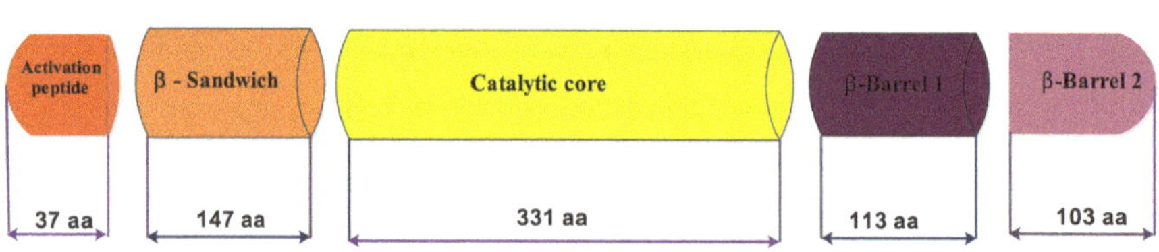

Fig. 13.1 Structure of factor XIII-A subunit. Factor XIII consists of an activation peptide that comprises the first 37 amino acids of the N-terminus, β-sandwich domain (R38–184), the catalytic core domain (R185–515), β-barrel 1 (R516–628), and final domain of factor XIII-A at the C-terminal of the protein β-barrel 2 (R629–731)

thrombin that cleaves between arginine 37 in activation peptide and glycine 38 in β-sandwich. Activation peptide is released in plasma, and this cleavage helps the stabilization of FXIII-A dimer. Cleavage of only one activation peptide is sufficient to complete the activation of FXIII-A_2 (Fig. 13.2) [2, 3].

Finally in the presence of Ca^{2+}, disassociation of FXIII-B and FXIII-A subunits occurs, and FXIII becomes fully activated. Activated FXIII catalyzes an acyl transfer reaction [2, 10].

FXIII-B is a 641-amino acid glycoprotein with a molecular weight of about 80 kDa. FXIII-B is composed of ten short tandem repeats called sushi domains. Each of these domains consists of about 60 amino acids. FXIII-B is carrier of FXIII-A in plasma, and in the absence of FXIII-B subunit, plasma level of FXIII-A subunit significantly is decreased. It seems that sushi one has a crucial role in FXIII-A_2B_2 heterotetramer formation [2, 3].

In addition to the well-known role of FXIII in coagulation cascade, it has several important roles in the body including angiogenesis, wound healing, bone metabolism, cardiac protection, and pregnancy maintenance [2, 3, 10]. FII, FVII, FXIII, and tissue factors all had relatively significant role on angiogenesis [2, 3]. It seems that FXIII performs this role by activation of TGF-β, which is a potent proangiogenic factor, and also by stimulation of neovascularization. Recurrent miscarriage is a common feature of congenital FXIII deficiency [7, 15]. Although the exact process of miscarriage in congenital FXIII deficiency is not known, FXIII accumulates in the placenta in the joining site of maternal and fetus tissues and helps in the cytotrophoblastic shell formation and stabilization of fibrinoid layer. In FXIII-A deficiency, the formation of cytotrophoblastic shell and fibrinoid layer is impaired and leads to placenta detachment and subsequently fetal loss [2, 14].

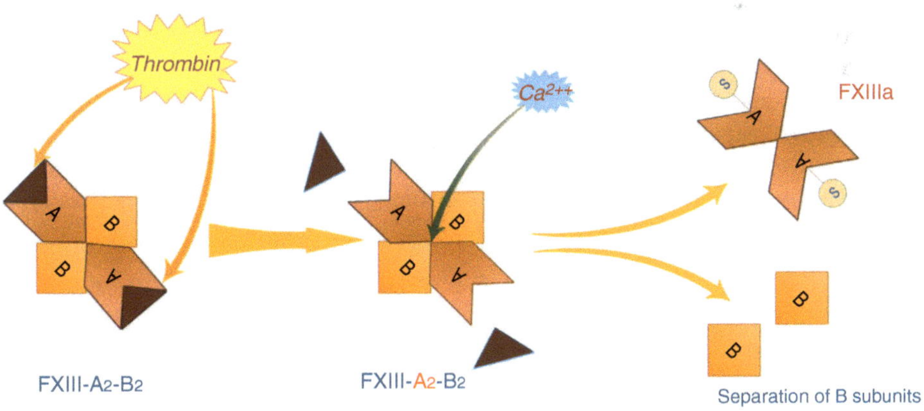

Fig. 13.2 Activation of factor (F) XIII ([2] with permission from publisher). For the activation of FXIII-A, the activation peptide should be cleaved by thrombin that cleaves between arginine 37 in activation peptide and glycine 38 in β-sandwich. Activation peptide is released in plasma and this cleavage helps the stabilization of FXIII-A dimer. In the next step, in the presence of Ca^{2+}, disassociation of FXIII-B and FXIII-A subunits occurs, and FXIII becomes fully activated

Impaired wound healing was reported in 20% of patients with congenital FXIII deficiency. It seems that the main issue which causes impaired wound healing is the impact of FXIII on collagen synthesis and its cross-linking that in some extent is performed by FXIII [5, 16, 17].

13.3 Congenital Factor XIII Deficiency

Congenital FXIII deficiency is an extremely rare hemorrhagic disorder with estimated incidence of 1 per 2 million in the general population. This disorder is inherited in autosomal recessive manner and therefore is more frequent in areas with high rate of consanguineous marriage [7]. Iran, especially southeast Iran, is such area that with high rate of consanguinity has the highest global incidence of this disorder. Patients with congenital FXIII deficiency represent a wide range of clinical manifestations notably umbilical cord bleeding (>80%) in the first days of life. Moreover patients have other life-threatening bleeds including umbilical cord bleeding, ICH, and recurrent pregnancy loss [5, 18]. Other bleeds such as hematoma, hemarthrosis, and epistaxis also can be observed among these patients. Due to the high rate of life-threatening bleeding, timely diagnosis and appropriate management of this disorder are crucial [18, 19]. Diagnosis of this disorder is a challenge worldwide, and FXIII functional assay is recommended as the first-line screening test, but clot solubility test remained as the only diagnostic test in many areas of the world [8, 19–21]. Due to the high rate of ICH in congenital FXIII deficiency, regular primary prophylaxis is mandatory for all severely affected patients from the time of diagnosis, even in the absence of severe clinical presentations. Patients with congenital FXIII deficiency can be managed by FFP and cryoprecipitate, as traditional choices, or by FXIII concentrate (Corifact™/Fibrogammin®P) or recombinant FXIII (rFXIII) (NovoThirteen, Tretten), as new therapeutic options. Due to the risk of transmission of blood-borne diseases with transfusion of FFP and cryoprecipitate, FXIII concentrate is the treatment of choice [18, 22]. But this plasma-derived component is not available everywhere, and in these areas, it is better to use viral inactivated blood component, especially FFP because viral inactivated form of cryoprecipitate is not available [2]. Although FXIII deficiency is

Table 13.1 Classification of factor XIII deficiency

		Plasma FXIII activity	Plasma FXIII-A_2B_2 antigen	Plasma FXIII-A antigen	Plasma FXIII-B antigen	Plt FXIII-A antigen
FXIII-A deficiency	Type I	↓↓↓	↓↓↓	↓↓↓	>30%	↓↓↓
	Type II	↓↓↓	↓N	↓N	>30%	↓↓↓
FXIII-B deficiency		↓↓	↓↓↓	↓↓	↓↓↓	N

accompanied with high rate of morbidity and mortality, with timely diagnosis and appropriate management, life-threatening diathesis can be significantly decreased or even can be alleviated [18, 19]. Based on FXIII functional and antigen assays, FXIII deficiency is classified to FXIII-A type I and type II and FXIII-B deficiency (Table 13.1) [23].

13.4 Worldwide Distribution of Congenital Factor XIII Deficiency

The precise distribution of FXIII deficiency in different geographical areas is not clear, and the exact number of patients, such many other inherited disorders in the world was not determined. Due to complications in diagnosis of disease, especially in areas with less equipped coagulation laboratories as well as lower incidence of bleeding in patients with mild and moderate FXIII deficiency, determining the exact distribution of the disease is difficult [8]. According to the World Federation of Hemophilia (WFH) survey in 2016, the total number of patients with FXIII deficiency was 1553 among 72 countries of the world that covered 90% of the world population. According to this survey, Iran with 593 patients has the largest number of patients with FXIII deficiency worldwide [18, 24]. In our recent study, the more precise number of patients with FXIII deficiency in Iran was determined, and it was clear that Iran has the largest global population of FXIII deficiency, and in Iran, Sistan and Baluchestan Province, southeast of Iran, with 410 affected patients has a great number of patients with FXIII deficiency [18]. Although Iran has the biggest population of FXIII deficiency, according to the WFH survey, the United States with 103 affected patients, has a large number of patients with FXIII deficiency (Fig. 13.3).

In a recent report of PRO-RBDD from 52 hemophilia treatment centers (HTCs), data of 573 patients with FXIII deficiency was released. In fact, due to the high number of precipitate countries in this project, this international network gives us some information about prevalence and distribution of the disease worldwide, although other main aims of the study are about frequency of bleeding episodes and management of bleeding and establishment of minimum coagulant activity level to prevent bleeding [24, 25]. In a worthwhile study, on 104 patients with FXIII deficiency with 24 nationalities living in 15 countries, an isolated Finnish population with an incidence of 1 per 650,000 inhabitants has the highest rate of FXIII deficiency in Europe. This high prevalence of FXIII deficiency in Finland was reported previously and has been attributed to be a consequence of the founder effect [26, 27]. According to the investigation of Vytautas Ivaskevicius et al., Switzerland had a prevalence of 14 unrelated families per 7.4 million inhabitants and Poland had 1 case per 6,000,000 residents (total population of 38 million) [27].

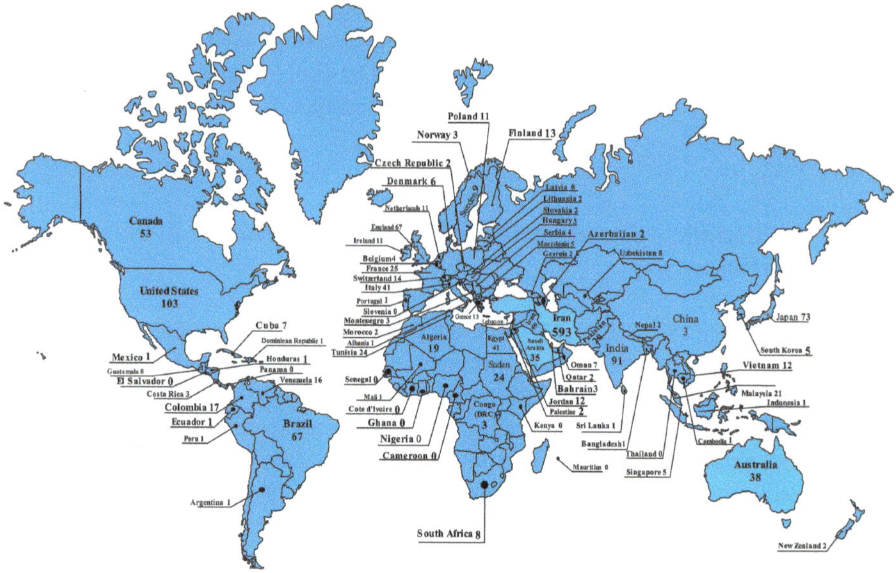

Fig. 13.3 The number of patients with congenital factor XIII deficiency in different countries. World Federation of Hemophilia (WFH) 2016 survey

13.5 Clinical Manifestations

Congenital FXIII deficiency is one of the most serious and severe congenital bleeding disorders with very high rate of life-threatening bleeding diathesis. Umbilical cord bleeding with a frequency of >80% is the most common presentation of congenital FXIII deficiency. This presentation is also frequent in congenital afibrinogenemia (~85%) [27–29]. Umbilical cord bleeding is a medical emergency that requires medical intervention [19, 29]. ICH is another severe presentation of congenital FXIII deficiency that is more frequent in this disorder than any other congenital bleeding disorder [19, 30]. The prevalence of ICH in congenital FVII, FXD, FVD, and FVIII deficiencies and afibrinogenemia is 15%, 7%, 5%, 4%, and 2%, respectively [30–32]. This diathesis, rarely, was reported in FII deficiency, von Willebrand disease (VWD) type 3, Glanzmann thrombasthenia, and gray platelet syndrome [32–37]. Without timely diagnosis and appropriate management of patients with congenital FXIII deficiency, ICH leads to death of about one third of patients with this disorder until the middle age [19, 30, 38]. ICH is the cause of 80% of death in congenital FXIII deficiency and in 15% of cases who experience this diathesis results in death [19]. Miscarriage is another common presentation of women with congenital FXIII deficiency. This presentation can be observed in both FXIII-A and FXIII-B deficiencies. The frequency of miscarriage is about 15% in FXIII-B deficiency, while this diathesis is more common in FXIII-A deficiency. Although, rarely successfully delivery can be observed in FXIII-A deficiency without replacement therapy, generally it is accepted that without replacement therapy unable to have successfully delivery [8, 14, 39, 40]. Different clinical presentations of patients with congenital FXIII deficiency according to four main studies were summarized in Table 13.2.

13.6 Molecular Basis

FXIII-A_2B_2 is encoded by two separated genes on 6p24–25 (FXIII-A subunit) and 1q31–32.1 (FXIII-B subunit) chromosomal regions. *F13A1* and *F13B* genes have 15 and 12 exons, respectively. A wide spectrum of normal gene variations was observed throughout two genes [41, 42]. Five common polymorphisms were observed in *F13A1* gene including Val34Leu, Tyr204Phe, Pro564Leu, Glu651Gln, and Val650Ile. Val34Leu polymorphism as the most common polymorphism is common among different populations except for Asian [2, 42]. Two common polymorphisms were reported in *F13B* gene including His95Arg and IVS11+144 (nt29756 C > G). In addition to these normal gene variations, a wide range of disease-causing mutations was observed in *F13A1* gene, while only 16 mutations were observed in *F13B* gene. A total of 156 mutations, mostly missense, were observed within *F13A1* gene [1, 43, 44] (Fig. 13.4).

These mutations are scattered throughout *F13A1* gene and mostly are specific to an especial family or ethnicity. Trp187Arg (c.559T>C) (according to HGVS: Trp188Arg, c.562 T>C), as the most common mutation of *F13A1* gene, only was

Table 13.2 Clinical manifestations of patients with congenital factor XIII deficiency

	Dorgalaleh et al (*n*: 190) (%)	Lak et al. (*n*: 93) (%)	Shetty et al. (*n*: 96) (%)	Ivaskevicius et al. (*n*: 104) (%)
Umbilical cord bleeding	82.5	73	73	56
Hematoma	53	58	–	49
Prolonged wound bleeding	31	–	–	–
Gum bleeding	17	48	13	–
Epistaxis	14	32	25	–
Ecchymosis	13	–	58	–
GI bleeding	–	10	–	6
Delayed postdental extraction bleeding	7	–	–	–
Intracranial bleeding	17	25	19	34
Post-circumcision bleeding	4	–	–	–
Hemarthrosis	4	55	7	36
Postsurgical bleeding	3	84	19	40
Miscarriage	10[a]	50	–	–
Menorrhagia	5	10	94	–

observed in a large number of Iranian patients. IVS5–1G>A and c.1984C>T were observed among different European countries [27, 41, 44]. c.1984C>T was also observed in Korea and India [45–47]. These mutations can be used for prenatal diagnosis (PND), in affected families. Trp187Arg, as the only disease-causing mutation of *F13A1* gene in southeast Iran, routinely is used for diagnosis of patients, pre-marriage and PND [2, 41, 44]. Most of *F13A1* gene mutations cause FXIII protein insatiability and intracellular degradation [2, 41, 44].

13.7 Diagnosis

Since FXIII deficiency is an autosomal recessive disorder with severe bleeding tendency, diagnosis of disorder could be made based on family history, clinical presentations, and an appropriate laboratory approach [8]. Diagnosis of congenital FXIII deficiency is a challenge worldwide, and FXIII deficiency is on of the most underdiagnosed bleeding disorders. In patients with congenital FXIII deficiency, all routine coagulation tests including prothrombin time (PT) and activated partial thromboplastin time (aPTT), thrombin time (TT), and bleeding time (BT) are normal, unless concomitant coagulopathy is present. For example, in systemic lupus erythematosus with lupus anticoagulant, both prolonged aPTT and decrease FXIII level due to autoantibody against FXIII may be present [2, 48]. Traditionally, clot solubility test is used for diagnosis of FXIII deficiency. Although clot solubility test is not further recommended for diagnosis of FXIII deficiency, a considerable number of laboratories over the world use this test as the only diagnostic test for detection of FXIII deficiency [7, 8, 49]. In this assay, patient's plasma is incubated with calcium with or without thrombin for 1 hour at room temperature (RT) or 37 °C. Then clot is suspended in a solubilizing agent most often urea 5M, acetic acid 2%, or monochloroacetic acid (MCA) 1% and incubated at 37 °C or RT, and then it is evaluated in regular intervals of 20 min, 1 h, and 24 h. In patients with FXIII deficiency, clot is dissolved within a few minutes to 1 h, while in normal individuals, clot is stable for 1 day or more [20].

Sensitivity and specificity of clot solubility test are affected by clotting agent and solubilizing agent. Although there are more sensitive combinations of clot solubility test including the combination of thrombin as clotting agent and acid acetic 2% as solubilizing agent, one of the least sensitive combinations and one of the most commonly used method worldwide includes urea 5M as solubilizing agent and calcium chloride as clotting agent. These common combinations are sensitive to 1–5% of plasma FXIII, while combination of thrombin and acetic acid is sensitive to 10% [20, 8]. Other combinations, such as calcium chloride with acetic acid and thrombin with urea, were reported to have intermediate sensitivity. Severe bleeding may occur even in the absence of abnormal clot solubility test. Since, clot solubility test is a qualitative assay, with low sensitivity and specificity, and is a poorly standardized test that can be affected by several factors including clotting agent, solubilizing agent, and fibrinogen concentration, FXIII and Fibrinogen subcommittee of the International Society on Thrombosis and Hemostasis (ISTH) recommended a

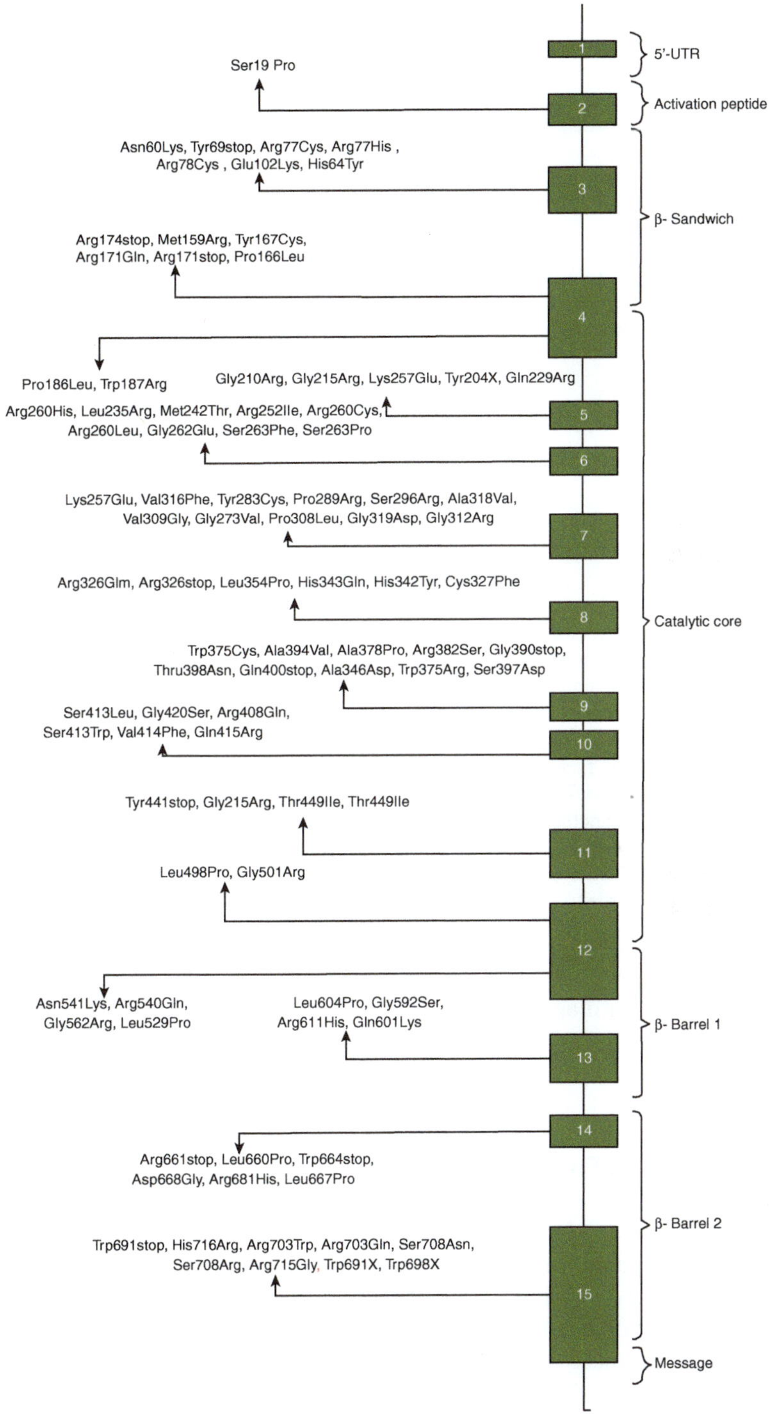

Fig. 13.4 *F13A1* gene missense mutations

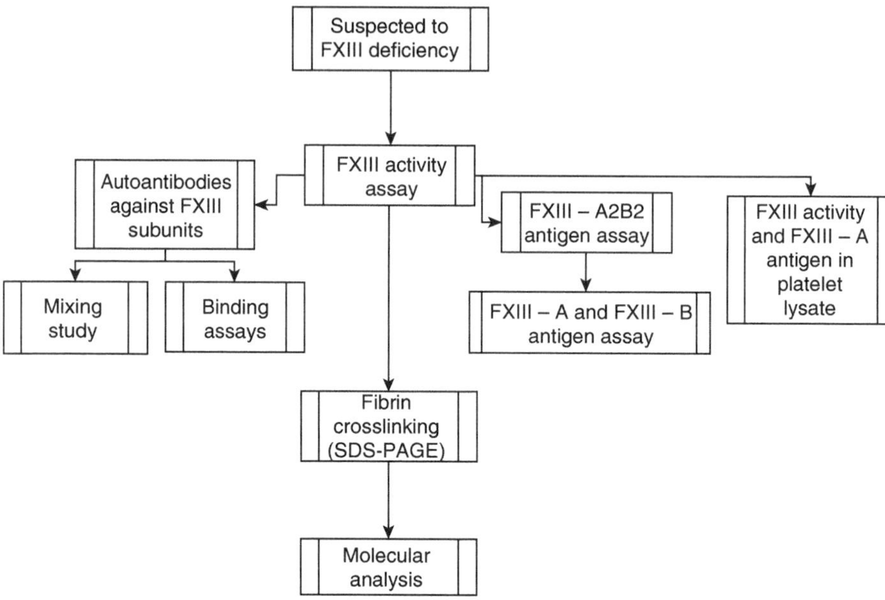

Fig. 13.5 International Society on Thrombosis and Hemostasis (ISTH) recommended algorithm for diagnosis and classification of factor XIII deficiency. factor XIII functional activity assay is recommended as the first-line screening test. If plasma factor XIII activity is decreased, the subtype of disorder can be determined by the measurement of plasma factor XIII-A_2B_2 antigen assay and measurement of FXIII activity and FXIII-A antigen in platelet lysate. If factor XIII-A_2B_2 antigen level is decreased, factor XIII-A_2 and factor XIII-B_2 should be measured. If the presence of inhibitor is suspected, mixing study for detection of neutralizing antibodies against factor XIII-A should be performed. For detection of non-neutralizing antibodies against factor XIII-A and factor XIII-B, binding assays should be done. For further evaluation of disorder, assessment of fibrin cross-linking by SDS-PAGE can be performed. Molecular analysis can be performed for final confirmation of the disorder

reliable algorithm for diagnosis and classification of FXIII deficiency. According to this algorithm, FXIII functional assay is recommended as the first-line screening test (Fig. 13.5) [23].

13.7.1 Factor XIII Functional Assay

Different methods were introduced for FXIII functional assay, including photometric assay, incorporation assay, and fluorometric assay. Each of these methods has some advantages and disadvantages; familiarity with these issues can help to have a proper and precise diagnosis of the disorder [2, 8, 50]. Several commercial kits are available based on these methods. Available FXIII functional assays are based on the measurement of end products of FXIII transglutaminase activity including the measurement of (1) ammonia released from a glutamine-containing substrate, (2) a substrate amine incorporated into a substrate protein, and (3) assessment of fibrin cross-linking. The ammonia release assays are the only available commercial FXIII functional assays [8, 23, 50]. These kinds of assays are quick, user friendly, and kinetic and can be used on coagulometer. One of the most common available photometric assays is Berichrom FXIII assay (Dade Behring, Marburg, Germany). In photometric assay, FXIII is activated by thrombin and calcium during lag phase of reaction, and transglutaminase activity of FXIII is measured [2, 20, 50]. In first step of reaction, FXIII catalyzed and acyl transfer reaction. In this reaction, carboxamide group of peptide-bound glutamine residue is acyl donor. It forms a thioacyl complex with the –SH group Cys314 of FXIII active site and ammonia is released [20]. In the second step of reaction, the thioester is broken, and the acyl acceptor primary amine through a peptide bond is bound to the glutamyl residue. Finally, released ammonia is measured. This measurement in Berichrom FXIII assay, is NADH, and in REA-chrom assay is a NADPH-dependent glutamate dehydrogenase (GlDH) reaction, and the rate of decrease of NADH or NADPH absorbance measured at 340 nm is directly proportional to the catalytic amount of FXIII (Table 13.3) [20, 50–52].

One of the most important point about ammonia release assay is the potential significant overestimation of FXIII activity between 2% and 14% without plasma blank that is more important in the low level of FXIII [8, 52, 53]. To overcome this problem, plasma blank is used in which an irreversible FXIII active site inhibitor such as iodoacetamide is used, and the obtained value from this blank is subtracted from the measured FXIII activity of the sample [8, 52–55]. Another problem with ammonia release assay is low sensitivity. In order to improve the sensitivity of this assay, it was recommended to increase plasma: reagent ratio and prolong measurement intervals [20].

13.7.2 Factor XIII Antigen Assay

FXIII antigen assay can be used for classification of FXIII deficiency. In most common type I of FXIII-A deficiency, concomitant decrease is observed in both FXIII activity and antigen assays, while in type II, FXIII antigen level is in normal range. With available commercial kits, FXIII-A, FXIII-B, and FXIII-A_2B_2 antigens can be measured [8, 20]. Reference interval of FXIII-A_2B_2 antigen is between 67% and 133%, and this range for FXIII activity is between 67% and 143% [2, 20]. Activity and antigen assays also can be performed on platelet lysate. Enzyme-linked immunosorbent assay (ELISA) is one of the most sensitive and reliable methods for the measurement of FXIII antigen level [19, 54]. According to Clinical and Laboratory Standards Institute (CLSI) guidelines, these three points should be considered for FXIII antigen assay [8, 54]:

(1) Non-complex FXIII-B should not interfere with FXIII-A_2B_2 antigen assay.
(2) When subunit assays are performed, both free and complex antigenic forms should react with anti-FXIII subunit antibodies with the same extent.
(3) Used assay should not be interfered by fibrinogen concentration.

Table 13.3 Qualitative and quantitative assays for diagnosis of factor XIII deficiency

Assay	Clotting	Solubilizing	Detection limit (%)	Advantage	Disadvantage
Clot solubility test	Thrombin	Acetic acid	10	1. Sensitive 2. Rapid	Low specificity
	$CaCl_2$	$CaCl_2$	0–3	1. Rapid 2. Easy	Low sensitivity
	$CaCl_2$	Urea	3–5	1. Rapid 2. Easy	No consensus about the sensitivity
Functional assay	Available kit	Country			
Amine release assays	Berichrom assay	Germany	<5	1. Quick 2. One-step kinetic 3. Easily automated 4. Good reproducibility	Low sensitivity
	REA-chrom assay	Hungary	<3		
	Technochrom assay	Austria	<5		
Amine incorporation assays	Commercial kit is not available but used in research and specialized laboratories			1. Highly sensitive	1. Time-consuming 2. Not automated 3. Poorly standardized 4. Affected by Val34Leu polymorphism

13.8 Management

13.8.1 Prophylaxis

Regular primary prophylaxis is mandatory for all patients with severe congenital FXIII deficiency, from the time of diagnosis, even in the absence of severe clinical presentations. The main reason for this decision is the high rate of life-threatening bleeds, notably ICH. Different choices were used for treatment of congenital FXIII deficiency, including whole blood (WB), FFP, and cryoprecipitate. Although, now, FXIII concentrate (Corifact™/Fibrogammin®P) and rFXIII (catridecacog, NovoThirteen, Tretten). A significant number of countries over the world only can use FFP and cryoprecipitate, most often due to economic affairs [56–62]. The main concern with regard to use of FFP and cryoprecipitate is the risk of transfusion-transmitted infectious. In spite of these issues, use of FXIII concentrate is growing, and today this plasma-derived component is the treatment of choice. It was accepted that for prevention of major bleeding, plasma FXIII level should be kept above 5%, and to remain patients asymptomatic, a goal of 10% of FXIII is desirable [58–61].

Although several prophylaxis programs were introduced, two main strategies are 10 IU/Kg FXIII concentrate (Fibrogammin P; CLS Behring, Marburg, Germany) and 40 IU/kg (Corifact; CLS Behring, Marburg, Germany) every 4 weeks [2, 56, 60, 63]. The first one was successfully used for a long time in a large number of Iranian patients with congenital FXIII deficiency. This regimen significantly reduces the rate of minor bleeds and deviates major bleeds. In the latter program, incidence of minor bleeds was lower than the former. In addition to prophylaxis dose of FXIII concentrate, patients may require on-demand treatment that means stopping of bleeding as soon as possible after onset of bleeding. These include treatment and management of acute bleeding, ICH, and dental management as well as successful delivery and major and minor surgeries [57, 63].

13.8.2 Management of Intracranial Hemorrhage

ICH is the most dreadful complication and the main cause of morbidity and mortality among patients with congenital FXIII deficiency. In addition to ICH, these patients may rarely experience extracranial hemorrhage (ECH) (~5%). ICH is the most common in congenital FXIII deficiency than any other congenital bleeding disorder [30]. Although the incidence of ICH is about 30%, as high as 60% were reported in neonatal period [30, 63]. Post-traumatic ICH is more frequent in neonatal period, while spontaneous ICH is more common in adults [19]. About one fifth of patients experience this diathesis recurrently in the absence of appropriate replacement therapy. The most common site of ICH is intraparenchymal (>90%), while subdural and epidural hemorrhages are rarely seen [30]. ICH is the main cause of death in congenital FXIII deficiency, and 80% of deaths are attributed to this life-threatening diathesis. ICH, in 15% of patients, leads to death, while in the majority of patients, it causes neurological complications. Although ICH is a very severe presentation of congenital FXIII deficiency, with timely diagnosis and appropriate management, the incidence of this diathesis can significantly decrease. Primary prophylaxis is very effective in preventing ICH, but traumatic ICH can occur even in patients under prophylaxis. For patients undergoing ICH, timely diagnosis is the key step to decrease debilitating consequences [19]. In patients with congenital FXIII deficiency with signs and symptoms of cranial hemorrhage including headache, vomiting, loss of consciousness, and visual disturbance, replacement therapy should be considered even before establishment of diagnosis [30, 64–66]. The mainstay of treatment of ICH in FXIII deficiency is replacement therapy, while the role of neurosurgery remained controversial. For patients with ICH, plasma FXIII level should be kept in normal range for at least 2 weeks. For this purpose, up to an alternate day dose before reducing replacement therapy to routine prophylaxis program may be required [30]. ICH leads to different neurological complications, including locomotor disability, mental disorders and visual disturbance, hearing problems, and speech and psychological impairments. Locomotor disability and psychological disabilities are the most common. Some of these patients experience severe neurological complications such as hemiplegia that disrupt their normal lifestyle. Due to the high rate of neurological complications, long-term neuropsychological evaluations should be considered for patients with congenital FXIII deficiency and ICH [19, 30, 67, 68].

13.8.3 Successful Delivery

Pregnancy loss is one of the main complications of women with congenital FXIII deficiency. This complication is more frequent in FXIII-A deficiency than FXIII-B deficiency. Reported frequency of pregnancy loss is between 30% and 100% for FXIII-A deficiency and 15% for FXIII-B deficiency, respectively. Although successful delivery without replacement therapy was observed among women with congenital FXIII deficiency, generally it is accepted that women with severe congenital FXIIID (<1%) are unable to have successful delivery without replacement therapy. These patients may experience recurrent pregnancy loss in the absence of replacement therapy, while appropriate management can lead to successful delivery in about all women (Fig. 13.6) [39, 69–73].

For successfully delivery, plasma FXIII level should be kept higher than 10%. Several strategies have been proposed for successful delivery. For instance, it was recommended that women get 250 IU FXIII concentrate (Corifact™/Fibrogammin®P) during the first 22 weeks of gestation and then 500 IU and finally 1000 IU before labor [39]. Another strategy successfully used on a large number of women is the administration of 10 IU/kg Fibrogammin P (Dade Behring, Marburg, Germany) every 4 weeks as routine prophylaxis, then 10 IU/kg every 2 weeks during pregnancy, and finally 10 IU/kg before labor [56, 72, 73].

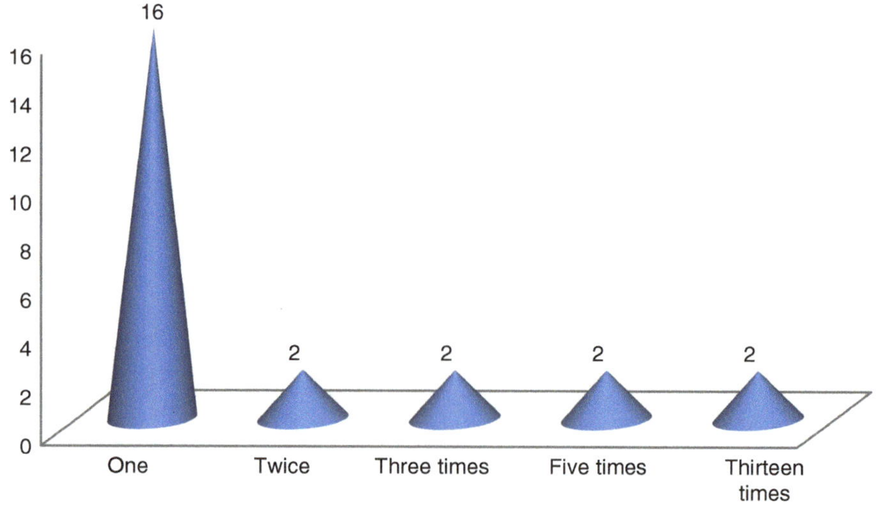

Fig. 13.6 Number of miscarriage in a study on the large number of women with congenital factor XIII deficiency

13.8.4 Management of Major and Minor Surgeries

Management of surgery is a challenge in congenital FXIII deficiency, and even a minor invasive procedure can lead to severe life-threatening hemorrhage. According to the United Kingdom Haemophilia Centre Doctors' Organization guideline [73–75]:

1. For minor surgery consider tranexamic acid 15–20 mg/kg or 1 g four times daily alone.
2. For major surgery, consider additional FXIII concentrate 10–40 IU/kg depending on the interval since the last prophylaxis and severity of bleeding.

Although it was also recommended that for major surgeries, patients should receive higher dose to keep plasma level higher than 5%, recent studies proposed more suitable recommendations. Patients should receive replacement therapy immediately before surgery [73, 74].

It was recommended to have a replacement therapy administrated immediately before surgery. For major surgeries, plasma FXIII level should increase to 50% before procedure, and in sophisticated and prolonged surgeries, plasma level of FXIII should increase to 100%. But even a FXIII level of 100% can not grangtee prevention of hemorrhge. For surgery, especially major and sophesticated surgeries, all steps of surgery should be performed with close monitoring of patients durring surery. It should kept in the mind that a unique protocol can not be used for all patients with FXIII deficiency and several factors can affect management of surgery. These factors including kind of surgery, durriation and complication of surgery. A suitable therpeutic therapeutic dose not only should lead to a safe surgery but also provoke normal postsurgery wound healing. In fact, for management of a surgery in congenital FXIII deficiency, all issues including the type and duration as well as complication of surgery should be considered [59, 75].

References

1. Duckert F. The fibrin stablizing factor, factor XIII. Blut. 1973;26(3):177–9.
2. Dorgalaleh A, Rashidpanah J. Blood coagulation factor XIII and factor XIII deficiency. Blood Rev. 2016;30(6):461–75.
3. Muszbek L, Bereczky Z, Bagoly Z, Komáromi I, Katona É. Factor XIII: a coagulation factor with multiple plasmatic and cellular functions. Physiol Rev. 2011;91(3):931–72.
4. Inbal A, Lubetsky A, Krapp T, Castel D, Shaish A, Dickneitte G, et al. Impaired wound healing in factor XIII deficient mice. Thromb Haemost. 2005;94(2):432–7.
5. Dardik R, Solomon A, Loscalzo J, Eskaraev R, Bialik A, Goldberg I, et al. Novel proangiogenic effect of factor XIII associated with suppression of thrombospondin 1 expression. Arterioscler Thromb Vasc Biol. 2003;23(8):1472–7.
6. Nahrendorf M, Hu K, Frantz S, Jaffer FA, Tung C-H, Hiller K-H, et al. Factor XIII deficiency causes cardiac rupture, impairs wound healing, and aggravates cardiac remodeling in mice with myocardial infarction. Circulation. 2006;113(9):1196–202.
7. Dorgalaleh A, Alavi SER, Tabibian S, Soori S, Moradi E, Bamedi T, et al. Diagnosis, clinical manifestations and management of rare bleeding disorders in Iran. Hematology. 2017;22:224–30.

8. Dorgalaleh A, Tabibian S, Hosseini S, Shamsizadeh M. Guidelines for laboratory diagnosis of factor XIII deficiency. Blood Coagul Fibrinolysis. 2016;27(4):361–4.
9. Diagnosis and management of congenital and acquired FXIII deficiencies. In: Muszbek L, Katona É, editors. Seminars in thrombosis and hemostasis. New York: Thieme Medical Publishers; 2016.
10. Muszbek L, Yee VC, Hevessy Z. Blood coagulation factor XIII: structure and function. Thromb Res. 1999;94(5):271–305.
11. Muszbek L, Adany R, Mikkola H. Novel aspects of blood coagulation factor XIII. I. Structure, distribution, activation, and function. Crit Rev Clin Lab Sci. 1996;33(5):357–421.
12. Shi DY, Wang SJ. Advances of coagulation factor XIII. Chin Med J. 2017;130(2):219–23.
13. Muszbek L, Adany R, Szegedi G, Polgar J, Kavai M. Factor XIII of blood coagulation in human monocytes. Thromb Res. 1985;37(3):401–10.
14. Asahina T, Kobayashi T, Okada Y, Goto J, Terao T. Maternal blood coagulation factor XIII is associated with the development of cytotrophoblastic shell. Placenta. 2000;21(4):388–93.
15. Coagulation factor deficiencies and pregnancy loss. In: Inbal A, Muszbek L, editors. Seminars in thrombosis and hemostasis. New York: Thieme Medical Publishers; 2003.
16. Andersson C, Kvist PH, McElhinney K, Baylis R, Gram LK, Pelzer H, et al. Factor XIII transglutaminase supports the resolution of mucosal damage in experimental colitis. PLoS One. 2015;10(6):e0128113.
17. Paye M, Nusgens BV, Lapiere CM. Factor XIII of blood coagulation modulates collagen biosynthesis by fibroblasts in vitro. Haemostasis. 1989;19(5):274–83.
18. Factor XIII deficiency in Iran: a comprehensive review of the literature. In: Dorgalaleh A, Naderi M, Hosseini MS, Alizadeh S, Hosseini S, Tabibian S, et al., editors. Seminars in thrombosis and hemostasis. New York: Thieme Medical Publishers; 2015.
19. Dorgalaleh A, Naderi M, Shamsizadeh M. Morbidity and mortality in a large number of Iranian patients with severe congenital factor XIII deficiency. Ann Hematol. 2016;95(3):451–5.
20. Dorgalaleh A, Tabibian S, Hosseini MS, Farshi Y, Roshanzamir F, Naderi M, et al. Diagnosis of factor XIII deficiency. Hematology. 2016;21(7):430–9.
21. Dorgalaleh A, Tabibian S, Shams M, Tavasoli B, Gheidishahran M, Shamsizadeh M. Laboratory diagnosis of factor XIII deficiency in developing countries: an Iranian experience. Lab Med. 2016;47:220.
22. Inbal A, Oldenburg J, Carcao M, Rosholm A, Tehranchi R, Nugent D. Recombinant factor XIII: a safe and novel treatment for congenital factor XIII deficiency. Blood. 2012;119(22):5111–7.
23. Kohler H, Ichinose A, Seitz R, Ariens R, Muszbek L. Diagnosis and classification of factor XIII deficiencies. J Thromb Haemost. 2011;9(7):1404–6.
24. Peyvandi F. Prospective data collection on patients with fibrinogen and factor XIII deficiencies: preliminary results of the PRO-RBDD project. Haemophilia. 2015;21:74–5.
25. Peyvandi F, Menegatti M, Palla R, Siboni SM, Boscarino M, Susan H, et al. Prospective data collection on patients with fibrinogen and factor XIII deficiencies: prelimary results of the PRO-RBDD project. Blood. 2014;124(21):2838.
26. Mikkola H, Syrjala M, Rasi V, Vahtera E, Hamalainen E, Peltonen L, et al. Deficiency in the A-subunit of coagulation factor XIII: two novel point mutations demonstrate different effects on transcript levels. Blood. 1994;84(2):517–25.
27. Ivaskevicius V, Seitz R, Kohler HP, Schroeder V, Muszbek L, Ariens RA, et al. International registry on factor XIII deficiency: a basis formed mostly on European data. Thromb Haemost. 2007;97(6):914–21.
28. De Moerloose P, Neerman-Arbez M. Treatment of congenital fibrinogen disorders. Expert Opin Biol Ther. 2008;8(7):979–92.
29. Anwar R, Minford A, Gallivan L, Trinh CH, Markham AF. Delayed umbilical bleeding—a presenting feature for factor XIII deficiency: clinical features, genetics, and management. Pediatrics. 2002;109(2):e32.
30. Intracranial hemorrhage: a devastating outcome of congenital bleeding disorders—prevalence, diagnosis, and management, with a special focus on congenital factor XIII deficiency. In: Alavi SER, Jalalvand M, Assadollahi V, Tabibian S, Dorgalaleh A, editors. Seminars in thrombosis and hemostasis. New York: Thieme Medical Publishers; 2017.

31. Singleton TC, Keane M. Diagnostic and therapeutic challenges of intracranial hemorrhage in neonates with congenital hemophilia: a case report and review. Ochsner J. 2012;12(3):249–53.
32. Tsuda T, Okamoto Y, Sakaguchi R, Katayama N, Ota K. Isolated factor VII deficiency diagnosed after a lifethreatening brain haemorrhage. J Int Med Res. 2000;28(6):318–23.
33. Viola L, Chiaretti A, Lazzareschi I, Pesaresi MA, Rossodivita A, Polidori G. [Intracranial hemorrhage in congenital factor II deficiency]. Pediatr Med Chir. 1995;17(6):593–4.
34. Espitia O, Ternisien C, Agard C, Boisseau P, Denis CV, Fouassier M. Use of a thrombopoietin receptor agonist in von Willebrand disease type 2B (p.V1316M) with severe thrombocytopenia and intracranial hemorrhage. Platelets. 2017;28:518–20.
35. Labarque V, Stain AM, Blanchette V, Kahr WH, Carcao MD. Intracranial haemorrhage in von Willebrand disease: a report on six cases. Haemophilia. 2013;19(4):602–6.
36. Yamahata H, Hirahara K, Tomosugi T, Yamada M, Ishii T, Uetsuhara K, et al. Acute epidural hematoma in a patient with Glanzmann's thrombasthenia: case report. Neurol Med Chir. 2010;50(10):928–30.
37. Gootenberg JE, Buchanan GR, Holtkamp CA, Casey CS. Severe hemorrhage in a patient with gray platelet syndrome. J Pediatr. 1986;109(6):1017–9.
38. Richard A, Matthew RP, Naif Z, Abraham J. Henry's clinical diagnosis and management by laboratory methods. 21st ed. Philadelphia: Saunders Elsevier; 2007. p. 1026–7.
39. Asahina T, Kobayashi T, Takeuchi K, Kanayama N. Congenital blood coagulation factor XIII deficiency and successful deliveries: a review of the literature. Obstet Gynecol Surv. 2007;62(4):255–60.
40. Sharief L, Kadir R. Congenital factor XIII deficiency in women: a systematic review of literature. Haemophilia. 2013;19(6):e349.
41. Dorgalaleh A, Assadollahi V, Tabibian S, Shamsizadeh M. Molecular basis of congenital factor XIII deficiency in Iran. Clin Appl Thromb Hemost. 2016. https://doi.org/10.1177/1076029616680473.
42. Ariëns RA, Lai T-S, Weisel JW, Greenberg CS, Grant PJ. Role of factor XIII in fibrin clot formation and effects of genetic polymorphisms. Blood. 2002;100(3):743–54.
43. Dorgalaleh A, Tabibian S, Bamedi T, Tamaddon G, Naderi M, Varmaghani B, et al. Molecular genetic analysis of ten unrelated Iranian patients with congenital factor XIII deficiency. Int J Lab Hematol. 2017;39:e33.
44. Biswas A, Ivaskevicius V, Seitz R, Thomas A, Oldenburg J. An update of the mutation profile of Factor 13 A and B genes. Blood Rev. 2011;25(5):193–204.
45. Jang M-A, Park YS, Lee K-O, Kim H-J. Novel and recurrent mutations in the F13A1 gene in unrelated Korean patients with congenital factor XIII deficiency. Blood Coagul Fibrinolysis. 2015;26(1):46–9.
46. Shanbhag S, Ghosh K, Shetty S. Genetic basis of severe factor XIII deficiency in a large cohort of Indian patients: identification of fourteen novel mutations. Blood Cell Mol Dis. 2016;57:81–4.
47. Kulkarni BP, Nair SB, Vijapurkar M, Mota L, Shanbhag S, Ali S, et al. Molecular pathology of rare bleeding disorders (RBDs) in India: a systematic review. PLoS One. 2014;9(10):e108683.
48. Lorand L, Velasco TV, Hill MJ, Hoffmeister J, Kaye JF. Intracranial hemorrhage in systemic lupus erythmatosus associated with an autoantibody against factor XIII. Thrombosis and haemostasis. 2002;88(06):919–23.
49. Jennings I, Kitchen S, Woods T, Preston F. Problems relating to the laboratory diagnosis of factor XIII deficiency: a UK NEQAS study. J Thromb Haemost. 2003;1(12):2603–8.
50. Diagnosis and management of congenital factor XIII deficiency, seminar in thromobsis and hemostasis. 2016;42(4):429–39.
51. Ajzner E, Muszbek L. Prophylactic and perioperative replacement therapy for acquired factor XIII deficiency: a rebuttal. J Thromb Haemost. 2004;2(11):2075–7.
52. Lawrie A, Green L, Mackie I, Liesner R, Machin S, Peyvandi F. Factor XIII–an under diagnosed deficiency–are we using the right assays? J Thromb Haemost. 2010;8(11):2478–82.
53. Cini M, Legnani C, Frascaro M, Pancani C, Cappelli C, Rodorigo G, et al. Measurement of factor XIII (FXIII) activity by an automatic ammonia release assay using iodoacetamide

blank-procedure: no more overestimation in the low activity range and better detection of severe FXIII deficiencies. Clin Chem Lab Med. 2016;54(5):805–9.
54. Ariëns R, Kohler H, Mansfield M, Grant P. Subunit antigen and activity levels of blood coagulation factor XIII in healthy individuals. Arterioscler Thromb Vasc Biol. 1999;19(8):2012–6.
55. Kárpáti L, Penke B, Katona É, Balogh I, Vámosi G, Muszbek L. A modified, optimized kinetic photometric assay for the determination of blood coagulation factor XIII activity in plasma. Clin Chem. 2000;46(12):1946–55.
56. Ichinose A, Asahina T, Kobayashi T. Congenital blood coagulation factor XIII deficiency and perinatal management. Curr Drug Targets. 2005;6(5):541–9.
57. Naderi M, Dorgalaleh A, Alizadeh S, Tabibian S, Hosseini S, Shamsizadeh M, et al. Clinical manifestations and management of life-threatening bleeding in the largest group of patients with severe factor XIII deficiency. Int J Hematol. 2014;100(5):443–9.
58. Fadoo Z, Merchant Q, Rehman KA. New developments in the management of congenital Factor XIII deficiency. J Blood Med. 2013;4(2):65–73.
59. Miloszewski K, Losowsky M. Proceedings: Factor XIII concentrate in the long term management of congenital factor XIII deficiency. Thromb Diath Haemorrh. 1975;34(1):323.
60. Nugent DJ. Prophylaxis in rare coagulation disorders—factor XIII deficiency. Thromb Res. 2006;118:S23–S8.
61. Meili E. Clinical course and management of severe congenital factor XIII deficiency. Hamostaseologie. 2002;22(1):48–52.
62. Lusher J, Pipe S, Alexander S, Nugent D. Prophylactic therapy with Fibrogammin® P is associated with a decreased incidence of bleeding episodes: a retrospective study. Haemophilia. 2010;16(2):316–21.
63. Nugent D. Corifact™/Fibrogammin® P in the prophylactic treatment of hereditary factor XIII deficiency: results of a prospective, multicenter, open-label study. Thromb Res. 2012;130:S12–S4.
64. Moerloose P, Schved JF, Nugent D. Rare coagulation disorders: fibrinogen, factor VII and factor XIII. Haemophilia. 2016;22(S5):61–5.
65. Davies J, Kadir R. Mode of delivery and cranial bleeding in newborns with haemophilia: a systematic review and meta-analysis of the literature. Haemophilia. 2016;22(1):32–8.
66. Kulkarni R, Lusher JM. Intracranial and extracranial hemorrhages in newborns with hemophilia: a review of the literature. J Pediatr Hematol Oncol. 1999;21(4):289–95.
67. Nagel K, Pai MK, Paes BA, Chan AK. Diagnosis and treatment of intracranial hemorrhage in children with hemophilia. Blood Coagul Fibrinolysis. 2013;24(1):23–7.
68. Naderi M, Zarei T, Haghpanah S, Eshghi P, Miri-Moghaddam E, Karimi M. Intracranial hemorrhage pattern in the patients with factor XIII deficiency. Ann Hematol. 2014;93(4):693–7.
69. Anwar R, Miloszewski KJ. Factor XIII deficiency. Br J Haematol. 1999;107(3):468–84.
70. Burrows R, Ray J, Burrows E. Bleeding risk and reproductive capacity among patients with factor XIII deficiency: a case presentation and review of the literature. Obstet Gynecol Surv. 2000;55(2):103.
71. Coopland A, Alkjaersig N, Fletcher AP. Reduction in plasma factor XIII (fibrin stabilizing factor) concentration during pregnancy. J Lab Clin Med. 1969;73(1):144–53.
72. Padmanabhan L, Mhaskar R, Mhaskar A, Ross C. Factor XIII deficiency: a rare cause of repeated abortions. Singap Med J. 2004;45(4):186–7.
73. Naderi M, Eshghi P, Cohan N, Miri-Moghaddam E, Yaghmaee M, Karimi M. Successful delivery in patients with FXIII deficiency receiving prophylaxis: report of 17 cases in Iran. Haemophilia. 2012;18(5):773–6.
74. Janbain M, Nugent DJ, Powell JS, St-Louis J, Frame VB, Leissinger CA. Use of Factor XIII (FXIII) concentrate in patients with congenital FXIII deficiency undergoing surgical procedures. Transfusion. 2015;55(1):45–50.
75. Mumford AD, Ackroyd S, Alikhan R, Bowles L, Chowdary P, Grainger J, et al. Guideline for the diagnosis and management of the rare coagulation disorders. Br J Haematol. 2014;167(3):304–26.

Part IV

Inherited Platelet Function Disorders

Glanzmann Thrombasthenia 14

Akbar Dorgalaleh, Man-Chiu Poon, and Yavar Shiravand

14.1 Introduction

Glanzmann thrombasthenia (GT) is a rare congenital bleeding disorder of platelet function with an estimated incidence of one per million in the general population. In regions where consanguineous marriage is common, the incidence may be as high as, or even higher than, 1 in 200,000 persons [1]. GT is caused by mutations in the *ITGA2B* and *ITGB3* genes that encode αIIbβ3 [glycoprotein (GP) IIb/IIIa], resulting in qualitative or quantitative integrin defects. As αIIbβ3 is critical in platelet aggregation, which is impaired in GT. The bleeding tendency is highly variable among affected patients, ranging from asymptomatic conditions to life-threatening hemorrhage. Patients with GT usually present with mucocutaneous bleeding early in life. Purpura, epistaxis, and gum bleeding are the most common clinical presentations; menorrhagia is one of the most common presentations among women with GT [2, 3]. Diagnosis of this disorder is based on clinical manifestations, family history, and appropriate laboratory assessment. In laboratory diagnosis, patients with GT have an impaired response to all physiological agonists but have normal response

A. Dorgalaleh (✉) · Y. Shiravand
Department of Hematology and Blood Transfusion, School of Allied Medicine, Iran University of Medical Sciences, Tehran, Iran

M.-C. Poon
Department of Medicine, University of Calgary Cumming School of Medicine, Calgary, AB, Canada

Department of Pediatrics, University of Calgary Cumming School of Medicine, Calgary, AB, Canada

Department of Oncology, University of Calgary Cumming School of Medicine, Calgary, AB, Canada

Southern Alberta Rare Blood and Bleeding Disorders Comprehensive Care Program, Foothills Medical Centre, Alberta Health Services, Calgary, AB, Canada
e-mail: mcpoon@ucalgary.ca

A. Dorgalaleh (ed.), *Congenital Bleeding Disorders*,
https://doi.org/10.1007/978-3-319-76723-9_14

to ristocetin. In flow cytometric analysis, αIIbβ3 (CD41/CD61) is decreased, but in the variant form of GT, nonfunctional αIIbβ3 is expressed in nearly normal amounts. A wide spectrum of mutations is identified in both *ITGA2B* and *ITGB3* genes, although more mutations affect *ITGA2B* [4]. The therapeutic options available for management of patients with GT include local and systemic measures and the use of antifibrinolytics, platelet concentrates, and recombinant human activated factor VII (rFVIIa). More advanced curative options are stem cell transplantation and gene therapy. Currently, platelet transfusion is the standard treatment of patients with GT, but local and antifibrinolytic agents can be used for mild bleeds. Repeated platelet transfusion can result in allo-immunization against platelet human leukocyte antigen (HLA) or αIIbβ3 antigens. HLA-matched leukocyte-reduced platelet concentrates, particularly from single donors, can minimize the risk of HLA allo-immunization. rFVIIa can be used for the management of patients with platelet antibodies and platelet refractoriness [1, 5–7].

14.2 Integrin αIIbβ3 (GPIIb/IIIa) Structure and Function

14.2.1 Biosynthesis Pathway

αIIbβ3 And αvβ3 are two members of the β3 subfamily, with a common β-subunit and 36% amino acid sequence identity of the α-subunits; they have a similar biosynthetic pathway. αIIbβ3 Consists of α- and β-subunits that are noncovalently bonded to each other. Initially, αIIb (GPIIb) is synthesized as a pro-αIIb moiety, which consists of light (L) and heavy (H) chains that are connected. β3 (GPIIIa) is produced as a single chain. β3 Undergoes *N*-linked glycosylation and complexes with pro-αIIb in the endoplasmic reticulum (ER). The heterodimers are then transported into the Golgi system. The intracellular transport, stability, and processing of the αIIb-subunit are dependent on the complex formation with β3. Almost all translated αIIb will complex with β3 and appear on the cell surface. Only 40% of the translated β3 binds to αIIb to form the αIIbβ3 complex; the other 60% remains inside the megakaryocytes. It is suggested that αIIb and the α-subunit (αv) of vitronectin receptors (αvβ3) compete for complex formation with the β3-subunit within the ER (Fig. 14.1) [7, 8].

14.2.2 Integrin αIIbβ3 (GPIIb/IIIa) Structure

The αIIbβ3 complex is the most abundant glycoprotein (GP) on the platelet surface, forming approximately 1% of the platelet's weight. Nearly 70% of αIIbβ3 is distributed randomly on the platelet surface; the remaining 30% is located between the closed canalicular membrane and the α-granule membrane. When platelets are suspended in a buffer containing calcium chelators, the αIIbβ3 structure changes, leading to separation of the monomeric subunits that can no longer support platelet

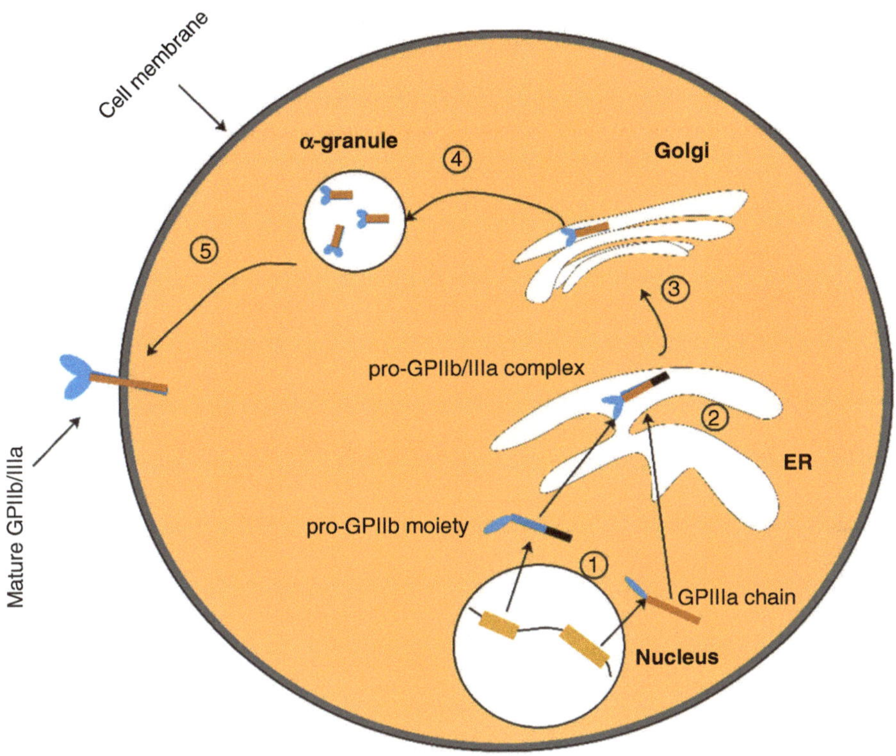

Fig. 14.1 Biosynthesis pathway of integrin αIIbβ3 (GPIIb/IIIa). (1) Two subunits of integrin αIIb (GPIIb) and β3 (GPIIIa) are encoded by the *ITGA2B* and *ITGB3* genes located on the long arm of chromosome 17. The synthesis of these subunits differs. GPIIb is synthesized as a pro-GPIIb moiety, which consists of a heavy (H) and a light (L) chain, but GPIIIa is synthesized as a single chain. (2) Within the endoplasmic reticulum (ER), the GPIIIa undergoes posttranslational glycosylation and make a complex with the pro-GPIIb moiety. In addition, high mannose *N*-linked oligosaccharide processing and degradation of uncompleted subunits occur in the ER. (3) The formed pro-GPIIb/IIIa (αIIbβ3) complex is transported into the Golgi apparatus. Further *N*-linked oligosaccharide processing and proteolytic cleavage of pro-αIIb occur in the Golgi complex. (4) After final processing, mature αIIbβ3 (GPIIb/IIIa) complexes are stored within the α-granules. (5) Mature αIIbβ3 (GPIIb/IIIa) complexes appear on the cell surface as needed. *Golgi* Golgi complex

aggregation response. Activation of platelets in the presence of strong agonists (thrombin and collagen) or weak agonists [adenosine diphosphate (ADP) and epinephrine] results in a conformation change of αIIbβ3 on the platelet surface to function as active fibrinogen receptors (Fig. 14.2) [8, 9].

14.2.2.1 αIIb (GPIIb) Subunit

ITGA2B, the gene encoding αIIb, spans 17.2 kb and consists of 30 exons. Located on the long arm of chromosome 17. αIIb, it has a molecular weight of 139 kDa and

Table 14.1 Characteristics of αIIbβ3 (GPIIb/IIIa) subunits

Characterization	Subunit	
	GPIIb	GPIIIa
Amino acids, *n*	1146	747
Glycosylation sites, *n*	5	6
Cysteine residues, *n*	17	56
Calcium-binding domains, *n*	4	1
Cytoplasmic domain length, *aa*	37	45
Transmembrane domain length, *aa*	23	22

n, Number; *aa*, Amino acid

consists of two polypeptide chains, L and H, which are bound through disulfide bonds. The H chain consists of 871 amino acids and has a molecular weight of 125 kDa; the L chain consists of 37 amino acids and has a molecular weight of 23 kDa. The L chain contains one transmembrane domain with 25 amino acids, whereas the H chain is entirely extracellular. About 15% of αIIb includes mannose-rich complex carbohydrates. The H chain of αIIb has a 12-amino-acid sequence containing the calcium/calmodulin-binding domain, which can bind γ-chain dodecapeptide sequences of fibrinogen. In addition, four calcium-binding sites exist on this chain (Table 14.1) [8–10].

14.2.2.2 β3 (GPIIIa)-Subunit

ITGB3, the gene encoding β3, spans 65 kb and consists of 15 exons. It is also located on the long arm of chromosome 17. The single-chain β3, with a molecular weight of 92 kDa, has 747 amino acids and contains a 26-amino-acid polypeptide in the *N*-terminal and a large external domain with 56 cysteine residues. The transmembrane domain and cytoplasmic tail of β3 consist of 29 and 41 amino acids, respectively. Carbohydrates account for about 15% of the β3 molecular weight (Table 14.1).

14.2.3 Ligand Binding to αIIbβ3

After platelet activation, the αIIbβ3 complex undergoes conformational changes and binds to fibrinogen and other physiological agonists such as ADP, adrenalin, thrombin, and platelet-activating factor (PAF). Each αIIbβ3 complex binds to one fibrinogen molecule. Upon ADP stimulation, approximately 15,400–82,500 (mean, 38,000) fibrinogen molecules can bind to αIIbβ3 (GPIIb/IIIa) complexes on the platelet surface. In addition to fibrinogen, other ligands can bind the platelet surface and activate the αIIbβ3 complex with a similar mechanism. These ligands include von Willebrand factor (VWF), fibronectin, and vitronectin. Amino acid sequences that mediate these interactions with αIIbβ3 are constructed of a sequence of three amino acids: arginine, glycine, and asparagine (RGD). RGD was initially identified as an adhesive sequence in fibronectin molecules and subsequently was also identified in fibrinogen, VWF, and vitronectin. Fibrinogen has two RDG sequences (at amino acid sequences 95–97 and 572–574) on its alpha chain, although other ligands only have one RDG sequence. The other important area in the fibrinogen molecule participating in αIIbβ3 interaction is the 12-peptide sequence (HHLGGAKQAGDV) located at the carboxylic tail of its gamma chain (Fig. 14.2). This dodecapeptide sequence is not found in other αIIbβ3-interacting adhesive molecules [8–12].

14.2.4 Signaling Pathway for αIIbβ3 (GPIIb/IIIa) Activation

αIIbβ3 is pivotal in platelet aggregation and platelet activation, and the acquisition of a capacity to bind soluble ligands is necessary for this function. Two main mechanisms, outside-in and inside-out signaling, are involved in αIIbβ3 affinity to ligands. The former is triggered by the ligands binding to the extracellular domains of αIIbβ3 and the latter is triggered by the factors binding to the cytoplasmic domains of αIIbβ3 following platelet activation.

The inside-out signaling generated by the activation of platelets leads to conformational changes of αIIbβ3 and alters the relative orientation of αIIb- and β3-subunits to one another. The biochemical events involved in the signaling pathway of αIIbβ3 (GPIIb/IIIa) are classified into the following processes: (1) binding of platelet agonists ADP, collagen, serotonin, thrombin, epinephrine, thromboxane A2 (TxA2), or PAF to their receptors on the platelet surface, which leads to platelet activation and

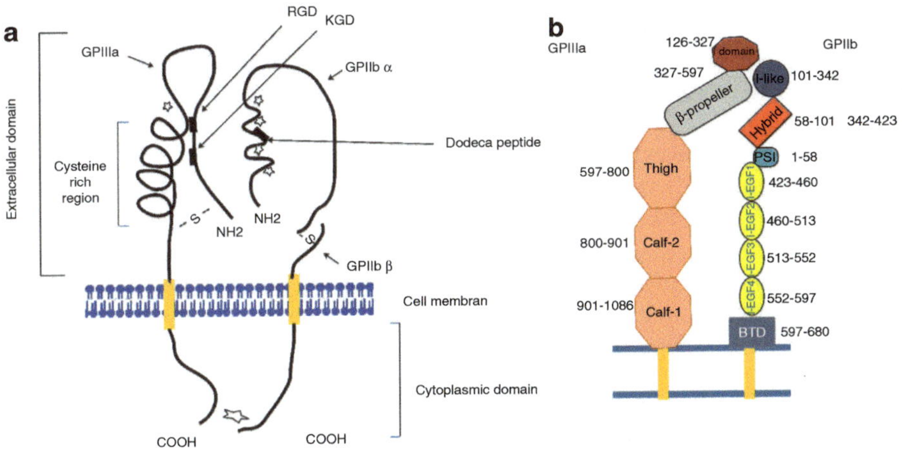

Fig. 14.2 (**a**) Structure of integrin αIIbβ3 (GPIIb/IIIa). (**b**) Domain structure of integrin αIIbβ3. *GP* glycoprotein. Dodecapeptide (DXDXD/NGXX/DXXD) is a fibrinogen-binding site on the αIIb (GPIIb) subunit. *GPIIbα* heavy chain of GPIIb, *GPIIb β* light chain of GPIIb, *RGD* Arg-Gly-Asp. This sequence is a fibrinogen-binding site on the GPIIIa subunit. *KGD* Lys-Gly-Asp. *BTD* β-tail domain, *IEGF1-4* integrin epidermal growth factor domain, *PSI* plexin-semaphorin-integrin domain, *hybrid* β-sandwich hybrid domain, *I-like* β I-like domain, *I* domain A-type domain, *β-propeller* N-terminal domain of GPIIIa; *thigh and calf-1-2*, cysteine-rich region and protease-resistant domains. *Star shape* indicates cation-binding sites

signal transduction via the agonist receptor cytoplasmic domains; (2) signal transduction from the agonist receptor cytoplasmic domain to the cytoplasmic domains of αIIbβ3; (3) signal transduction from αIIbβ3 cytoplasmic domains to its extracellular domains leads to integrin conformational changes and increased integrin affinity; (4) platelet-activating secondary signal leads to cytoplasmic granular release.

The various platelet agonists [ADP, PAF, lysophosphatidic acid (LPA), TxA2, serotonin, and thrombin] transmit signaling through the G proteins. G proteins consist of three subunits, α, β, and γ, in a heterotrimeric complex that binds the G-protein-coupled receptors (GPCRs). GPCRs are a large family of seven-transmembrane domain receptors on the cell surface. Based on α-subunit similarity, G proteins have been divided into four subfamilies: Gq, G12, Gi, and Gs. Binding of ligands to the G protein results in the conversion of the inactive GDP-bound form to the active GTP-bound form of the α-subunit, and separation of the β/γ complex from the activated α-subunit. The activated α-subunit and β/γ complex can interact with downstream targets in the G-protein signaling pathway. A number of changes induced by the platelet agonists include platelet deformation, granule content release, clot contraction, and platelet adherence to the vascular endothelial cells. All these events are considered as a result of the following biological processes (Fig. 14.3):

1. G proteins activate phospholipase C (PLC) and A2 (PLA2), which leads to the production of secondary messengers including diacylglycerol (DAG), inositol triphosphate (IP3), and arachidonic acid (AA).
2. The assembled integrin activates serine/threonine kinase and phosphatases, which lead to phosphorylation/dephosphorylation of cytoplasmic proteins such as lipid kinase (phosphatidyl inositol 3 and 4 kinase, PI3 and PI4k).
3. PLC converts phosphatidylinositol 4,5-bisphosphate (PIP2) to DAG, and IP3 leads to the entrance of calcium from outside the cell and the endoplasmic reticulum (ER) into the cytoplasm.
4. Phosphokinase C (PKC) phosphorylates Ras-proximate-1/guanosine diphosphate (Rap1/GDP), which has been bound to the cytoplasmic tail of αIIb. Calcium- and DAG-regulated guanine nucleotide exchange factor 1 (CalDAG/GEF1) serve as cofactors for this function.
5. Activation of antiporter of Na^+/K^+ leads to elevation of cytoplasm pH as well as phosphorylation of pleckstrin through PKC.
6. Rap1/GDP interacts with the Rap1–GTP-interacting adaptor molecule (RIAM).
7. RIAM recruits talin 1 and kindlin-3, which interact with the cytoplasmic tail of β3.
8. The rearrangement of cytoskeletal proteins leads to the conformational change in extracellular domains of both αIIb and β3, which enables αIIbβ3 to bind other ligands.

Talin 1, with a molecular weight of 270 kDa, is one of the cytoskeletal proteins that connect the cytoplasmic domains of integrin β-subunit to actin

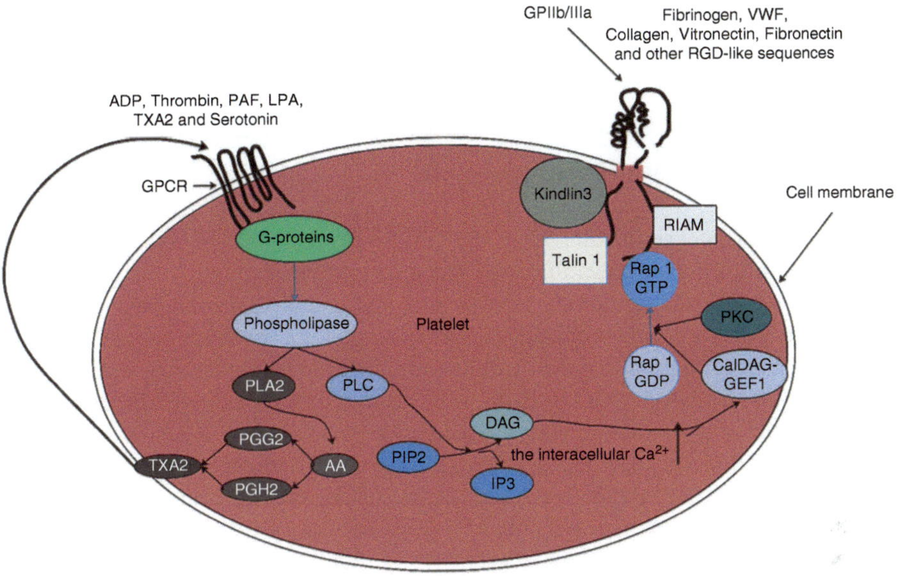

Fig. 14.3 The molecular mechanisms involved in the signaling pathway of integrin αIIbβ3 (GPIIb/IIIa). The G-protein-mediated signaling pathway is critical in the activation of αIIbβ3, which is initiated by binding of ADP and some other agonists such as thrombin, PAF, TXA2, and serotonin to their receptors. The downstream molecules of G-protein-mediated signaling such as phospholipase A2 (PLA2) and phospholipase C (PLC) cooperate in this activation. The downstream molecules including calcium- and DAG-regulated guanine nucleotide exchange factor 1 (CalDAG/GEF1), Ras-proximate-1/guanosine diphosphate, Rap1/GTP (Rap1/GDP), Rap1-GTP-interacting adaptor molecule (RIAM), and protein kinase C (PKC) are considered as important molecules in the activation of αIIbβ3. *ADP* adenosine diphosphate, *PAF* platelet-activating factor, *LPA* lysophosphatidic acid, *TxA2* thromboxane A2, *GPCR* G-protein-coupled receptors, *AA* arachidonic acid, *PGG2* prostaglandin G2, *PGH2* prostaglandin H2, *PIP2* phosphatidylinositol biphosphate, *DAG* diacyglycerol, *IP3* inositol trisphosphate, *VWF* von Willebrand factor, *RGD* arginine, glycine, and asparagine

filaments. Talin 1 is composed of a talin-H (a globular N-terminal head domain) and talin-R (a flexible C-terminal domain). Talin-H binds the NPLY motif of the integrin β-subunit, which initiates a conformational change in the extracellular domains of integrin αIIbβ3. The interaction between talin 1 and the cytoplasmic domains of integrin β-subunit is a key element in αIIbβ3 activation [8, 13–16].

Kindlin-3 is an integrin co-activator that binds the cytoplasmic domains of the integrin β-subunit and contributes to αIIbβ3 activation. Kindlin-3 binds the NITY motif of the integrin β-subunit. The integrin-binding protein and calcium-binding protein then interact with the cytoplasmic domains of integrin β-subunit and cooperate with kindlin-3 and talin 1 in activation of αIIbβ3. When αIIbβ3 is activated, it can bind with high affinity to fibrinogen and VWF. These ligands serve as bridges between adjacent platelets to form platelet aggregates [15, 17].

The importance of the αIIbβ3 signaling pathways for primary hemostasis is reflected by the recent description that patients with mutations in CalDAG/GEF1 and Kindlin-3 have thrombasthenia-like bleeding symptoms [3].

14.3 Integrin αIIbβ3 Antagonists

The binding of integrin αIIbβ3 to ligands results in cross-linking between adjacent platelets, resulting in aggregation and subsequent clot formation. Although platelet aggregation and clot formation are considered as a natural mechanism to prevent bleeding following tissue damage, uncontrolled platelet aggregation can result in thrombus formation, giving rise to varied morbidity. Such overactivation and aggregation can be prevented by antagonists targeting the αIIbβ3 receptor. There are three groups of such inhibitors: abciximab, eptifibatide, and tirofiban. Abciximab, an irreversible noncompetitive inhibitor, is a Fab fragment of chimeric monoclonal antibody 7E3 that binds to the αIIbβ3 and inhibits cell–ligand interactions. Eptifibatide and tirofiban are antagonists that bind to the α-subunit of αIIbβ3 in a competitive reversible manner. Tirofiban contains the RGD sequence; in eptifibatide, the arginine residue of the RGD motif is replaced by lysine amino acid [18, 19].

14.4 Glanzmann Thrombasthenia

GT is a rare autosomal recessive bleeding disorder that most often presents with spontaneous mucocutaneous bleeding early in life. The bleeding tendency is highly variable among affected patients, ranging from an asymptomatic condition to potentially life-threatening bleeds. Purpura, epistaxis, gum hemorrhage, and menorrhagia are the most common clinical presentations. However, other severe life-threatening bleeds such as intracranial hemorrhage (ICH) can also be observed, albeit more rarely. Generally, the severity of bleeding decreases with age. This finding is contrary to the Bernard–Soulier syndrome (BSS) in which the bleeding tendency is worsened in adult age. Most patients are diagnosed early in life with mucocutaneous bleeding. Timely diagnosis and appropriate management of the disorder are crucial. Diagnosis of GT can be based on clinical presentations, physical examinations, family history, and appropriate laboratory assessments. For patients without a family history of GT, the differential diagnosis that should be considered includes malignancies and autoantibody-induced acquired GT. All routine coagulation tests are normal in GT except for a prolonged bleeding time (BT)/closure time [platelet function analyzer (PFA), 100/200]. Confirmatory investigations will show the distinct feature with impaired aggregation response to all physiological agonists, although ristocetin-induced platelet agglutination is normal. Flow cytometry analysis reveals a decrease of αIIbβ3 (CD41/CD61) in GT but may be quantitatively normal (but dysfunctional) in variant GT forms (Table 14.2) [1–3].

GT is caused by mutations in αIIbβ3 (GPIIb/IIIa) encoded by two separate genes, *ITGA2B* (for αIIb) and *ITGB3* (for β3). A wide spectrum of mutations has

Table 14.2 Classification and characteristics of Glanzmann thrombasthenia

Type	Percent	Platelet integrin $\alpha IIb\beta 3$ expression	Platelet integrin $\alpha IIb\beta 3$ (%) (flow cytometry)	Platelet aggregation[a]	Platelet agglutination[b]	BT/CT (PFA-100/200)	Clot retraction
Type I	~75%	Undetectable or trace	<5	Absent	Normal	Prolonged	Absent
Type II	~15%	Significantly reduced	5–20	Absent	Normal	Prolonged	Subnormal
Variant	~10%	Nearly normal	>20	Absent/abnormal	Normal	Prolonged	Variable

[a]Thrombin, collagen, or adenosine diphosphate and epinephrine
[b]Ristocetin
BT bleeding time, *CT* closure time, *PFA-100/200* platelet function analyzer-100/200
Adapted from Poon et al. [1] with permission from the publisher

been identified, more so in *ITGA2B* than *ITGB3*. Family-specific mutations can be used for carrier detection and prenatal diagnosis (PND) in the affected family. Mutation analysis is also useful in identifying αIIbβ3 mutations that may be at risk for the development of αIIbβ3 allo-immunization following platelet transfusion [20].

14.4.1 Clinical Manifestations

Patients with GT have a variable bleeding tendency: some patients have quite mild bleeding symptoms whereas others experience life-threatening hemorrhages. Bleeding symptoms usually occur in homozygotes and double heterozygotes, although heterozygotes with about a half-normal concentration of αIIbβ3 usually are asymptomatic. Rare exceptions are GT with gain-of-function αIIbβ3 mutations inherited autosomal dominantly [3, 21]. These patients usually have macrothrombocytopenia.

Although the disorder usually manifests early in life, some cases may not be diagnosed until much later. The majority of GT patients are diagnosed before the age of 5 years with recurrent epistaxis and gingival bleeds. In the majority of patients, bleeding symptoms may be sufficiently severe to require blood transfusion. With increasing age, the bleeding tendency in GT is generally decreased, but the incidence of severe bleeds is not. The bleeding symptoms in GT are mostly mucocutaneous, with purpura, epistaxis, gum bleeding, and menorrhagia nearly constant features of this disorder, whereas gastrointestinal (GI) bleeding and hematuria are less frequent bleeding symptoms. There is no correlation or little relationship between platelet αIIbβ3 concentration (hence GT types) and the severity of hemorrhagic tendency. Some patients with an undetectable level of αIIbβ3 may have a mild bleeding phenotype whereas others with an αIIbβ3 level of 10% to 15% may have severe life-threatening hemorrhagic manifestations. It seems that the absence of αvβ3 in vascular cells can contribute to the severity of bleeding symptoms (Table 14.3) [2, 8, 22].

There is also a poor relationship between the underlying *αIIbβ3* gene defect and severity of bleeding tendency, and the bleeding tendency can be variable even among family members. In males, diagnosis of the disorder may occur after excessive post-circumcision bleeding, whereas in women diagnosis may be delayed until menarche, when severe menorrhagia requires management that may include blood transfusion. Delivery is a special concern in women with GT, as these women are at risk of severe life-threatening hemorrhage at this time.

Single-nucleotide polymorphisms (SNPs) may be associated with a decrease or increase in the bleeding tendency. *ITGA2* C807T SNP, associated with higher density of α2β1, has been shown to confer a milder phenotype of GT. Although GT is a severe bleeding disorder, the prognosis is generally good if careful supportive care is provided [25].

Table 14.3 Clinical manifestations of patients with Glanzmann thrombasthenia

Bleeding symptoms	Iranian (*n* = 382) (%) [22]	France (*n* = 177)[a] (%) [23]	Pakistan (*n* = 162) (%) [24]	GTR (*n* = 216) (%) [1]
Epistaxis	50	73	62.5	79
Gingival bleeding	23	55	56.4	62
Ecchymosis, easy bruising, purpura, petechiae	15	86	76.6	43
Hematuria	–	6	8	7
Gastrointestinal bleeding	4.7	12	7.4	23#
Hematoma	4.7	1	–	13
Menorrhagia	12.9	98	70	74
Post-circumcision bleeding	3.6	–	43.4	5
Postsurgical bleeding	2.8	–	–	–
Post-trauma bleeding	–	–	47.2	–
Bleeding at injection sites	2	–	–	1.4
Umbilical cord bleeding	0.3	–	5.5	–
Excessive bleeding at delivery	0.5	–	–	74
Central nervous system bleeding	0.3	2	–	1.8
Hemarthrosis	0.3	3	–	6

[a]Data from 113 patients from the literature and 64 patients from France
GTR Glanzmann's Thrombasthenia Registry, *n* number; #; 23% for general GI bleeding (additional 6% for hemorrhoidal bleeding); 13% for muscle hematoma (additional 38% for subcutaneous hematoma); bleeding from vaccination injection site

14.4.2 Molecular Basis

GT is an extremely rare bleeding disorder that is inherited in an autosomal recessive manner as the result of mutations in the *ITGA2B* and *ITGB3*. Mutations in both genes have been identified in different populations including the French Gypsy, Japanese, African, American, Iranian, Chinese, and mixed Caucasian [2, 8, 22].

ITGA2B gene encodes the alpha chain of the αIIbβ3 complex consisting of heavy (H) and light (L) chains connected by disulfide bonds. *ITGB3* encodes the beta chain of the αIIbβ3 complex. The *ITGA2B* gene comprises 30 exons that are transcribed to a 3.1-kb mRNA and then translated to a precursor protein with 1146 amino acids. The *ITGB3* gene consisting of 15 exons is transcribed to a 2.3-kb mRNA and is translated to a 747-amino-acid precursor protein. Unlike the alpha chain (αIIb), which is restricted to the megakaryocyte lineage, the beta chain (β3) is distributed in a wide range of tissues (Figs. 14.4 and 14.5) [8].

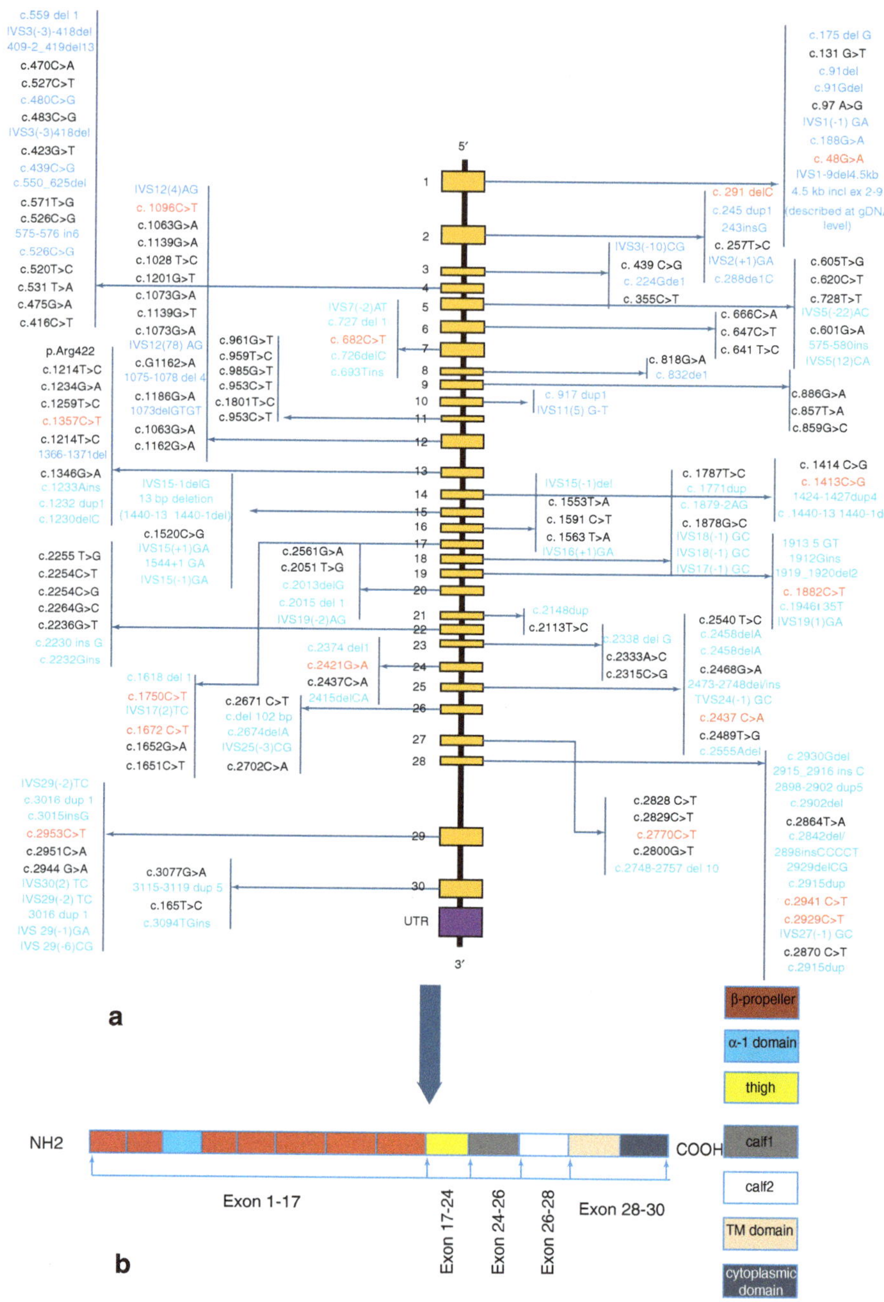

Fig. 14.4 (**a**) Schematic representation of *ITGA2B* gene structure, which is composed of 30 exons with genetic abnormalities that lead to Glanzmann thrombasthenia. Approximately 221 mutations, including 92 missense (in *black letters*), 88 frameshift (in *blue letters*), and 23 nonsense (in *red letters*) mutations have now been reported to the Glanzmann thrombasthenia database (https://glanzmann.mcw.edu/ (accessed July 2017)). (**b**) Domain structure of GPIIb. *UTR* untranslated region, *inv* inversion, *del* deletion, *ins* insertion, *dup* duplication

14.4.2.1 The *ITGA2B* and *ITGB3* Gene Mutations

Missense, nonsense, and frameshift mutations are common causes of GT. Based on mutation locations, they have different effects on αIIbβ3; for example, c.433G>T (D145Y) and c.2332T>C (S778P) mutations in *ITGB3* gene involve the Fg-binding site and signaling pathway of the β3-subunit of αIIbβ3. More than 300 mutations have now been reported in GT patients [3, 26, 27]. A continually updated list of the *ITGA2B* and *ITGB3* mutations can be found on https://glanzmann.mcw.edu/. Depending on the nature of the mutations, patients may have total absent expression of αIIbβ3 (type I GT), decreased αIIbβ3 (type II GT), or qualitatively defective αIIbβ3 (variant GT). Causative mutations of some variants of GT are listed in (Table 14.4).

Mutations causing GT occur worldwide, but because the rate of consanguineous marriages is significantly higher in certain ethnic groups such as Iranian, Jewish, Jordanian, Iraqi, and Palestinian, the disease is expected to be more prevalent in these ethnics [2, 22].

14.4.2.2 Mutations Affecting the αIIb-Subunit

More GT-causing mutations affect the *ITGA2B* gene than the *ITGB3* gene. A prevalent GT-causing mutation in the Israeli-Arab population is the 13-bp deletion of the *ITGA2B* gene, which leads to a six-amino-acid deletion of the αIIb-subunit of the αIIbβ3 complex. This was the founder mutation; it involves the acceptor splice site of exon 4, resulting in a lack of expression of the αIIbβ3 complex [28]. Certain important causative mutations occurring in *ITGA2B* gene include the following.

KW-Milwaukee Patient

A large homozygote deletion (IVS1→9del4.5kb) in exon 1 of *ITGA2B* gene leads to premature termination of mRNA that translates into a shortened αIIb-subunit consisting of 88 amino acids. This aberrant αIIb-subunit is not able to complex with the β3-subunit for expression on the platelet surface [8].

SK I and SK II Patient

Two nonsense mutations in the *ITGA2B* gene, and more common in the Japanese population, include the c.1750C>T mutation in exon 17, resulting in the p.Arg584 stop amino acid substitution (SK I patient), and IVS25(-3) C>G mutation in exon 26 (SK II patient). These mutations lead to the absence of an αIIb proteolytic cleavage site and decrease the expression of αIIbβ3 on the platelet surface [8, 29].

LM Patient

A missense mutation in exon 13 (c.1346G>A) leads to p.Gly418Asp and involves the fourth calcium-binding site in the αIIb-subunit. The integrin αIIbβ3 is formed but not expressed on the platelet surface [8].

Table 14.4 Glanzmann thrombasthenia (GT) variant causative mutations and their effect on phenotypic characteristics of disease

Exon	AAS	Mutation	Subunit	Genotype	Phenotype	Bleeding	Aggregation	Leads to
4	Y174H	c.520T>C	αIIb	Hetero	Missense	Mild	Absent	The residual alteration of β-propeller domain
5	T207I	c.620C>T	αIIb	Homo	Missense	Severe	Absent	The residual alteration of β-propeller domain
30	R1026Q	c.3077G>A	αIIb	Hetero	Missense	Mild	Reduced	Thrombocytopenia
4	D145Y	c.433G>T	β3	Homo	Missense	Severe	Absent	Alteration of Fg-binding site
5	R240Q	c.719G>A	β3	Homo	Missense	Severe	Absent	Unstable integrin/alteration of Ca^{2+}-binding site
4	S188L	c.563C>T	β3	Homo	Missense	Severe	Absent	Refractory integrin poorly expressed
6	L288P	c.863 T >C	β3	Hetero	Missense	Moderate	Absent	Production of an unstable integrin
15	S778P	c.2332T>C	β3	Hetero	Missense	Mild	Absent	Signaling alteration of β3 CT
14	R750X	c.2248C>T	β3	Homo	Nonsense	Severe	Absent	Signaling alteration of β3 CT
11	C575R	c.1723T>C	β3	Homo	Missense	Severe	Absent	Production of a constitutively active receptor
11	C586R	c.1756 T>C	β3	Homo	Missense	Moderate	Much reduced	Production of a constitutively active receptor
14	L718P	c.2231T>C	β3	Hetero	Frame shift	Severe	Much reduced	Aggregation and secretory defects

AAS amino acid substitution, *Hetero* heterozygous, *Homo* homozygous, *Del* deletion, *Fg* fibrinogen, *CT* cytoplasmic tail

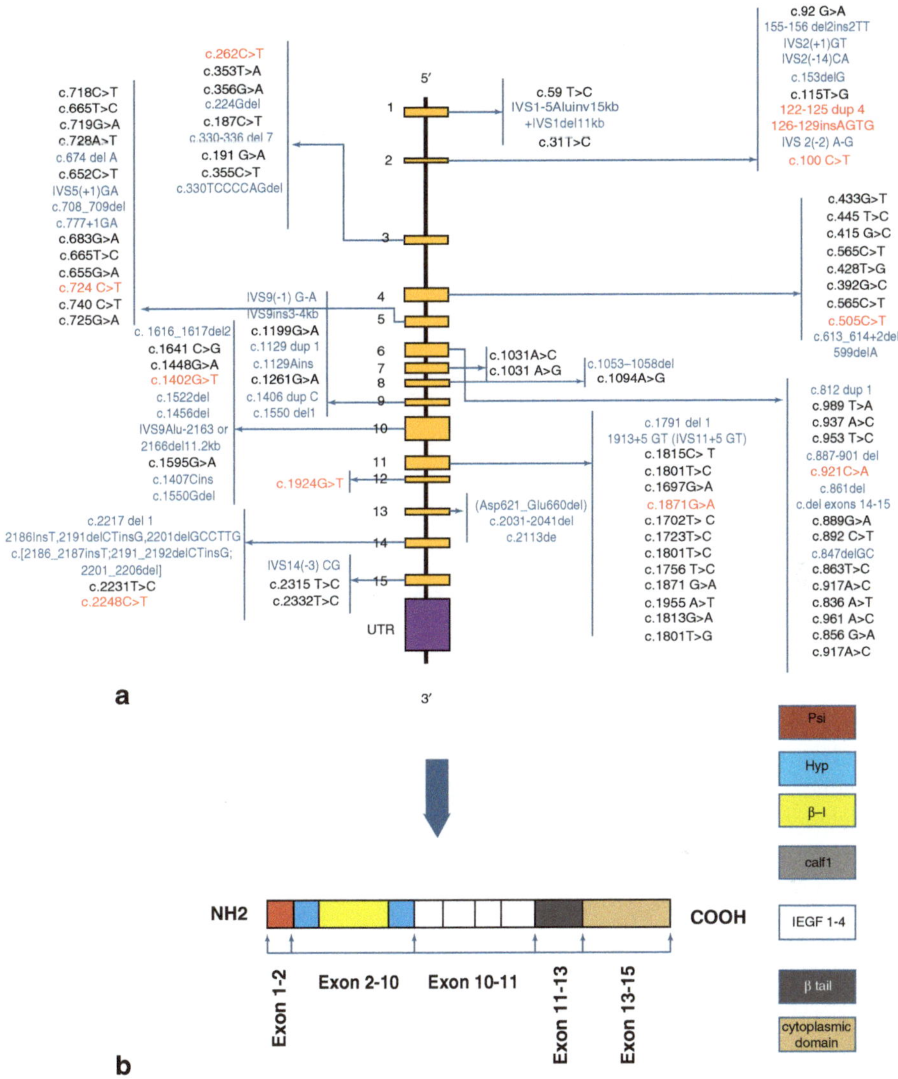

Fig. 14.5 (**a**) Schematic representation of the *ITGB3* gene structure, which is composed of 15 exons with genetic abnormalities that lead to Glanzmann thrombasthenia. Approximately 134 mutations, including 62 missense (in *black letters*), 47 frameshift (in *blue letters*), and 11 nonsense (in *red letters*) mutations have now been reported to the Glanzmann thrombasthenia database (https://glanzmann.mcw.edu/ (accessed July 2017)), (**b**) Domain structure of GPIIIa. *UTR* untranslated region, *inv* inversion, *del* deletion, *ins* insertion, *dup* duplication

UP Patient

A missense mutation, c.818G>A, in exon 8 of the *ITGA2B* gene leads to p.Gly273Asp, which involves the first calcium-binding site in the αIIb-subunit. The abnormal αIIb-subunit complexes with the β3-subunit, but the formed complex is not transported from the ER to the Golgi apparatus, and αIIbβ3 are hence not expressed on the platelet surface [8].

KJ Patient

A homozygote missense mutation, c.1037G>A, in exon 12 that leads to p.Arg327His occurs in the ligand-binding site in the αIIb-subunit; this represents one of the mutations affecting the β-propeller domain that are found in German patients. Platelets of these patients show a decreased level of integrin αIIbβ3 [3, 8].

The β-propeller domain is considered a mutation-rich domain of the integrin αIIb-subunit, which is critical in the biogenesis of the αIIbβ3 complex. The GT database (https://glanzmann.mcw.edu/ (accessed July 2017)) showed that in this domain there are about 131 different mutations include 62 missense, 43 frameshift, 13 nonsense, and 13 others.

14.4.2.3 Mutations Affecting the β3-Subunit

Mutations such as inversion, deletion, frameshift, and splice-site can change the ability and stability of β3 to make a complex with αIIb. Examples of causative mutations in *ITGB3* genes include the following.

Strasbourg I Variant

A homozygous mutation, c.718C>T, in exon 5 leads to p.Arg214Trp in the β3-subunit. This mutation, occurring in the ligand-binding site of the β3-subunit, was reported in the French population. In contrast to other GT patients, the affected patients showed an absence of platelet aggregation in response to ristocetin [8].

ET Variant

A missense mutation, c.719G>A, in exon 5 of the *ITGB3* gene leads to the p.Arg214Glnin in the β3-subunit, which was reported in Australia's population [3, 8].

Cam Variant

A homozygous missense mutation in the β3-subunit, c.433G>T, in exon 4 of *ITGB3* leads to p.Asp119Tyr. This mutation, involving the ligand-binding site and the calcium-binding site of the β3-subunit, was reported in the Guam population. The mutant αIIbβ3 is not able to bind RGD-containing ligands [3, 8].

14.4.3 Diagnosis

Because a considerable number of patients with GT may present with severe life-threatening bleeds, early and timely diagnosis of the disorder is crucial for their appropriate management. Diagnosis of GT can be based on family history, clinical presentations, and appropriate physical examination as well as suitable laboratory assessments. In such autosomal recessive bleeding disorders, a positive family history is a very important diagnostic clue that can help provide a rapid diagnosis for the patient. In a patient with history of excessive bleeding and a positive family history of GT, more direct and specific tests can be used. On the other hand, in those patients without a family history of GT, but with signs of primary hemostasis disorders, more general tests could be used. Clinical presentations are other important clues for the diagnosis of GT. Most patients with GT present early in life with mucocutaneous bleeding. Purpura, petechia, and easy bruising are common physical signs. All routine coagulation tests including activated partial thromboplastin time (aPTT), prothrombin time (PT), and thrombin time (TT) are normal in GT, except for a prolongation of the bleeding time (BT)/closure time. BT lacks specificity and is an invasive procedure, and is now more or less replaced by closure times as assayed by the platelet function analyzer 100/200 (PFA-100/200). PFA-100/200 as a screening test for primary hemostasis including GT has good sensitivity but it is not specific. Platelet count is usually normal with normal platelet morphology in patients with GT (except for the rare patients with macrothrombocytopenia associated with gain-of-function mutations that are usually inherited autosomal dominantly) [3, 21]. Clot retraction also is affected in GT, being absent in type I, with less than 5% αIIbβ3, and decreased in type II, with 5% to 20% αIIbβ3, and in 'variant' (or type III) GT with normal or near-normal (60–100%) expression of dysfunctional receptors (Table 14.2). This test is not widely available and is no longer required for the diagnosis of GT, as it is not specific and is also impaired in Stormorken syndrome and Wiskott–Aldrich syndrome (WAS). Platelet aggregation studies are most important in the diagnosis of GT. GT platelets typically have an absent to markedly diminished aggregation response to physiological agonists, but platelet agglutination response to ristocetin and VWF is present as the GPIb receptors on the GT platelets are normal. Flow cytometry is an effective and powerful instrument for quantitative assessment of platelet integrin αIIbβ3 and is important for the proper classification of GT. It is, however, an expensive method and requires technical expertise. αIIbβ3 is involved in uptake of fibrinogen from the peripheral blood stream to platelet storage granules, so that fibrinogen in the α-granules is absent in type I GT. Expression of functional integrin αIIbβ3 is also necessary for proper release of the platelet δ-granule contents, and abnormality in release of these granular contents may be observed in GT.

According to the Platelet Physiology Subcommittee of the International Society on Thrombosis and Haemostasis (ISTH) guidelines; the first step for diagnosis of inherited platelet function disorders (IPFDs) should include blood smear examination and light transmission aggregometry (LTA) using a limited number of agonists as well as assessment of platelet granules release and flow cytometric analysis of major platelet glycoproteins (Fig. 14.6) [30–32].

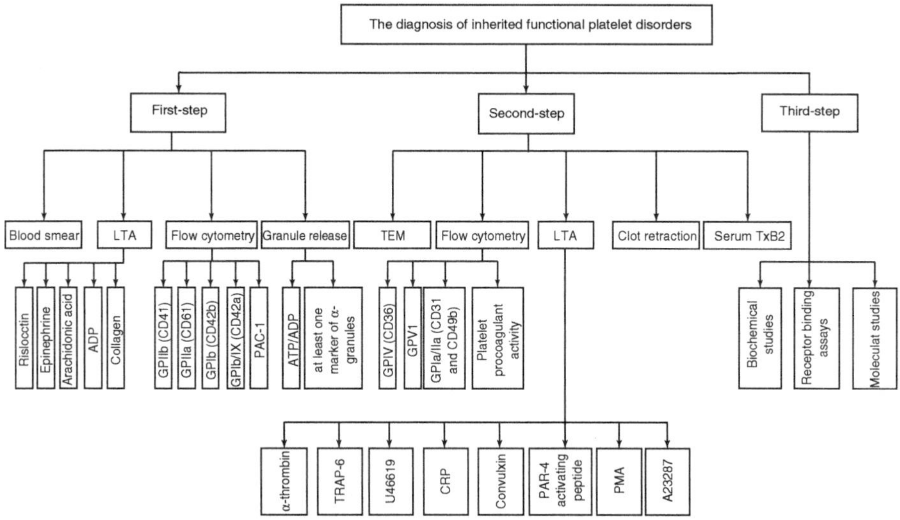

Fig. 14.6 ISTH-suggested algorithm for diagnosis of inherited platelet function disorders. *ISTH* International Society on Thrombosis and Haemostasis, *LTA* light transmission aggregometry, *TEM* transmission electron microscopy, *ADP* adenosine diphosphate

14.4.3.1 Platelet Function Testing

Bleeding time (BT) is the traditional platelet function test for investigation of primary hemostasis. However, this test is invasive, time consuming, and is not well standardized because it is affected by operator technique, patient variables, and conditions including age, gender, and skin temperature and thickness. BT is now largely replaced by closure times assessed by PFA-100/200 that is very sensitive to severe platelet function disorders such as GT and BSS. PFA-100/200 requires a citrated blood sample that is dispensed by the operator into a test reservoir. The sample is aspirated at high shear rates through a membrane coated with collagen/epinephrine (C/EPI) or collagen/adenosine diphosphate (C/ADP). These agonists trigger adhesion and aggregation of platelets, leading to the occlusion of an aperture in the test cartridge. The time of occlusion of the aperture is considered as the endpoint of the test and is reported as 'closure time' (CT) (Fig. 14.7) [30, 33].

Although PFA-100/200 is sensitive in the detection of GT, it is nonspecific and is affected by a considerable number of variables, including platelet count and hematocrit.

Platelet aggregometry is one of the most widely used test procedures for assessing platelet function and was suggested by the Platelet Physiology Subcommittee of the ISTH as a first-line screening test for platelet function disorders. Two types of instruments are available, including (1) light transmission aggregometry (LTA) and (2) whole blood aggregometry (WBA).

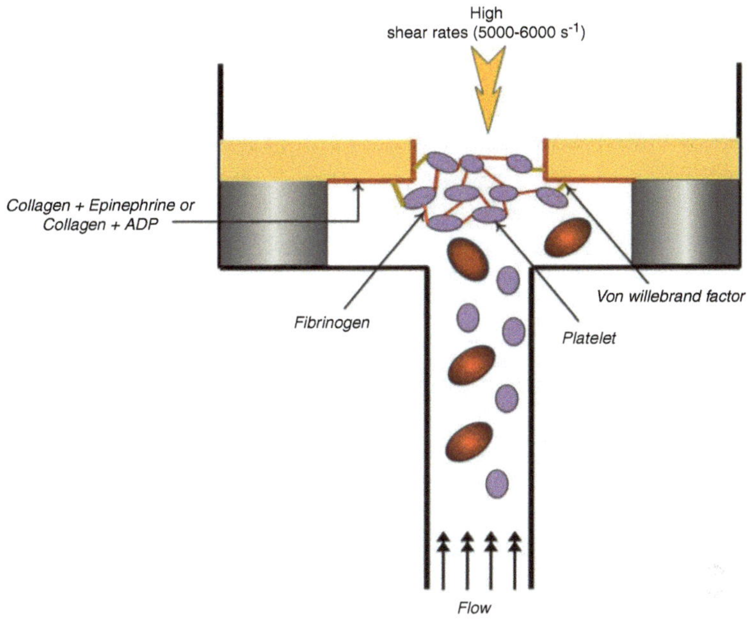

Fig. 14.7 Platelet function analysis (PFA). In this assay, the citrated blood sample is aspirated at high shear rate and primary hemostasis is triggered by a membrane coated with collagen/epinephrine (C/EPI) or collagen/adenosine diphosphate (C/ADP). Activation of primary hemostasis leads to occlusion of an aperture in the test cartridge

LTA is the most widely used method and is considered the gold standard method for the detection of GT. GT is the only disorder with the absence of platelet aggregation to all physiological agonists including ADP, collagen, thrombin, and arachidonic acid but with normal response to the antibiotic ristocetin (Fig. 14.8). In this assay, the citrated blood sample is centrifuged to obtain platelet-rich plasma (PRP). Platelet aggregation is monitored by measuring changes in light absorbance. This method, however, has several disadvantages that include the need for sample preparation and the large amount of blood sample required. The test procedure is also time consuming and is poorly standardized.

Although platelet aggregation is severely decreased or absent in GT, agonist-induced platelet shape change is normal in GT.

The lumiaggregometer is a modification of the traditional LTA that analyzes platelet secretion in parallel with platelet aggregation. The method is based on bioluminescent determination of adenosine triphosphate (ATP). ATP released from platelets reacts with firefly luciferin and luciferase, leading to light emission. In lumiaggregometry, strong agonists such as thrombin, collagen, and thrombin receptor-activating peptide (TRAP) can induce platelet secretion. A key feature can be used for differential diagnosis between platelet secretion and storage pool disorders. Platelet aggregation as well as lumiaggregometry can now be performed with

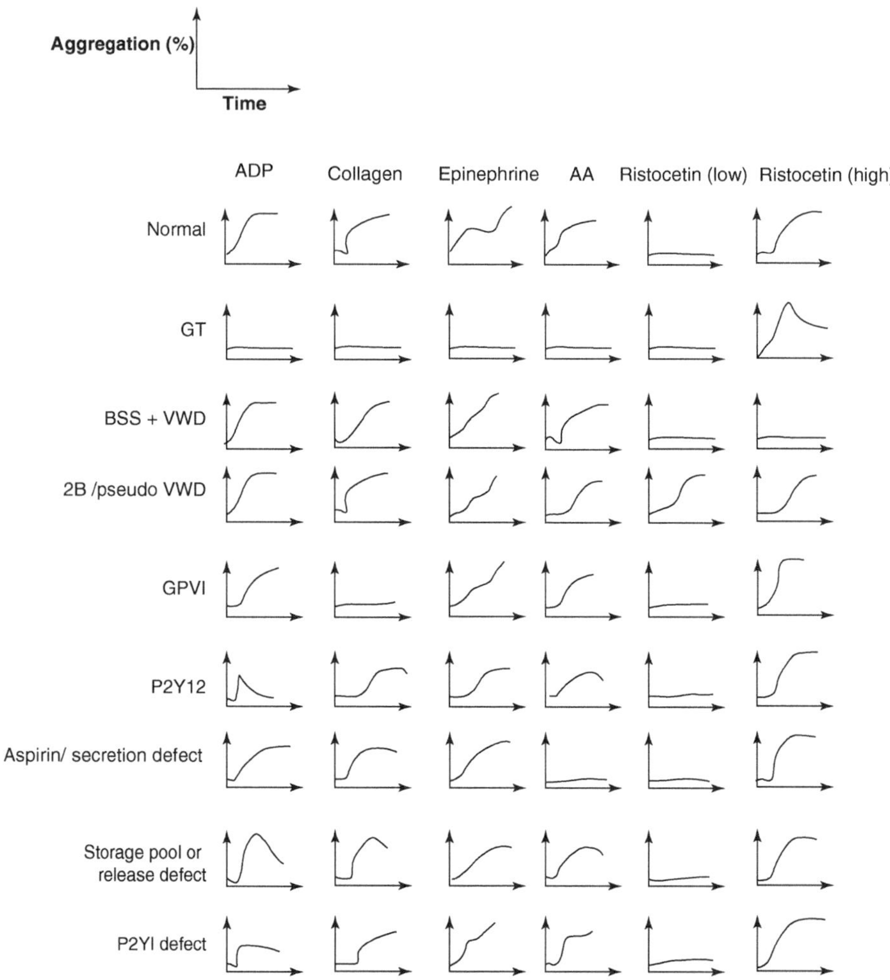

Fig. 14.8 In platelet aggregation studies, patients with Glanzmann thrombasthenia have distinct features that include absent aggregation response to all physiological agonists such as adenosine diphosphate (ADP), arachidonic acid (AA), epinephrine, and collagen, although response to ristocetin is normal. This aggregation pattern is different from other platelet disorders

whole blood. For whole blood aggregation (WBA), whole blood is diluted 1:1 with saline. Platelet response to an agonist is then measured using an electrode immersed in the blood sample. Several agonists including collagen, ADP, thrombin, ristocetin, and arachidonic acid (AA) are used to obtain information on the platelet activation pathway. Again, GT platelets show no aggregation to agonists such as collagen, ADP, thrombin, ristocetin, and AA, but ristocetin aggregation is observed. The main advantage of WBA by multiple electrode aggregometry (MEA) over LTA is the elimination of the time-consuming step of blood centrifugation to prepare PRP and

PPP. In addition, platelet aggregation is assessed in a more native environment in presence of other blood cells minimizing artificial change in platelets, thus improving their functional analysis [30, 33, 34].

14.4.3.2 Flow Cytometry

Flow cytometry is an effective, powerful, and reliable instrument for the determination of platelet phenotype. This test requires a minimum amount of blood sample. A sample of approximately 5 μl from a patient with normal platelet count (150–400 × 10^9/l) is sufficient for the appropriate 5000–10,000 platelet analysis events. Flow cytometry analysis can be performed on whole blood, PRP, or washed platelets. Commonly, PRP is used for calcium flux analysis and washed platelets are used for activation studies using strong agonists. What sample type should be used is determined by the antibody and antagonist used for the assay. In general, whole blood is preferred as the platelets are tested in the more native environment with minimal manipulation and minimal artificial changes, as well as minimal loss of the platelet subpopulation. Sodium citrate is the anticoagulant of choice for flow cytometric analysis for GT platelets. EDTA can induce the disassociation of integrin αIIbβ3 on the platelet surface and should be avoided [30, 33].

Flow cytometric analysis using monoclonal antibodies specific for αIIb (CD41) and β3 (CD61) is reliable for the rapid diagnosis of GT resulting from a deficiency of αIIbβ3. In new patients, deficiency of αIIbβ3 always should be confirmed by flow cytometry using monoclonal antibodies. This method can also be used to determine the homozygous and heterozygous states in these patients based on the level of αIIbβ3 expression on platelet surface [25]. In heterozygous patients with GT, it is possible to determine the level of αIIbβ3 expression in different populations of platelets and therefore one can determine if the bleeding phenotype is related to a decrease in expression of integrin αIIbβ3 in the entire platelet population or in a special platelet population [25].

In patients suspected of GT, additional studies should be done for patients with normal or near-normal platelet αIIbβ3 levels to exclude the possibility of variant GT with dysfunctional αIIbβ3. These patients with variant GT will have abnormal platelet aggregation to physiological agonists, as indicated earlier. Diagnosis of variant GT can also be made by the inability of stimulated platelet to bind either to procaspase-activating compound (PAC-1), a monoclonal antibody specific for activated αIIbβ3, or fluorochrome-labeled fibrinogen (FITC-fibrinogen). PAC-1 specifically recognizes the integrin αIIbβ3 epitope on activated platelets for fibrinogen binding. TRAP is a common agonist that can be used to activate platelets. In addition, different monoclonal antibodies (e.g., CD41a, clone HIP8) can specifically bind to the resting form of integrin αIIbβ3 but will lose their binding affinity when integrin αIIbβ3 is activated. Today, the availability of commercial platelet flow cytometry kits facilitates the routine use of flow cytometry for diagnosis of platelet function disorders. These kits contain both the detecting antibodies as well as the agonists such as TRAP [30, 35].

14.4.4 Differential Diagnosis

In a considerable number of patients, the diagnosis of GT is overlooked, being overshadowed by the more common acquired platelet function disorders with their common clinical presentations and laboratory findings. For this reason, it is essential to perform proper physical examination looking for such common findings as purpura and ecchymoses. We should obtain an appropriate medical history on unprovoked bruising or bleeding episodes or on severe bleeds after minor trauma. A history on use of medication capable of interfering platelet function should be obtained. In isolated cases without family history, leukemia-associated chromosomal rearrangements and the presence of autoantibodies against integrin αIIbβ3 should be considered as a part of the differential diagnosis. Acquired autoantibodies against integrin αIIbβ3 can sufficiently block the platelet function to induce a thrombasthenia-like state [36, 37].

14.4.5 Treatment

Although GT is one of the most severe IPFDs, the prognosis of this disorder is good if appropriate management is provided. The goal of treatment in GT is not only to treat bleeds but also to prevent the occurrence of bleeds and their bleed-related complications to improve the patient's quality of life. Management in a comprehensive care center with multidisciplinary expertise on bleeding disorders similar to the management of hemophilia is preferred [38].

On-demand therapy is normally provided in patients with GT, and most of these patients experience blood transfusion in their life. The management approach includes local and adjunctive measures as well as systemic hemostatic agents. Mild bleeds can be managed by local measures and/or antifibrinolytic drugs. But when use of these agents is not successful, when more severe bleeding occurs, or when surgical intervention is required, systemic hemostatic agents such as platelet transfusion or rFVIIa can be used. Platelet transfusion is currently the standard treatment in GTR. However, repeated platelet transfusion may result in allo-immunization against HLA and/or integrin αIIbβ3 antigens and cause refractoriness to future platelet transfusion. To decrease HLA allo-immunization, HLA-compatible single-donor apheresis platelet concentrates are preferred for patients with platelet disorders, but these may not always be readily available. In addition, the risk of blood-borne infectious agent transmission is a major concern in use of human blood products. rFVIIa is increasingly used for management of patients with GT. rFVIIa is approved in the European Union for management of patients with GT and antibodies against platelet HLA and/or integrin αIIbβ3 with refractoriness to platelets; in the United States, this therapeutic agent is approved for the management of patients refractory to platelet transfusion. In Canada, it is approved for clinical refractoriness and/or antibodies against platelets or when platelets are not immediately available [1, 37, 38].

Thus, the following therapeutic options are available for patients with GT:

1. Local measures and/or antifibrinolytic drugs
2. Systemic hemostatic management
3. Curative treatment options

14.4.5.1 Local Measures and Antifibrinolytic Drugs

Mild to moderate bleeding episodes can be managed by conservative measures, such as application of local pressure or local use of topical thrombin or fibrin sealants. Antifibrinolytic agents such as tranexamic acid or epsilon-aminocaproic acid are often effective in the management of bleeding.

Epistaxis is one of the most common bleeding symptoms in GT, especially in children. The most important measures to control epistaxis include compression, topical thrombin, antifibrinolytics, and nasal packing, preferably absorbable gelfoam packing. In severe epistaxis that is not controlled with these conservative measures, platelet transfusion and/or rFVIIa can be used. In severe cases, in surgical procedures such as electrocautery, laser coagulation, and septoplasty, arterial ligation can be used to control bleeding. It is also important to counsel GT patients to refrain from conditions that may predispose them to trauma and bleeding. Antiplatelet agents (e.g., aspirin and NSAIDs) should be avoided [1, 8, 37].

14.4.5.2 Systemic Hemostatic Management

When local measures are not successful in stopping hemorrhagic episodes, systemic hemostatic management can be used, including transfusion of platelet concentrate and administration of rFVII [1, 39].

14.4.5.3 Platelet Concentrate

Currently, platelet transfusion is the standard treatment for the control of severe hemorrhagic episodes and for management of surgical procedures. Platelet transfusion has two main concerns, including the risk of blood-borne infectious disease transmission and allo-immunization against HLA or αIIbβ3 antigens. Allergic reaction- and transfusion-related acute lung injury (TRALI) are other risks of platelet transfusion. To minimize the risk of HLA-allo-immunization against platelets, patients preferably should receive HLA-matched leukocyte-reduced platelet concentrates, particularly from a single donor. In GT patients with bleeding, the effectiveness of platelet transfusion is monitored clinically for bleeding cessation. In those with baseline normal platelet count, monitoring of platelet count for platelet increment is not perfect but can give an estimation of platelet recovery. In GT patients with a deficiency of integrin αIIbβ3, monitoring the increase in platelets bearing αIIbβ3 by flow cytometry (if available) can be used. It should be noted that this method cannot predict treatment efficacy of the increased platelets, especially in those patients with allo-immunization against platelets. Furthermore, GT platelets have been shown to interfere with the function of transfused donor platelets so that sufficient platelets should be given to overcome interference for proper hemostasis [39–41].

Platelet Refractoriness

About 50% of patients with nonimmune thrombocytopenia develop anti-HLA following repeated transfusion of platelet concentrate. The risk is 10% to 15% when leukocyte-reduced platelet concentrate is used.

With repeated platelet transfusion in patients with GT, allo-antibodies developing against the platelet glycoproteins αIIbβ3 and/or the HLA antigens are common. Thus, platelet refractoriness is a major problem in GT patients. Platelet refractoriness is defined as repeated failure to achieve suitable responses to platelet transfusions. In patients with HLA antibodies and platelet refractoriness, HLA-matched platelets should be used. In nonimmune patients, the risk of HLA allo-immunization can also be lessened by transfusion of HLA-matched platelets and the use of leukocyte-depleted blood components. It is important that hemostatic response to platelet transfusions is monitored in GT patients. Clinical improvements in bleeding and laboratory evaluation of platelet function including the use of flow cytometry are monitoring options in GT. Another alternative treatment option for platelet refractory patient with or without platelet antibodies (to HLA and/or αIIbβ3) is rFVIIa.

Because of the risk of allo-immunization from repeated platelet transfusions, it has been suggested that rFVIIa be considered as the first-line treatment or prevention of bleeding in GT patients at risk for the development of anti-αIIbβ3. In this context, genetic information of patients can be very helpful. Patients with GT and disease-causing mutations that result in an absent expression of αIIbβ3 expression on platelets (e.g., mutations leading to premature termination of αIIb or β3) have been shown to be more susceptible to anti-αIIbβ3 development and therefore platelet refractoriness. Thus, genetic findings can be used to help in the decision whether platelet transfusion or rFVIIa should be used in nonimmune GT patients [1, 8, 37, 42].

14.4.5.4 Activated Recombinant Factor VII

rFVIIa (NovoSeven/Niastase, Novo Nordisk, Bagsvaerd, Denmark) is produced via recombinant DNA technology in baby hamster kidney (BHK) cells. In the production process no human proteins or derivatives are present, so that human pathogen transmission is not a risk. rFVIIa was used successfully in platelet function disorders for the first time in 1996 in a 2-year-old boy with GT with epistaxis not responsive to conservative management. Since then, there have been many reports of successful use of rFVIIa in GT and other platelet function disorders. In 2014, the U.S. Food and Drug Administration (FDA) approved rFVIIa for the treatment of bleeding episodes and perioperative management in adults and children with GT who are refractory to platelet transfusions, with or without platelet allo-antibodies. As indicated earlier, for patients with type I GT, especially those with severe mutations resulting in the total absence of αIIbβ3 expression, the suggestion is that rFVIIa be preferred to platelet transfusion to prevent αIIbβ3 allo-immunization, reserving platelets to be used effectively for emergent life/limb-threatening situations and major surgical procedures. A generic version of rFVIIa was developed by AryoGen (Tehran, Iran) and was first licensed by the Ministry of Health and Medical Education of Iran. AryoSeven is similar to NovoSeven in post-injection rFVIIa activity and in clinical efficacy. This Iranian biogeneric rFVIIa is currently used by several thousand patients with hemophilia with inhibitors, acquired hemophilia, congenital FVII deficiency, and Glanzmann's thrombasthenia in different countries. In pregnant women, anti-αIIbβ3 may be transferred across the placenta to result in thrombocytopenia and bleeding in the fetus or the neonates. Thus, platelet transfusion should be avoided during pregnancy, and in women of reproductive age as well as in prepubertal girls. rFVIIa can be used instead for their management of bleeding and surgical procedures [43–45].

The recommended dose of rFVII is as follows:

Bleeding episodes: 90 μg/kg q2–6 h until hemostasis is achieved

Perioperative management:

1. 90 μg/kg immediately before surgery and repeat q2 h for the duration of procedure
2. 90 μg/kg q2–6 h to prevent postoperative bleeding

Mechanism of Action of rFVIIa

Physiologically, FVIIa exerts its hemostatic action after forming a complex with tissue factor (TF). In a normal person, at the site of vascular injury, the FVII–TF complex induces activation of FX and FIX that results in initial thrombin production and subsequently activation of several clotting factors (e.g., FV, FVIII, FXI) as well as platelets. Activated platelets at the injury site support further coagulation activation that leads to sufficient thrombin generation (thrombin burst). This proper amount of thrombin generates a fibrin clot and induces hemostasis. In GT, because of the lack of αIIbβ3 receptor for fibrinogen binding, thrombin generation is not sufficient to induce platelet aggregate formation and to support the thrombin burst at the vascular injury site. Therefore, GT platelets have reduced thrombin generation capacity. High-dose rFVIIa improves hemostasis via a TF-independent mechanism. rFVIIa in pharmacological dosage binds to the negatively charged phospholipid surface exposed on activated platelets and is able to activate FX to FXa, which eventually results in a burst of thrombin generation, enhancing hemostasis and improving GT platelet adhesion and aggregation. Increased thrombin generation by high-dose rFVIIa has also been shown to improve fibrin clot structure in GT plasma. It is also suggested that rFVIIa activates platelets, resulting in an increase in phosphatidyl serine exposure on the platelet surface and an increase in hemostatically active platelet-derived circulating microparticles [43–46].

14.4.5.5 Surgical Management

Surgery is an important hemostatic challenge in patients with IPFDs, including GT, and can be accompanied by life-threatening hemorrhage. Currently, the standard therapeutic option for surgical interventions is also transfusion of platelet concentrate. Before a surgical procedure, patients with IPFD should be screened for platelet antibodies. In those patients with current or history of platelet antibodies or refractoriness, rFVIIa, together with (or without) anti-fibrinolytic agents is preferred rather than platelet concentrate. As in the treatment of bleeding, HLA-matched and leukocyte-depleted platelet concentrate is the best therapeutic choice whether HLA antibodies are present or not. If HLA-matched platelet concentrate is not available, random donor platelet concentrate can be used in patients without HLA antibodies or platelet refractoriness [37, 47].

Minor Surgery

Minor surgeries including dental extraction in patients with GT and platelet refractoriness or anti-platelet antibodies can be successfully managed using rFVIIa. rFVIIa is usually given preoperatively and, depending on procedure type and severity of bleeding, may be continued for the first 12–24 h.

rFVIIa use in platelet refractory patients is recommended by the United Kingdom Haemophilia Centre Doctors' Organisation for minor surgical prophylaxis including dental extractions. If platelet transfusion is required, HLA-matched leukocyte-depleted platelets is preferred. A rFVIIa dose of 90–140 μg/kg at ≤2.5-h intervals for two or more doses can be successfully used for the prevention of bleeding in minor surgeries. Anti-fibrinolytics should be started preoperatively and may be continued for 1 to 2 weeks [1, 37, 47].

Major Surgery

Successful management of major surgeries in patients with GT requires a suitable communication among the surgeons, the hemophilia center, and the transfusion laboratory. Anti-fibrinolytics may be needed in some cases and should be started preoperatively and continued for 7–14 days. Platelet transfusion remain the standard of care in nonimmune GT patients. rFVIIa is recommended for allo-immunized patients (particularly with platelet refractoriness) undergoing major procedures: rFVIIa at ≥90 μg/kg in ≤2.5-h intervals should be used, at least at the beginning. The clinical condition of the patient will determine the number and duration of subsequent doses [1, 37, 47].

14.4.5.6 Hematopoietic Stem Cell Transplantation (HSCT)

Effective treatments are available for patients with GT that include the use of platelet concentrates and rFVIIa. Nonetheless, there are patients who continue to have severe and recurrent bleeding episodes despite adequate management and have very poor quality of life. For these patients, hemopoietic stem cell transplantation (HSCT) may represent a necessary curative therapy. The first successful HSCT was reported in the literature in 1985 on a 4-year old boy with anti-αIIbβ3 [48]. So far, 47 patients with GT who received HSCT between 1981 and 2016 have been registered with the Center for International Blood and Marrow Transplantation Research (CIBMTR). As of December 2016, 83% of these patients were alive (9% dead and 9% missing for follow-up) (preliminary data obtained from the Statistical Center of the CIBMTR; the analysis has not been reviewed or approved by the Advisory or Scientific Committees of the CIBMTR). Sources of stem cells include bone marrow, cord blood, and peripheral blood. The conditioning regimens include both myeloablative and nonmyeloablative types [1, 49, 50].

14.4.5.7 Gene Therapy

Gene therapy for GT is in the experimental phase, but there are important preclinical reports in animal models. Hodivala-Dilke et al. reported the first animal model (mice) of GT with *ITGB3* gene knockout. These GT mice had prolonged bleeding time (BT) and absence of clot retraction compared to heterozygous and normal animals. The platelet function of these mice was corrected after transplantation of hematopoietic cells with a lentivirus vector encoding integrin β3. In a dog model of GT (dogs from the Great Pyrenees with a genetic defect in *ITGA2B* gene, including insertion of 14 nucleotides in *ITGA2B* exon 13), gene therapy resulted in expression of integrin αIIbβ3 that stabilized to about 10% in three dogs after 2, 4, and 5 years, respectively. Although this level of integrin αIIbβ3 (GPIIb/IIIa) is similar to that in human GT type II, the dogs had decreased cutaneous bruising and shortened BT. Induced pluripotent stem cell (iPSC) was generated from two patients with type 1 GT. Insertion of human αIIb cDNA together with the GP1ba promoter led to a high level of αIIb mRNA expression in the iPSC-derived megakaryocytes (MK), and these MK cells responded to agonist stimulation, suggesting recovery in the expression and activation of integrin αIIbβ3. All these studies can be considered as a very important advance in gene therapy that may eventually be applicable to humans GT [1, 51, 52].

References

1. Poon MC, Di Minno G, d'Oiron R, Zotz R. New insights into the treatment of Glanzmann thrombasthenia. Transfus Med Rev. 2016;30(2):92–9.
2. Nurden AT, Pillois X, Nurden P. Understanding the genetic basis of Glanzmann thrombasthenia: implications for treatment. Expert Rev Hematol. 2012;5(5):487–503.
3. Nurden AT, Fiore M, Nurden P, Pillois X. Glanzmann thrombasthenia: a review of ITGA2B and ITGB3 defects with emphasis on variants, phenotypic variability, and mouse models. Blood. 2011;118(23):5996–6005.
4. Srivastava A, Usher S, Nelson EJ, Jayandharan G, Shaji RV, Chandy M, et al. Prenatal diagnosis of Glanzmann thrombasthenia. Natl Med J India. 2003;16(4):207–8.
5. Wang ZY, Ruan CG. Current state and prospect in treatment of Glanzmann's thrombasthenia. Zhonghua Xue Ye Xue Za Zhi. 2016;37(5):430–1.
6. Fang J, Hodivala-Dilke K, Johnson BD, Du LM, Hynes RO, White GC 2nd, et al. Therapeutic expression of the platelet-specific integrin, alphaIIbbeta3, in a murine model for Glanzmann thrombasthenia. Blood. 2005;106(8):2671–9.
7. Seligsohn U. Glanzmann thrombasthenia: a model disease which paved the way to powerful therapeutic agents. Pathophysiol Haemost Thromb. 2002;32(5–6):216.
8. Kato A. The biologic and clinical spectrum of Glanzmann's thrombasthenia: implications of integrin alpha IIb beta 3 for its pathogenesis. Crit Rev Oncol Hematol. 1997;26(1):1–23.
9. Bennett JS. Structure and function of the platelet integrin alphaIIbbeta3. J Clin Invest. 2005;115(12):3363–9.
10. Calvete JJ. Platelet integrin GPIIb/IIIa: structure–function correlations. An update and lessons from other integrins. Proc Soc Exp Biol Med. 1999;222(1):29–38.
11. Suzuki H. Structure and function of platelet alpha IIb beta 3 integrin. Rinsho Byori. 1997;104(Suppl):60–72.

12. Cierniewski CS. Structure and function of integrin receptors based on platelet receptor for fibrinogen. Postepy Biochem. 1994;40(1):45–54.
13. Estevez B, Du X. New concepts and mechanisms of platelet activation signaling. Physiology (Bethesda). 2017;32(2):162–77.
14. Liu J, Das M, Yang J, Ithychanda SS, Yakubenko VP, Plow EF, et al. Structural mechanism of integrin inactivation by filamin. Nat Struct Mol Biol. 2015;22(5):383–9.
15. Nieswandt B, Varga-Szabo D, Elvers M. Integrins in platelet activation. J Thromb Haemost. 2009;7((suppl 1):206–9.
16. Ma YQ, Qin J, Plow EF. Platelet integrin alpha(IIb)beta(3): activation mechanisms. J Thromb Haemost. 2007;5(7):1345–52.
17. Xu Z, Chen X, Zhi H, Gao J, Bialkowska K, Byzova TV, et al. Direct interaction of kindlin-3 with integrin alphaIIbbeta3 in platelets is required for supporting arterial thrombosis in mice. Arterioscler Thromb Vasc Biol. 2014;34(9):1961–7.
18. Mandava P, Thiagarajan P, Kent TA. Glycoprotein IIb/IIIa antagonists in acute ischaemic stroke: current status and future directions. Drugs. 2008;68(8):1019–28.
19. Goto S, Tamura N, Ishida H. Ability of anti-glycoprotein IIb/IIIa agents to dissolve platelet thrombi formed on a collagen surface under blood flow conditions. J Am Coll Cardiol. 2004;44(2):316–23.
20. Fiore M, Firah N, Pillois X, Nurden P, Heilig R, Nurden AT. Natural history of platelet antibody formation against alphaIIbbeta3 in a French cohort of Glanzmann thrombasthenia patients. Haemophilia. 2012;18(3):e201–E209.
21. Kashiwagi H, Kunishima S, Kiyomizu K, Amano Y, Shimada H, Morishita M, et al. Demonstration of novel gain-of-function mutations of alphaIIbbeta3: association with macrothrombocytopenia and glanzmann thrombasthenia-like phenotype. Mol Genet Genomic Med. 2013;1(2):77–86.
22. Toogeh G, Sharifian R, Lak M, Safaee R, Artoni A, Peyvandi F. Presentation and pattern of symptoms in 382 patients with Glanzmann thrombasthenia in Iran. Am J Hematol. 2004;77(2):198–9.
23. George JN, Caen JP, Nurden AT. Glanzmann's thrombasthenia: the spectrum of clinical disease. Blood. 1990;75(7):1383–95.
24. Borhany M, Fatima H, Naz A, Patel H, Shamsi T. Pattern of bleeding and response to therapy in Glanzmann thrombasthenia. Haemophilia. 2012;18(6):e423–5.
25. Simou M, Kouskouni E, Vitoratos N, Economou E, Creatsas G. Polymorphisms of platelet glycoprotein receptors and cell adhesion molecules in fetuses with fetal growth restriction and their mothers as detected with pyrosequencing. In Vivo. 2017;31(2):243–9.
26. Nurden AT, Pillois X, Wilcox DA. Glanzmann thrombasthenia: state of the art and future directions. Semin Thromb Hemost. 2013;39(6):642–55.
27. Franchini M, Favaloro EJ, Lippi G. Glanzmann thrombasthenia: an update. Clin Chim Acta. 2010;411(1-2):1–6.
28. Rosenberg N, Hauschner H, Peretz H, Mor-Cohen R, Landau M, Shenkman B, et al. A 13-bp deletion in alpha(IIb) gene is a founder mutation that predominates in Palestinian-Arab patients with Glanzmann thrombasthenia. J Thromb Haemost. 2005;3(12):2764–72.
29. Newman PJ, Seligsohn U, Lyman S, Coller BS. The molecular genetic basis of Glanzmann thrombasthenia in the Iraqi-Jewish and Arab populations in Israel. Proc Natl Acad Sci U S A. 1991;88(8):3160–4.
30. Albanyan A, Al-Musa A, Al Nounou R, Al Zahrani H, Nasr R, AlJefri A, et al. Diagnosis of Glanzmann thrombasthenia by whole blood impedance analyzer (MEA) vs. light transmission aggregometry. Int J Lab Hematol. 2015;37(4):503–8.
31. Fiore M, Nurden AT, Vinciguerra C, Nurden P, Pillois X. Rapid diagnosis of the French gypsy mutation in Glanzmann thrombasthenia using high-resolution melting analysis. Thromb Haemost. 2010;104(5):1076–7.
32. French DL, Coller BS, Usher S, Berkowitz R, Eng C, Seligsohn U, et al. Prenatal diagnosis of Glanzmann thrombasthenia using the polymorphic markers BRCA1 and THRA1 on chromosome 17. Br J Haematol. 1998;102(2):582–7.

33. Awidi A, Maqablah A, Dweik M, Bsoul N, Abu-Khader A. Comparison of platelet aggregation using light transmission and multiple electrode aggregometry in Glanzmann thrombasthenia. Platelets. 2009;20(5):297–301.
34. McGlasson DL, Fritsma GA. Whole blood platelet aggregometry and platelet function testing. Semin Thromb Hemost. 2009;35(2):168–80.
35. Nagy B Jr, Debreceni IB, Kappelmayer J. Flow cytometric investigation of classical and alternative platelet activation markers. eJIFCC. 2013;23(4):124–34.
36. Yazici ZM, Celik M, Yegin Y, Gunes S, Kayhan FT. Glanzmann's thrombasthenia: a rare case of spontaneous bilateral hemotympanum. Braz J Otorhinolaryngol. 2015;81(2):224–55.
37. Solh T, Botsford A, Solh M. Glanzmann's thrombasthenia: pathogenesis, diagnosis, and current and emerging treatment options. J Blood Med. 2015;6:219–27.
38. Srivastava A, Brewer AK, Mauser-Bunschoten EP, Key NS, Kitchen S, Llinas A, et al. Guidelines for the management of hemophilia. Haemophilia. 2013;19(1):e1–e47.
39. Poon M-C, Di Minno G, Zotz R, d'Oiron R. Glanzmann's thrombasthenia: strategies for identification and management. Expert Opin Orphan Drugs. 2017;5(8):641–53.
40. Al-Battat S, Rand ML, Bouskill V, Lau W, Blanchette VS, Kahr WHA, et al. Glanzmann thrombasthenia platelets compete with transfused platelets, reducing the haemostatic impact of platelet transfusions. Br J Haematol. 2018;181(3):410-3.
41. Jennings LK, Wang WC, Jackson CW, Fox CF, Bell A. Hemostasis in Glanzmann's thrombasthenia (GT): GT platelets interfere with the aggregation of normal platelets. Am J Pediatr Hematol Oncol. 1991;13(1):84–90.
42. Chitlur M, Rajpurkar M, Recht M, Tarantino MD, Yee DL, Cooper DL, et al. Recognition and management of platelet-refractory bleeding in patients with Glanzmann's thrombasthenia and other severe platelet function disorders. Int J Gen Med. 2017;10:95–9.
43. Rajpurkar M, Chitlur M, Recht M, Cooper DL. Use of recombinant activated factor VII in patients with Glanzmann's thrombasthenia: a review of the literature. Haemophilia. 2014;20(4):464–71.
44. Franchini M. The use of recombinant activated factor VII in platelet disorders: a critical review of the literature. Blood Transfus. 2009;7(1):24–8.
45. Poon MC, Zotz R, Di Minno G, Abrams ZS, Knudsen JB, Laurian Y. Glanzmann's thrombasthenia treatment: a prospective observational registry on the use of recombinant human activated factor VII and other hemostatic agents. Semin Hematol. 2006;43(1 suppl 1): S33–6.
46. Allen GA, Hoffman M, Roberts HR, Monroe DM 3rd. Recombinant activated factor VII: its mechanism of action and role in the control of hemorrhage. Can J Anaesth. 2002;49(10):S7–S14.
47. Gopalakrishnan A, Veeraraghavan R, Panicker P. Hematological and surgical management in Glanzmann's thrombasthenia: a case report. J Indian Soc Pedod Prev Dent. 2014;32(2):181–4.
48. Bellucci S, Devergie A, Gluckman E, Tobelem G, Lethielleux P, Benbunan M, et al. Complete correction of Glanzmann's thrombasthenia by allogeneic bone-marrow transplantation. Br J Haematol. 1985;59(4):635–41.
49. Ramzi M, Dehghani M, Haghighat S, Nejad HH. Stem cell transplant in severe Glanzmann thrombasthenia in an adult patient. Exp Clin Transplant. 2016;14(6):688–90.
50. Wiegering V, Winkler B, Langhammer F, Wolfl M, Wirbelauer J, Sauer K, et al. Allogeneic hematopoietic stem cell transplantation in Glanzmann thrombasthenia complicated by platelet alloimmunization. Klin Padiatr. 2011;223(3):173–5.
51. Fang J, Jensen ES, Boudreaux MK, Du LM, Hawkins TB, Koukouritaki SB, et al. Platelet gene therapy improves hemostatic function for integrin alphaIIbbeta3-deficient dogs. Proc Natl Acad Sci U S A. 2011;108(23):9583–8.
52. Wilcox DA, White GC 2nd. Gene therapy for platelet disorders: studies with Glanzmann's thrombasthenia. J Thromb Haemost. 2003;1(2311):2300–11.

Bernard-Soulier Syndrome

15

Bahare Ghasemi and Akbar Dorgalaleh

15.1 Introduction

Bernard-Soulier syndrome (BSS) is a rare inherited platelet function disorder characterized by thrombocytopenia, giant platelets (macrothrombocytopenia), and abnormal bleeding tendency. The hallmark of BSS is a deficiency or dysfunction of the von Willebrand factor (VWF) receptor, also known as glycoprotein (GP) Ib-IX-V complex (CD42a-d) that is required for normal primary hemostasis [1]. The GPIb-IX-V complex is a crucial receptor for normal hemostasis, and it is necessary for adherence of platelets to the exposed vascular subendothelium via binding to VWF at the site of vascular injury, especially at high shear flow rates [2–4]. BSS is caused by mutations in *GPIBA*, *GPIBB*, or *GP9* genes coding GPIbα, GPIbβ, and GPIX, respectively [5, 6].

BSS is most often inherited in autosomal recessive manner (biallelic form), and therefore this disorder is more frequent in areas with high rate of consanguinity. However, autosomal dominant pattern of inheritance was also reported for this disorder (monoallelic form) [3, 7].

Although BSS usually presents early in life with different bleeding diathesis, late diagnosis in adulthood is not rare. Mucocutaneous bleeds such as easy bruising, purpura, epistaxis, gingival bleeding, and also menorrhagia are common among these patients. Severe post-dental hemorrhage, post-surgical bleeding, and post-traumatic hemorrhage can occur among these patients. Bleeding tendency among these patients is variable, even among member of a family [1, 3, 6, 7]. Routine and specific assessments can be used for timely diagnosis of BSS. In complete blood count (CBC), thrombocytopenia presents, and in peripheral blood smear (PBS) examination, large and giant platelets are seen. Bleeding time (BT) and closure time (CT) in platelet function analyzer-100/200 (PFA-100/200) are prolonged, and

B. Ghasemi · A. Dorgalaleh (✉)
Department of Hematology and Blood Transfusion, School of Allied Medicine,
Iran University of Medical Sciences, Tehran, Iran

A. Dorgalaleh (ed.), *Congenital Bleeding Disorders*,
https://doi.org/10.1007/978-3-319-76723-9_15

ristocetin-induced platelet agglutination (RIPA) is absent. In BSS, RIPA is not corrected with addition of normal plasma as a source of VWF. Flow cytometric analysis of GPIb-IX-V can be used for precise diagnosis, and molecular analysis can be used for confirmation of the disorder [2, 7–9].

Treatment for BSS involves both general supportive cares and specific therapy for bleeding. Patients with BSS should be guided to avoid activities carrying bleeding risk and intake antiplatelet medication. Patients with serious bleeding may require platelet and red blood cell (RBC) transfusion. Administration of antifibrinolytic drugs, recombinant activated factor VII (FVII), and hormones (in female patients) also may be effective in the management of bleeding symptoms. In patients with life-threatening bleeding, stem cell transplantation may be considered [1, 3, 10–15].

15.2 Glycoprotein Ib-IX-V Complex

15.2.1 Structure and Function

The GPIb-IX-V complex is a crucial platelet receptor that participates in primary hemostasis, where platelets adhere to exposed subendothelium at the site of vascular injury. This complex uniquely expresses on platelet/megakaryocyte lineage, and it is the second most abundant GP on platelet surface. There are approximately 25,000 copies of the GPIb-IX-V complex on platelet surface [2, 3, 16–18].

GPIb-IX-V complex consists of four subunits including GPIbα (CD42b) that binds covalently with disulfide bonds to two GPIbβ (CD42c) subunits and non-covalently associated with GPIX (CD42a) and GPV (CD42d). The four distinct genes are responsible for coding of four subunits of the GPIb-IX-V complex including *GPIBA* (chromosome 17p13), *GPIBB* (chromosome 22q11.21), *GP9* (chromosome 3q21), and *GP5* (chromosome 3q29) that encode GPIbα, GPIbβ, GPIX, and GPV, respectively. Concomitant and proper expression of GPIbα, GPIbβ, and GPIX subunits are required for appropriate and efficient expression of the GPIb-IX-V complex on the cell surface [1, 3, 9, 10, 16, 19, 20].

Lack of each subunit except for GPV that has a weak association with the complex leads to impaired expression of this complex. GPIbα is the most important subunit of GPIb-IX-V complex because it contains the binding site on N-terminal region for adhesive ligands such as VWF, thrombospondin, β2 glycoprotein I (β2 GPI), coagulation factors (FXI, FXII, high molecular weight kininogen (HMWK), and thrombin), and counter receptor on activated endothelial cell and platelets (P-selectin) or white blood cells (macrophage-1 antigen (Mac-1) or integrin $\alpha_M\beta 2$). Moreover, GPIbα has binding site for 14-3-3ζ, a signaling protein and filamin A, a cytoskeletal protein, in its cytoplasmic domain [1–3, 9, 16, 19, 21, 22].

All four subunits of the GPIb-IX-V complex are type I transmembrane protein. These subunits belong to the leucine-rich repeat (LRR) superfamily of proteins. Each subunit of the complex has one large N-terminal extracellular domain, a transmembrane helix, and a relatively short C-terminal cytoplasmic domain. Moreover,

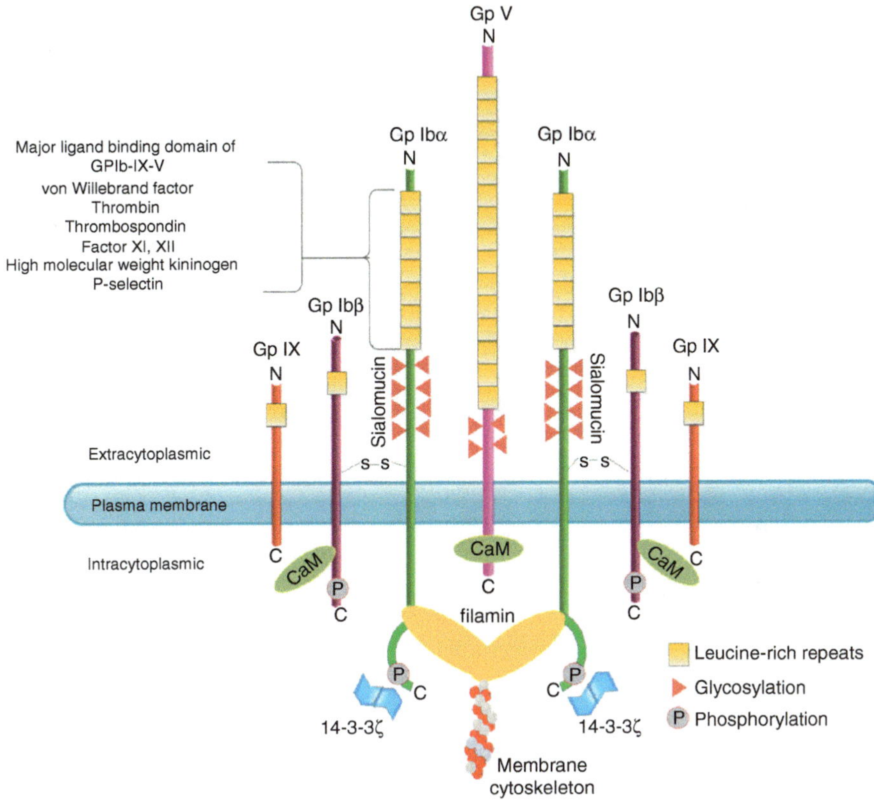

Fig. 15.1 Glycoprotein (GP) Ib-IX-V complex composed of four distinct subunits: GPIbα, GPIbβ, GPIX, and GPV. GPIbα with disulfide bonds linked to two GPIbβ subunits and non-covalently associated with GPIX and GPV. Each subunit belongs to the leucine-rich repeat (LRR) glycoprotein superfamily and contains a single transmembrane domain separating an extracellular N-terminal from an intracellular C-terminal. GPIbα is the major subunit and contains ligand-binding site on its extracellular domain for adhesive ligands such as von Willebrand factor, thrombospondin, and P-selectin. This complex via cytoplasmic domain associated with cytoskeletal elements such as filamin A, adapter and signaling proteins such as 14-3-3ζ and calmodulin. *N* N-terminal, *C* C-terminal, *P* phosphorylated residues, *CaM* calmodulin

GPIbα has a highly glycosylated region (sialomucin) in its extracellular domain. The LRR sequences are approximately 24 amino acids in length. These sequences are located on N-terminal domain of each GP. The LRR sequences are required for stability of each subunit and correct assembly of the GPIb-IX-V complex (Fig. 15.1) [2, 9, 12, 16, 17, 23, 24].

The main function of the GPIb-IX-V complex is binding via GPIbα to VWF A1-domain that its attachment to exposed subendothelial collagen results in adhesion of platelets at the site of vascular damage (please refer to Chap. 3). Interaction between GPIb-IX-V complex and VWF induces signal transduction. Direct or indirect interaction of cytoplasmic tail of GPIb-IX-V subunits with signaling proteins

Table 15.1 Characteristics of the glycoprotein Ib-IX-V subunits

Subunit	Number of amino acids	Molecular weight	Number of leucine-rich repeat	Gene location	Function
GPIbα	610	135 kDa	7	17p13	Major ligand-binding subunit/receptor for VWF, thrombin, thrombospondin, β2 GPI, factor XI, factor XII, HMWK, Mac-1, P-selectin. Interaction with filamin A and 14-3-3ζ via cytoplasmic tail
GPIbβ	181	26 kDa	1	22q11.21	Structurally important for GPIbα efficient expression on the plasma membrane. Interaction with calmodulin via cytoplasmic tail
GPIX	160	20 kDa	1	3q21	Structurally important for GPIbα efficient expression on the plasma membrane
GPV	544	82 kDa	15	3q29	Regulation of platelet-collagen interactions. Substrate for active thrombin. Interaction with calmodulin via cytoplasmic tail

GP glycoprotein, *kDa* kilodalton, *VWF* von Willebrand factor, *HMWK* high molecular weight kininogen, *Mac-1* macrophage-1 antigen, *β2 GPI* β2 glycoprotein I

such as calmodulin, 14-3-3ζ, phosphoinositide(PI) 3-kinase, TNF receptor-associated factor 4 (TRAF4), and Src family kinase (Lyn and Syc) leads to degranulation, calcium flux and rearrangement of cytoskeletal proteins, activation of integrin αIIbβ3 (GPIIb/IIIa), and platelet aggregation. Another function of GPIb-IX-V complex is the maintenance of platelet normal shape via interaction between the GPIbα cytoplasmic tail and actin-binding protein filamin A that this association links the GPIb-IX-V complex with the platelet membrane skeleton. The GPIb-IX-V complex also has role in inflammation and thrombosis because of its interaction with counter receptor including P-selectin on activated endothelial cells and platelets and Mac-1 on leukocytes [1–3, 9, 10, 12, 17, 19].

The GPIb-IX-V complex is an important receptor on platelet surface for coagulation activity due to its binding site for coagulation factors such as thrombin, FXI, FXII, and HMWK that is located on N-terminal region of GPIbα (Table 15.1) [2, 9, 10].

15.3 Bernard-Soulier Syndrome (BSS)

BSS is a rare inherited platelet function disorder presents early in life with moderate to severe bleeding diathesis. Estimated incidence of disorder is 1 per 1 million in the general population, but due to mild bleeding phenotype in a number of patients and also due to misdiagnosis, the expected prevalence of disorder is higher. The incidence is also higher in areas with high rate of consanguineous marriages. Moreover, the calculated frequency of carrier for BSS based on Hardy-Weinberg law is 1 per 500 individuals in the general population [1, 3, 6, 12, 14, 25, 26].

BSS was first described by Jean Bernard and Jean Pierre Soulier, two French hematologists in 1948. They described a young man with severe bleeding episodes, prolonged BT, and low platelet count with extremely large platelets. They named this disorder "hemorrhagiparous thrombotic dystrophy". Weiss and his colleagues in 1974 demonstrated that BSS platelets are unable to adhere to rabbit aortic subendothelium. Nurden and Caen in 1975 observed that one of the important platelet surface GP was absent in BSS platelets, and finally they found that this absent GP is GPIb-IX-V complex [1, 10, 12, 27, 28].

Platelets from patients with BSS have quantitative or qualitative defect in GPIb-IX-V complex that leads to disability of platelets to adhere to exposed subendothelium at the site of vascular injury (adhesion defect). At the time of vascular injury, the VWF via its A3 domain binds to the exposed subendothelium collagen. Collagen-bound VWF expresses a binding site for platelets. Platelets through GPIbα, a major subunit of the GPIb-IX-V complex, bind to the VWF-A1 domain. This process is the first step in primary hemostasis that leads to platelet adhesion to the subendothelium and subsequent platelet activation and platelet plug formation at the site of vascular damage (please refer to Chap. 1) [10, 17, 29–33].

The GPIb-IX-V complex is a crucial platelet receptor that has several functions. This receptor has different ligands such as VWF, thrombospondin, β2 GPI, coagulation factors (FXI, FXII, thrombin, and HMWK), and counter receptor on activated endothelial cells and platelets (P-selectin) or leukocytes (integrin $\alpha_M\beta 2$ or Mac-1; CD11b/CD18). Defect in the GPIb-IX-V complex can result in several complications because of different functions of this receptor, for instance, its role in regulation of platelet size, shape, and platelet formation as well as its function in hemostasis and its interaction with other cells [2, 3, 10, 11].

15.4 Molecular Basis

The GPIb-IX-V complex formation requires products of four distinct genes including *GPIBA*, *GPIBB*, *GP9*, and *GP5*. The products of these genes assemble within maturing megakaryocytes (MK) in the bone marrow and then express on the platelet surface [5, 7, 30, 34, 35].

Genes encoding GPIbα, GPIbβ, GPIX, and GPV subunits are located on chromosomes 17p13 (*GPIBA*), 22q11.21 (*GPIBB*), 3q21 (*GP9*), and 3q29 (*GP5*), respectively [1, 6].

These genes share some structural features like other genes belong to the LRR superfamily. They have simple, compact, and intron-depleted structure. Moreover, promoter of these genes has similar regulatory elements including binding sites for transcription factors such as GATA-1 and Ets. Three out of four genes including *GPIBA*, *GPIBB*, and *GP5* contain two exons and one intron, whereas *GP9* gene consists of three exons and two introns. In these genes the coding sequence also

Table 15.2 Main features of two main forms of Bernard-Soulier syndrome

Disorder	Inheritance	Thrombocytopenia	Platelet morphology	Bleeding tendency	Level of the GPIb-IX-V complex on the surface of platelet	RIPA
Biallelic form	AR	Moderate to severe	Giant platelet	Moderate to severe	Very low or absent	Absent
Monoallelic form	AD	Mild	Large platelet	Mild	Normal or slightly reduced	Normal or slightly reduced

RIPA ristocetin-induced platelet agglutination, *AR* autosomal recessive, *AD* autosomal dominant, *GP* glycoprotein

resides in one exon except for *GPIBB*. The *GPIBB* gene contains an intron 10 bases after the start codon [1, 3, 9, 12, 34, 36, 37].

Different mutations may occur in GPIbα, GPbβ, and GPIX genes and give rise to impaired biosynthesis and expression of the GPIb-IX-V complex on the platelet surface and subsequently lead to BSS. No BSS causing mutation has been reported in *GP5* gene so far. This is consistent with weak association of the GPV subunit with other subunits of the GPIb-IX-V complex as well as the lack of the requirement of GPV for the other subunit expression [1, 2, 16, 30, 38–44].

BSS is most often caused by mutations at both alleles of *GPIBA*, *GPIBB*, and *GP9* genes that cause biallelic forms of BSS (autosomal recessive). There are few mutations that occur in one allele of *GPIBA* or *GPIBB* genes and result in monoallelic BSS (autosomal dominant) (Table 15.2) [9, 21, 45, 46].

On the basis of the last cohort study that was performed on 211 families with BSS in 2014, 112 different mutations have been described including 45, 39, and 28 variants in *GPIBA*, *GPIBB*, and *GP9* genes, respectively. These mutations are heterogeneous including missense, nonsense, and frameshift insertion/deletion. These mutations cause GPIb-IX-V complex to be unstable, truncated, or dysfunctional [9–11, 17, 47, 48].

Missense mutations are common genetic defects in BSS that occur in GPIbβ and GPIX subunits more frequently than GPIbα subunit. Missense mutations usually hamper subunits folding and lead to unstable complex formation with severe decreased expression of the GPIb-IX-V complex on the platelet surface. Missense mutations can also affect functional domains with normal or slightly decreased expression of a dysfunctional GPIb-IX-V complex on the platelet surface [1, 9, 14, 16, 49].

Nonsense mutations lead to truncated subunits with lack of transmembrane domain. Frameshift insertion/deletion mutations lead to the production of a novel protein with altered sequence from native protein. No splicing defects have been detected that is due to the simple and compact structure of the genes coding different subunits of GPIb-IX-V complex (Fig. 15.2) [1, 9, 16, 42, 44, 50–52].

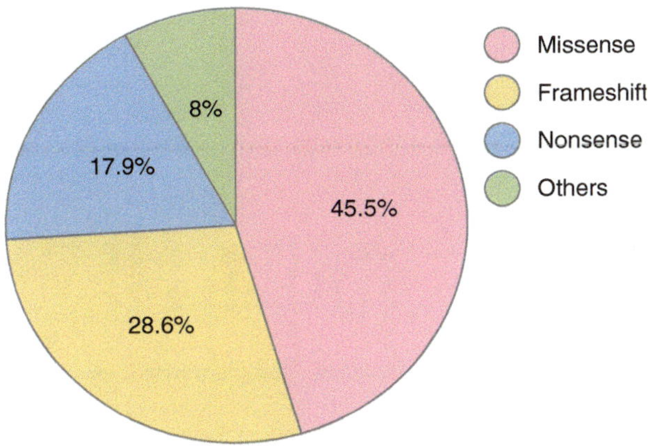

Fig. 15.2 The distribution of different mutations in Bernard-Soulier syndrome (BSS). One hundred and twelve different disease causing mutations have been identified in patients with BSS, so far. Fifty-one out of one hundred twelve are missense, which are the most common genetic defects in BSS. Thirty-two frameshift and twenty nonsense mutations have also been reported. Other rare genetic abnormalities including in frame alternation and defect in start codon and promoter region have also been reported

The majority of mutations affect more frequently extracellular domain than transmembrane and cytoplasmic domains. There are some rare mutations that affect the promoter and signal peptide of the genes. For instance, one mutation (g.-160C>G) affects the promoter region of the *GPIBB* gene and disrupts the GATA-1 binding site [3, 9, 30, 42, 44, 50, 51]. In addition, GPIbβ defect can occur in patients with DiGeorge/velocardiofacial syndrome that is caused by microdeletion within chromosome 22q11.2, which in this region contains the *GPIBB* gene; thus, these patients are obligatory carriers of BSS (Fig. 15.3) [3, 11, 17, 20, 22, 23, 32, 46, 53, 54].

Most of disease causative mutations in BSS are loss-of-function mutations that disrupt complex and trafficking through the endoplasmic reticulum and Golgi apparatus and prevent localization of complex on the cell surface. There are some rare gain of function mutations in the *GPIBA* gene, which cause platelet-type von Willebrand disease (VWD) that is different from BSS and characterized by spontaneously binding of plasma VWF to platelets that give rise to clearance of plasma VWF, and this disorder is similar to type 2B VWD (please refer to Chap. 3) [1, 3, 7, 30, 35, 47, 53, 55, 56].

Most of BSS causing mutations are unique and restricted to a single patient or family, but there are some exceptions such as Asn45Ser mutation in *GP9* gene which was reported in Caucasian families from northern and central European countries due to founder effect (please refer to Chap. 1) [1, 17, 30].

Patients with the classic form of BSS (biallelic form) are homozygous or compound heterozygous for the causative mutations. BSS carriers (heterozygote individuals in biallelic BSS) who only have one mutant allele are usually asymptomatic, and their platelets express about half the normal levels of the functional GPIb-IX-V

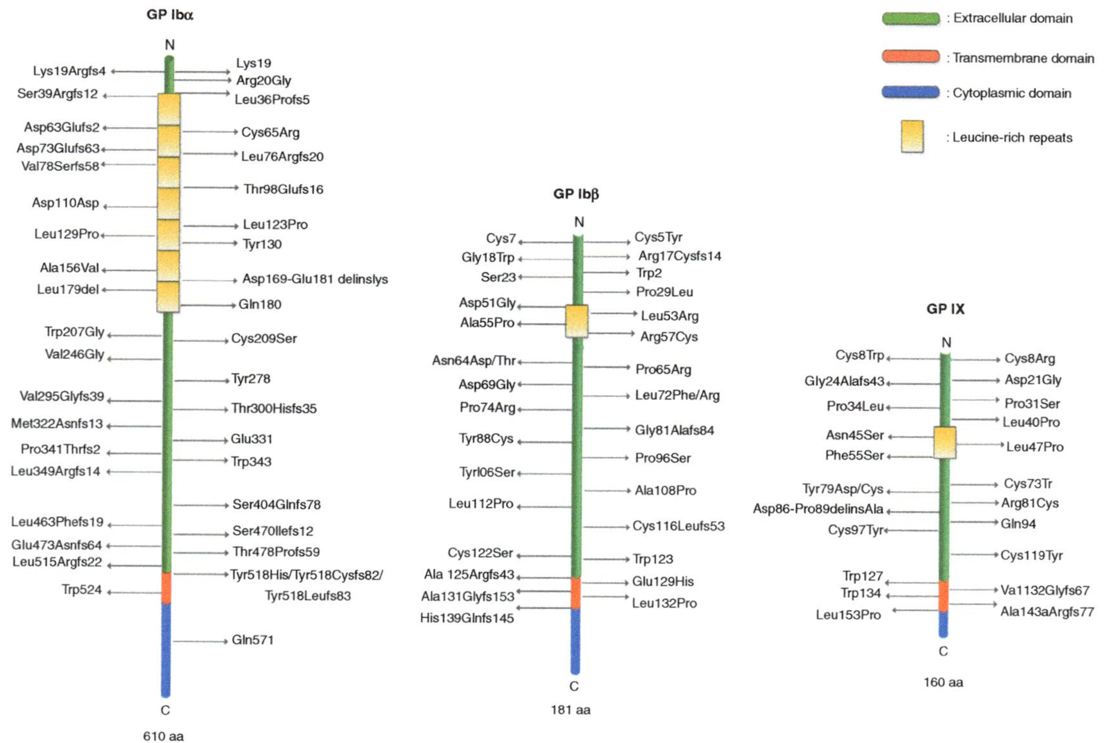

Fig. 15.3 Different mutations throughout GPIbα, GPIbβ, and GPIX subunits associated with Bernard-Soulier syndrome. Most of the mutations hit the extra-cellular domains of glycoproteins. *GP* glycoprotein, *N* N-terminal, *C* C-terminal

complex. However, some BSS carriers may show mild to moderate bleeding tendency. Most BSS carriers have lower platelet count than healthy individuals, and they have slightly enlarged platelets. Furthermore, there are a few monoallelic mutations in *GPIBA* and *GPIBB* genes that exert a type of dominant effect and give rise to a milder form of BSS (monoallelic form) [3, 9, 12, 14, 20, 34, 48, 54, 55, 57–60].

A monoallelic form of BSS with autosomal dominant manner of inheritance is Bolzano variant that mostly occurs among Italian population. In this variant, Ala156Val mutation occurs in *GPIBA* gene (located within the sixth LRR) results in macrothrombocytopenia. Platelets of Bolzano variant have normal level of GPIb-IX-V complex, but they are unable to bind to VWF. Therefore, there is a functional defect in this complex. Moreover, the binding of thrombin to GPIbα is normal in Bolzano variant [1–3, 10, 12, 34, 55].

Another autosomal dominant variant of BSS is associated with a substitution in the conserved region of GPIbα (Leu57Phe) on LRR domains. This variant is characterized by macrothrombocytopenia and expression of the dysfunctional GPIbα subunit. The GPIbα shows susceptibility to proteolysis in this variant. In aggregometry study response to ristocetin is also slightly reduced [3, 12, 52].

Furthermore, other monoallelic mutations with dominant effects including p.Asn57His and p.Tyr70Asp in *GPIBA* gene and also p.Arg42Cys and p.Tyr113Cys in *GPIBB* gene have been reported in few patients. These mutations are responsible for mild macrothrombocytopenia [5, 46, 48, 55, 61].

15.5 Clinical Manifestations

BSS is moderate to severe bleeding disorder, usually presents in infancy or early in childhood with abnormal more profound bleeding tendency. Bleeding tendency is more severe than predicted from platelet count because platelets have a functional defect in BSS. Bleeding mostly occurs in mucocutaneous tissues and includes easy bruising, epistaxis, petechiae, purpura, and gingival bleeding. The severity of bleeding increases later in the life that is unlike Glanzmann thrombasthenia (GT) in which with age the severity of bleeding is decreased (see Chap. 14). In female patients during puberty, menorrhagia may become an important issue. Other presentations such as hematuria, gastrointestinal (GI) and genitourinary bleedings may also occur. Severe and life-threatening bleeding may occur in hematologic stress conditions such as surgical procedures, tooth extraction, trauma, and delivery. Joint bleeding, intracranial hemorrhage (ICH), and deep visceral bleeding are rare presentations of this disorder. Consistent with heterogeneous molecular defects in BSS, the severity and frequency of bleeding episodes differ among patients even in patients with the same mutation and from the same family [1, 3, 7, 12, 13, 29, 55, 58, 61–63].

Although BSS carriers (heterozygous patients in biallelic BSS) are usually asymptomatic, some carriers may show mild to moderate bleeding tendency [3, 9, 14, 59].

Table 15.3 Clinical manifestations of patients with Bernard-Soulier syndrome

Clinical manifestations	Naz et al. (*n*:7) (%)	Toogeh et al. (*n*:97) (%)	Afrabiasi et al. (*n*:7) Presentation/ follow-up (%)	Hadjati et al. (*n*:15) (%)	Sanchez-Guiu et al. (*n*:8) (%)
Epistaxis	100	63.9	28/57	80	100
Petechiae and purpura	–	1	–/29	6.6	–
Ecchymosis	–	7.2	–/29	–	–
Bleeding from minor wounds	–	–	–	–	13
Gum bleeding	100	15.5	15/28	60	38
Gastrointestinal bleeding	–	4.1	–/42	–	33
Post-dental extraction bleeding	–	–	15/–	–	57
Post-surgical bleeding	–	–	–	6.6	71
Menorrhagia	–	11.3	–	–	100
Post-partum hemorrhage	–	–	–	–	75
Hematoma	100	3	–	6.6	–
Hemarthrosis	–	–	–	–	–
Post-vaccination bleeding	–	–	42/–	–	–
Bruises	100	–	–	–	–
Cerebral bleeding	–	1	–	–	–

N number of patients

Patients with the autosomal dominant disorder that is also known as monoallelic BSS have a milder phenotype than the biallelic form of the disease. These patients such as Bolzano variant usually have no or minor bleeding diathesis (Table 15.3) [35, 47, 55].

15.6 Diagnosis

Initially, BSS is characterized by macrothrombocytopenia and abnormal bleeding tendency. These features are not restricted to BSS, and therefore diagnosis of BSS can be challenging. It should keep in mind that in spite of this issue, diagnosis of BSS in comparison with other mild IPFD is straightforward and is not a sophisticated process. Overall, diagnosis of inherited macrothrombocytopenia is difficult and time-consuming because these disorders are rare and required specific laboratory tests [9, 11, 55, 64–66].

The first step in the diagnosis of individual who suspected to BSS is obtaining a detailed clinical history, particularly history of unexpected mucocutaneous bleeding. Initial laboratory assessments should include CBC and precise examination of PBS. In patients with BSS, these tests revealed variable degree of thrombocytopenia (30–150 × 10^9/L) and presence of large or giant platelets in blood film that can be as large as red blood cells. Presence of giant platelets is a significant finding in BSS. Since cell counters usually count cells by their size (impedance system), therefore giant platelets may count as erythrocyte. So evaluation of blood smear for detection of giant platelet and manual counting for accurate platelet count is mandatory by an expert hematologist [1, 3, 9–13, 29, 32, 54, 55, 65, 67].

The precise mechanism of macrothrombocytopenia in BSS is still unclear. Different studies suggested that macrothrombocytopenia could be related to decreased platelet life span, impaired megakaryopoiesis, and defective proplatelet formation as well as a defect in the interaction between the GPIb-IX-V complex and platelet membrane skeleton. Nevertheless, some studies demonstrated both decreased and normal platelet survival in patients with BSS. Electron microscopy studies determined the aberrant development and vacuolated demarcation membrane system (DMS) in bone marrow MK from patients with BSS and a murine model of BSS. This abnormality indicates impaired megakaryopoiesis in BSS that may contribute to the formation of giant platelets and thrombocytopenia. Moreover, in vitro studies suggested that the GPIbα is critical for platelet formation, because block of this subunit by monoclonal antibodies or cleavage of its extracellular domain by metalloproteinase Mocarhagin inhibited proplatelet formation in human MK. This finding was also confirmed by study on BSS murine model and patients with BSS. Therefore, defect in GPIbα is responsible for impaired proplatelet formation with production of platelet macrocytosis and thrombocytopenia. In addition, immunofluorescence studies revealed that α-tubulin distribution within proplatelets was deranged, so alteration of α-tubulin distribution was involved in impaired proplatelet formation. The GPIb-IX-V complex via cytoplasmic domain of GPIbα interacts with the cytoskeletal protein, filamin A. The GPIbα-filamin A interaction regulates platelet size, shape change and adhesion to ligands. Therefore, impaired interaction between GPIbα and filamin A can cause giant platelet formation, and this impaired interaction is consistent with the increased membrane deformability seen in BSS platelets [2, 3, 10–12, 17, 20–22, 34, 54, 55, 60, 68–70].

BT is moderately (5–10 min) to severely (>20 min) prolonged in patients with BSS. BT is a simple and quick in vivo test that it evaluates primary hemostasis by assessment of function of platelets and plasma VWF. BT is less reproducible, invasive, nonspecific and not enough sensitive to detect many mild platelets disorders. As a result, the use of BT is decreased today and largely is replaced by PFA-100/200, although BT is still used for evaluation of primary hemostasis, particularly in laboratories without other platelet function tests [1, 12, 29, 31, 71–73].

Closure time (CT) that is the time of occlusion of an aperture in the test cartridge in PFA-100/200 instrument is also prolonged in patients with BSS on both collagen/adenosine diphosphate (ADP) and collagen/epinephrine cartridges. This test is an in vitro measure of the bleeding time, in which a small volume (0.8 ml per cartridge) of citrated whole blood is aspirated at high shear rate through the capillary and disposable cartridge consists of a microscopic aperture in a membrane coated with platelet agonists, collagen/ADP, or collagen/epinephrine. These agonists result in platelet activation, adhesion, aggregation, and platelet plug formation leading to occlusion of the aperture (CT). CT is influenced by platelet count, hematocrit, and VWF level, so in individuals with hematocrit under 25% and platelet count under 50×10^9/L, the result should be interpreted carefully. Furthermore, the concentration of sodium citrate that is used as an anticoagulant in this test can affect the CT. The use of sodium citrate 3.8% leads to more reliable results. Although the PFA-100/200 results are useful for screening of abnormality in primary hemostasis such as VWD and some platelet function disorders, this test is not very sensitive to detection of mild platelet function disorders. However, the sensitivity of this test is high for some severe IPFD such as BSS and GT, but low specificity is a constant issue with PFA-100/200 [11, 13, 17, 29, 31, 65, 72–76].

Another laboratory hallmark of platelets in BSS is isolated defect in RIPA that unlike the defect in VWD, this pattern is not corrected by addition of normal plasma as a source of VWF (please refer to Chap. 3) (Fig. 15.4). Platelet aggregation in response to other agonists such as ADP, collagen, arachidonic acid, and epinephrine is normal. Additionally, BSS platelets show decreased aggregation in response to low dose (but not high dose) of thrombin [1–3, 10, 13, 20, 22, 25, 29, 77, 78].

Light transmission aggregometry (LTA) is a gold standard and key method for diagnosis of platelet function disorders. In this method the ability of platelet aggregation in response to different agonists such as ADP, collagen, arachidonic acid, epinephrine, and ristocetin is assessed based on changing in optical density of a stirring sample of citrated platelet-rich plasma (PRP) in a cuvette at 37 °C following to addition of agonists. The change in optical density is measured by a

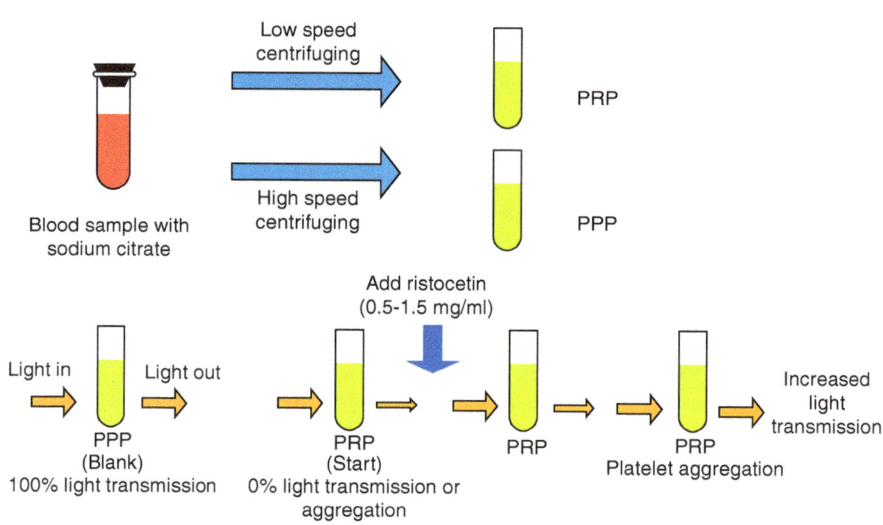

Fig. 15.4 Principle of the ristocetin-induced platelet agglutination (RIPA). RIPA test is usually performed by using platelet-rich plasma (PRP) and a turbidimetric aggregometer. In this assay, a beam of light passes through two cuvettes, one containing platelet-poor plasma (PPP) and the other containing PRP. PPP is used as a blank and is determining 100% light transmission. The starting PRP is used as a sample to be analyzed and is determined 0% light transmission or 0% aggregation. Adding ristocetin as an agonist induces platelet aggregation through promoting binding VWF to glycoprotein Ibα. Platelet aggregation leads to increase light transmission

photometer. If platelets are able to aggregation, the increase of light transmission is observed. In this method, platelet-poor plasma (PPP) can be used to define 100% light transmission. Before testing, PRP should be kept at room temperature (RT) for 15 min. The rate of aggregation (%/min) and maximal percentage of aggregation (%) are parameters that are measured after a fixed period of time (usually 6–10 min). However, this method is very useful for diagnosis of platelet function disorders; it has some disadvantages including manual sample processing, time-consuming, large blood volume, and difficulty in obtaining PRP in children and in patients with severe thrombocytopenia. Moreover, the results of LTA can be influenced by some pre-analytical and analytical variables such as blood sampling conditions, platelet count, presence of hemolysis, lipemia, sample processing, and use of different concentrations of agonists (Fig. 15.5) [11, 65, 71–74, 78–85].

Another platelet function assay is whole blood aggregometry (WBA) or impedance platelet aggregometry. This method monitors changes in electrical impedance between two metal electrodes when platelet aggregation occurs in response to agonists. Adhesion of activated platelets to the surface of electrodes and subsequently aggregation of platelets in response to agonists lead to increase in electrical impedance that is reported in Ohms. WBA is performed on citrated whole blood, and platelet function is assessed with other blood elements and under more physiological condition than LTA. Moreover, WBA needs smaller amount of sample than LTA and does not require sample manipulation. The results of WBA can be influenced by platelet count, hematocrit, type of anticoagulant, and delay in testing [65, 71, 72, 82, 84, 85].

The provisional diagnosis of BSS based on aggregometry with the rare exception can be primarily confirmed by flow cytometry analysis. Flow cytometry using a panel of specific monoclonal antibodies that specially recognize the subunits of the GPIb-IX-V complex (CD42a-d) can reveal absent or severe reduction of complex on the surface of resting platelets [1, 3, 11–13, 29, 55, 64, 79, 80].

In Bolzano variant of BSS, platelets express normal or slightly reduced level of the GPIb-IX-V complex on their surface, but this complex cannot bind to VWF, and there is a functional abnormality in this complex. Flow cytometry analysis can identify BSS carriers (in biallelic BSS) who express about half of functional GPIb-IX-V complex on their platelet surface [2, 20, 60, 73].

Flow cytometry, a laser-based method, is very valuable method because it is rapid, reliable, and sensitive and required a small amount of blood, so it is suitable choice in pediatrics. This method is independent of platelet count thus is suitable test for assessment of platelet function in patients with thrombocytopenia. Flow cytometry can also assess platelet count and platelet size as well as reticulated platelets. Moreover, another advantage of flow cytometry is less manipulation of the sample. On the other hand, this assay is expensive and requires well-educated operator [11, 13, 71, 73, 74, 85–89].

Flow cytometry analysis could be performed on citrated whole blood, washed platelets, or PRP. Whole blood analysis is better because PRP and washed platelets requiring additional preparation may cause platelet activation. Another advantage of

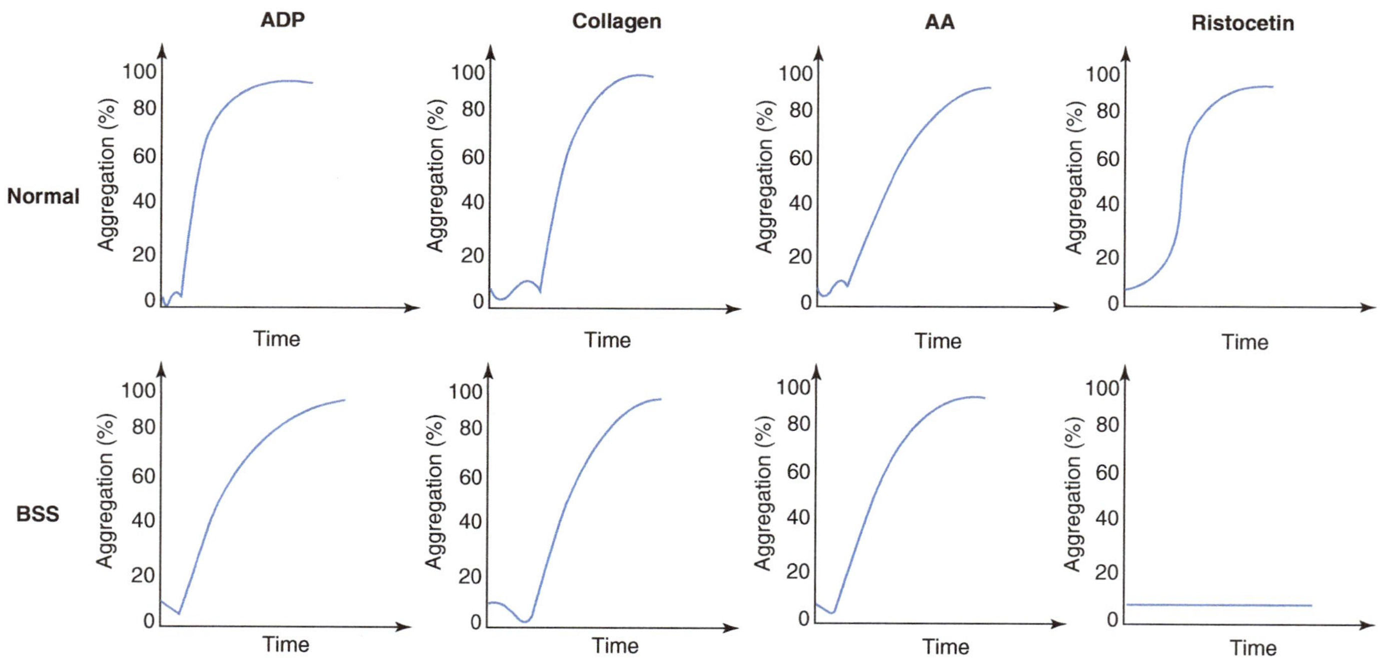

Fig. 15.5 Light transmission aggregometry results in a normal sample and Bernard-Soulier syndrome (BSS). BSS platelets manifest isolated aggregation defect in response to ristocetin. *BSS* Bernard-Soulier syndrome, *ADP* adenosine diphosphate, *AA* arachidonic acid

whole blood in this test is the assessment of platelet function with other blood elements and in more closely to in vivo conditions. Sodium citrate is used as an anticoagulant in flow cytometry analysis [71, 87].

In BSS, coagulation tests and clot retraction test should be normal. A significantly reduction in prothrombin consumption and thrombin generation tests is observed in patients with BSS due to defective binding of FXI and thrombin to GPIbα. Some additional tests can be performed in specialized centers for confirmation of BSS including sodium dodecyl sulfate-polyacrylamide gel electrophoresis (SDS-PAGE) and immunoblotting for analysis of platelets GP with the use of specific antibodies. Finally, molecular genetic testing for detection of causative mutations in *GPIBA*, *GPIBB*, and *GP9* genes can be performed for confirmation of the disorder and determination of underlying mutation(s) [1–3, 11, 12, 17, 52, 54, 75, 90].

Some important issues should be considered in platelet function testing including blood sampling conditions, blood collecting, and sample processing. Sample for platelet study should be collected in resting and fasting patients who have refrained from smoking, physical activity, antiplatelet drugs, and caffeine intake, because these conditions can affect platelet function. Patients should be avoided to intake medications that can affect platelet function for 7–10 days before testing. Blood sample should be collected with minimal tourniquet pressure by 19–21 gauge (*G*) needle into tube containing sodium citrate. Blood sample should properly be mixed with anticoagulant by three to six times inverting. Sodium citrate is a common anticoagulant used for platelet function testing. The ethylenediaminetetraacetic acid (EDTA) can inhibit binding of natural ligands, and it also makes dissociation of the integrin αIIbβ3 (GPIIb/IIIa) from platelet surface, so in platelet function studies, EDTA should be avoided. Samples should be kept in RT and avoiding from shaking and vibration of samples tubes, and analysis should be performed within 30 min to 2 h after blood collection [65, 72, 87, 89].

15.7 Differential Diagnosis

Since primary findings of BSS are not specific, diagnosis of BSS may be challenging. A considerable number of patients with BSS are not diagnosed early in childhood, and the average age at diagnosis is 16 years in this disorder. BSS is most often misdiagnosed as immune thrombocytopenic purpura (ITP) because both have macrothrombocytopenia. Differential diagnosis is important for avoiding futile treatments such as steroid therapy and splenectomy [1, 3, 9, 12, 17, 25].

BSS should also be differentiated from other inherited macrothrombocytopenia such as May-Hegglin, Sebastian, Fechtner, and Epstein's syndrome (myosin heavy chain 9 (MYH9)-related syndromes) and Gray platelet syndrome (GPS). Examination of PBS can be helpful in distinguishing of these syndromes. In MYH9-related syndromes, examination of PBS is very important for detection of bright-blue cytoplasmic inclusions (Dohle body-like inclusion) in granulocytes. In these syndromes unlike BSS platelet aggregation in response to ristocetin and thrombin is normal. In blood smear of GPS, large gray to gray-blue platelets are present. Platelet aggregometry in patients with GPS shows variable results. GPS platelets in aggregometry studies show reduced response to collagen as well as thrombin, while response to ristocetin is normal or slightly reduced (please refer to Chap. 16) [3, 17, 25, 29, 31, 54].

Moreover, BSS should be discriminated from VWD because these disorders may have similar clinical symptoms including mucocutaneous bleeding. In platelet aggregometry test, absent agglutination with ristocetin is observed in both BSS and VWD. In BSS unlike VWD addition of normal plasma as a source of VWF cannot correct the test (Table 15.4) (please refer to Chap. 3) [1, 25, 29].

15.8 Management

Bleeding diathesis in patients with BSS is variable; thus, management of these patients should individually be performed. Therapeutic approaches in BSS include both general and specific treatments. The majority of patients don't need a regular treatment, and patients should be warned to prevent trauma, contact sports, and intake of antiplatelet drugs such as aspirin. Patients should maintain proper dental hygiene to prevent invasive dental procedures. Minor and local bleeding such as gum bleeding and epistaxis can be managed by local measures including fibrin sealants, gelatin sponges, and compression with gauze soaked with tranexamic acid. Iron deficiency anemia may present due to chronic bleeding episodes or menorrhagia and should be treated. Patients with severe bleeding require medical interventions including red blood cell and platelet transfusion, but these treatments have several risks such as developing alloantibodies against human leukocyte antigens (HLA) and missing platelet GP and also have the risk of infection transmission. Therefore, these patients should be HLA typed and should receive HLA-compatible platelet units as well as leukocyte-depleted blood products. Moreover, these patients should be vaccinated against hepatitis A and B, due to risk of transfusion-transmitted infections. Prophylactic transfusion of platelet and blood before surgery may also be required. To stop bleeding, administration of antifibrinolytic drugs such as tranexamic acid and aminocaproic acid or recombinant activated FVII (rFVIIa) may be helpful. In females with menorrhagia, management of patients depends on severity of bleeding. The first treatment for menorrhagia is administration of antifibrinolytic agents, and in most severe cases that failed to control bleeding, oral contraceptives and hormone supplementation are suggested. Management of pregnancy and child birth in women with BSS can be challenging, and severe bleeding during delivery and post-partum may occur. In these women bleeding should be controlled by platelet transfusion, antifibrinolytic drugs, and desmopressin. In rare patients with life-threatening bleeds, hematopoietic stem cell transplantation may be considered. BSS can also be candidate for gene therapy in the future (Table 15.5) [1, 11–15, 17, 32, 52, 56, 73, 91–93].

Table 15.4 Laboratory features of some inherited macrothrombocytopenias

Disorder	Platelet count	Platelet morphology	Platelet aggregation					
			Arachidonic acid	ADP	Collagen	Thrombin	Epinephrine	Ristocetin
Bernard-Soulier syndrome	Decreased	Large and giant platelets	Normal	Normal	Normal	Normal (but not in low dose of thrombin)	Normal	Absent
MYH9-related disorders	Decreased	Giant platelets	Normal	Normal	Normal	Normal	Normal or impaired	Normal
Gray platelet syndrome	Decreased	Large platelets	Impaired	Variable	Impaired	Variable	Variable	Variable

ADP adenosine diphosphate, *MYH9* myosin heavy chain 9

Table 15.5 Management of Bernard-Soulier syndrome

Treatment modality	Indication	Recommended dose
Desmopressin (DDAVP)	Mild bleeding, before major procedures, after significant trauma, menorrhagia Minor procedure such as dental extractions	0.3 μg/kg (IV) diluted in 20–50 ml saline over 30 min Intranasal spray; 150 μg per dose for a child under 50 kg in weight, 300 μg per dose in an adult
Antifibrinolytic agents (tranexamic acid, aminocaproic acid)	Minor bleedings such as epistaxis and gingival bleeding, menorrhagia, minor surgical procedures, oral/nasal surgery, in invasive procedures are used in conjunction with another therapy such as desmopressin and platelet transfusion	Tranexamic acid: 15–25 mg/kg three times per day orally, 10–15 mg/kg (IV) three times per day Aminocaproic acid: 100 mg/kg (IV) over 15 min 60–80 mg/kg three to four times a day orally
Platelet transfusion	Severe bleedings such as severe menorrhagia and severe epistaxis, surgical procedures, after significant trauma	Depend on patient's clinical condition 10–15 ml/kg in children One adult therapeutic dose is equivalent to four to six single donor units
Female hormones	Menorrhagia (when does not response to initial therapies such as antifibrinolytic agents)	High-dose conjugated estrogen for 24–48 h (IV) followed by high doses of oral estrogen-progestin and high dose of progesterone such as norethisterone 5 mg every 4 h

DDAVP 1-deamino-8-d-arginine vasopressin, *IV* intravenous

References

1. Lanza F. Bernard-Soulier syndrome (hemorrhagiparous thrombocytic dystrophy). Orphanet J Rare Dis. 2006;1(1):46.
2. Berndt MC, Andrews RK. Bernard-Soulier syndrome. Haematologica. 2011;96:355.
3. Kunishima S, Kamiya T, Saito H. Genetic abnormalities of Bernard-Soulier syndrome. Int J Hematol. 2002;76(4):319–27.
4. Afrabiasi A, Artoni A, Karimi M, Peyvandi F, Ashouri E, Mannucci P. Glanzmann thrombasthenia and Bernard–Soulier syndrome in south Iran. Int J Lab Hematol. 2005;27(5):324–7.
5. Savoia A, Pastore A, De Rocco D, Civaschi E, Di Stazio M, Bottega R, et al. Clinical and genetic aspects of Bernard-Soulier syndrome: searching for genotype/phenotype correlations. Haematologica. 2011;96(3):417–23.
6. Ali S, Ghosh K, Shetty S. Novel genetic abnormalities in Bernard-Soulier syndrome in India. Ann Hematol. 2014;93(3):381–4.
7. Boeckelmann D, Hengartner H, Greinacher A, Nowak-Göttl U, Sachs U, Peter K, et al. Patients with Bernard-Soulier syndrome and different severity of the bleeding phenotype. Blood Cell Mol Dis. 2017;67:69.
8. Takata Y, Kanaji T, Moroi M, Seki R, Sano M, Nakazato S, et al. Platelets with a W127X mutation in GPIX express sufficient residual amounts of GPIbα to support adhesion to von Willebrand factor and collagen. Int J Hematol. 2012;96(6):733–42.
9. Savoia A, Kunishima S, De Rocco D, Zieger B, Rand ML, Pujol-Moix N, et al. Spectrum of the mutations in Bernard–Soulier syndrome. Hum Mutat. 2014;35(9):1033–45.
10. Andrews RK, Berndt MC. Bernard–Soulier syndrome: an update. Semi Thromb Hemost. 2013;39:656.
11. Diz-Küçükkaya R. Inherited platelet disorders including Glanzmann thrombasthenia and Bernard-Soulier syndrome. Hematology Am Soc Hematol Educ Program. 2013;2013(1):268–75.
12. López JA, Andrews RK, Afshar-Kharghan V, Berndt MC. Bernard-soulier syndrome. Blood. 1998;91(12):4397–418.
13. Alamelu J, Liesner R. Modern management of severe platelet function disorders. Br J Haematol. 2010;149(6):813–23.
14. Kirchmaier CM, Pillitteri D. Diagnosis and management of inherited platelet disorders. Transfus Med Hemother. 2010;37(5):237–46.
15. Seligsohn U. Treatment of inherited platelet disorders. Haemophilia. 2012;18(Suppl 4):161–5.
16. Li R, Emsley J. The organizing principle of the platelet glycoprotein Ib–IX–V complex. J Thromb Haemost. 2013;11(4):605–14.
17. Diz-Kücükkaya R, López JA. Inherited disorders of platelets. Hematol Oncol Clin North Am. 2013;27(3):613–27.
18. Hayward CP, Rao A, Cattaneo M. Congenital platelet disorders: overview of their mechanisms, diagnostic evaluation and treatment. Haemophilia. 2006;12(Suppl 3):128–36.
19. Andrews R, Gardiner E, Shen Y, Whisstock J, Berndt M. Glycoprotein Ib–IX–V. Int J Biochem Cell Biol. 2003;35(8):1170–4.
20. Balduini CL, Iolascon A, Savoia A. Inherited thrombocytopenias: from genes to therapy. Haematologica. 2002;87(8):860–80.
21. Favier R, Raslova H. Progress in understanding the diagnosis and molecular genetics of macrothrombocytopenias. Br J Haematol. 2015;170(5):626–39.
22. Rabbolini DJ, Morel-Kopp MC, Stevenson W, Ward CM. Inherited macrothrombocytopenias. Semin Thromb Hemost. 2014;40:774.
23. Kunishima S, Imai T, Kobayashi R, Kato M, Ogawa S, Saito H. Bernard–Soulier syndrome caused by a hemizygous GPIbβ mutation and 22q11. 2 deletion. Pediatr Int. 2013;55(4):434–7.
24. Gardiner EE, Andrews RK. Platelet receptor expression and shedding: glycoprotein Ib-IX-V and glycoprotein VI. Transfus Med Rev. 2014;28(2):56–60.
25. Pham A, Wang J. Bernard-Soulier syndrome: an inherited platelet disorder. Arch Pathol Lab Med. 2007;131(12):1834–6.

26. Naz A, Jamal MY, Amanat S, Najmuddin A, Patel H, Raziq F, et al. Autosomal recessive inherited bleeding disorders in Pakistan: a cross-sectional study from selected regions. Orphanet J Rare Dis. 2017;12(1):66.
27. Weiss HJ, Tschopp TB, Baumgartner HR, Sussman II, Johnson MM, Egan JJ. Decreased adhesion of giant (Bernard-Soulier) platelets to subendothelium. Further implications on the role of the von Willebrand factor in hemostasis. Am J Med. 1974;57:920.
28. Nurden AT, Caen JP. Specific roles for platelet surface glycoproteins in platelet function. Nature. 1975;255(5511):720–2.
29. Carubbi C, Masselli E, Nouvenne A, Russo D, Galli D, Mirandola P, et al. Laboratory diagnostics of inherited platelet disorders. Clin Chem Lab Med. 2014;52(8):1091–106.
30. Shlebak A, Poles A, Manning R, Almuhareb S, De La Funte J, Mitchell M, et al. A novel homozygous c. 800C> G substitution in GP1BA exon 2 in a Kuwaiti Family with Bernard-Soulier Syndrome. Acta Haematol. 2015;134(3):193–8.
31. Matthews DC. Inherited disorders of platelet function. Pediatr Clin. 2013;60(6):1475–88.
32. Simon D, Kunicki T, Nugent D. Platelet function defects. Haemophilia. 2008;14(6):1240–9.
33. Andrews RK, Berndt MC. Platelet adhesion: a game of catch and release. J Clin Invest. 2008;118(9):3009.
34. Nurden AT, Nurden P. Inherited defects of platelet function. Rev Clin Exp Hematol. 2001;5(4):314–34.
35. Gothwal M, Sandrock-Lang K, Zieger B. Genetics of inherited platelet disorders. Hamostaseologie. 2014;34(2):133–41.
36. Roth GJ, Yagi M, Bastian LS. The platelet glycoprotein Ib-V-IX system: regulation of gene expression. Stem Cells. 1996;14(S1):188–93.
37. Yagi M, Edelhoff S, Disteche CM, Roth GJ. Human platelet glycoproteins V and IX: mapping of two leucine-rich glycoprotein genes to chromosome 3 and analysis of structures. Biochemistry. 1995;34(49):16132–7.
38. Clemetson KJ. Platelet glycoproteins and their role in diseases. Transfus Clin Biol. 2001;8(3):155–62.
39. Okoli S, Madan B, Mwirigi A, Moore G, Drew A, Mitchell M, et al. A diagnostic dilemma: variant Bernard-Soulier syndrome, a difficult clinical and genetic diagnosis. Haemophilia. 2015;21(6):e510–3.
40. Freson K, Wijgaerts A, Van Geet C. Update on the causes of platelet disorders and functional consequences. Int J Lab Hematol. 2014;36(3):313–25.
41. Zieger B, Jenny A, Tsakiris D, Bartsch I, Sandrock K, Schubart C, et al. A large Swiss family with Bernard-Soulier syndrome. Hamostaseologie. 2009;29(2):161–7.
42. Salles II, Feys HB, Iserbyt BF, De Meyer SF, Vanhoorelbeke K, Deckmyn H. Inherited traits affecting platelet function. Blood Rev. 2008;22(3):155–72.
43. Kenny D, Morateck PA, Gill JC, Montgomery RR. The critical interaction of glycoprotein (GP) Ibβ with GPIX—a genetic cause of Bernard-Soulier syndrome. Blood. 1999;93(9):2968–75.
44. McEwan PA, Yang W, Carr KH, Mo X, Zheng X, Li R, et al. Quaternary organization of GPIb-IX complex and insights into Bernard-Soulier syndrome revealed by the structures of GPIbβ and a GPIbβ/GPIX chimera. Blood. 2011;118(19):5292–301.
45. Miller JL. Glycoprotein analysis for the diagnostic evaluation of platelet disorders. Semin Thromb Hemost. 2009;35:224.
46. Noris P, Perrotta S, Bottega R, Pecci A, Melazzini F, Civaschi E, et al. Clinical and laboratory features of 103 patients from 42 Italian families with inherited thrombocytopenia derived from the monoallelic Ala156Val mutation of GPIbα (Bolzano mutation). Haematologica. 2012;97(1):82–8.
47. Rao AK, Songdej N. Parsing the repertoire of GPIb-IX-V disorders. Blood. 2017;129(4):403–4.
48. Sivapalaratnam S, Westbury SK, Stephens JC, Greene D, Downes K, Kelly AM, et al. Rare variants in GP1BB are responsible for autosomal dominant macrothrombocytopenia. Blood. 2017;129(4):520–4.
49. Sánchez-Guiu I, Antón AI, Padilla J, Velasco F, Lucia JF, Lozano M, et al. Functional and molecular characterization of inherited platelet disorders in the Iberian Peninsula: results from a collaborative study. Orphanet J Rare Dis. 2014;9(1):213.

50. Lanza F, De La Salle C, Baas MJ, Schwartz A, Boval B, Cazenave JP, et al. A Leu7Pro mutation in the signal peptide of platelet glycoprotein (GP) IX in a case of Bernard–Soulier syndrome abolishes surface expression of the GPIb–V–IX complex. Br J Haematol. 2002;118(1):260–6.
51. HadjKacem B, Elleuch H, Trigui R, Gargouri J, Gargouri AF. The same genetic defect in three Tunisian families with Bernard Soulier syndrome: a probable founder Stop mutation in GPIbbeta. Ann Hematol. 2010;89(1):75–81.
52. Nurden A. Qualitative disorders of platelets and megakaryocytes. J Thromb Haemost. 2005;3(8):1773–82.
53. Nurden A, Nurden P. Advances in our understanding of the molecular basis of disorders of platelet function. J Thromb Haemost. 2011;9(Suppl 1):76–91.
54. Kunishima S, Saito H. Congenital macrothrombocytopenias. Blood Rev. 2006;20(2):111–21.
55. Balduini C, Savoia A, Seri M. Inherited thrombocytopenias frequently diagnosed in adults. J Thromb Haemost. 2013;11(6):1006–19.
56. Nurden A, Freson K, Seligsohn U. Inherited platelet disorders. Haemophilia. 2012;18(Suppl 4):154–60.
57. Ali S, Shetty S, Ghosh K. A novel mutation in GP1BA gene leads to mono-allelic Bernard Soulier syndrome form of macrothrombocytopenia. Blood Coagul Fibrinolysis. 2017;28(1):94–5.
58. Bragadottir G, Birgisdottir ER, Gudmundsdottir BR, Hilmarsdottir B, Vidarsson B, Magnusson MK, et al. Clinical phenotype in heterozygote and biallelic Bernard-Soulier syndrome—a case control study. Am J Hematol. 2015;90(2):149–55.
59. Savoia A, Balduini CL, Savino M, Noris P, Del Vecchio M, Perrotta S, et al. Autosomal dominant macrothrombocytopenia in Italy is most frequently a type of heterozygous Bernard-Soulier syndrome. Blood. 2001;97(5):1330–5.
60. Balduini A, Malara A, Pecci A, Badalucco S, Bozzi V, Pallotta I, et al. Proplatelet formation in heterozygous Bernard-Soulier syndrome type Bolzano. J Thromb Haemost. 2009;7(3):478–84.
61. Pecci A, Balduini CL. Lessons in platelet production from inherited thrombocytopenias. Br J Haematol. 2014;165(2):179–92.
62. Toogeh G, Keyhani M, Sharifian R, Safaee R, Emami A, Dalili H. A study of Bernard-Soulier syndrome in Tehran, Iran. Arch Iran Med. 2010;13(6):549.
63. Gh T. Quantitative immunophemotyping of platelet surface glycoproteins among Iranian patients with Bernard-Soulier syndrome. Iran J Blood Cancer. 2014;7(1):3–9.
64. Gresele P. Diagnosis of inherited platelet function disorders: guidance from the SSC of the ISTH. J Thromb Haemost. 2015;13(2):314–22.
65. Israels S. Laboratory testing for platelet function disorders. Int J Lab Hematol. 2015;37(Suppl 1):18–24.
66. Gresele P, Harrison P, Bury L, Falcinelli E, Gachet C, Hayward C, et al. Diagnosis of suspected inherited platelet function disorders: results of a worldwide survey. J Thromb Haemost. 2014;12(9):1562–9.
67. Krishnegowda M, Rajashekaraiah V. Platelet disorders: an overview. Blood Coagul Fibrinolysis. 2015;26(5):479–91.
68. Li J, Dai K, Wang Z, Cao L, Bai X, Ruan C. Platelet functional alterations in a Bernard-Soulier syndrome patient with filamin A mutation. J Hematol Oncol. 2015;8(1):79.
69. Balduini A, Malara A, Balduini CL, Noris P. Megakaryocytes derived from patients with the classical form of Bernard-Soulier syndrome show no ability to extend proplatelets in vitro. Platelets. 2011;22(4):308–11.
70. Strassel C, Eckly A, Léon C, Petitjean C, Freund M, Cazenave J-P, et al. Intrinsic impaired proplatelet formation and microtubule coil assembly of megakaryocytes in a mouse model of Bernard-Soulier syndrome. Haematologica. 2009;94(6):800–10.
71. Paniccia R, Priora R, Liotta AA, Abbate R. Platelet function tests: a comparative review. Vasc Health Risk Manag. 2015;11:133.
72. Lordkipanidzé M. Platelet function tests. Semin Thromb Hemost. 2016;42:258.
73. Bolton-Maggs PH, Chalmers EA, Collins PW, Harrison P, Kitchen S, Liesner RJ, et al. A review of inherited platelet disorders with guidelines for their management on behalf of the UKHCDO. Br J Haematol. 2006;135(5):603–33.

74. Choi J-L, Li S, Han J-Y. Platelet function tests: a review of progresses in clinical application. Biomed Res Int. 2014;2014:456569.
75. Cox K, Price V, Kahr WH. Inherited platelet disorders: a clinical approach to diagnosis and management. Expert Rev Hematol. 2011;4(4):455–72.
76. Hayward C, Harrison P, Cattaneo M, Ortel T, Rao A. Platelet function analyzer (PFA)-100® closure time in the evaluation of platelet disorders and platelet function. J Thromb Haemost. 2006;4(2):312–9.
77. Hartman MJ, Caccamese JF, Bergman SA. Perioperative management of a patient with Bernard-Soulier syndrome for third molar surgery. Oral Surg Oral Med Oral Pathol Oral Radiol Endod. 2007;103(5):626–9.
78. Frontroth JP, Favaloro EJ. Ristocetin-induced platelet aggregation (RIPA) and RIPA mixing studies. Methods Mol Biol. 2017;1646:473–94.
79. Gresele P, Bury L, Falcinelli E. Inherited platelet function disorders: algorithms for phenotypic and genetic investigation. Semin Thromb Hemost. 2016;42:292.
80. Podda G, Femia EA, Pugliano M, Cattaneo M. Congenital defects of platelet function. Platelets. 2012;23(7):552–63.
81. Knöfler R, Streif W. Strategies in clinical and laboratory diagnosis of inherited platelet function disorders in children. Transfus Med Hemother. 2010;37(5):231–5.
82. Koltai K, Kesmarky G, Feher G, Tibold A, Toth K. Platelet aggregometry testing: molecular mechanisms, techniques and clinical implications. Int J Mol Sci. 2017;18(8):1803.
83. Frontroth JP. Light transmission aggregometry. Methods Mol Biol. 2013;992:227–40.
84. McGlasson DL, Fritsma GA. Whole blood platelet aggregometry and platelet function testing. Semin Thromb Hemost. 2009;35:168.
85. Rechner A. Platelet function testing in clinical diagnostics. Hamostaseologie. 2011;31(2):79.
86. Rubak P, Nissen PH, Kristensen SD, Hvas A-M. Investigation of platelet function and platelet disorders using flow cytometry. Platelets. 2016;27(1):66–74.
87. Linden MD. Platelet flow cytometry. Methods Mol Biol. 2013;992:241–62.
88. Michelson AD, Barnard MR, Krueger LA, Frelinger A, Furman MI. Evaluation of platelet function by flow cytometry. Methods. 2000;21(3):259–70.
89. Saboor M, Moinuddin M, Ilyas S. New horizons in platelets flow cytometry. Malays J Med Sci. 2013;20(2):62.
90. Macêdo MB, de MM Brito J, da Silva Macêdo P, Brito JA. Primigravida with Bernard-Soulier syndrome: a case report. BMC Res Notes. 2015;8(1):178.
91. Prabu P, Parapia L. Bernard–Soulier syndrome in pregnancy. Int J Lab Hematol. 2006;28(3):198–201.
92. Uotila J, Tammela O, Mäkipernaa A. Fetomaternal platelet immunization associated with maternal Bernard-Soulier syndrome. Am J Perinatol. 2008;25(4):219–23.
93. Valera MC, Kemoun P, Cousty S, Sie P, Payrastre B. Inherited platelet disorders and oral health. J Oral Pathol Med. 2013;42(2):115–24.

Gray Platelet Syndrome (GPS) 16

Hojat Shahraki, Akbar Dorgalaleh, and Barbara J. Bain

16.1 Introduction

Gray platelet syndrome (GPS) is a rare, mostly autosomal recessive inherited bleeding disorder that is categorized as a platelet storage pool disease (SPD). The most common finding of this disorder is a decreased number of platelet α-granules [1–4]. This disorder was first described by Raccuglia [2] in 1971 when petechiae, bruising, thrombocytopenia, and abnormalities of the megakaryocytes (MKs) and platelets (absence of granules and an odd gray appearance) were observed in a patient.

Because of a misdiagnosis of autoimmune thrombocytopenic purpura, patients with GPS manifestations have been treated with corticosteroids and eventually splenectomy. This treatment caused a transient increase of platelets, but the platelet abnormalities and prolonged bleeding time persisted [2, 3].

Platelet vacuoles are abundant, and platelet adenosine triphosphate and platelet lipids, especially phosphatidyl serine, are significantly reduced. Raccuglia called this condition gray platelet disease [2] and further biochemical studies in 1980 [5] revealed the absence of α granules in this first reported patient.

GPS is an extremely rare bleeding disorder, and fewer than 100 individuals have been reported worldwide to date [3, 6–9]. Molecular studies led to identification of

H. Shahraki
Department of Laboratory Sciences, School of Allied Medicine,
Zahedan University of Medical Sciences, Zahedan, Iran

A. Dorgalaleh
Department of Hematology and Blood Transfusion, School of Allied Medicine,
Iran University of Medical Sciences, Tehran, Iran

B. J. Bain (✉)
Department of Haematology, Faculty of Medicine, Imperial College of Science,
Technology and Medicine, St Mary's Hospital Campus, London, UK
e-mail: b.bain@imperial.ac.uk

A. Dorgalaleh (ed.), *Congenital Bleeding Disorders*,
https://doi.org/10.1007/978-3-319-76723-9_16

mutations in the neurobeachin-like2 (*NBEAL2*) gene on the petite (p) arm of chromosome 3 in 2011 [8–10], but other studies reported X-linked inheritance in other patients with mutations in *GATA1* and also an autosomal dominant pattern of inheritance with mutation in the growth factor-independent 1B transcriptional repressor (*GFI1B*) gene [11–13]. For the diagnosis of GPS, hematological and biochemical tests, platelet aggregation studies, platelet lysate analysis, and flow cytometry can be helpful, but the best method or gold standard is transmission electron microscopy, which can confirm the absence of platelet α-granules [6, 9, 10, 14, 15].

16.2 Structure and Function of Platelet Inclusions

Inclusions in platelet cytoplasm are generally variable, but these inclusions differ remarkably in number and content. Each type of platelet cytoplasmic inclusion or microstructure is crucial in platelet function. These inclusions and microstructures include the following.

Mitochondria Mitochondria are very important in metabolic processes such as cellular respiration and energy transfer.

Open Canalicular System The open canalicular system (OCS) membrane structure is physically connected to the platelet surface and allows platelets to communicate with the extracellular matrix (ECM). The presence of the OCS is necessary for exchanging requisite platelet materials.

In addition, the OCS is crucial in the secretion of platelet materials into the surrounding medium, and indeed it is considered as a link between platelets and their environment [14, 16].

Dense Tubular System The dense tubular system (DTS) originates from the rough endoplasmic reticulum and, in contrast to the OCS, it is not attached to the surface of the platelet and is not considered as a platelet membrane channel. The DTS fills crucial functions in platelet metabolic processes and the storage of calcium and other metabolic enzymes, similarly to mitochondria. As about 30% of total platelet calcium is inside this system, the DTS is vital in the activation and regulation processes of platelets [14, 17].

Dense Granule These small, nonprotein granules (200–300 nm) are, with the secretion of their contents, crucial in platelet recruitment and aggregation. Because they are electron dense and heavy, they are known as dense granules. They contain significant amounts of adenine nucleotides such as adenosine triphosphate and ade-

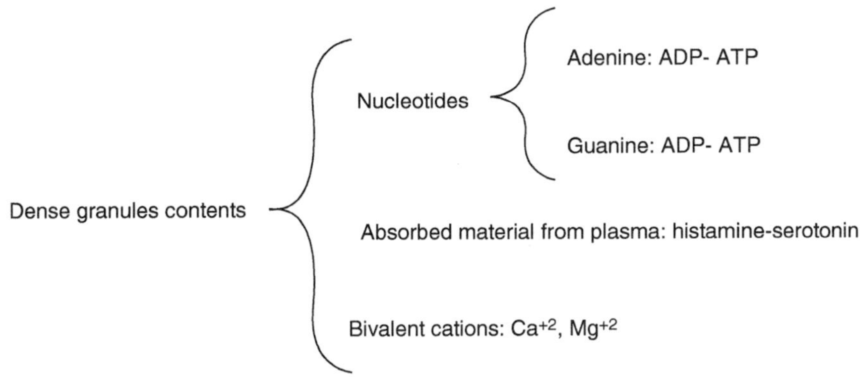

Fig. 16.1 Dense granule contents include nucleotides (ADP and ATP), plasma absorbed materials (serotonin and histamine), and bivalent cations (calcium and magnesium). *ATP* adenosine triphosphate, *ADP* adenosine diphosphate

nosine diphosphate (ADP), as well as some amines such as serotonin, histamine, and bivalent cations (Fig. 16.1) [1].

α-Granules α-Granules are large protein structure granules (200–500 nm) that are known to be the most important platelet granules. Their structure is more diverse than that of dense granules and they also are more abundant than the dense granules. The protein contents of these granules are required for hemostasis, inflammation, and wound healing [1]. Two important specific platelet proteins are beta-thromboglobulin (βTG) and platelet factor 4 (PF4), which are located in the α-granules. Moreover, large adhesive glycoproteins (fibronectin, von Willebrand factor (VWF), thrombospondin), coagulation factors (fibrinogen, factor V, factor VII, factor XIII), cellular mitogens [epidermal growth factor (EGF), transforming growth factor-beta (TGF-β), platelet-derived growth factor (PDGF)], protease inhibitors (alpha2-macroglobulin, alpha2-antiplasmin), immunoglobulins (IgG, IgA), and albumin are present in α-granules [17–19]. Some α-granule proteins such as PF4 and βTG are synthesized in MKs, then packaged in special vesicles and transported to the α-granules. Other proteins such as immunoglobulins and albumin are passively absorbed from plasma, whereas the endocytosis of fibrinogen into MKs and platelets is mediated by integrin αIIbβ3 (GPIIb/IIIa) (CD41/CD61). Because α-granules contain essential proteins and biomaterials, deficiency or loss of the α-granules has a major effect on platelet function (Fig. 16.2) [14, 15, 41].

Lysosome Lysosomes are between α-granules and dense granules in size, and they contain proteases and glycohydrolases. These organelles participate in clearance of unnecessary platelet aggregates [17].

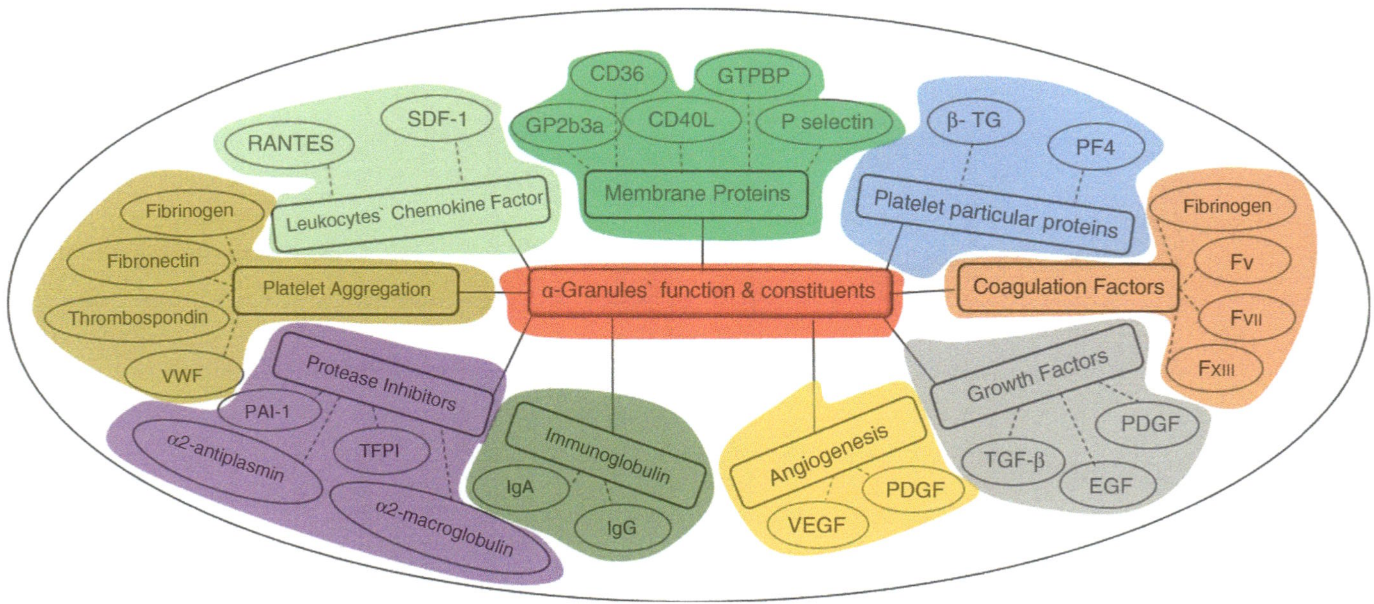

Fig. 16.2 α-Granule function and constituents. *PF4* platelet factor 4, *PDGF* platelet-derived growth factor, *EGF* epidermal growth factor, *TGF-beta* transforming growth factor-β, *VEGF* vascular endothelial growth factor, *IgG* immunoglobulin G, *IgA* immunoglobulin A, *TFPI* tissue factor pathway inhibitor, *PAI-1* plasminogen activator inhibitor-1, *VWF* von Willebrand factor, *RANTES* C-C motif chemokine ligand 5, *GTPBP* GTP-binding proteins

16.3 Molecular Basis

For many years, the only way to diagnose GPS was by observing a decrease or deficiency of platelet α-granules by examination of a blood film, followed by electronic microscopy but after 2000, molecular studies were significantly developed to reveal that GPS is usually inherited in an autosomal recessive manner (Table 16.1).

Table 16.1 The most important molecular investigations in gray platelet syndrome (GPS) patients

Name (year)	Technique	Result
Mori et al. (1984)	TEM-LTA	Determination of autosomal dominant manner in GPS
Hyman et al. (2003)	DNA microarray	Increase of cytoskeletal protein expression
Nurden et al. (2004)	Flow cytometry	Severe deficiency of GP VI
Benit et al. (2005)	Sanger sequencing	No sign of mutation in HZF gene in GPS patients
De Candia et al. (2006)	Sanger sequencing–immunofluorescence microscopy	Reduction of platelet aggregation => no response of platelet to thrombin, PAR1-AP, or PAR4-AP
Tubman et al. (2007)	Sanger sequencing—linkage analysis	X-linked GPS caused by a *GATA1* (Arg21, Gln mutation)
Gunay-Aygun et al. (2010)	Using genome wide linkage analysis—homozygosity mapping	Determination of GPS causative gene location in an 9.4 Mb interval on chromosome 3p
Fabbro et al. (2011)	SNP arrays–homozygosity mapping	Reduction of 9.4 Mb interval to 1.7 Mb
Albers et al. (2011	Next generation sequencing (exome sequencing)	Mutations in GPS causative gene "*NBEAL2*"
Kahr et al. (2011)	Next-generation sequencing (RNA sequencing)	Mutations in GPS causative gene "*NBEAL2*"
Gunay-Aygun et al. (2011)	Proteomic analysis	Mutations in GPS causative gene "*NBEAL2*"
Depperman et al. (2013)	Fluorescent labeling of α-granule—TEM—recombination	Knocking out of *NBEAL2* gene in rat and observation of clinical manifestations of GPS
Monteferraria et al. (2013)	Sequencing—linkage analysis	Mutations in GPS causative gene "*GFI1B*"
Guerrero et al. (2014)	TEM-qPCR–sequencing	Knocking out of *NBEAL2* gene in rat and observation of clinical manifestations of GPS
Rensing-Ehl et al. (2015)	Homozygosity mapping–whole exome sequencing	Mimic autoimmune lymphoproliferative syndrome by GPS
Di Buduo et al. (2016)	TEM—cloning–flow cytometry	GPS MK with *NBEAL2* mutations cultured for the first time
Tomberg et al. (2016)	Whole exome sequencing	8bp deletion in *NBEAL2* gene (GPS mice)
Bottega et al. (2017)	Flow cytometry–sequencing	Novel mutation of *NBEAL2*

TEM transmission electron microscopy, *LTA* light transmission aggregometry, *cDNA* complementary deoxyribonucleic acid, *GP* glycoprotein, *qPCR* quantitative polymerase chain reaction, *HZF* hematopoietic zinc finger, *SNP* single nucleotide polymorphism, *MK* megakaryocyte

In 2010, a study using genome-wide linkage analysis and haplotype analysis was conducted on 25 patients with GPS, and eventually the position of the causative gene was determined to be within a span of 9.4 Mb on chromosome 3p21.1-3p22.1 [6]. Then, in 2011, in a study with utilization of homozygosity, mapping showed this interval to be reduced from 9.4 Mb to 1.7 Mb [7]. These two studies were very important in recognition of the causative gene defect in GPS. Finally, it was shown by next-generation sequencing (NGS) that causative mutations in *NBEAL2* are responsible for most cases of GPS [9]. For confirmation of this finding, the *NBEAL2* gene was knocked out in zebrafish, resulting in abrogated platelet formation [940, 42, 45]. In addition, further studies confirmed the role of *NBEAL2* mutation in the pathogenesis of GPS [8, 1044, 47]. This gene is located at 3p21.31 and has 56 exons. Beige and Chédiak–Higashi (BEACH) domain and multiple WD40 domains are two important domains of the *NBEAL2* protein that appear to be important for membrane protein trafficking. Other BEACH domain proteins are NBEA, NBEAL2, LRBA, and LYST [8, 10].

The pathogenetic mechanism of Chédiak–Higashi syndrome (CHS) is dysregulation of lysosomal trafficking caused by truncation or loss of BEACH and multiple WD40 domains by a mutation in the *LYST* gene. Recent studies have shown that NBEAL2 protein is required for vesicular trafficking development and platelet α-granule formation. More than 35 mutations that lead to GPS have been identified in the *NBEAL2* gene [22, 2346].

GPS is a heterogeneous disorder, and three forms of genetic inheritance have been reported (autosomal recessive, X-linked, autosomal dominant). For example, a mutation in location 759 of the *GATA1* gene (Arg216Glu) was identified in one family in 2007, and it was proposed that GATA1 is an upstream regulator of genes involved in platelet α-granule biogenesis (Fig 16.3) [11].

In another study on eight patients with GPS in Japan, an autosomal dominant pattern of inheritance was proposed for this disorder [12]. Then, in 2013 Monteferrairo et al. nominated mutations of *GFI1B* as responsible for autosomal dominant GPS. They suggested that GFI1B had an important role in the development of MKs and platelets [13]. In 2016, a study on cultured MKs from GPS patients found that MK differentiation from human hematopoietic progenitor cells is not affected by *NBEAL2* mutations, and the following was noted [21]:

1. The α-granule content of human MKs is decreased in patients with GPS.
2. Emperipolesis can occur in human MKs of patients with GPS.
3. Mutation in *NBEAL2* has no effect on calcium signaling.
4. Impaired pro-platelet formation is seen in human MKs of GPS.

It seems that advances in genetic science and new approaches such as NGS in the next few years will help us to a better understanding of the precise molecular mechanism of GPS.

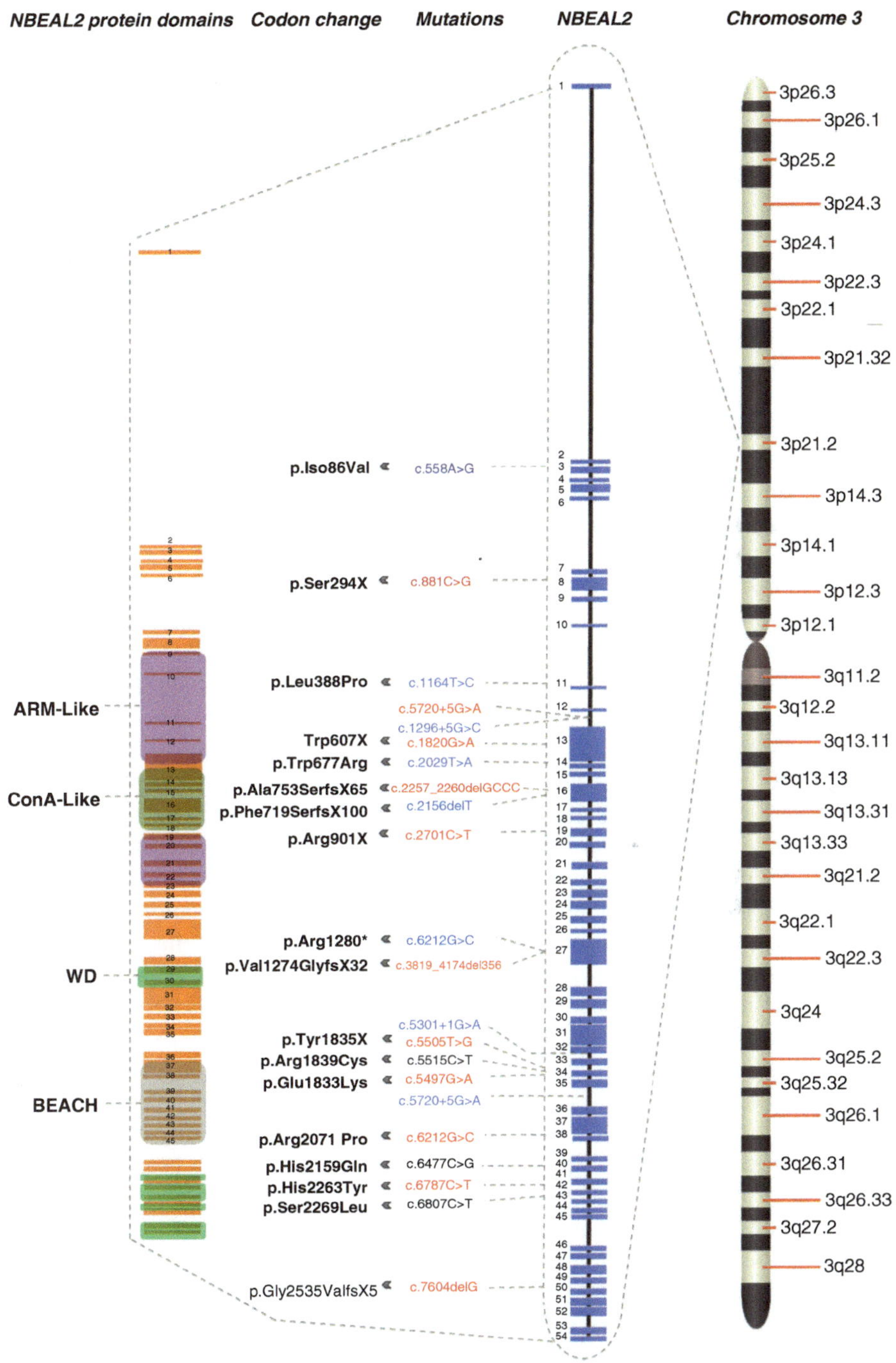

Fig. 16.3 *NBEAL2* gene mutations that are responsible for gray platelet syndrome (GPS)

16.4 Clinical Manifestations

Clinical manifestations of GPS are heterogeneous, but patients usually present with mild bleeding such as petechiae and easy bruising although severe bleeds are less often observed. In a study on 21 individuals from 14 families, 42% of patients with GPS experienced life-threatening bleeds, which revealed the variability in the clinical manifestations of this disorder [6]. Similarly to other inherited platelet function disorders (IPFDs), spontaneous mucocutaneous bleeding can be observed among these patients. Splenomegaly with a frequency of about 80% to 90% is another finding of GPS [3, 6]. The defects in platelet α-granules allow their constituents, such as growth factors and mitogens (PDGF, TGF-β, ECGF, EGF), to leak into the ECM of the bone marrow, causing increased reticulin deposition and collagen formation [14, 20, 24]. It is noteworthy that rarely extramedullary hematopoiesis can be observed in patients with GPS and splenomegaly [4].

16.5 Laboratory Diagnosis

Although the diagnosis of some severe IPFDs such as Glanzmann thrombasthenia (GT) and Bernard–Soulier syndrome (BSS) is straightforward, diagnosis of most other IPFDs is sophisticated and requires a correct laboratory approach and advanced instruments and diagnostic tests. For the diagnosis of mild IPFDs such as GPS, a complete family history, appropriate clinical studies, and physical examinations in addition to the correct laboratory approach can help in timely diagnosis and appropriate management. IPFDs may present with spontaneous or posttraumatic hemorrhage (mostly skin, mucocutaneous, and nose bleeding) but contrariwise muscle and joint bleeding are less common [25]. Splenomegaly is another presentation of GPS that can be observed on physical examination of the patient [3, 23]. In addition to physical examination, assessment of clinical manifestations, and a family history, an appropriate laboratory approach is crucial in timely diagnosis of these disorders. For the diagnosis of GPS, both routine and specific laboratory assays are useful. The International Society on Thrombosis and Haemostasis (ISTH) proposed a reliable algorithm for diagnosis of IPFDs (see Chap. 11).

1. *Primary tests*:
    - *Complete Blood Count (CBC)* is very important in laboratory assessment of patients with GPS. In these patients, the platelet count is usually less than 100×10^9/L and therefore patients have thrombocytopenia. Mean platelet volume (MPV) is significantly raised, and therefore macrothrombocytopenia is a significant finding of this disorder [3].
    - *Prothrombin Time (PT) and Activated Partial Thromboplastin Time (aPTT)*: These tests are normal in GPS because there is no abnormality of coagulation factors [3, 6].
    - *Peripheral Blood Smear (PBS)*: Peripheral blood smear examination is necessary because cell counters usually underestimate the number of platelets in the presence of macrothrombocytopenia. In Wright's or May–Grünwald–

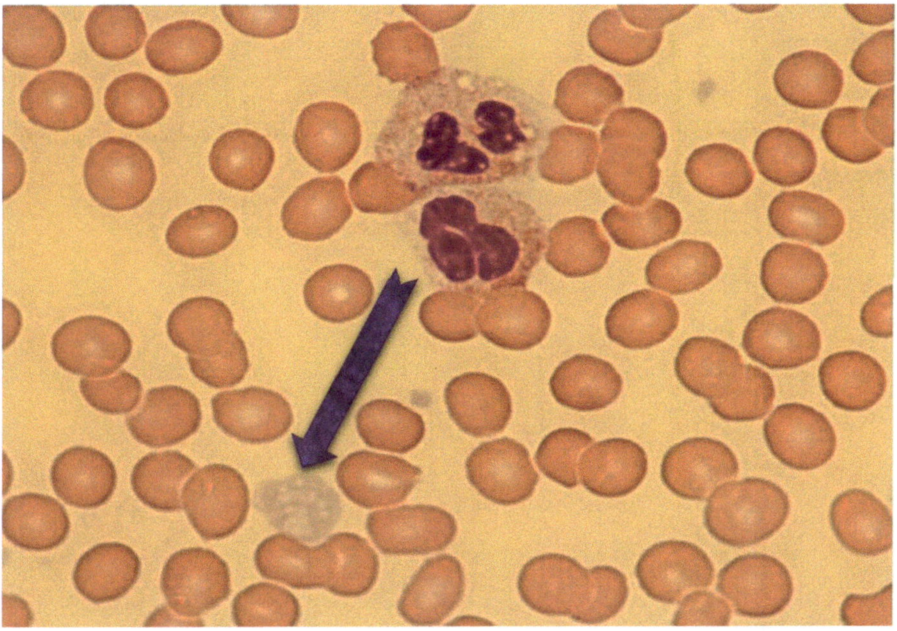

Fig. 16.4 Peripheral blood smear of a patient with gray platelet syndrome (GPS). In patients with GPS, one of the most important features is presence of odd pale large gray vacuolar platelets in peripheral blood smear (*arrow*)

Giemsa staining, the size and appearance of platelets are important diagnostic clues because they are gray or pale and large (Fig. 16.4) [5, 19].

- *Bleeding Time (BT)*: This factor is usually prolonged in GPS, but the test is not necessary. Although thrombocytopenia may be corrected by corticosteroid therapy and splenectomy, prolonged BT persists [2].

2. *Platelet Special Tests*:
   - *Transmission Electron Microscopy*: This technique is regarded as the gold standard for the diagnosis of GPS. Because of defects in platelet α-granule packaging and leakage of their constituents (PF4, βTG, fibrinogen, fibronectin, and PDGF) into the ECM, platelets and MKs become hypogranular because of the loss or decrease of α-granule content, and subsequently they will become gray [14]. Loss of α-granules causes many vacuoles to appear in these cells, which can assist in diagnosis of the disorder. The numbers of mitochondria, dense bodies, peroxisomes, and lysosomes are surprisingly normal (Table 16.2) [14, 26].
   - *Light Transmission Aggregation (LTA)*: This test is for checking of platelet function. Platelet-rich plasma (PRP) samples and primary agonists (epinephrine, ADP, collagen, arachidonic acid, and ristocetin) are used for platelet aggregation analysis. Platelet responses to agonists are heterogeneous in GPS patients, but generally they are normal for ADP, epinephrine, arachidonic

Table 16.2 The most important characteristics of platelet storage pool deficiency (PSPD)

Disorder	Abbreviation	Gene (chromosome)	Platelet defect	Peripheral blood		Bleeding tendency	Clinical manifestation	TEM	Inheritance manner
				Size	Decrease of platelet number				
Gray platelet syndrome	GPS	*NBEAL2* (3p21.1)	Platelet aggregation and secretion defects and subsequently platelet function disorders (alpha granules)	Large (pale)	Mild	Mild to moderate	Mild bleeding such as petechiae, also splenomegaly, myelofibrosis, extramedullary hematopoiesis, increased serum vitamin B_{12}	Decrease of alpha granules	Mostly autosomal recessive
Quebec platelet disorder	QPD	*PLAU* (10q22)	Defects of platelet uPA and subsequently platelet function disorders (alpha granules)	Normal	Mild to normal	Mild	Skin and mucosal, delayed bleeding, marked increase of uPA, abnormal proteolysis of platelet α-granule constituents	Decrease of alpha granules	Autosomal dominant

Hermansky–Pudlak syndrome	HPS	*HPS* (10q24.2), *ADTB3A* (q14.9), *HPS3* (3q24), *HPS* (22q12.1), *HPS* (11p15.1), *HPS6* (10q24.32), *DTNBP1* (6p22.3), *Bloc153* (19q13.32)	Defects of lysosomal regulating proteins and subsequently platelet function disorders (dense granules)	Normal	Mild to normal	Mild	Oculocutaneous albinism, photophobia, nystagmus, immunodeficiency, bleeding disorders	Decrease of dense granules	Autosomal recessive
Griscelli syndrome	GS	*MYO5A* (15q21), *RAB27A* (15q21.3), *MLPH* (2q37.3)	Platelet degranulation and secretion defects and subsequently platelet function defects (dense granules)	Normal	Mild to normal	Mild	Albinism, hemophagocytosis, mental retardation, immunodeficiency, hepatosplenomegaly	Decrease of dense granules	Autosomal recessive
Thrombocytopenia absent radius	TAR	*RBM8A* (1q21.1)	Platelet development defects and subsequently incorrect platelet function	Normal	Severe for infants	Moderate to severe	Skeletal abnormalities including absent radius, thrombocytopenia, defective platelet function, nose bleeding	Decrease of dense granules	Autosomal recessive

(continued)

Table 16.2 (continued)

Disorder	Abbreviation	Gene (chromosome)	Platelet defect	Peripheral blood		Bleeding tendency	Clinical manifestation	TEM	Inheritance manner
				Size	Decrease of platelet number				
Wiskott-Aldrich syndrome	WAS	*WAS* (Xp1.23)	Abnormal release of platelet constituents and subsequently platelet function defects (dense granules)	Small	Severe	Moderate to severe	Eczema, immunodeficiency, small platelets with thrombocytopenia	Decrease of dense granules	X-linked
Chédiak–Higashi syndrome	CHS	*CHS1* (1q42.1-42.2)	Lysosomal regulation proteins defects and subsequently functional defects of platelets (dense granules)	Normal	Normal	Mild	Oculocutaneous albinism, bleeding disorders, immunodeficiency	Decrease of dense granules	Autosomal recessive

TEM transmission electron microscopy, *uPA* urokinase plasminogen activator acid, and ristocetin and deficient in response to thrombin and collagen. Because of dissimilarity of information, it is important to know that the purpose of this test is to differentiate GPS from other IPDFs [3].

- *Assessment of Platelet Lysates*: As the platelet α-granule content is markedly decreased or absent in GPS, analysis of their constituents can be useful because PF4 and βTG are decreased in platelets (α-granules) and increased in plasma. Suitable samples for this test are eluted platelets. Also, applicable techniques are enzyme-linked immunosorbent assay (ELISA) for assessment of PF4, βTG, fibronectin, and fibrinogen, and Western blot for thrombospondin-1 (TSP-1) analysis.
- *Flow Cytometry*: Because some platelet surface proteins are reduced in GPS, analysis of platelet α-granule membranes and platelet membrane glycoproteins can be useful. Citrated whole blood combined with a peripheral blood smear (PBS) is ideal for this test. In addition, flow cytometry is practical for specific analysis of fibrinogen receptor, fibronectin receptor, and P-selectin (CD62) [3, 2739]. Low numbers and abnormal distribution of secretory compartment components (alkaline phosphatase, CD35, CD11b/CD18) of hypogranular neutrophils were also observed [28].
- *Analysis of Vitamin B_{12}*: About half of GPS patients showed considerably increased serum vitamin B_{12} concentration. Assay of B_{12} has therefore been recommended [6].
- *Bone Marrow Analysis*:

  Myelofibrosis: Laboratory investigations have revealed an increased amount of reticulin and bone marrow collagen fibrosis in patients with GPS, probably because of leakage of platelet α-granule mitogens (PDGF, TGF-β, ECGF, VEGF) into the surrounding bone marrow environment [14, 24].

  Emperipolesis: Existence of an intact cell within the cytoplasm of another cell is a phenomenon called emperipolesis, which occurs in less than 2% of the bone marrow MKs of normal people but involves about 38–65% of the MKs in GPS patients. The bone marrow microenvironment is not considered to be the main source of emperipolesis in GPS; rather, MKs and intrinsic cellular defects are the most important [21, 29].

3. *Molecular Analysis*:

   Because GPS is genetically heterogeneous, it is necessary to proceed to molecular and genetic tests, choosing a suitable panel of genes and using an appropriate protocol for molecular analysis. Because this condition is most often inherited in an autosomal recessive manner, most molecular approaches are based on this kind of inheritance. Assessment of the *NBEAL2* gene by NGS is a suitable choice for those patients suspected to have an autosomal recessive inheritance pattern [8–10]. NGS is a powerful technology and has improved our ability to determine the molecular basis of genetic disorders. Utilization of Sanger sequencing was common for a long time but it was time consuming and not cost-effective, so with the advent of NGS a momentous evolution in mutation detection was the rapid and simultaneous analysis of large groups of candidate genes. Now, NGS enables us to scrutinize *NBEAL2* and other suspected genes (Fig. 16.5) [27].

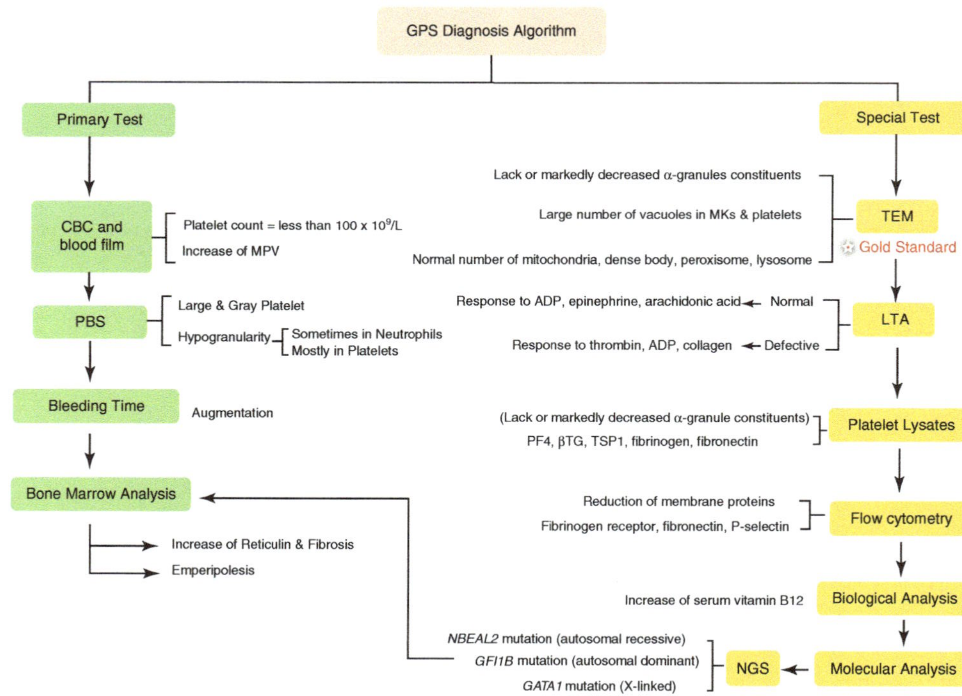

Fig. 16.5 Gray platelet syndrome diagnosis algorithm. Primarily, CBC is measured for GPS diagnosis and reduction of platelet numbers (less than 100×10^9/L). Also, increased MPV is observed in GPS patients. BT usually shows significant increment, and large gray or pale platelets are present in PBS. We suspect GPS after checking these tests. Using the TEM method to assess lack or decrease of α-platelet granules and the increase of platelet vacuoles and megakaryocytes is recognized as diagnostic for GPS. LTA results are different, but generally the response to ADP and epinephrine is normal; however, for collagen and ADP, abnormal response has been reported. Platelet lysates such as PF4 and BTG and fibrinogen are significantly reduced, and also granule membrane proteins such as fibrinogen receptor show reduction by flow cytometry. Vitamin B_{12} is increased at times and, by using molecular methods such as NGS, eventually we should evaluate mutations of NBEAL2 as the genetic cause of GPS. BM analysis is important in primary and special GPS tests because of the evidence of fibrosis elevation and emperipolesis in GPS. *CBC* complete blood count, *MPV* mean platelet volume, *BT* bleeding time, *PBS* peripheral blood smear, *TEM* transmission electron microscopy, *LTA* light transmission aggregation, *NGS* next-generation sequencing

16.6 Management of Patients with Gray Platelet Syndrome

There is no specific therapy for GPS, and the best management is medical support and on-demand management. Thrombocytopenia must be assessed precisely, and drugs such as aspirin that reduce platelet function should not be prescribed [3]. Platelet transfusion can be beneficial for some patients but it may cause allo-immunization, so donors and recipients should be HLA matched. If surgery is required, 1-deamino-8-D-arginine vasopressin (DDAVP) is a suitable choice to reduce the risk of bleeding [30]. Except in patients with significant splenomegaly, splenectomy is not recommended because it has no significant effect on platelet numbers. Therefore, supportive care and on-demand management of the disease is the treatment of choice for these patients [3, 23, 27].

16.7 Conclusion

IPDFs are a heterogeneous group of disorders, often with similar clinical presentations and requiring sophisticated laboratory diagnosis. Although the diagnosis of severe IPFDs such as GT and BSS is straightforward, proper and timely diagnosis of mild IPFDs is difficult and requires advanced laboratory assessment. In spite of this, physical examination, family history, assessment of clinical presentations, and basic laboratory tests including blood count and blood film examination are crucial in diagnosis of this disorder and lead to the diagnosis in a considerable number of these patients.

16.8 Quebec Platelet Disorder (QPD)

Quebec platelet disorder (QPD) is an IPFD with autosomal dominant pattern of inheritance that is characterized by mucocutaneous and delayed (almost 12–24 h after injury) bleeding, joint bleeding, markedly increased platelet urokinase plasminogen activator (uPA), and abnormal proteolysis and degradation of platelet α-granule constituents [31–33].

The general prevalence of the disorder is 1 per million but it is higher, 1 per 300,000 individuals, in Canada (Quebec). Initially QPD was described as factor V (FV) Quebec [34]. One important constituent of α-granules is platelet FV and its binding protein multimerin, which may function as a carrier protein for platelet FV, its attachment to platelets, membrane transportation, and platelet α-granule secretion. In QPD, platelet uPA concentration and activity are augmented (more than 100 times normal) and subsequently plasmin and enhanced fibrinolysis lead to proteolysis and abnormal degradation of platelet α-granule constituents (multimerin, fibronectin, fibrinogen, P-selectin, thrombospondin, osteonectin, and VWF) [35, 36].

The platelet count is reduced or normal ($80–250 \times 10^9$/l) in QPD, and BT is prolonged. UPA, uPA-plasminogen activator inhibitor 1 (uPA-PAI-1), and plasmin-α2 anti-plasmin inhibitor (PAP) are increased in platelets but they are normal in plasma [31, 36]. In aggregometry analysis, platelet aggregation is impaired in response to epinephrine. Tandem duplication of *PLAU* (on chromosome 10q22), encoding urinary plasminogen activator, and leading to upregulation, is the probable genetic mechanism of QPD [37, 38].

The best approach to QPD diagnosis is analysis of platelet α-granule constituents, especially FV and multimerin, and then measurement of platelet uPA by Western blot and antigen assay [36]. Finally, NGS can be applied for recognition of mutations of *PLAU*. QPD patients do not respond to platelet or plasma transfusion, but fibrinolytic system inhibitors such as tranexamic acid and amino caproic acid are effective [32, 33].

References

1. Holmsen H, Weiss HJ. Secretable storage pools in platelets. Annu Rev Med. 1979;30(1):119–34.
2. Raccuglia G. Gray platelet syndrome: a variety of qualitative platelet disorder. Am J Med. 1971;51(6):818–28.
3. Nurden AT, Nurden P. The gray platelet syndrome: clinical spectrum of the disease. Blood Rev. 2007;21(1):21–36.
4. Jantunen E, Hänninen A, Naukkarinen A, Vornanen M, Lahtinen R. Gray platelet syndrome with splenomegaly and signs of extramedullary hematopoiesis: a case report with review of the literature. Am J Hematol. 1994;46(3):218–24.
5. Gerrard JM, Phillips DR, Rao G, Plow EF, Walz DA, Ross R, et al. Biochemical studies of two patients with the gray platelet syndrome. Selective deficiency of platelet alpha granules. J Clin Invest. 1980;66(1):102.
6. Gunay-Aygun M, Zivony-Elboum Y, Gumruk F, Geiger D, Cetin M, Khayat M, et al. Gray platelet syndrome: natural history of a large patient cohort and locus assignment to chromosome 3p. Blood. 2010;116(23):4990–5001.
7. Fabbro S, Kahr WH, Hinckley J, Wang K, Moseley J, Ryu G-Y, et al. Homozygosity mapping with SNP arrays confirms 3p21 as a recessive locus for gray platelet syndrome and narrows the interval significantly. Blood. 2011;117(12):3430–4.
8. Kahr WH, Hinckley J, Li L, Schwertz H, Christensen H, Rowley JW, et al. Mutations in NBEAL2, encoding a BEACH protein, cause gray platelet syndrome. Nat Genet. 2011;43(8):738–40.
9. Albers CA, Cvejic A, Favier R, Bouwmans EE, Alessi M-C, Bertone P, et al. Exome sequencing identifies NBEAL2 as the causative gene for gray platelet syndrome. Nat Genet. 2011;43(8):735–7.
10. Gunay-Aygun M, Falik-Zaccai TC, Vilboux T, Zivony-Elboum Y, Gumruk F, Cetin M, et al. NBEAL2 is mutated in gray platelet syndrome and is required for biogenesis of platelet [alpha]-granules. Nat Genet. 2011;43(8):732–4.
11. Tubman VN, Levine JE, Campagna DR, Monahan-Earley R, Dvorak AM, Neufeld EJ, et al. X-linked gray platelet syndrome due to a GATA1 Arg216Gln mutation. Blood. 2007;109(8):3297–9.
12. Mori K, Suzuki S, Sugai K. Electron microscopic and functional studies on platelets in gray platelet syndrome. Tohoku J Exp Med. 1984;143(3):261–87.
13. Monteferrario D, Bolar NA, Marneth AE, Hebeda KM, Bergevoet SM, Veenstra H, et al. A dominant-negative GFI1B mutation in the gray platelet syndrome. N Engl J Med. 2014;370(3):245–53.
14. Breton-Gorius J, Vainchenker W, Nurden A, Levy-Toledano S, Caen J. Defective alpha-granule production in megakaryocytes from gray platelet syndrome: ultrastructural studies of bone marrow cells and megakaryocytes growing in culture from blood precursors. Am J Pathol. 1981;102(1):10.

15. Levy-Toledano S, Caen J, Breton-Gorius J, Rendu F, Cywiner-Golenzer C, Dupuy E, et al. Gray platelet syndrome: alpha-granule deficiency. Its influence on platelet function. J Lab Clin Med. 1981;98(6):831–48.
16. White JG. Interaction of membrane systems in blood platelets. Am J Pathol. 1972;66(2):295.
17. Rendu F, Brohard-Bohn B. The platelet release reaction: granules' constituents, secretion and functions. Platelets. 2001;12(5):261–73.
18. Berman C, Yeo E, Wencel-Drake JD, Furie B, Ginsberg M, Furie B. A platelet alpha granule membrane protein that is associated with the plasma membrane after activation. Characterization and subcellular localization of platelet activation-dependent granule-external membrane protein. J Clin Invest. 1986;78(1):130.
19. White JG. Ultrastructural studies of the gray platelet syndrome. Am J Pathol. 1979;95(2):445.
20. Hyman T, Huizing M, Blumberg PM, Falik-Zaccai TC, Anikster Y, Gahl WA. Use of a cDNA microarray to determine molecular mechanisms involved in grey platelet syndrome. Br J Haematol. 2003;122(1):142–9.
21. Di Buduo CA, Alberelli MA, Glembostky AC, Podda G, Lev PR, Cattaneo M, et al. Abnormal proplatelet formation and emperipolesis in cultured human megakaryocytes from gray platelet syndrome patients. Sci Rep. 2016;6:23213.
22. Savoia A. Molecular basis of inherited thrombocytopenias. Clin Genet. 2016;89(2):154–62.
23. Gresele P, Bury L, Falcinelli E. Inherited platelet function disorders: algorithms for phenotypic and genetic investigation. Semin Thromb Hemost. 2016;42:292.
24. Caen J, Deschamps J, Bodevin E, Bryckaert M, Dupuy E, Wasteson A. Megakaryocytes and myelofibrosis in gray platelet syndrome. Nouv Rev Fr Hematol. 1986;29(2):109–14.
25. Golebiewska EM, Poole AW. Platelet secretion: from haemostasis to wound healing and beyond. Blood Rev. 2015;29(3):153–62.
26. Cramer EM, Vainchenker W, Vinci G, Guichard J, Breton-Gorius J. Gray platelet syndrome: immunoelectron microscopic localization of fibrinogen and von Willebrand factor in platelets and megakaryocytes. Blood. 1985;66(6):1309–16.
27. Nurden A, Nurden P. Inherited disorders of platelet function: selected updates. J Thromb Haemost. 2015;13(suppl 1):S2.
28. Drouin A, Favier R, Massé J-M, Debili N, Schmitt A, Elbim C, et al. Newly recognized cellular abnormalities in the gray platelet syndrome. Blood. 2001;98(5):1382–91.
29. Larocca LM, Heller PG, Podda G, Pujol-Moix N, Glembotsky AC, Pecci A, et al. Megakaryocytic emperipolesis and platelet function abnormalities in five patients with gray platelet syndrome. Platelets. 2015;26(8):751–7.
30. Pfueller S, Howard M, White J, Menon C, Berry E. Shortening of bleeding time by 1-deamino-8-arginine vasopressin (DDAVP) in the absence of platelet von Willebrand factor in gray platelet syndrome. Thromb Haemost. 1987;58(4):1060–3.
31. Kahr WH, Zheng S, Sheth PM, Pai M, Cowie A, Bouchard M, et al. Platelets from patients with the Quebec platelet disorder contain and secrete abnormal amounts of urokinase-type plasminogen activator. Blood. 2001;98(2):257–65.
32. McKay H, Derome F, Haq MA, Whittaker S, Arnold E, Adam F, et al. Bleeding risks associated with inheritance of the Quebec platelet disorder. Blood. 2004;104(1):159–65.
33. Blavignac J, Bunimov N, Rivard GE, Hayward CP. Quebec platelet disorder: update on pathogenesis, diagnosis, and treatment. Semin Thromb Hemost. 2011;37:713.
34. Tracy PB, Giles AR, Mann KG, Eide LL, Hoogendoorn H, Rivard GE. Factor V (Quebec): a bleeding diathesis associated with a qualitative platelet factor V deficiency. J Clin Invest. 1984;74(4):1221.
35. Diamandis M, Veljkovic DK, Maurer-Spurej E, Rivard GE, Hayward CP. Quebec platelet disorder: features, pathogenesis and treatment. Blood Coagul Fibrinolysis. 2008;19(2):109–19.
36. Hayward CP, Rivard GE. Quebec platelet disorder. Expert Rev Hematol. 2011;4(2):137–41.
37. Paterson AD, Rommens JM, Bharaj B, Blavignac J, Wong I, Diamandis M, et al. Persons with Quebec platelet disorder have a tandem duplication of PLAU, the urokinase plasminogen activator gene. Blood. 2010;115(6):1264–6.

38. Diamandis M, Paterson AD, Rommens JM, Veljkovic DK, Blavignac J, Bulman DE, et al. Quebec platelet disorder is linked to the urokinase plasminogen activator gene (PLAU) and increases expression of the linked allele in megakaryocytes. Blood. 2009;113(7):1543–6.
39. P. Nurden, (2004) Severe deficiency of glycoprotein VI in a patient with gray platelet syndrome. Blood 104 (1):107-114
40. L. BÉNIT, E. M. CRAMER, J. M. MASSÉ, I. DUSANTER-FOURT, R. FAVIER, (2005) Molecular study of the hematopoietic zinc finger gene in three unrelated families with gray platelet syndrome. Journal of Thrombosis and Haemostasis 3 (9):2077-2080
41. E. DE CANDIA, A. PECCI, G. CIABATTONI, R. DE CRISTOFARO, S. RUTELLA, Z. YAO-WU, I. LAZZARESCHI, R. LANDOLFI, S. COUGHLIN, C. L. BALDUINI, (2007) Defective platelet responsiveness to thrombin and protease-activated receptors agonists in a novel case of gray platelet syndrome: correlation between the platelet defect and the -granule content in the patient and four relatives . Journal of Thrombosis and Haemostasis 5 (3):551-559
42. Carsten Deppermann, Deya Cherpokova, Paquita Nurden, Jan-Niklas Schulz, Ina Thielmann, Peter Kraft, Timo Vögtle, Christoph Kleinschnitz, Sebastian Dütting, Georg Krohne, Sabine A. Eming, Alan T. Nurden, Beate Eckes, Guido Stoll, David Stegner, Bernhard Nieswandt, (2013) Gray platelet syndrome and defective thrombo-inflammation in Nbeal2-deficient mice. Journal of Clinical Investigation 123 (8):3331-3342
43. Davide Monteferrario, Nikhita A. Bolar, Anna E. Marneth, Konnie M. Hebeda, Saskia M. Bergevoet, Hans Veenstra, Britta A.P. Laros-van Gorkom, Marius A. MacKenzie, Cyrus Khandanpour, Lacramiora Botezatu, Erik Fransen, Guy Van Camp, Anthonie L. Duijnhouwer, Simone Salemink, Brigith Willemsen, Gerwin Huls, Frank Preijers, Waander Van Heerde, Joop H. Jansen, Marlies J.E. Kempers, Bart L. Loeys, Lut Van Laer, Bert A. Van der Reijden, (2014) A Dominant-Negative Mutation in the Gray Platelet Syndrome. New England Journal of Medicine 370 (3):245-253
44. J. A. Guerrero, C. Bennett, L. van der Weyden, H. McKinney, M. Chin, P. Nurden, Z. McIntyre, E. L. Cambridge, J. Estabel, H. Wardle-Jones, A. O. Speak, W. N. Erber, A. Rendon, W. H. Ouwehand, C. Ghevaert, (2014) Gray platelet syndrome: proinflammatory megakaryocytes and Â -granule loss cause myelofibrosis and confer metastasis resistance in mice. Blood 124 (24):3624-3635
45. A. Rensing-Ehl, U. Pannicke, S.-Y. Zimmermann, M. R. Lorenz, B. Neven, I. Fuchs, U. Salzer, C. Speckmann, A. Strauss, E. Maass, B. Collet, A. Enders, R. Favier, M. C. Alessi, F. Rieux-Laucat, B. Zieger, K. Schwarz, S. Ehl, (2015) Gray platelet syndrome can mimic autoimmune lymphoproliferative syndrome. Blood 126 (16):1967-1969
46. Kärt Tomberg, Rami Khoriaty, Randal J. Westrick, Heather E. Fairfield, Laura G. Reinholdt, Gary L. Brodsky, Pavel Davizon-Castillo, David Ginsburg, Jorge Di Paola, Christian Schulz, (2016) Spontaneous 8bp Deletion in Nbeal2 Recapitulates the Gray Platelet Syndrome in Mice. PLOS ONE 11 (3):e0150852
47. Roberta Bottega, Elena Nicchia, Caterina Alfano, Ana C. Glembotsky, Annalisa Pastore, Debora Bertaggia-Calderara, Bettina Bisig, Michel A. Duchosal, Guillermo Arbesú, Lorenzo Alberio, Paula G. Heller, Anna Savoia, (2017) Gray platelet syndrome: Novel mutations of the NBEAL2 gene. American Journal of Hematology 92 (2):E20-E22